Comprehensive Coronary Care

Nigel I. Jowett MBBS MRCS LRCP MD FRCP

Consultant Physician and Cardiologist,
Pembrokeshire and Derwen NHS Trust,
and Director, Heart-Start, Pembrokeshire, Wales, UK

David R. Thompson BSc MA PhD MBA RN FRCN FESC

Professor of Cardiovascular Nursing, University of Leicester, Leicester, UK

FOREWORD

Roger Boyle CBE FRCP FRCPE FESC

Professor and National Director for Heart Disease and Stroke,
Department of Health, London, UK

FOURTH EDITION

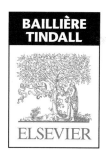

BAILLIÈRE TINDALL

ELSEVIER

EDINBURGH   LONDON   NEW YORK   OXFORD   PHILADELPHIA   ST LOUIS   SYDNEY   TORONTO   2007

BAILLIÈRE
TINDALL
ELSEVIER

An imprint of Elsevier Limited

First edition 1989
Second edition 1995
Third edition 2003
Fourth edition 2007

ISBN 978 0 7020 2859 5

British Library Cataloguing in Publication Data
A catalogue record for this book is available from the British Library

Library of Congress Cataloging in Publication Data
A catalog record for this book is available from the Library of Congress

Note
Medical knowledge is constantly changing. Standard safety precautions must be followed, but as new research and clinical experience broaden our knowledge, changes in treatment and drug therapy may become necessary or appropriate. Readers are advised to check the most current product information provided by the manufacturer of each drug to be administered to verify the recommended dose, the method and duration of administration, and contraindications. It is the responsibility of the practitioner, relying on experience and knowledge of the patient, to determine dosages and the best treatment for each individual patient. Neither the Publisher nor the authors assume any liability for any injury and/or damage to persons or property arising from this publication.

The Publisher

 ELSEVIER your source for books, journals and multimedia in the health sciences

www.elsevierhealth.com

The publisher's policy is to use paper manufactured from sustainable forests

Printed in China

Comprehensive Coronary Care

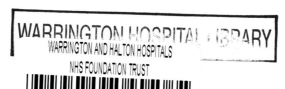

DEDICATION

One man is as good as another until he has written a book.

From: *The Letters of Benjamin Jowett, Volume 1,*
edited by E.A. Abbott and L. Campbell (1899)

Dedicated to Sheena, Alex and Luci, and Rose, Luke and Jack, who have continued to support us
whilst we have been bettering ourselves.

For Elsevier

Publisher: Steven Black
Development Editor: Katrina Mather
Project Manager: Anne Dickie
Design Direction: George Ajayi
Illustrators: Chartwell and Graeme Chambers
Illustration Manager: Gillian Richards

Contents

Foreword

This fourth edition is a very welcome development for the many readers of this important textbook on coronary care. It is well suited to a wide readership, being in tune with the multidisciplinary team approach that is such an important part of modern emergency care.

The publication of this edition is extremely timely. Across the globe, we are heading for a pandemic of coronary heart disease (CHD). CHD not only remains the commonest cause of death and a major cause of long-term disability but is also spreading rapidly in concert with the epidemic of obesity and diabetes. In the developed world, the impact of these negative factors has been offset by improvements in treatment and lifestyle, but in some of the less developed and most populated areas of the world, death rates are rising and are expected to continue to do so exponentially. In total, there are 54 million deaths every year worldwide, of which 17 million (31%) are cardiovascular in origin. Of these, 44% are due to CHD and 31% to stroke. Nearly 80% of these cardiovascular deaths occur in countries defined as 'low income' (*The World Health Report 2003: Shaping the future*. Geneva, WHO). By 2002, over one-third of all deaths from CHD worldwide occurred in China, Russia and India. It is inevitable, then, that coronary care will remain a major part of emergency care for a long time yet.

A quarter of a century ago, the only real tools available in coronary care units (CCUs) were opiates and defibrillators. Now, however, CCU staff face the formidable challenge of a complex array of treatment options that need tailoring to individual patients. First, they must keep pace with the burgeoning evidence base of effective interventions. Excellence in care requires not only an up-to-date knowledge of the latest technologies and when to apply them but also a systematic approach to ensure that simple things are done correctly all the time. But as coronary care staff strive to offer optimal care to every acutely ill patient, as indicated by the latest clinical trial or guideline, they still have to ensure that patients and carers are fully informed and cared for in a thoughtful and considerate yet honest fashion.

Excellence also requires teamwork. Success in providing top-quality care is dependent on skilled, informed and professional personnel that work as a team, spanning all the various disciplines along the patient's path before, during and after admission to hospital. The case mix has also changed. Admissions of patients with acute coronary syndromes now outnumber those with ST elevation myocardial infarction. So the daily agenda now extends beyond accurate diagnosis and eligibility for thrombolysis to a more complex decision matrix including triage, risk-stratification and the choice of a much wider range of interventions than would have seemed possible only a decade ago.

In these rapidly changing times, it is imperative that the staff who care for patients suffering from CHD are kept fully informed and up to date.

This text, the fourth edition, makes a major contribution to preparing staff for the task ahead. Written by an experienced team, combining medical and nursing expertise with extensive clinical and research experience, this book will make an important addition to every CCU library. It will inspire and encourage our industrious and committed staff to explore the evidence base ever more thoroughly in the pursuit of excellence and further improvements in care.

Roger Boyle CBE
February 2007

Preface to the fourth edition

It is nearly 20 years since we were working in coronary care at Leicester General Hospital and decided that it was time someone wrote a practical book for all those working in such units, and not just the doctors or nurses. In that pre-thrombolytic era, management of heart attacks was straightforward and mostly passive. CCU still stood for the coronary (rather than cardiac) care unit, 'mega-trials' and evidence-based medicine were only just emerging, and no-one had heard of acute coronary syndromes or PCI (percutaneous coronary intervention). Already, we are on to the fourth edition of *Comprehensive Coronary Care* as a result of the multiple revisions needed to keep pace with the rapid advances in acute cardiac care. Whilst we thought that thrombolysis was likely to remain the greatest advance in the modern era, we are currently witnessing the rise of primary angioplasty that could bring even greater benefits to our heart attack patients. Hopefully, we will soon see this become normal treatment for acute coronary thrombosis, rather than being rationed to a lucky minority. As we progress through the 21st century, the traditional role and design of CCUs will have to change to provide specialist care for all presentations of acute coronary syndromes, and we will have to develop new ways of managing this large group of patients to improve outcomes. In addition, developments in pre-hospital care, public access defibrillation, PCI, off-pump cardiac surgery, and new rehabilitation/secondary prevention programmes, along with new international resuscitation guidelines, should help give our patients a second chance.

Nigel I. Jowett
David R. Thompson
February 2007

Preface to the first edition

The role of coronary care has changed markedly since its inception in the early 1960s, and it now has an extended importance for patients with other manifestations of coronary artery disease, and for those with critical cardiac dysfunction who require intensive care and cardiovascular monitoring. This book is intended as an up-to-date guide to the current practice of 'cardiac intensive care', and to provide a basis for further exploration of the subject. Because we believe that such practice is not the sole domain of either nursing or medical staff we have tried to utilise an integrated approach, suitable for all those concerned with patient management on the coronary care unit. Some of our material extends outside the traditional boundaries of coronary care, but we think it important that it is appreciated how the patients come to be there, and what may happen to them after they leave.

Whilst we hope that nurses never lose sight of their primary caring role, in reality much of their work in the area of coronary care involves a high degree of medical and technical expertise, and our book reflects this. We have assumed that nurse-readers have a basic understanding of primary nursing, the nursing process, nursing theories and conceptual models, and only salient features are mentioned in the text.

Leicester 1989
Nigel I. Jowett
David R. Thompson

Chapter 1

An introduction to coronary care

The emergence of cardiovascular disease (CVD) as a major cause of disability and death was first seen in North America, Europe and Australia in the early part of the twentieth century, and was described as an 'epidemic' when numbers of affected patients peaked in the 1960s and early 1970s.

There were two main reasons why cardiovascular disease had become so common. First, improvements in general heath in these countries allowed this 'new' disease to emerge. Deaths from infectious diseases and nutritional deficiencies had nearly been eliminated and, with the end of the Second World War, populations were living long enough to die of other causes, specifically heart disease. In recognition of this, the International Classification of Diseases (ICD) introduced a new disease category called *arterio-sclerotic heart disease*, to replace the previous non-specific diagnosis of *myocardial degeneration*. This revision enabled more accurate death certification and, in one year (1948–1949), coronary disease death rates appeared to increase by about 25%. Cardiovascular disease is still the commonest chronic illness in both developed and developing countries, causing the most deaths and having the greatest impact on morbidity. Approximately one-third of the total deaths worldwide are cardiovascular in origin, 43% from coronary heart disease and 32% from stroke, and while industrialised countries have made huge advances in the management of CVD, many new populations are experiencing a substantial increase in the different manifestations of CVD. Unless current trends are halted or reversed, over a billion people will die from CVD in the first half of this century, mostly in developing countries, where much of the life will be lost in middle age (Murray & Lopez, 1997).

In the UK, CVD currently costs the country nearly £26 billion annually, 57% from direct health costs, 24% through loss of production and 19% from informal care of those with the disease. Globally, 78% of cardiovascular deaths occur in lower and middle income countries that are unable to finance healthcare adequately (Yusuf et al, 2001).

There are at least three contributory factors that have led to this spread of CVD from industrialised to developing countries. First, just as was seen at the start of the CVD epidemic in the western world, life expectancy in developing countries is increasing because of reduced mortality from other causes, especially infectious diseases. Populations are living longer to die from other causes. Secondly, in some populations, genetic factors may be conferring susceptibility to coronary disease, particularly in those people from Southern Asia. This is unlikely to result from a direct genetic cause of coronary disease, but more likely a genetic predisposition towards associated risk factors such as hypertension, obesity and metabolic influences, particularly diabetes (Jowett, 1984). Finally, while globalisation can clearly bring benefits in alleviating poverty and facilitating infective disease control, there are adverse consequences through the promotion of tobacco products, refined foods and high-calorie drinks that often replace healthier traditional foods. Many countries have now adopted the western lifestyle of unhealthy diets, lack of exercise and smoking. While sales of cigarettes in the USA are at the lowest point for 50 years, worldwide sales of tobacco continue to climb (5500 billion cigarettes sold in 2000), with more than a third being smoked in China. It is estimated that smoking-related mortality in India will have increased from 1% in 1990 to 13% by 2020 and, in most Latin American countries, continued high levels of smoking with unfavourable changes in nutrition (including obesity), physical activity and less effective control of hypertension has meant that the reduction in coronary heart disease (CHD) is much less than in other western countries, such as North America and Canada (Rodríguez et al, 2006).

In the United Kingdom, diseases of the heart and circulatory system are still the main cause of death, and more than one in three people die from CVD, half from CHD and a quarter from stroke (Allender et al, 2006). In 2004, there were just over 216 000 cardiovascular deaths, of which more then 105 000 were from CHD (Fig. 1.1A and B). Someone in the UK suffers a heart attack every 5 minutes.

The World Health Organization MONICA project monitored the trends and determinants of CVD across 38 populations in 21 countries from the mid-1980s to the mid-1990s (Tunstall-Pedoe et al, 1994), and showed that coronary heart mortality was falling in most populations studied (Fig. 1.2). But whereas in the UK there were 68 230 fewer deaths from CHD between 1981 and 2000, mortality rates did not fall as quickly as in other countries,

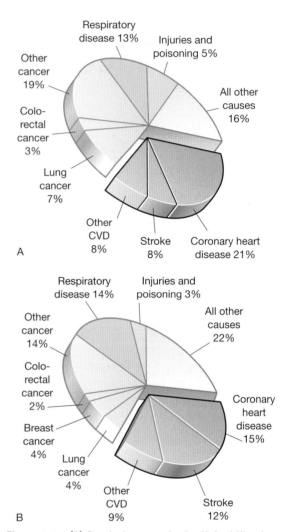

Figure 1.1 (A) Deaths by cause in the United Kingdom (2004), men. (B) Deaths by cause in the United Kingdom (2004), women. Data from the Office for National Statistics, London (HMSO).

meaning that death here is still among the highest in the world (Fig. 1.3). Mortality is higher in Scotland and the north of England compared with the south, areas where the incidence of acute myocardial infarction is also higher. CHD is also more prevalent in certain ethnic minorities, particularly South Asians living in the UK (Wild & McKeigue, 1997). People born in India, Bangladesh, Pakistan or Sri Lanka are approximately 50% more likely to die prematurely from CHD than the

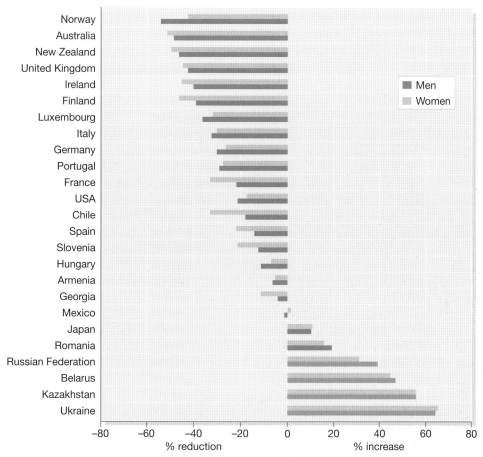

Figure 1.2 Changes in coronary heart disease mortality rates in selected countries (1990–2000) for men and women aged 35–74 years. Data from the World Health Organization, 2004.

general population (Fig. 1.4). The reasons for this are not known, but risk factors such as diabetes and smoking are more common in these populations, and members of Asian communities also tend to present later, with more advanced disease, suggesting sociological influences.

PREVENTION OF CARDIOVASCULAR DISEASE

Cardiovascular disease is not inevitable, and most is preventable. The development of atherosclerosis and its consequences is closely linked to factors that have their roots in social and physical environments. This is commonly referred to as 'lifestyle', which for most in the western world

means an unhealthy diet, taking little or no exercise, smoking cigarettes and becoming obese. Many precipitants of atherosclerosis are established from an early age and, as exposure to the number of cardiovascular risk factors increases, so does the severity of asymptomatic coronary and aortic atherosclerosis in young people. Fatty atherosclerotic streaks may be found in the blood vessels of up to half of children under 15 years of age (Berenson et al, 1998).

The INTERHEART study has confirmed that it is the same lifestyle risk factors that account for most heart attacks in all populations around the world (Yusuf et al, 2004). This applies to both men and women of all ages and on every continent, where smoking and abnormal blood lipid concentrations

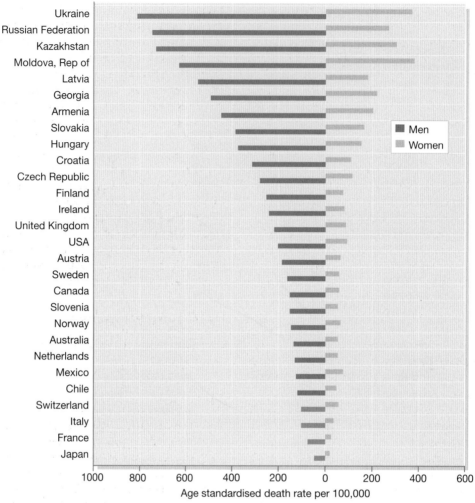

Figure 1.3   Death rates from coronary heart disease in selected countries for men and women aged 35–74 years (2000). Data from the World Health Organization, 2004.

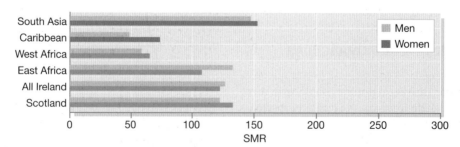

Figure 1.4   Standardised mortality ratios for CHD by sex and country of birth, 1989–1992, England and Wales. Data from the Office for National Statistics, London (HMSO).

account for two-thirds of the overall risk of coronary disease. The other major contributors are hypertension, diabetes, abdominal obesity, lack of exercise, excess alcohol, lack of vegetables and fruit in the diet and psychosocial factors, such as stress and depression. Stopping smoking, taking more exercise and eating a healthier diet could reduce the risk of myocardial infarction by 80%, regardless of age, sex or country of origin.

Traditionally, cardiovascular management strategies have focused on treating those with symptoms or those who have had a cardiovascular event, but about a half of heart attacks, and a third of fatal heart attacks, occur in patients with no prior evidence of coronary disease (Deedwania, 2001). The division between 'primary' and 'secondary' prevention is therefore arbitrary, as individuals with atherosclerosis all have the same underlying disease process, regardless of whether or not they have symptoms. Modern CVD prevention needs to focus equally on those with known atherosclerotic disease, as well as asymptomatic individuals at high risk of developing symptomatic atherosclerotic disease. Foremost among these are patients with diabetes.

Diabetes is one of the major contributors to ill-health and premature mortality worldwide. All patients with diabetes mellitus are at risk of vascular disease, and those with type 2 diabetes are at a substantially increased risk of CHD, being perhaps two to four times in men and three to five times in women compared with non-diabetics. Currently, it is estimated that at least 1 in 20 deaths in the world is attributable to the complications of diabetes and, in adults aged 35–64 years, the proportion is over 1 in 10. The prevalence of type 2 diabetes is predicted to double over the next 25 years, mostly in developing countries, and related cardiovascular complications will predominantly affect people in their most economically productive years. Again, this is not inevitable. A prediabetic state can be defined in many individuals well before the disease emerges, presenting an opportunity for intervention to prevent or delay the onset of diabetes and reduce the future burden of CVD (Scarpello, 2004).

Death rates from CHD have been falling in the UK since the late 1970s and, for people under 65 years, they have fallen by 44% in the last 10 years.

Most of this reduction has not come from new medical and surgical treatments, but from risk factor control in the population and in the individual, particularly in the reduction of smoking, blood cholesterol and blood pressure (Unal et al, 2005). Widespread risk factor modification may also have produced a shift from major cardiovascular events to less severe manifestations of disease at presentation (Rosengren et al, 2005). In British men, there are now fewer heart attacks, but the incidence of diagnosed angina has increased (Lampe et al, 2005). Greater awareness and treatment of cardiovascular risk factors, with more widespread prescription of drugs such as statins and beta-blockers, may be bringing about a more benign onset of symptomatic heart disease rather than sudden death or acute transmural myocardial infarction (Go et al, 2006).

PRESENTATION OF CHD

Coronary disease usually presents in one of two ways.

Chest pain

The most common presentation of CHD is chest pain (Suttcliffe et al, 2003), about a half presenting with stable angina and a quarter with myocardial infarction (Table 1.1). For those presenting with acute coronary disease, ST elevation myocardial infarction is becoming less common, being replaced by unstable angina or myocardial infarction without ST elevation on the presenting electrocardiogram (ECG). Over half of men and two-thirds of women with coronary disease are

Table 1.1 Presentation of coronary heart disease in adults, Bromley Health Authority, UK (data from Suttcliffe et al, 2003).

Presentation	Men	Women
Angina	41%	52%
Unstable angina	13%	13%
Myocardial infarction	32%	22%
Sudden death	14%	13%

now presenting with an undamaged left ventricle, so there is considerable potential to reduce morbidity and mortality of CHD.

Unfortunately, the initial diagnosis of CHD is often difficult, and it is sometimes not possible to differentiate between cardiac and non-cardiac pain at presentation. Chest pain is a very common symptom in the community and, although most underlying causes are benign, it may cause concern in both patients and doctors. There are approximately 345 000 new cases of angina annually in the UK, and predicting the clinical course from symptoms alone is difficult. Stable angina may progress to myocardial infarction or death in about 2% of cases every year (Daly et al, 2006). In addition, certain patients present with unusual symptoms of coronary ischaemia, and the diagnosis may be missed. Women often present with 'atypical' chest pain, while the elderly may not get any chest discomfort at all, and simply complain of shortness of breath (Then et al, 2001). Rapid-access chest pain clinics may provide swift reassurance or timely intervention, and can reduce hospital admissions and associated costs (McManus et al, 2002). Most patients assessed in these clinics do not have a cardiac cause for their symptoms, and prompt reassurance is beneficial for both general practitioner (GP) and patient alike. Negative investigations (either non-invasive or invasive) identify a low-risk population, no matter what the final diagnosis is. In contrast, patients who are not investigated or who have inconclusive tests are at the same level of risk of death or myocardial infarction as those with established coronary disease (Daly et al, 2006).

In our chest pain clinic, fewer than a third of those assessed have cardiac or other important chest pain. We are able to reassure and discharge over half these patients immediately, and only 10–15% require a further outpatient appointment to complete their treatment.

Sudden cardiac death

While most patients present alive to medical services with their first symptoms of coronary disease, sudden cardiac death (SCD) may be the first and final sign of CHD, and is responsible for about two-thirds of all sudden deaths (Zheng et al, 2001).

SCD describes a natural death due to a cardiac cause where individuals appear fit and well at one moment and then collapse, to die in less than an hour and often immediately. In the majority of cases, it is not possible to determine whether death has been caused by a primary ventricular dysrhythmia, or whether cardiac arrest has occurred as a result of an acute coronary arterial occlusion. Even if a post-mortem examination is carried out, the reason for death may still not be clear. The probability of finding an acute coronary lesion (a ruptured atheromatous plaque with thrombosis) at post mortem ranges widely, depending on the duration of prodromal symptoms before death. The presence of an occlusive thrombus in a coronary artery is only seen in about a third of sudden cardiac deaths, although an additional 43% have a non-occlusive thrombus (Davies, 1992). Plaque fissuring is seen in some cases but, as this is a random and recurrent event, it may be found in people who die from unrelated causes. Hence, a quarter of sudden deaths cannot be confirmed as acute coronary thrombosis and, where there is no other obvious cause, deaths are usually attributed to malignant ventricular dysrhythmias. Most of these patients have coronary disease, but there are other conditions that associate with SCD, including cardiomyopathy, aortic stenosis, the long Q–T syndrome and anomalous origins of the coronary arteries. Advances in electrophysiological cardiology have highlighted groups of patients at risk of SCD, who are candidates for implantation of automatic cardiodefibrillators (see Chapter 13).

There are of course other mechanisms that may associate with sudden death, such as aortic dissection, subarachnoid haemorrhage or massive pulmonary embolism, but only a minority of cases of SCD occur in the absence of coronary artery disease or chronic heart failure.

PREHOSPITAL CORONARY CARE

Despite all the recent advances in acute cardiac care, the majority of deaths from coronary disease occur in the prehospital phase, and most victims do not survive long enough to receive medical help, let alone benefit from all the new evidence-based interventions. Data from the Augsburg myocardial infarction register in Germany found that the 28-day case fatality in 3729 cases of acute myocardial infarction was 58% (Lowel et al, 1995). Of these, 28% had died within 1 hour of the onset of symptoms, 40% by 4 hours and 51% by 24 hours. In other words, most deaths resulting from acute myocardial infarction occurred in the first 24 hours, and the majority before hospital admission. Most of those who died outside hospital were alone at the time of death and, despite the involvement of emergency medical services, only 1 in 10 was seen alive by a doctor.

While improvements in acute coronary care have resulted in a fall in hospital mortality and improved long-term survival, the impact on deaths in the community has been marginal. Prehospital care has changed little in recent decades, and the proportion of cardiac deaths occurring out of hospital continues to rise, because in-hospital mortality continues to fall (Norris, 1998). Those of us working in hospital practice must realise that our view of acute myocardial infarction is based on caring for survivors of a devastating clinical event that has already taken its major toll. Opportunities for further reducing death from heart attack lie mainly outside hospital, and the optimal interventions linking the victim of sudden cardiac arrest with survival have been referred to as the 'chain of survival'.

The four links in this chain are:

- early recognition of cardiac arrest with a prompt call for help;
- early cardiopulmonary resuscitation (to buy time);
- early defibrillation (to restart the heart);
- post-resuscitation care (to restore quality of life).

The first link (early recognition) not only applies to those who have already suffered a cardiac arrest, but also to those who may do so because of critical illness or a sudden change in their medical status (prearrest recognition). The central links in the chain of survival integrate life support with defibrillation as the fundamental components of early resuscitation in an attempt to restore life. The final link, post-resuscitation care, concentrates on preserving the function of vital organs, particularly of the brain and heart.

Bystander resuscitation

In the UK Heart Attack Study (Norris, 1998), three-quarters of heart attack deaths in people aged less than 75 years occurred outside hospital. Eighty per cent of these cardiac arrests occurred in the home, half of which were witnessed. Only 20% of cases collapsed in a public place, although in contrast, nearly all of these were witnessed (Norris, 2005). Resuscitation attempts were twice as likely to take place when the arrest occurred in the public place rather than at home (41% vs. 22%), and survival was consequently better (8% vs. 2%).

For patients who suffer sudden cardiac arrest following acute coronary occlusion, the initial rhythm is usually ventricular fibrillation, although if resuscitation is not attempted early enough, this will deteriorate into asystole. Less commonly, cardiac arrest is initially caused by heart block or asystole, mostly as a consequence of thrombosis in the right coronary artery. In patients recovering from acute myocardial infarction, sudden death is usually ventricular tachycardia or ventricular fibrillation related to the infarcted and scarred myocardium, but may also be induced by a new episode of ischaemia or a combination of both.

Even the best emergency response schemes do not have the capability to deliver defibrillation within the first vital minutes following cardiac arrest outside hospital, and the use of *first responders* to deliver prompt cardiopulmonary resuscitation (CPR) and defibrillation using automatic external defibrillators (AEDs) has become widespread. First responders are individuals who have been trained to act independently within a physician-controlled system, and include members of the emergency services (ambulance personnel, firemen, police), airline cabin crew, families of high-risk patients and other targeted lay personnel.

CPR by the first on the scene (*bystander resuscitation*) extends the period for successful resuscitation, and provides a bridge to first defibrillation. At any point in time between collapse and first defibrillation, bystander CPR at least doubles the chance of survival. As ventricular fibrillation is the initial rhythm in the majority of cases, defibrillation is the best treatment, and will be effective in over 90% of cases if applied within 1 minute. If applied more than 10 minutes after collapse, the rhythm will usually have become unshockable. First responders do not need extensive or complex training to deploy modern AEDs (Hallstrom et al, 2000).

In the UK, 12 000 people suffer a cardiac arrest in a public place every year, and the British Heart Foundation has pioneered the Heart-Start project to teach basic resuscitation skills until an AED can be brought to the patient. Traditional CPR with intermittent chest compressions and ventilation is not crucial in the early period after cardiac arrest, and simple chest compressions alone can be an effective bridge to defibrillation.

With the recognition that as many as 1000 lives were being lost every year from cardiac arrest in commercial aircraft, AEDs were acquired by several airlines, with appropriate training of cabin staff. In a report on a 64-month period on Qantas airlines, AEDs were recorded as being used 63 times for monitoring an acutely ill passenger and 46 times for treating cardiac arrest. Long-term survival for victims in ventricular fibrillation was achieved in 26%. AEDs are likely to become standard on most airlines in the near future and, with appropriate crew training, will be helpful in the management of cardiac emergencies (Page et al, 1998).

Another example of successful AED placement came from the USA, where defibrillation by security guards in Las Vegas casinos resulted in 56 of 105 (53%) patients who collapsed with ventricular fibrillation surviving (Valenzuela et al, 2000). In those defibrillated within 3 minutes of collapse, the survival rate was 74%. On average, the conventional emergency response team arrived nearly 10 minutes after the patient collapsed, when survival, even with early CPR, would be predicted to be around 5–10%.

The main problem for first responder/AED programmes is that the rescuer needs to arrive not just earlier than the emergency medical services (EMS), but early enough to have an influence on successful cardioversion (Groh et al, 2001). Implementation of community-based lay responder programmes is feasible, although they require substantial resources and commitment (Richardson et al, 2005). It is early recognition, early CPR and early defibrillation that all contribute to increased survival from out-of-hospital cardiac arrest. With longer delays, the survival curve flattens, and a few minutes' gain in time will have little impact when a first responder does not improve on the paramedic response time. First responders need to continually practice their response, know how to link with the local EMS system, and the whole structure must be subject to continuous audit (Hazinski et al, 2005). The Department of Health has already funded the installation of around 700 AEDs in public places around the country, including railway stations, shopping centres and airports, where ambulance data have shown there to be an appreciable risk of cardiac arrest (Department of Health, 1999; Davies et al, 2002). More than 6000 people have received training in basic life support skills and the use of an AED, and the national defibrillator programme aims to increase this further in the coming years.

Given that only a fifth of prehospital arrests occur in public places, and fewer than 2% of prehospital arrests occur in public places in which the frequency of arrests exceeds one every 10 years (Pell et al, 2002), the overall impact of the national defibrillator programme on sudden cardiac death is limited. On the other hand, 80% of all sudden cardiac deaths occur in people with known cardiovascular disease, usually within 18 months of hospital discharge following acute myocardial infarction. Individuals assessed to be at very high risk of arrest can be provided with implantable cardioverter defibrillators (NICE, 2006) and, as most episodes of cardiac arrest occur at home, family members could be targeted for instruction in basic life support and provided with automated external defibrillators.

DELAYS IN ACTIVATION OF THE EMERGENCY MEDICAL SERVICES

The major obstacle to prompt assessment of patients with symptoms of a heart attack is the delay in the call for help. Around 50% of patients who are eligible for reperfusion do not make medical contact until 3 hours after the onset of symptoms (Hasdai et al, 2002). The reasons for this are complex, and include the severity of the symptoms, as well as the patient's age, sex and level of education (Gurwitz et al, 1997). Delay is more frequent where:

- Symptoms are mild.
- The patient is at home rather than in a public place.
- The patient called the GP first.
- The patient lives in a rural area.
- A family member is present.
- The patient is elderly.
- The patient is female.
- Symptom onset is at night (18.00–06.00 hours).

Education of high-risk patients should be most beneficial, as nearly half of all myocardial infarcts occur in those with a history of cardiovascular disease but, surprisingly, a prior history of myocardial infarction or angina does not shorten the delay in seeking help (Table 1.2). Public educational campaigns have not helped to reduce delays, perhaps because of inconsistency of advice, and television portrayal of acute cardiac events has not helped to dispel the myth that a heart attack is an easily recognised and dramatic event (Ruston et al, 1998). In the real world, intermittent chest pain is the most common prodromal symptom in the majority of patients (Table 1.3) and, in many, the onset of pain is gradual rather than sudden. In about a quarter of non-fatal myocardial infarctions, the symptoms are unrecognised, particularly where the patient is elderly or has diabetes.

Minimising the delay in coming under medical care for those with an evolving myocardial

infarction reduces the chance of death from ventricular fibrillation, and maximises the potential benefit from reperfusional strategies to salvage the myocardium at risk. Although regional and international circumstances vary, about 50% of patients with ST elevation myocardial infarction will present via the emergency medical services, rather than by attending the emergency department or the GP surgery. The ambulance service has a major role in assessing and stabilising the patient before starting a diagnostic work-up that may enable prehospital interventions to limit or abort significant myocardial infarction.

EMERGENCY MEDICAL SERVICE (EMS) RESPONSE

Early advanced life support by a well-trained and well-equipped emergency response team is probably the most important link in the *chain of survival*. If the initial call from a patient with chest pain is to a general practitioner (GP), it is better that the patient is triaged by telephone, with a direct call for a properly equipped ambulance crew, rather than arranging for a home visit. Most GPs do not wish to give thrombolytic therapy, and their involvement often results in substantial delays in definitive treatment (Prasad et al, 1997). Where GPs are able to offer a first-response thrombolytic

Table 1.3 Premonitory symptoms in 100 sequential cases of myocardial infarction admitted to our coronary care unit.

Symptoms[a]	Percentage
Angina	
New	11
Old	17
Chest pain	26
Emotional stress	19
Dyspnoea	13
Lethargy	10
Palpitations	4
None	46

a Note that some symptoms were multiple.

Table 1.2 Time between onset of symptoms and call for medical help in 200 patients admitted to our coronary care unit, with and without previous myocardial infarction (MI) or angina.

Time (h)	Previous MI/angina	No previous MI/angina
0–3	28	42
3–6	34	19
6–24	21	23
> 24	17	18
Total	100	100

service, the 'call-to-needle' time may be well within the National Service Framework target of 60 minutes, particularly if the patient lives more than 30 minutes from the hospital (Rawles et al, 1998). In the absence of such a system, an infrastructure of transportation that responds to emergency calls is vital, particularly in rural or remote areas, to ensure rapid access to effective prehospital and hospital care. GPs should have practice policies for responding rapidly to patients with chest pain, and those patients at high risk of acute myocardial infarction and their family should be aware of the practice policy.

NHS Direct provides advice to people calling about suspected heart attacks and arranges for the ambulance service to send appropriately trained and equipped crew immediately. In most countries, access to the EMS is achieved by means of a single dedicated telephone number, such as 999 in the UK or 911 in the USA. A uniform European public access telephone number of '112' has been proposed by the European Society of Cardiology, but this has not been widely accepted.

The EMS response interval, which measures the time taken for the ambulance to reach the patient from the time of the call, is generally the shortest of all the delays in getting treatment under way. All patients with chest pain or collapse require an emergency (category A) response from the emergency services to reach the patient within 8 minutes, in a vehicle containing a defibrillator and staff trained in its use, a target being reached in 80% of calls in England. Recent enthusiasm for improving the speed of delivery of thrombolytic treatment may hide the major benefit of a rapid response, i.e. getting a defibrillator to the patient. It was the importance of rhythm monitoring and prompt defibrillation that revolutionised the management of acute coronary patients and led to the establishment of coronary care units when it was first suggested nearly 50 years ago (Julian, 1961).

Pantridge and Geddes (1967) extended this important part of treatment for heart attack victims by taking the coronary care unit to the patient. Their mobile unit was staffed by a physician and a nurse, and demonstrated that many patients could be saved by early recognition and treatment of the complications of acute myocardial infarction. Of course, in these early times, there was no

treatment for coronary thrombosis, so much of the mortality benefit was from haemodynamic stabilisation and prompt defibrillation in the patient's home ('stay-and-stabilise'). The idea of prehospital cardiac care spread to other countries but, as physician manned units are a limited resource, doctors were replaced by paramedics who had been trained to diagnose and treat the early complications of acute myocardial infarction, including cardiac arrest. The presence of a physician before hospitalisation is still perceived as being important in many healthcare systems, although often impractical, and has been one limitation to widespread implementation of prehospital fibrinolysis programmes (Welsh et al, 2005).

The main goals in assessing and treating patients with acute chest pain by the EMS are:

- haemodynamic stabilisation;
- formulating a diagnosis;
- relieving symptoms;
- preventing complications and permanent organ damage.

The diagnostic procedure in patients with acute chest pain aims to identify high-risk patients for 'fast track' management, and to differentiate other patients in whom there is little suspicion of a life-threatening disorder. The recognition that chest pain is likely to have a cardiac origin is of major importance, as an evolving myocardial infarction requires immediate treatment. In hospital, this is made easier by the availability of skilled multidisciplinary staff and investigative tools. Prehospital diagnosis of an acute coronary syndrome is based only on the clinical history and a single (often suboptimal) ECG recording, but can still be reasonably accurate. Acquiring a 12-lead ECG prior to hospital admission reduces in-hospital delays, as can direct communication between the ambulance and the admitting coronary care unit staff. Prehospital ECG telemetry with relayed information on the expected time of arrival, the patient's condition, haemodynamic status and cardiac rhythm can reduce the door-to-needle time for thrombolysis by as much as two-thirds (Weaver et al, 1993).

Peripheral intravenous access should be achieved at the outset, and the administration of nitrates, analgesics and oxygen may help to limit the size of the infarction. Clopidogrel 300 mg should be given in combination with aspirin 300 mg as soon as possible to all patients with suspected acute coronary syndromes (NICE, 2005).

Prehospital thrombolysis

Delays in establishing reperfusion in patients with coronary thrombosis and ST elevation myocardial infarction are inevitable for many reasons, and are mostly due to a deferred call for medical help. The United Kingdom Heart Attack Study reported that only 2% of patients were receiving thrombolytic therapy within 1 hour following the onset of symptoms when therapy is of most value (UKHAS, 1998). While the overall treatment value of aspirin with fibrinolysis therapy is quoted as 50 lives saved per 1000 patients treated, most of this benefit occurs in those treated within this first 'golden hour' (Boersma et al, 1996). By 4–6 hours, this falls to around 20 patients per 1000 (Anti-thrombotic Trialists' Collaboration, 2002). Reducing delay in providing thrombolytic treatment has been a major goal for primary and secondary care in recent years, and various strategies for prehospital thrombolysis and 'fast track' procedures in emergency departments have been proposed (Hill, 2005).

Prehospital thrombolysis is now commonplace, although implementation was based on very scant evidence. An overview of prehospital thrombolysis (Morrison et al, 2001) showed a 17% reduction in 30-day mortality with only about 1 hour being saved. Many of the individual trials were too small to show statistical significance and included very heterogeneous strategies, with administration of thrombolytics by GPs, cardiologists, paramedics or nurses. Conclusions from this widely referenced meta-analysis were greatly influenced by the GREAT trial (1992) that was not primarily designed to look at outcomes, but the feasibility and safety of prehospital thrombolysis. Claims that this trial proved the efficacy of prehospital treatment are weak because patients were up to 50 miles from the base hospital, where there was very poor door-to-needle times (over 90 minutes), resulting in a difference of 135 minutes between the two groups. The GPs responsible for thrombolysis were only performing this once per year, which

limited skill retention. Most GPs gave up prehospital thrombolysis after the trial had finished. Skill retention is still a problem for paramedic crews, unless thrombolysis can be concentrated in the hands of a few specialist crews. In urban areas, there will be greater numbers of patients allowing more experience. However, the journey to hospital in cities will be much shorter, so there is not so much to be gained from prehospital intervention. Prehospital thrombolysis would seem to be of greater value in rural areas, where the journey time is likely to cause the major delay in treatment (Rawles et al, 1998), although in rural communities, ambulances are more spread out, and there is little opportunity to concentrate the experience in the hands of smaller number of specialist crews. Furthermore, the GREAT trial showed that prehospital intervention 'tied up' ambulances and their specialist crews for longer than usual and impacted on ambulance availability in getting to other category A calls.

In the two most recent trials of prehospital fibrinolysis (Bonnefoy et al, 2002; Wallentin et al, 2003), a median time for call to treatment of 2 hours was achieved. However, it was an experienced physician who made decisions on thrombolysis, either in the ambulance or via telemetry, a situation that is not practicable in many areas where rapid transmission to hospital may still be the best method of management ('scoop-and-run'). Practically speaking, prehospital treatment should be given at least an hour sooner if it is going to make any difference, and anything less than this probably makes hospital treatment equally effective. With the diminishing numbers of ST elevation infarcts, it may be more logical to divert resources into developing a rapid response and transport system to get patients to the place where they may receive optimal therapy in the shortest time. This has obvious benefits for patients who are able to receive reperfusion by primary angioplasty.

Primary angioplasty

While thrombolysis is the commoner form of initial therapy for acute ST elevation myocardial infarction, reperfusion is gradual and incomplete in most cases; the occluded artery will be opened in only about half the cases. Up to 1 in 10 patients may have contraindications to thrombolysis (French et al, 1996), and patients who do not receive or are ineligible for thrombolysis are at high risk of death (Brown et al, 1999).

Primary (direct) angioplasty will mechanically disrupt the thrombus and restore patency in over 90% of cases of acute coronary thrombosis and, in turn, limits the size of the infarct and is associated with less post-infarct angina and heart failure. In addition, where there is no thrombolysis, there is no excess risk of bleeding. Randomised trials comparing primary percutaneous coronary intervention (PCI) with thrombolytic therapy have shown that the PCI strategy can save lives in both the short and the long term (Keeley et al, 2003). Outcome varies according to the expertise of the operator and centre, and PCI must be delivered promptly by an experienced team to achieve equivalent results (Van deer Warf et al, 2003). As for thrombolysis, time should always be kept to a minimum. Increasing 'door-to-balloon' times are associated with sharp increases in mortality, and there is also a 'golden hour' for primary PCI, although this probably extends to 90 minutes (Juliard et al, 2003). Each additional 30-minutes delay in the initiation of treatment is associated with a 7.5% increased risk of dying (De Luca et al, 2004). If thrombolysis can be given within 3 hours of the onset of symptoms, mortality is no higher than that associated with primary angioplasty. After 3 hours, primary angioplasty is preferable (Widimsky et al, 2000; Steg et al, 2003). In the controversy over whether primary angioplasty or thrombolysis is better, we should not forget that approximately one-third of patients fail to receive either (Eagle et al, 2002).

Although the current NHS infrastructure does not lend itself to primary angioplasty in most areas (Hartwell et al, 2005), in regions where a primary PCI centre can easily be reached, and an accurate prehospital diagnosis is possible, patients should be taken to the centre rather than the nearest hospital. Bypassing non-interventional hospitals may shorten delays by as much as 1 hour, although it is hoped that many larger district general hospitals will eventually be able to offer emergency PCI services (Qaisar et al, 2005). Taking the patient directly to the catheter laboratory rather than via the emergency department or coronary care unit (CCU)

may also reduce time to intervention. Currently, about 2000 patients in the UK are being treated with primary angioplasty annually, compared with only 390 cases in 2003/4.

Where preparation of the catheter laboratory is associated with delays, a strategy of *facilitated PCI* has been utilised. This involves fibrinolysis *en route* to the interventional hospital, followed by PCI as soon as possible. The PRAGUE study examined three strategies for patients presenting with acute ST elevation myocardial infarction to a district hospital without on-site catheterisation facilities – immediate thrombolysis, thrombolytic therapy during transfer for PCI, and transfer for primary angioplasty. Death, reinfarction or stroke was most frequent in those treated by thrombolysis alone. The best outcome was for those transferred for primary angioplasty, and results for facilitated angioplasty were intermediate (Widimsky et al, 2000). The ASSENT-4 PCI trial was terminated prematurely because of higher in-hospital mortality in those undergoing facilitated PCI rather than those who had direct angioplasty (ASSENT-4 PCI investigators, 2006).

The EMS–hospital interface

The EMS–hospital interface must ensure continuity between prehospital and in-hospital management of patients with acute coronary syndromes. Patients are usually taken to the emergency department, but these days should be taken directly to the CCU or catheter laboratory, but all diagnostic information obtained before presentation must be available to the receiving team to avoid unnecessary duplication of investigations delaying intervention. Where the diagnosis is not clear, admitting all patients with high-risk chest pain directly to the CCU for evaluation is the preferred option, although beyond the capability of many hospitals. If patients are seen first in the emergency department or admitted directly to a medical assessment unit (MAU), a system for rapid triage is needed to ensure that the appropriate cases get urgent treatment at the earliest opportunity. Protracted delays in reaching a therapeutic decision may occur if the history is atypical or if the ECG shows non-specific abnormalities. Much depends on the experience of the receiving physician as seeking a second opinion from a cardiologist may cause further delay. Where junior medical staff experience difficulty in the interpretation of an ECG, direct transmission by fax machines for opinion from the CCU may be useful. Adopting this practice in our hospital halved our door-to-needle times for thrombolysis.

For patients who do not have the advantage of prehospital thrombolysis, 'fast tracking' systems can be effective in reducing door-to-needle times for patients eligible for thrombolysis. Using 'thrombolysis pathways' may be particularly helpful (Cannon et al, 1999). The primary method of screening for an acute coronary syndrome is by a standard resting 12-lead electrocardiogram. It is then possible to separate patients presenting with a possible acute coronary syndrome as:

- *fast track*: acute coronary syndrome with an ECG showing ST elevation or bundle branch block;
- *intermediate track*: probable acute coronary syndrome (normal ECG or other changes);
- *slow track*: unlikely to be acute coronary syndrome (normal ECG).

Fast track patients should preferably be managed on the CCU, and reducing the in-hospital delay in getting these patients to the CCU has been a major task in recent years. The triage system should preferably bypass routine assessment by the on-call general medical team. Even if they are not fast tracked, patients with acute coronary syndromes are best managed on CCUs rather than on general medical wards, because the chances of resuscitation are two or three times higher. In addition, patients admitted to medical wards are often not considered soon enough for thrombolytic therapy or for other secondary interventions (Lawson-Matthew et al, 1994). Reductions in hospital mortality have mainly been achieved by faster admission procedures, infarct limitation with thrombolysis and primary angioplasty, and enhanced therapies for cardiogenic shock and heart failure.

The UK myocardial infarction national audit programme (MINAP) reports that 86% of cases of ST elevation myocardial infarction patients in England now receive thrombolysis within a door-to-needle time of 30 minutes, compared with 44%

in 2001 (Royal College of Physicians of London, 2004). This has become possible by better organisation of fast track procedures, direct CCU admission and bolus thrombolytic therapy either before hospital or in the emergency department.

Chest pain units

About 500 000 patients attend emergency departments in the UK each year with chest pain, and 20–30% of all medical admissions are because of acute chest pain. A normal initial ECG associates with a low mortality and morbidity, but does not exclude an acute coronary syndrome (Herlitz et al, 1998). In those patients known to have coronary disease, there is a 4% risk of progression to acute myocardial infarction but, if there is no previous history, the risk is only 1–2% (Lee & Goldman, 2000). It must be remembered that there may be other important diagnoses than an acute coronary syndrome that may not affect the ECG, such as aortic dissection or pulmonary embolism. Optimal management of non-fast track patients may be continued in a dedicated chest pain assessment unit (Farkouh et al, 1998).

Chest pain assessment units (CPUs) allow a more conclusive cardiac evaluation, often avoiding unnecessary hospital admission. The design and location of such units differs, but continues to evolve. They may form part of the CCU or the MAU or be located within the emergency department. Importantly, they must be readily accessible and have suitably trained physicians and nurses, with adequate monitoring and resuscitation facilities. The use of critical care pathways is particularly suited to allow an early decision about the presence or absence of an acute coronary syndrome, and may help to reduce variation in care, decrease resource utilisation, improve guideline compliance and, potentially, improve quality of care (Every et al, 2000). They may also prevent high-risk patients from being sent home. Between 2% and 4% of patients (usually women) with evolving myocardial infarction are discharged from emergency departments with a diagnosis of non-cardiac chest pain because of an atypical history and normal ECG (Pope et al, 2000).

After initial triage, either in the ambulance or in the emergency department using the history and a

12-lead ECG, those patients who do not have an obvious acute coronary syndrome are admitted to the CPU. Here, patients are monitored and serial cardiac biomarkers and ECGs are obtained. Continuous 12-lead ECG recording is very helpful, so that transient ECG changes are not missed. Rapid access to cardiac biomarker assays is particularly valuable, and near-patient testing may be especially helpful. If all tests are negative, the patient may undergo further evaluation, perhaps including stress testing or echocardiography. Those patients who have a recurrence of chest pain, a positive serum biomarker value, a significant ECG change or a positive stress test result are admitted for inpatient evaluation. Those with negative tests are usually discharged with outpatient follow-up if appropriate.

Randomised trials support the introduction of CPUs as a safe and effective method for the evaluation of low- to intermediate-risk chest pain patients (Goodacre, 2000). The ROMEO study showed that, by using a pathway for ruling out myocardial ischaemia (with troponin assay followed by exercise testing), the median admission time could be reduced to 23 hours without any adverse events occurring among discharged patients (Taylor et al, 2002).

The role of the modern coronary care unit

Before CCUs existed, treatment of acute myocardial infarction took place on general medical wards and was directed towards the healing of the infarct and the prevention of cardiac rupture. This usually involved prolonged periods of bedrest and intensive nursing support to prevent any minor degree of exertion. Thromboembolic complications were frequent, and the enthusiasm for positive inotropic agents such as digoxin and noradrenaline (norepinephrine) to support the failing heart probably contributed to a hospital mortality of around 25–30%. With the recognition of the importance of rhythm monitoring, cardiopulmonary resuscitation and prompt defibrillation, the management of coronary patients was revolutionised (Julian, 1961). The first purpose-built coronary care unit was opened on 20 May 1962 by Hughes Day in Kansas City, and others quickly followed in

Toronto, Sydney, New York, and Philadelphia (Day, 1972). From then on, medical and public demand led to the development of many similar units, so that by the early 1970s, most large hospitals had facilities for monitoring the acute coronary patient, either as part of a general ward or on a separate intensive care unit. Following establishment of coronary care units, in-patient mortality approximately halved probably secondary to the recognition and appropriate treatment of serious dysrhythmias (Julian, 1987).

Until relatively recently, the management of acute myocardial infarction was still essentially supportive, and it is only 20 years since the GISSI trial (1986) showed that we could actively treat the coronary thrombosis with streptokinase. The Clinical Trial Service Unit in Oxford then went on to design many similar 'megatrials', initially of thrombolysis (ISIS-1 Collaborative Group, 1988), but later using other cardiac interventions that have revolutionised coronary care. Because of the GISSI and ISIS studies, thrombolysis became routine therapy for acute myocardial infarction in the late 1980s, and every acute hospital needed to develop a coronary care facility.

Design and organisation of the coronary care unit

The design and layout of the coronary care unit has to be a compromise between desirability and practicality. A separate unit within the hospital complex is desirable, but there are advantages in locating the unit adjacent to other critical care areas, such as high dependency or intensive care units. Close access to exercise stress testing, echocardiography and a pacing room with catheter laboratory (if available) is useful. Accommodating patients in individual rooms often seems advantageous, so that they are unaware of other patients' problems and are protected from the high drama of cardiac arrests. However, while this design may allow privacy and promote rest, it makes no allowance for direct vision of the patient by the staff. Constant visual observation is a prime consideration in acute coronary care and, apart from its main role of spotting early signs of distress, may contribute towards the patients' overall feeling of well-being. Without this, patients may feel isolated, and fearful about not being discovered if they were to collapse. Most units offer a combination of open plan and side-rooms.

Patient bed areas must be large enough to accommodate staff and equipment and probably no smaller than 10 m². Each bed should have piped oxygen and suction and must be of suitable design for manoeuvring in case of cardiac arrest. Bed design has improved over the years, and electric 'profiling' beds have many useful features including adjustability for height, autocontouring controls, rapid Trendelenburg/reverse Trendelenburg controls, easily removable head and footboards and collapsible built-in side-rails. Two handles under the head section activate a rapid, cushioned release to flatten the bed should cardiac arrest occur, and the sleep surface is rigid enough to enable effective chest compressions.

Equipment should be located on the walls and fixed securely. Bedside monitors need to be connected to a central station to allow constant cardiac monitoring (Jowett, 1997). There should be sufficient natural (and artificial) light, with window views to the outside world, so that the patient does not become unduly disorientated. The ability to see a clock is particularly helpful in this respect. Noise insulation and air-conditioning are important for comfort and to promote rest. A separate procedure room away from the main unit is desirable for elective cardioversion and temporary pacing. Provision should be made for interviewing relatives in private and should be additional to a normal visitors' waiting room. Staff rest rooms are useful for periods of relaxation. A lecture room could also be included in CCU design, equipped with projection facilities and audiovisual aids, for continuing medical education and rehabilitation group meetings.

The benefits of these discrete cardiac units seems to have been maintained despite their changing role and the way in which we manage, not just acute myocardial infarction, but heart failure, dysrhythmias and cardiogenic shock. Mortality is three times less in patients cared for on a CCU by specialist staff rather than on general wards (Rotstein et al, 1999). This has led to a dichotomy of care, with relatively small numbers of patients (usually with ST elevation myocardial infarction) receiving specialist care on well-staffed CCUs,

whereas other patients with acute coronary syndromes are cared for on admission units or other medical wards. Most cardiac care units still have between four and eight beds and, while this has been sufficient for the management of patients with ST elevation myocardial infarction, it has become a relatively small number given the increasing referrals of others with acute coronary syndromes and other types of cardiovascular instability. An analysis by the MINAP group found that, although 84% of patients with ST elevation myocardial infarction were cared for on the CCU, over half of those with non-ST elevation myocardial infarction were admitted elsewhere, despite the known associated high mortality and morbidity of the latter syndrome (Quinn et al, 2005).

To ensure equity of care for all patients presenting with acute coronary syndromes, the traditional 'stand-alone' CCU will have to change, particularly in those hospitals where additional cardiac beds are not close by. A single, larger facility encompassing assessment, therapy and stepdown may be the way in which the modern cardiac care unit will develop in the future. Use of critical care pathways in the management of the various coronary syndromes, heart failure or common rhythm disturbances may help with continuity of care when the patient leaves the unit (Reinhart, 1995).

Modern management of acute coronary syndromes has continued to develop with the understanding of the pathophysiology of myocardial infarction, risk factors and newly acquired evidence-based interventions (Box 1.1), which have dramatically reduced 6-month mortality in patients with acute coronary syndromes (Mukherjee et al, 2004). Routine use of fibrinolytic therapy, aspirin, statins and angiotensin-converting enzyme (ACE) inhibitors has reduced the overall mortality from CHD in men by 72% and in women by 56% (Tunstall-Pedoe et al, 2000).

Stepdown units

As the risk of primary ventricular fibrillation is highest in the first few hours following myocardial infarction, there is little need for uncomplicated cases to remain on the CCU for longer than a day or two. Some patients can be transferred

Box 1.1 Summary results of cardiovascular drug trials.

ASPIRIN for ALL suspected acute myocardial infarction or unstable angina (+ LONG–TERM aspirin after leaving hospital)

Benefit: 24 lives/1000 (+ definite EXTRA from LONG TERM; increased benefits when given early with clopidogrel in unstable angina – 28 fewer coronary events/1000 patients treated)

FIBRINOLYTICS for patients with bundle branch block or ST elevation with aspirin

Benefit: 50–60 lives prevented/1000 treated in first hour (rapid loss of benefit to only 20 deaths/1000 prevented if treated 4–6 h after symptom onset)

BETA-BLOCKERS, STARTED WHEN STABLE and continued LONG TERM

Benefit: about 7 lives/1000 in first month (+ 10–20 EXTRA per year from LONG TERM + 21 fewer reinfarctions)

ACE INHIBITORS, STARTED EARLY (except in shock or persistent hypotension) and continued LONG TERM, especially in those with left ventricular dysfunction

Benefit: about 5–8 lives/1000 in first month (perhaps 14 lives/1000 in high-risk groups + EXTRA from LONG TERM in those with left ventricular dysfunction, perhaps 40 cardiac events/1000 treated)

STATINS – LONG TERM

Benefit: 20% reduction in major coronary events, coronary revascularisation and stroke per mmol/L reduction in LDL cholesterol over 5 years. 14 deaths/1000 treated for each mmol/L LDL reduction

ACE, angiotensin-converting enzyme; LDL, low-density lipoprotein.
NB. Heparin, magnesium, calcium antagonists, nitrates: little or no net benefit (and little difference between different fibrinolytic agents).

within the first 24 hours after admission if they do not have risk factors such as a history of previous infarction, persistent ischaemic pain, heart failure, hypotension or haemodynamically compromising ventricular dysrhythmias. It is unlikely that such patients will require transfer back to the CCU or will die in the hospital. However, those patients who survive to discharge remain at risk of further cardiovascular events, long-term survival being most closely related to age and left ventricular function.

Patients with high-risk features such as post-infarction angina should be referred for angiography without further investigation and not transferred to stepdown. For low-risk patients, early ambulation and discharge from hospital is encouraged. Low-level activities such as toileting, assisted bathing and light ambulation should be used to prevent physiological deconditioning,

which may occur in as little as 6 hours if the patient is kept in the supine position. Early mobilisation will prevent the complications caused by bedrest, particularly thromboembolic disorders, and will additionally reduce depression and physical weakness. A protocol for encouraging the patient quickly back to normal activity (Table 1.4) may be best undertaken on a stepdown unit, where the use of telemetry to monitor cardiac rhythm in the presence of immediate and practised resuscitation facilities is of advantage. An additional benefit of stepdown units is that early (phase I) rehabilitation and education can take place with all the patients together, as a form of group therapy, perhaps with their family being present. Inclusion of partners during teaching also increases learning and retention. In these days of shorter hospital stays, discharge planning needs to be started promptly by a skilled multidisciplinary team as

Table 1.4 Typical physical activity plan following acute myocardial infarction.

Time	Activity
Day 1	Bed/chair rest
Day 2	Sit out of bed or chair; discharge from CCU
Day 3	Walk around ward and to toilet
Day 4	Try stairs
Day 5–7	Submaximal exercise stress test Discharge home
Day 7–14	Exercise within home and garden
Day 14–28	Gradual increased walking outside home (20–30 min, once or twice daily)
Day 28	Symptom-limited exercise stress test Enrol in rehabilitation programme (phase III) Recommence driving (in line with DVLA regulations)
Day 36	Outpatient review Return to work

soon as possible after hospital admission and continue through the early discharge period (phase II rehabilitation). The decreasing length of hospital stays has raised concerns about adequate opportunity for appropriate patient education, although short educational sequences have been shown to produce outcomes comparable to lengthy sessions. Patient education effectively decreases emotional distress, increases knowledge and changes behaviour following a heart attack. Patients often need information about risk factors and self-management techniques (e.g. what to do if they get chest pain) rather than information about the disease itself. Innovative presentation styles using programmed instruction and audiovisual techniques can produce benefits comparable to individual educational sessions. Not all patients may be ready to learn during hospitalisation, and methods of accommodating them are needed. Use of a single folder for all educational materials may provide consistency and identify goals achieved and those that remain. Staffing of stepdown units by coronary care-trained nurses allows patients to benefit from continuity of care, as well as uniformity

of approach. Such units may ensure that all discharge plans are in place, such as medication plan and risk factor control, with arrangements for exercise stress testing and rehabilitation.

REHABILITATION

A heart attack is usually a devastating experience for most patients, particularly for younger victims who often have never been ill before. Like all major illnesses, a myocardial infarction has a physical, psychological and behavioural impact on the patient and their families. While most patients make a good cardiological recovery, some degree of chronic invalidism is common, often affecting their vocation, hobbies, social life and sexual activity. Psychosocial dysfunction is common, including depression, anger, anxiety disorders and social isolation. Of the 30–50% of patients who fail to return to work following their heart attack, only a few fail to do so for physical reasons. While the usual goal is to return patients to full normal activities, including work, within 6–8 weeks, this period may be too long. A 2-week target may not be unreasonable in low-risk patients, particularly for those in sedentary occupations, and may prevent elements of cardioneurosis (Kovoor et al, 2006).

The term *cardiac rehabilitation* refers to co-ordinated, multifaceted interventions designed to optimise a cardiac patient's physical, psychological and social functioning. In addition, it aims to stabilise, slow or even reverse the progression of coronary heart disease, thereby reducing morbidity and mortality. Cardiac rehabilitation services were originally directed at patients who had recently had a myocardial infarction or had undergone coronary artery bypass graft surgery, but they are now usually extended to those who have undergone percutaneous coronary interventions or valvular surgery. Rehabilitation also has a major role in improving outcome for patients with heart failure (Piña et al, 2003).

Exercise-based cardiac rehabilitation after myocardial infarction can promote recovery and reduce the chances of death (Taylor et al, 2004). There is also a trend towards fewer non-fatal myocardial infarctions and revascularisation procedures. The quality of life may also be improved for these patients by the relief of stress and anxiety and other measures to prevent cardiac neurosis.

Rehabilitation after an acute coronary syndrome should be part of an integrated treatment programme, and conform to the guidelines and standards laid out by the British Association of Cardiac Rehabilitation (BACR UK) in an agreed way across primary, secondary and tertiary care (Thompson et al, 1996). Rehabilitation services are often poorly developed and underutilised in many areas (Thompson et al, 1997) and, apart from financial constraints limiting the provision of adequate services, there is a low referral rate, particularly of women, older adults and those from ethnic minorities. In rural areas, there are often geographical limitations that restrict accessibility to the programme site.

Cardiac rehabilitation programmes differ in organisation, but most comprise sections on exercise and relaxation, with discussion and education. In addition to exercise training, comprehensive rehabilitation programmes include secondary prevention components aiming to reduce risk factors through nutritional counselling, weight management and promoting adherence to prescribed drug therapy. The last is particularly important as audits of lifestyle, risk factors and therapeutic management of patients with established coronary disease show poor adherence. The EUROASPIRE II Group survey (2001) of patients from 15 European countries in the convalescent phase following acute myocardial infarction found that 21% were still smoking cigarettes, 31% were still obese, 50% had raised blood pressure and 58% had raised serum total cholesterol. Prescription of evidence-based drugs was also suboptimal, with only 86% taking aspirin, 63% taking beta-blockers, 38% ACE inhibitors and 61% lipid-lowering agents. Hence, there remains considerable potential to reduce recurrent coronary disease through the implementation of proven interventions.

The needs of the cardiac patient vary, and thus require the expertise of a diverse team rather than doctor and nurse alone. Other team members may include physiotherapists, pharmacists, dieticians, occupational therapists and social workers. Nursing staff with cardiology training can play a significant role in family education and the physical rehabilitation of the patient, and their input is increasing in counselling sessions, exercise programmes and relaxation classes (Thompson, 1994). The formal rehabilitation programme is run on an outpatient basis (phase III) and extended into the long term to maintain health and functional ability (phase IV).

Effective communication between the coronary care team and the primary care members cannot be overemphasised, and the British Heart Foundation Cardiac Liaison Nurse scheme enables patients to be seen within a week of discharge to ensure continuing education and risk factor modification. Their work complements that of the rehabilitation team, impacting on both phase II and phase IV. These posts have an invaluable role in forging links between primary, secondary and tertiary care.

Palliative care

Good symptom control, psychological support and open communication about disease outcomes should be offered to all patients suffering from heart disease. Palliative care is normal in cancer medicine but, until recently, there has been little research into the needs of patients dying from other illnesses associated with a poor prognosis. Few non-cancer patients receive hospice, inpatient, home or day care. Chronic heart failure, in particular, can become a debilitating, terminal illness in many patients despite maximal medical therapy, with symptoms limiting daily life, including lethargy, anorexia, marked breathlessness and poor exercise capacity. Cardiac cachexia is common. The palliative approach shifts the focus of care from curing this debilitating disease to managing symptoms and incorporating treatment based on patient quality of life and survival goals (Quaglietti et al, 2005). Palliative care should be available for all heart failure patients who are not candidates for cardiac transplantation or mechanical support.

Staffing of coronary care

The staffing and organisation of the CCU is of great importance. Nursing staff ratios usually depend upon local conditions, but should be at least 1.5 times those of general medical wards. Minimum standards for all staff should include the capability to assess the acutely ill patient, the ability to apply immediate life support and an understanding of modern cardiac drugs and procedures.

The style of management will vary from unit to unit, but most function better where decisions are democratic rather than autocratic. This is more likely to encourage individual initiative, and helps to reduce stress levels in staff members on the unit, which would otherwise be transmitted to the patient. A consultant in cardiovascular medicine usually undertakes administrative duties, but it is desirable that selection and training of staff, unit policy and therapy are subject to discussion by all senior staff on the unit.

Patients are usually investigated and treated by two groups of doctors, trainee physicians and their supervising consultants. While the consultants direct the management of the patients, the junior medical staff are responsible for the day-to-day care of the patients on the unit. As patients on these units require constant supervision, it is usually not possible for this to be undertaken on a 24-hours basis by medical staff, and the responsibility has fallen to the nursing staff, which has extended the role of nursing that has evolved considerably during the last decade. Nurses were pivotal to the success of CCUs at their inception, and cardiac nurses have developed a much broader remit that includes working with cardiac patients in a variety of settings and with a range of knowledge and skills that encompass not only acute but also chronic disease management (Thompson & Stewart, 2002). The term 'cardiac nurse' was initially applied to those who were highly trained and technically skilled in the management of acute conditions in the cardiac care unit or in the post-operative intensive care setting. This has been redefined to encompass nurses working in a wider variety of settings in primary and secondary care, including the provision of rehabilitation and support for people with heart failure (Hatchett & Thompson, 2002).

Until recently, nurses have tended to rely on others for guidance and direction, rather than assuming the role of decision-maker. New initiatives have given cardiac care nurses the opportunity to undertake a wider range of clinical tasks to improve patient care, including requesting diagnostic investigations, making and receiving direct referrals, admitting and discharging patients for specified conditions and, within agreed protocols, managing patient caseloads (Department of Health, 2002). With the increased duties and responsibilities, the traditional doctor–nurse relationship is altered, which often proves awkward to the uninitiated (Jowett, 1986).

Some responsibilities have been widely criticised as not so much enhancing nursing roles, but rather filling gaps left by a failure to employ sufficient medical staff. The European working hours directive has effectively halved the working hours of junior medical staff, a gap that has not yet been filled by appropriate recruitment. Many nurses will no doubt be eager to undertake extended roles, but should not lose touch with their primary nursing role, nor be seduced into inappropriate tasks or areas where there has been insufficient training and supervision. With these new roles come new responsibilities. This includes frequent updating by reading relevant literature and keeping informed of professional issues and clinical practice. The medical profession is obliged to take compulsory, rather than optional, study leave for continuing professional development. The recent reforms in nurse education must ensure that this is an obligatory, and not an optional, part of patient care. In addition, audit, research and its clinical application are a normal part of medical training, and should no longer be the sole domain of the medical staff.

THE FUTURE

For people under 65 years, cardiac deaths have fallen by 44% in the last 10 years, and most fatalities are now occurring in the elderly. Modern therapy for CHD means that more people are surviving myocardial infarction, and it appears that death is being postponed rather than being prevented. There is no cure for the underlying pathology of atherosclerosis, and even modern drug therapies are largely ineffective in reversing the pathological process of atherosclerosis once it is advanced. Revascularisation delays, but does not prevent, events.

With more people surviving an initial heart attack, the medical caseload for the consequences of coronary disease will increase dramatically in the coming years. In addition, many more patients with acute coronary syndromes are now being classified as having had a myocardial infarction, based on more sensitive and specific markers of myocardial necrosis (Luepker et al, 2003).

Overall, there are about 2.68 million people who either have angina or have had a heart attack in the UK, and over 662 000 cases of heart failure. Using data from morbidity statistics from UK general practice, there are about 341 500 newly diagnosed cases of angina and 65 000 cases of new heart failure every year. Both angina and heart failure are more common in men but, importantly, both increase steeply with age. Changing demographics (more elderly persons) will also increase the total number of people with cardiovascular disease over the next few decades.

In 1999, the UK government set out a national strategy in 'Saving Lives: Our Healthier Nation', which, with another document entitled 'Smoking Kills', formed an ambitious series of linked complementary health policies (Department of Health, 1999). The National Service Framework (NSF) for Coronary Heart Disease was published in March 2000 and set national standards of care for coronary heart disease prevention and therapy to improve health, reduce variations in management and promote fast, high-quality services (Department of Health, 2000). The 12 standards cover:

- reducing heart disease in the population;
- preventing coronary heart disease in high-risk patients;
- treating acute coronary syndromes;
- investigating and treating angina;
- managing heart failure;
- revascularisation;
- rehabilitation.

A new section on 'Arrhythmias and sudden cardiac death' was published in February 2005, and the Arrhythmia Alliance (a heart rhythm charity) has brought together healthcare professionals, commissioners and their allies to promote cardiac pacing, implantable defibrillators, catheter ablation and other treatments for dysrhythmias.

Clinical governance has helped to implement these standards, and the National Institute for Health and Clinical Excellence (NICE) has provided clinical guidelines to ensure that, where appropriate, interventions are evidence based and cost-effective. The Healthcare Commission has the task of monitoring the implementation of the NSF.

A progress report from the Department of Health in 2004 ('Winning the War on Heart Disease') concluded that the NSF for Coronary Heart Disease has been a stimulus for improvements in the delivery of cardiac care since it was launched. Treatment of heart attack patients is now faster, and bypass surgery is being carried out faster and in increasing numbers. Much still needs to be done, particularly in preventing cardiovascular disease, improved care of patients with heart failure and better access to cardiac rehabilitation. Comprehensive coronary care is not just what we do on the coronary care unit, but encompasses prevention, early diagnosis, treatment and rehabilitation of all those with the various manifestations of coronary heart disease. Such an integrated approach should mean that the government target of reducing the death rate from coronary heart disease and stroke in people under 75 by at least 40% by 2010 is achievable.

References

Allender S, Peto V, Scarborough P et al (2006) *Coronary Heart Disease Statistics*. London: British Heart Foundation. Statistics database: www.heartstats.org.

Anti-thrombotic Trialists' Collaboration (2002) Collaborative meta-analysis of randomised trials of anti-platelet therapy for prevention of death, myocardial infarction, and stroke in high-risk patients. *British Medical Journal* 324: 71–86.

ASSENT-4 PCI investigators (2006) Primary versus tenecteplase-facilitated percutaneous coronary intervention in patients with ST-segment elevation acute myocardial infarction: a randomised trial. *Lancet* 367: 569–578.

Berenson GS, Srinivasan SR, Bao W et al (1998) Association between multiple cardiovascular risk factors and atherosclerosis in children and young adults. *New England Journal of Medicine* 338: 1650–1656.

Boersma E, Maas ACP, Simoons ML (1996) Early thrombolytic treatment in acute myocardial infarction: reappraisal of the Golden Hour. *Lancet* 348: 771–775.

Bonnefoy E, Lapostolle F, Leizorovicz A et al (2002) Primary angioplasty versus prehospital fibrinolysis in acute myocardial infarction: a randomised study. *Lancet* 360: 825–829.

Brown N, Melville M, Gray D et al (1999) Relevance of clinical trial results in myocardial infarction to clinical practice: comparison of four years outcome in participants of thrombolytic trials, patients receiving routine thrombolysis and those deemed ineligible for thrombolysis. *Heart* 81: 598–602.

Cannon CP, Johnson EB, Cermignani M et al (1999) Emergency department thrombolysis critical pathway reduces door-to-drug times in acute myocardial infarction. *Clinical Cardiology* 22: 17–20.

Daly CA, De Stavola B, Sendon JL et al (2006) Predicting prognosis in stable angina – results from the Euro heart survey of stable angina: prospective observational study. *British Medical Journal* 332: 262–265.

Davies MJ (1992) Anatomic features in victims of sudden coronary death. *Circulation* 85(suppl 1): 19–24.

Davies CS, Colquhoun M, Graham S et al (2002) Public Access Defibrillation: the establishment of a national scheme for England. *Resuscitation* 52: 13–21.

Day HW (1972) History of coronary care units. *American Journal of Cardiology* 30: 405–407.

Deedwania P (2001) Global risk assessment in the pre-symptomatic patient. *American Journal of Cardiology* 88 (suppl J): 17J–22J.

De Luca G, Suryapranata H, Ottervanger JP et al (2004) Time delay to treatment and mortality in primary angioplasty for acute myocardial infarction: every minute of delay counts. *Circulation* 109: 1223–1225.

Department of Health (1999) *Saving Lives: Our Healthier Nation*. London: The Stationery Office.

Department of Health (2000) *National Service Framework for Coronary Heart Disease*. London: The Stationery Office.

Department of Health (2002) *The Nursing Contribution to the Provision of Comprehensive Critical Care for Adults*. London: The Stationery Office.

Eagle KA, Goodman SG, Avezum A et al (2002) Practice variation and missed opportunities for reperfusion in ST elevation myocardial infarction: findings from the GRACE registry. *Lancet* 359: 373–377.

EUROASPIRE II Group (2001) Lifestyle and risk factor management and use of drug therapies in coronary patients from 15 countries. Principal results from EUROASPIRE II. *European Heart Journal* 22: 554–572.

Every NR, Hochman J, Becker R et al for the Committee on Acute Cardiac Care, Council on Clinical Cardiology, American Heart Association (2000) Critical pathways. *Circulation* 101: 461–464.

Farkouh ME, Smars PA, Reeder GS et al (1998) A clinical trial of a chest pain observation unit for patients with unstable angina. Chest Pain Evaluation in the Emergency Room (CHEER) Investigators. *New England Journal of Medicine* 339: 1882–1888.

French JK, Williams BF, Hart HH et al (1996) Prospective evaluation of eligibility for thrombolytic therapy in acute myocardial infarction. *British Medical Journal* 312: 1637–1641.

GISSI (1986) Effectiveness of intravenous thrombolytic treatment in acute myocardial infarction. Gruppo Italiano per lo Studio della Streptochinasi nell'Infarto Miocardico. *Lancet* 1: 397–402.

Go AS, Irribarren C, Chandra M et al (2006) Statin and beta-blocker therapy and the initial presentation of coronary heart disease. *Annals of Internal Medicine* 144: 229–238.

Goodacre SW (2000) Should we establish chest pain observation units within the UK? A systematic review and critical appraisal of the literature. *Journal of Accident and Emergency Medicine* 17: 1–6.

GREAT Group (1992) Feasibility, safety, and efficacy of domiciliary thrombolysis by general practitioners: Grampian Region Early Anistreplase Trial. *British Medical Journal* 305: 548–553.

Groh WJ, Newman MM, Beal PE et al (2001) Limited response to cardiac arrest by police equipped with automated external defibrillators: lack of survival benefit in suburban and rural Indiana – the police as responder automated defibrillation evaluation (PARADE). *Academic Emergency Medicine* 8: 324–330.

Gurwitz JH, McLaughlin TJ, Willison DJ et al (1997) Delayed hospital presentation in patients who have had acute myocardial infarction. *Annals of Internal Medicine* 126: 593–599.

Hallstrom A, Cobb L, Johnson E et al (2000) Cardiopulmonary resuscitation by chest compression alone or with mouth-to-mouth ventilation. *New England Journal of Medicine* 342: 1546–1553.

Hartwell D, Colquitt J, Loveman E et al (2005) Clinical effectiveness and cost-effectiveness of immediate angioplasty for acute myocardial infarction: systematic review and economic evaluation. *Health Technology Assessment (Winchester UK)* 9: 1–99, iii–iv.

Hasdai D, Behar S, Wallentin L et al (2002) A prospective survey of the characteristics, treatments and outcomes of patients with acute coronary syndromes in Europe and the Mediterranean basin: The Euro Heart Survey of Acute Coronary Syndromes. *European Heart Journal* 23: 1190–1201.

Hatchett R, Thompson DR (2002) *Cardiac Nursing: a Comprehensive Guide*. Edinburgh: Churchill Livingstone.

Hazinski MF, Idris AH, Kerber RE et al (2005) Lay rescuer automated external defibrillator ('Public Access Defibrillation') programs. *Circulation* 111: 3336–3340.

Herlitz J, Karlson BW, Lindqvist J et al (1998) Predictors and mode of death over 5 years amongst patients admitted to the emergency department with acute chest pain or other symptoms raising suspicion of acute myocardial infarction. *Journal of Internal Medicine* 243: 41–48.

Hill P (2005) Developing a chest pain team to fast track AMI patients. *Nursing Times* 10: 34–35.

ISIS-1 Collaborative Group (1988) Mechanisms for the early mortality reduction produced by beta-blockade started early in acute myocardial infarction. *Lancet* 1: 921–923.

Jowett NI (1984) *Recombinant DNA Gene-specific Probes and the Genetic Analysis of Diabetes Hyperlipidaemia and Coronary Heart Disease*. London: University of London.

Jowett NI (1986) The junior doctor on the intensive care unit. *Intensive Care Nursing* 1: 177–179.

Jowett NI (1997) *Cardiovascular Monitoring*. London: Whurr.

Julian DG (1961) Treatment of cardiac arrest in acute myocardial ischaemia and infarction. *Lancet* ii: 840–844.

Julian DG (1987) The history of coronary care units. *British Heart Journal* 57: 497–502.

Juliard JM, Feldman LJ, Golmard JL et al (2003) Relation of mortality of primary angioplasty during acute myocardial infarction to door-to-thrombolysis in myocardial infarction (TIMI) time. *American Journal of Cardiology* 91: 1401–1405.

Keeley EC, Boura J, Grines CL (2003) Primary angioplasty versus intravenous thrombolytic therapy for acute myocardial infarction: a quantitative review of 23 randomised trials. *Lancet* 361: 13–20.

Kovoor P, Lee AK, Carrozzi W et al (2006) Return to full normal activities including work at two weeks after acute myocardial infarction. *American Journal of Cardiology* 97: 952–958.

Lampe FC, Morris RW, Walker M et al (2005) Trends in rates of different forms of diagnosed coronary heart disease, 1978 to 2000: prospective, population based study of British men. *British Medical Journal* 330: 1046.

Lawson-Matthew PJ, Wilson AT, Woodmansey PA et al (1994) Unsatisfactory management of patients with acute myocardial infarction admitted to general medical wards. *Journal of the Royal College of Physicians of London* 28: 49–51.

Lee TH, Goldman L (2000) Evaluation of the patient with acute chest pain. *New England Journal of Medicine* 342: 1187–1195.

Lowel H, Lewis M, Keil U et al (1995) Time trends of acute myocardial infarction morbidity, mortality, 28-day-case fatality and acute medical care: results of the Augsburg myocardial infarction register from 1985 to 1992. *Zeitschrift für Kardiologie* 84: 596–605.

Luepker, RV, Apple FS, Christenson RH et al (2003) Case definition for acute coronary heart disease in epidemiology and clinical research studies. *Circulation* 108: 2543–2549.

McManus RJ, Mant J, Davies MK et al (2002) A systematic review of the evidence for rapid access chest clinics. *International Journal of Clinical Practice* 56: 4–5.

Morrison LJ, Verbeek PR, McDonald AC et al (2001) Mortality and pre-hospital thrombolysis for acute myocardial infarction. A meta-analysis. *Journal of the American Medical Association* 283: 2686–2692.

Mukherjee D, Fang J, Chetcuti S et al (2004) Impact of combination evidence-based medical therapy on mortality in patients with acute coronary syndromes. *Circulation* 109: 745–749.

Murray CJL, Lopez AD (1997) Alternative projections of mortality and disability by cause 1990–2020; global burden of disease study. *Lancet* 349: 1498–1504.

NICE (2005) Clopidogrel and modified release dipyridamole in the prevention of occlusive vascular events. Technology Appraisal No. 90. www.nice.org.uk.

NICE (2006) Arrhythmia – implantable cardioverter defibrillators (ICDs). Review No. 95. www.nice.org.uk.

Norris RM on behalf of the UK Heart Attack Study (UKHAS) Collaborative Group (1998) Fatality outside hospital from acute coronary events in three British health districts 1994–95. *British Medical Journal* 316: 1065–1070.

Norris RM on behalf of the UK Heart Attack Study (UKHAS) Collaborative Group (2005) Circumstances of out of hospital cardiac arrest in patients with ischaemic heart disease. *Heart* 91: 1537–1540.

Page RL, Hamdan MH, McKenas DK (1998) Defibrillation aboard a commercial aircraft. *Circulation* 97: 1429–1430.

Pantridge JF, Geddes JS (1967) A mobile intensive care unit in the management of myocardial infarction. *Lancet* ii: 271–273.

Pell JP, Sirel JM, Marsden AK et al (2002) Potential impact of public access defibrillators on overall survival following out of hospital cardiopulmonary arrest. *British Medical Journal* 325: 515–517.

Piña IL, Epstein CS, Balady GJ et al (2003) American Heart Association Committee on exercise, rehabilitation, and prevention. Exercise and heart failure: a statement from the American Heart Association committee on exercise, rehabilitation, and prevention. *Circulation* 107: 1210 –1225.

Pope JH, Aufderheide TP, Ruthazer R et al (2000) Missed diagnosis of acute cardiac ischaemia in the emergency department. *New England Journal of Medicine* 342: 1163–1170.

Prasad N, Wright A, Hogg KJ et al (1997) Direct admission to the coronary care unit by the ambulance service for patients with suspected myocardial infarction. *Heart* 78: 462–464.

Qaisar S, Fellows M, Whitlam H et al (2005) Introduction of primary percutaneous coronary intervention for ST elevation myocardial infarction in a district general hospital. *British Journal of Cardiology* 12: AIC56–59.

Quaglietti S, Pham M, Froelicher V (2005) A palliative care approach to the advanced heart failure patient. *Current Cardiology Reviews* 1: 45–52.

Quinn T, Weston C, Birkhead J et al (2005) Redefining the coronary care unit: study of patients admitted to hospital in England and Wales in 2003. *Quarterly Journal of Medicine* 98: 797–802.

Rawles J, Sinclair C, Jennings K et al (1998) Audit of pre-hospital thrombolysis by general practitioners in peripheral practices in Grampian. *Heart* 80: 231–234.

Reinhart SI (1995) Uncomplicated myocardial infarction: a critical path. *Cardiovascular Nursing* 31: 1–7.

Richardson LD, Gunnels MD, Groh WJ et al (2005) Implementation of community-based public access defibrillation in the PAD trial. *Academic Emergency Medicine* 12: 688–697.

Rodríguez T, Malvezzi M, Chatenoud L et al (2006) Trends in mortality from coronary heart and cerebrovascular diseases in the Americas: 1970–2000. *Heart* 92: 453–460.

Rosengren A, Wallentin L, Simoons M et al (2005) Cardiovascular risk factors and clinical presentation in acute coronary syndromes. *Heart* 91: 1141–1147.

Rotstein Z, Mandelzweig L, Lavi B et al (1999) Does the coronary care unit improve prognosis of patients with acute myocardial infarction? *European Heart Journal* 20: 813–818.

Royal College of Physicians of London (2004) *How the NHS Manages Heart Attacks. Third Public Report of the Myocardial Infarction National Audit Project (MINAP).* London: Clinical Effectiveness and Evaluation Unit, RCP.

Ruston A, Clayton J, Calnan M (1998) Patients' action during their cardiac event: qualitative study exploring differences and modifiable factors. *British Medical Journal* 316: 1060–1065.

Scarpello JHB (2004) Will prevention of type 2 diabetes reduce the future burden of cardiovascular disease? *British Journal of Cardiology* 11: 249–254.

Steg PG, Bonnefoy E, Chabaud S et al (2003) Impact of time to treatment on mortality after prehospital fibrinolysis or primary angioplasty: data from the CAPTIM randomized clinical trial. *Circulation* 108: 2851–2856.

Suttcliffe SWJ, Fox KF, Wood DA et al (2003) Incidence of angina, myocardial infarction and sudden cardiac death – a community register. *British Medical Journal* 326: 20.

Taylor C, Forrest-Hay A, Meek S (2002) ROMEO: a rapid rule out strategy for low risk chest pain. Does it work in a UK emergency department? *Emergency Medicine Journal* 19: 395–399.

Taylor RS, Brown A, Ebrahim S et al (2004) Exercise-based rehabilitation for patients with coronary heart disease: systematic review and meta-analysis of randomized trials. *American Journal of Medicine* 116: 682–697.

Then KL, Rankin JA, Fofonoff DA (2001) Atypical presentation of acute myocardial infarction in 3 age groups. *Heart and Lung* 30: 285–293.

Thompson DR (1994) Cardiac rehabilitation services: the need to develop guidelines. *Quality in Health Care* 3: 169–172.

Thompson DR, Stewart S (2002) Nurse-directed services: how can they be made more effective? *European Journal of Cardiovascular Nursing* 1: 6–9.

Thompson DR, Bowman GS, Kitson AL et al (1996) Cardiac rehabilitation in the United Kingdom: guidelines and audit standards. *Heart* 75: 89–93.

Thompson DR, Bowman GS, Kitson AL et al (1997) Cardiac rehabilitation services in England and Wales: a national survey. *International Journal of Cardiology* 59: 299–304.

Tunstall-Pedoe H, Kuulasmaa K, Amouyel P et al (1994) Myocardial infarctions and coronary deaths in the World Health organisation MONICA project. Registration procedures, event rates, and case fatality rates in 38 populations from 21 countries in four continents. *Circulation* 90: 583–612.

Tunstall-Pedoe H, Vanuzzo D, Hobbs M et al (2000) Estimation of contribution of changes in coronary care to improving survival, event rates, and coronary heart disease mortality across the WHO MONICA Project populations. *Lancet* 355: 688–700.

Unal, B, Critchley MA, Capewell S (2005) Modelling the decline in coronary heart disease deaths in England and Wales, 1981–2000: comparing contributions from primary prevention and secondary prevention. *British Medical Journal* 331: 614–617.

United Kingdom Heart Attack Study (UKHAS) Collaborative Group (1998) Effect of time from onset of coming under care on fatality of patients with acute myocardial infarction: effect of resuscitation and thrombolytic treatment. *Heart* 80: 114–120.

Valenzuela TD, Roe D, Nichol G et al (2000) Outcomes of rapid defibrillation by security officers after cardiac arrest in casinos. *New England Journal of Medicine* 343: 1206–1209.

Van deer Warf F, Ardissino D, Betriu A (2003) Management of acute myocardial infarction in patients presenting with ST segment elevation. The task force on the management of acute myocardial infarction of the European Society of Cardiology. *European Heart Journal* 24: 28–66.

Wallentin L, Goldstein P, Armstrong PW et al (2003) Efficacy and safety of tenecteplase in combination with the low-molecular-weight heparin enoxaparin or unfractionated heparin in the pre-hospital setting: the Assessment of the Safety and Efficacy of a New Thrombolytic Regimen (ASSENT)-3 PLUS randomised trial in acute myocardial infarction. *Circulation* 108: 135–142.

Weaver WD, Cerqueira M, Hallstrom AP et al (1993) Prehospital-initiated vs. hospital-initiated thrombolytic therapy. The Myocardial Infarction Triage and Intervention Trial. *Journal of the American Medical Association* 270: 1211–1216.

Welsh RC, Chang W, Goldstein P et al (2005) Time to treatment and the impact of a physician on pre-hospital management of acute ST elevation myocardial infarction: insights from the ASSENT-3 PLUS trial. *Heart* 91: 1400–1406.

Widimsky P, Groch L, Zelizko M et al (2000) Multicentre randomized trial comparing transport to primary angioplasty vs immediate thrombolysis vs combined strategy for patients with acute myocardial infarction presenting to a community hospital without a catheterization laboratory. The PRAGUE study. *European Heart Journal* 21: 823–831.

Wild S, McKeigue P (1997) Cross-sectional analysis of mortality by country of birth in England and Wales, 1970–92. *British Medical Journal* 314: 705–710.

World Health Organization (2004) *WHO Statistics Annual.* Geneva: WHO.

Yusuf S, Reddy S, Ounpuu S et al (2001) Global burden of cardiovascular diseases: Part I: general considerations, the epidemiologic transition, risk factors, and impact of urbanization. Review. *Circulation* 104: 2746–2753.

Yusuf S, Hawken S, Ounpuu S et al (2004) Effect of potentially modifiable risk factors associated with myocardial infarction in 52 countries (the INTERHEART study): case–control study. *Lancet* 364: 937–952.

Zheng ZJ, Croft JB, Giles WH et al (2001) Sudden cardiac death in the United States, 1989 to 1998. *Circulation* 104: 2158–2163.

Chapter 2

Anatomy, physiology and pathology

THE ANATOMY OF THE HEART

The heart is a hollow muscular organ located behind the costal cartilages in the middle mediastinum. The size of the heart corresponds quite accurately with the size of the patient's clenched fist and weighs about 280–340 g. The heart lies obliquely in the chest resembling an inverted cone, with the base facing upwards and the apex pointing downwards, forwards and to the left (Fig. 2.1). The inferior surface sits on the central tendon of the diaphragm. About two-thirds of the heart lies to the left, and one-third to the right, of the median plane. The apex of the heart may be felt in the fifth intercostal space in the mid-clavicular line (the apex beat).

At the junction of the upper one-third and lower two-thirds of the heart, a deep oblique *atrioventricular groove* passes round the heart, separating the atria from the ventricles. From this, two other grooves extend towards the apex, anteriorly (the *anterior interventricular groove*) and posteriorly (the *posterior interventricular groove*). These mark the position of the *interventricular septum*, which separates the right and left ventricles internally. The junction of the posterior interventricular and posterior atrio-ventricular (AV) grooves is known as the *crux*. Internally at this junction, the *interatrial septum* joins the interventricular septum.

A tough, fibrous pericardium encloses the heart and prevents any sudden cardiac distension. Within the fibrous pericardium and extending on to the surface of the heart is a thin, delicate membrane, the *serous pericardium*. The outer parietal layer lines the inner surface of the pericardium, and the inner visceral layer (*epicardium*) covers the outer surface of the heart and the adjoining portions of the great vessels. Where the great vessels pass through the fibrous pericardium, the two layers of the serous pericardium are reflected back and become continuous with one another. Between the two layers is a potential space, the *pericardial cavity*. This normally contains a small amount of fluid secreted by the serous pericardium, which acts as a lubricant to facilitate movement of the heart within the pericardial cavity.

The fibrous pericardium blends with the tunica adventitia of the great vessels and is firmly attached to the central tendon of the diaphragm below, and to the back of the sternum by the sterno-pericardial ligaments.

The chambers and valves of the heart

The heart consists of four chambers: two *atria* above and two *ventricles* below (Fig. 2.2). The right

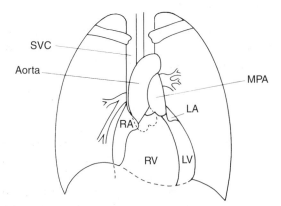

Figure 2.1 Anterior view of the heart. RA, right atrium; LA, left atrium; RV, right ventricle; LV, left ventricle; MPA, main pulmonary artery; SVC, superior vena cava.

and left sides of the heart are separated by an interatrial septum and an interventricular septum. The main valves of the heart are the *mitral* and *aortic* valves on the left side of the heart, and the *tricuspid* and *pulmonary* valves on the right side of the heart. They are complex avascular structures and are very strong. During a normal lifetime, they will open and close some 2700 million times.

The right atrium

The right atrium lies to the right of and slightly behind the right ventricle and anterior and to the right of the left atrium. It forms the lower right lateral heart border on the chest radiograph.

The right atrium is a thin-walled (2 mm) chamber that receives the venous return to the heart from the two largest veins in the body, the *superior* and *inferior venae cavae*. The right atrium also drains blood from the large *coronary sinus* that lies in the posterior AV groove. The location of the coronary sinus sometimes makes passage of pacing wires and electrodes used during electrophysiological studies difficult, particularly if trans-septal puncture is needed to position electrodes in the left atrium. Small cardiac veins sometimes also drain directly into the right atrium, as do two anterior

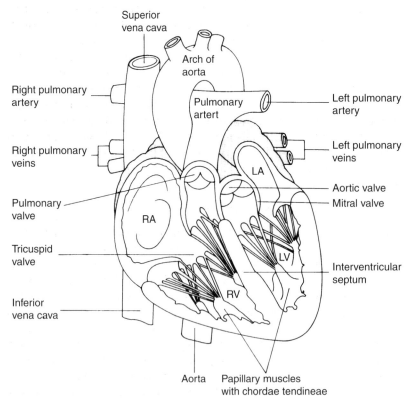

Figure 2.2 The internal anatomy of the heart. RA, right atrium; LA, left atrium; RV, right ventricle; LV, left ventricle.

cardiac veins. Thebesian veins (venae cordis minimae) are responsible for about a third of all venous drainage of the heart and pass directly into all chambers of the heart, mostly on the right.

The inferior vena cava passes through the diaphragm at the level of eighth thoracic vertebra and immediately enters the right atrium. The superior vena cava passes into the upper part of the right atrium. The opening of the superior vena cava is valveless, but the inferior vena cava and the opening of the coronary sinus have rudimentary valves that are remnants of the embryonic *sinus venosus*. The *Eustachian valve* lies at the entrance of the inferior vena cava, and the *Thebesian valve* guards the opening of the coronary sinus.

The inner surfaces of the posterior and septal walls are smooth, while the surfaces of the lateral wall and the right atrial appendage are composed of parallel muscle fibres known as the *pectinate muscles*. Posteriorly, they end on a longitudinal elevation (the *crista terminalis*), which runs from the right side of the opening of the superior vena cava to the right side of the orifice of the inferior vena cava. This is marked externally on the surface of the right atrium by a shallow groove, the *sulcus terminalis*. On the interatrial septum is a depression known as the *fossa ovalis*, a remnant of the septum primum.

The Chiari network is a congenital remnant of the right valve of the sinus venosus. It has been found in up to 4% of autopsy studies and, although of little clinical consequence, it often causes concern when seen on echocardiography, being confused with thrombus, vegetations or tumour. It appears as coarse strands connected to the Eustachian and Thebesian valves and attached to the crista terminalis. Unusually large strands may prolapse through the tricuspid valve during atrial systole. There is an association with a patent foramen ovale.

The tricuspid valve perforates the floor of the right atrium, and has three triangular cusps named septal, anterior and posterior. Between the valve orifice and the opening of the inferior vena cava is the coronary sinus, which is protected by a small valve that prevents blood flowing into the sinus during atrial systole. The AV node lies between this orifice and the septal cusp of the tricuspid valve.

The right ventricle

The right ventricle is the most anteriorly located chamber, lying directly beneath the sternum, with its inferior border being located beneath the xiphoid process. The crescent-shaped chamber has a relatively thin outer wall (3–5 mm), which is approximately one-third the thickness of the left ventricular wall. The pulmonary trunk rises from a smooth cone-shaped area (conus arteriosus or infundibulum) at the base of the ventricle. Blood entering the infundibulum is ejected superiorly and to the right, through the pulmonary valve and into the pulmonary artery. The pulmonary valve has three semi-lunar cusps named anterior, right and left. On the inner surface of the right ventricular wall are a number of irregular projections of raised interweaving muscle bundles (*trabeculae carneae*). The *papillary muscles* project into the ventricular cavity to become continuous with the *chordae tendineae*, which are attached to the free border of the cusps of the tricuspid valve. Contraction of the ventricle not only opposes the tricuspid valve cusps, but also prevents the valve being pushed back into the atrium, by maintaining tension on the chordae tendineae. A large, rounded muscle bundle, the *moderator band*, crosses the cavity of the right ventricle from the interventricular septum to the anterior wall. This conveys part of the right bundle branch of conducting tissue to the ventricular muscle. The right ventricle receives venous blood from the right atrium during ventricular diastole and expels it against low resistance (around 25 mmHg pressure) into the pulmonary circulation during ventricular systole.

The left atrium

The left atrium is the most posterior chamber and lies to the midline behind the right ventricle. It is the only cardiac chamber not normally visible on the chest radiograph. The left atrium receives blood from the four large valveless pulmonary veins, arranged in pairs on each side. The chamber is roughly cuboidal in shape and somewhat smaller than the right atrium, with slightly thicker walls (about 3 mm). A small conical pouch (the *auricle* or *left atrial appendage*) projects from the upper left corner. The left atrial appendage (LAA) is the only trabeculated structure in the left atrium because, unlike the right atrium, the left atrium has no crista terminalis. While sometimes regarded as just a minor extension of the atrium, the LAA is the usual source of cardiac emboli (90%). Surgical excision or percutaneous occlusion of the LAA is sometimes performed in patients with chronic or paroxysmal atrial fibrillation who are at high risk of developing thromboembolic events of stroke, but who are not candidates for long-term anticoagulation with warfarin.

The left atrial aspect of the septum is roughened, marking the site of the fetal foramen ovale. *In utero*, the foramen ovale serves as a channel for right-to-left shunting of oxygenated maternal blood. Once the pulmonary circulation is established after birth, left atrial pressure increases, allowing closure of the foramen ovale, which is followed by anatomical closure of the septum primum and septum secundum within 12 months. If closure fails or is incomplete, a *patent foramen ovale* remains, with a flap-like opening between the atrial septa primum and secundum allowing continuity with the right atrium. This may be demonstrable on between 10% and 15% of the adult population with contrast echocardiography. At autopsy, there is a 27% prevalence of probe-patent foramen ovale.

In the floor of the left atrium is the circular left atrio-ventricular orifice, guarded by the mitral valve, so called because it possesses two unequal triangular cusps (large anterior and small posterior), arranged like a bishop's mitre.

The left ventricle

The left ventricle receives blood from the left atrium during ventricular diastole and ejects blood against high resistance into the systemic circulation during ventricular systole. It forms the lower left lateral cardiac border when viewed from the front, and lies posteriorly and to the left of the right ventricle, and below and to the left of the left atrium.

The chamber is conical, and its apex lies approximately in the fifth intercostal space within the mid-clavicular line. As it normally expels blood against a much higher resistance than the right ventricle, the walls of the left ventricle are much more muscular than those of the right ventricle (8–12 mm). The interventricular septum is also thick and muscular, except for a small membranous area just behind the medial papillary muscle of the tricuspid valve that is occasionally malformed (membranous ventriculo-septal defect – VSD). The septum separates the two ventricles, and its upper portion also separates the right atrium from the left ventricle. The interventricular septum bulges to the right because the walls of the left ventricle are much thicker than those of the right ventricle. Upper septal hypertrophy is often related to degenerative change with ageing (sigmoid septum). Such septal angulation appears to form a localised bulge in the anterior septum where the proximal portion of the ventricular septum is bent, impinging into the outflow tract, an appearance sometimes confused with hypertrophic cardiomyopathy (Prasad et al, 1999).

Below and posteriorly, the left ventricle communicates with the left atrium through the left atrio-ventricular orifice and the mitral valve. The two papillary muscles are much larger than those of the right ventricle and, from these, chordae tendineae are attached to both cusps of the mitral valve. Above and anteriorly, the left ventricle opens into the aorta. The smooth outflow tract is called the aortic vestibule and corresponds to the membranous part of the interventricular septum. The aortic valve is in continuity with the mitral valve by a fibrous, double-looped band, shaped like a figure 8. The aortic valve has three semilunar cusps (right, left and non-coronary), which are stronger than those of the pulmonary valve. At the origin of each aortic cusp, the walls of the aorta show a slight dilatation or *sinus*. The right coronary artery arises from the right aortic sinus and the left coronary artery from the left aortic sinus, the orifice of each artery arising above the level of the cusp. These three aortic sinuses are known collectively as the *sinuses of Valsalva*. The *aortic root* is composed of the aortic annulus, the sinuses of Valsalva, the sino-tubular junction (sometimes called the supra-aortic ridge) and the ascending aorta. The 'normal' aortic diameter depends upon body surface area and age. The mean (SD) normal value for the aortic annulus in men is 2.6 (0.3) cm and in women is 2.3 (0.2) cm, and for the proximal ascending aorta 2.9 (0.3) cm and 2.6 (0.3) cm respectively. The upper normal limit for the ascending aorta is 2.1 cm/m^2. The aortic diameter gradually increases over time at an expected rate over 10 years of between 1 and 2 mm. This is greater for patients with an aorta that is larger than normal. A value beyond 4 cm is regarded as an aneurysm, a lower value as ectasia. As the normal value for the descending aorta is 1.6 cm/m^2, aneurysm is present when a value of 3 cm is exceeded.

The tissues of the heart

The main mass of the heart consists of muscular tissue (the *myocardium*), which is lined by the *endocardium* and covered by the visceral layer of serous pericardium (the *epicardium*). Blood and lymphatic vessels, nerves and specialised conducting tissues lie within the myocardial mass. The tough pericardium holds and protects the heart.

The epicardium

The epicardium consists of a single layer of mesothelial cells covering a thin layer of loose connective tissue, which contains elastic fibres, small blood vessels and nerves. In places, it is separated from the myocardium by a layer of adipose tissue, which carries the coronary blood vessels.

The myocardium

The myocardium is composed of specialised involuntary cardiac muscle. Individual myocardial cells are grouped in bundles in a connective tissue framework, which carries small blood and lymphatic vessels and autonomic nerve fibres. The density of capillaries in cardiac muscle cells is much greater than in skeletal muscle, because of its higher blood requirements. The myocardium is thickest towards the apex and thins towards the base.

The myocardium consists of a network of muscle fibres that show transverse and longitudinal striation and which branch and connect with each other. The ends of the cells are in very close contact with adjacent cells, and the 'joints' can be seen as thick dark striations called *intercalated discs*. Because of the close relationship of one muscle fibre with the next, once contraction starts in any part, it cannot remain localised and spreads throughout the entire network of muscle cells. The atrial muscle is thinner and less complicated than ventricular muscle. It has a short refractory period that allows a rapid rate of contraction.

The endocardium

The endocardium is in continuity with the lining of the blood vessels (endothelium). It is much thinner than the epicardium and consists of a lining of endothelial cells, a middle layer of dense connective tissue containing many elastic fibres and an outer layer of loose connective tissue, in which there are small blood vessels and specialised conducting tissue. The heart valves are formed by folds of endocardium, thickened by a core of fibrous tissue extending in from the tissue of the sulcus. The endocardium and myocardium are firmly bound together by connective tissue.

The pericardium

The outer layer of the pericardium blends with adventitia of the aorta, the pulmonary trunk, the superior vena cava and the central tendon of the diaphragm. Within this tough sac, there are two layers of serous pericardium in continuity with each other. One layer is applied to the heart (visceral layer) and the other to the inner surface of the pericardium (parietal layer).

The conducting system

In addition to the purely contractile muscle fibres of the atria and ventricles, the heart possesses certain specialised muscle cells that form the conducting system. These cells contain a few contractile fibres, but their ability to initiate and conduct electrical impulses within the heart is used to produce myocardial contraction. The conducting system comprises:

- the sinus node;
- the atrio-ventricular (AV) node;
- the AV bundle of His;
- the right and left bundle branches;

● the peripheral ramifications of the bundle branches (Purkinje fibres).

The sino-atrial node

The sino-atrial (SA) node is the normal site of initiation of the heartbeat. It is situated at the junction of the superior vena cava with the right atrium (Fig. 2.3). The top end of the crista terminalis marks this junction internally. The node is spindle-shaped, about 20 mm in length and about 3 mm in width. The framework of the node is collagenous, interlaced by bundles of small conduction fibres. There are numerous autonomic nerve endings in the node, with parasympathetic fibres derived from the right vagus nerve. The blood supply is via the nodal artery, which arises from the right coronary artery in 55% of people. Blood supply otherwise comes from the left coronary artery (42%) or from both left and right coronary arteries.

Conduction between the SA and AV nodes was thought to occur through conduction between normal atrial myocytes, but bands of specialised myocytes (rather like Purkinje fibres) lie between the SA node and the AV node called *internodal tracts*. Three discrete internodal tracts have been described:

1 An anterior tract leaves the anterior surface of the SA node, passes to the interatrial septum and then splits into two bundles, one passing to the left atrium and the other posteriorly to the AV node.

2 A middle tract leaves the posterior surface of the SA node and passes around the orifice of the inferior vena cava to reach the interatrial septum and then inferiorly to the AV node.

3 A posterior tract also leaves the posterior surface of the SA node and passes through the crista terminalis and around the valve of the inferior vena cava to reach the posterior surface of the AV node.

The atrio-ventricular (AV) junction

There is no muscular continuity between the atria and the ventricles except through the conducting tissue of the *atrio-ventricular node* and *AV bundle* (*of His*) that together comprise the *AV junction*. The aortic and mitral valves have strong fibrous rings that prevent the orifices from stretching and making the valves incompetent. These rings are continuous with a dense fibro-cartilaginous mass, sometimes called the *heart skeleton*. This framework affords a firm anchorage for the attachment of the atrial and ventricular musculature, as well as the valvular tissue. The pulmonary valve does not have a ring, and that of the tricuspid valve is only partially formed.

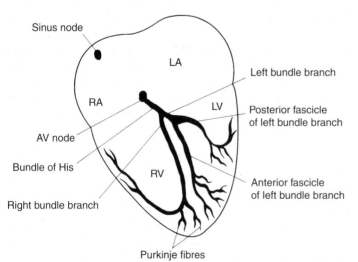

Figure 2.3 The conducting tissues of the heart.

The AV node

The AV node lies between the opening of the coronary sinus and the posterior border of the membranous interventricular septum. The node is divided into a transitional zone and a compact portion. Its function is to cause a delay in transmission of the cardiac impulse from the atria to the ventricles, so that the atria have time to expel their contents into the ventricles before systole.

The AV node has a structure similar to that of the sinus node, but there is much less collagen in the framework, and the conduction fibres are thicker and shorter than those in the SA node. There is a rich autonomic nerve supply, the parasympathetic fibres being derived from the left vagus nerve. The blood supply is from a specific nodal artery, which arises from the right coronary artery in 86% of cases, from the left circumflex artery in 12% and from both arteries in the remainder.

The AV bundle

The AV bundle extends from the AV node along the posterior margin of the membranous portion of the interventricular septum to the crest of the muscular septum.

Here, it bifurcates into the *right* and *left bundle branches*. The AV bundle is oval or triangular in cross-section with fibres that run parallel to one another, unlike the fibres of the sinus and AV nodes, which interweave. The connective tissue surrounding the bundle prevents depolarisation of the ventricular myocardium in direct contact with it during its course through the interventricular septum.

The AV bundle and the proximal few millimetres of both bundle branches are supplied by the terminal branch of the AV nodal artery and from the septal branches of the left anterior descending artery.

The bundle branches

The right and left bundle branches extend subendocardially along both sides of the interventricular septum. The right bundle is a cord-like structure that passes down the right side of the interventricular septum towards the apex, lying more deeply beneath the endocardium than the left main bundle.

It then runs in the free edge of the moderator band to reach the base of the anterior papillary muscle, where it ramifies among the right ventricular musculature.

The left bundle branch is an extensive sheet of fibres that passes down the left side of the interventricular septum. The initial part of the left bundle is fan-shaped and breaks up into two interconnecting left and right hemi-fascicles (see Fig. 2.3). The terminal branches of the bundle branches are the *Purkinje fibres*, which ramify within the ventricular myocardium. Septal arteries from the left anterior descending artery supply the bundle branches.

The coronary circulation

The heart and proximal portion of the great vessels receive their blood supply from two *coronary arteries*, which originate from the sinuses of Valsalva (Fig. 2.4). When healthy, the coronary arteries are capable of autoregulation to maintain coronary blood flow at levels appropriate to the needs of the tissues. These arteries are the only source of blood supply to the myocardium (end vessels), which is why coronary occlusion usually has such devastating effects.

The coronary arteries run over the outer surface of the heart (*epicardial coronary arteries*), but occasionally dip into the myocardium. Although all major epicardial coronary arteries may do this, involvement of the left anterior descending artery is the most common. During systole, the intramuscular segment of the vessel is compressed, a condition referred to as *milking* or *myocardial bridging*. In most instances, bridging is of little clinical significance, but severe bridging of the left anterior descending coronary artery can associate with myocardial ischaemia or sudden death. Bridging is recognised during angiography by arterial compression during systole, which reverses during diastole.

The epicardial vessels finally penetrate the myocardium to form a dense vascular network that is usually connected to the venous circulation via the cardiac capillaries. Interarterial coronary connections between different branches of the same coronary artery or between different coronary arteries may be present, and the heart may also

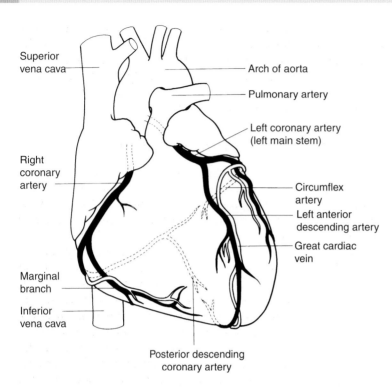

Figure 2.4 The coronary circulation.

Superior vena cava

Arch of aorta

Pulmonary artery

Left coronary artery (left main stem)

Right coronary artery

Circumflex artery

Left anterior descending artery

Great cardiac vein

Marginal branch

Inferior vena cava

Posterior descending coronary artery

---

receive perfusion from the bronchial arteries, the internal thoracic arteries and the mediastinal vessels. These 'auto bypasses' may explain the high clinical tolerance reported in some cases of severe coronary artery disease.

The right coronary artery (RCA)

The right coronary artery arises from the right coronary sinus above the right cusp of the aortic valve, and runs an extensive course around the orifice of the tricuspid valve. In the first few millimetres, it is submerged in adipose tissue of the epicardium below the right atrial appendage (the Rindfleisch fold). The first branch of the RCA is the conus branch, which courses anteriorly to supply the muscular right ventricular outflow tract. The RCA runs forward to the atrio-ventricular groove, usually giving off a small branch to the SA node (60% of cases). The main artery follows the sulcus downwards and round the inferior margin of the heart, giving off an acute marginal branch to supply the right ventricular wall, and usually a lateral atrial branch. The length of the RCA is variable.

It may terminate at the border of the heart or at the crux. In most people (85%), the RCA winds around the heart, and then passes down in the posterior interventricular groove as the *posterior descending coronary artery*, which supplies the inferior wall, ventricular septum and the postero-medial papillary muscle. Frequently, a transverse branch continues in the posterior AV groove, supplying branches of the left atrium before anastomosing with the circumflex branch of the left coronary artery. Branches of the RCA supply the conducting tissues, the right ventricle and the inferior (diaphragmatic) surface of the left ventricular wall.

The left coronary artery

The left coronary artery arises from the left posterior sinus of the aorta, runs to the left behind the pulmonary trunk and then forwards by the left atrial appendage to the AV groove. Here, this short left main stem (LMS) divides into two branches: the *left anterior descending* branch (otherwise known as the anterior interventricular artery) and a *circumflex* branch. Occasionally, the LMS divides into three branches, the third branch being known as the diagonal branch of the left anterior descending artery or the *ramus intermedius*.

The left anterior descending (LAD) artery descends in the anterior interventricular groove to the apex of the heart, where it turns back to ascend a short distance up the posterior interventricular groove, anastomosing with the posterior interventricular branch of the RCA. The LAD gives off two types of branches, septals and diagonals. Septals originate from the LAD at right angles to the surface of the heart, perforating and supplying the interventricular septum. Diagonals run along the surface of the heart and supply the lateral wall of the left ventricle and the antero-lateral papillary muscle.

The circumflex branch of the left coronary artery (LCx) gives rise to the sinus nodal artery in 40% of individuals, but then runs a variable course. In some patients, it terminates almost immediately but, more usually, it passes round the left margin of the heart in the AV groove under the left atrial appendage, supplying branches to the left atrium and the left surface of the heart (obtuse marginal arteries). The first obtuse marginal (OM_1) branch serves as the boundary between the proximal and distal portions of the LCx. Thus, the portion of the artery prior to the origin of OM_1 is known as the proximal LCx, while the segment just below the OM_1 is the distal LCx.

In 10% of individuals, the circumflex artery continues all the way round the mitral orifice, giving rise to the posterior descending artery. This is called a left-dominant coronary artery system (see below).

Coronary dominance

The term *coronary dominance* is used to describe the coronary artery that supplies the inferior (diaphragmatic) surface of the heart, and not the artery that supplies the greater part of the myocardium. Hence, the artery that supplies the posterior descending artery (and the postero-lateral arteries) determines the coronary dominance. If the RCA supplies both these arteries, the circulation can be classified as 'right-dominant'. If the LCx supplies both these arteries, the circulation is classified as

'left-dominant'. If the RCA supplies the posterior descending artery and the LCx supplies the postero-lateral artery, the circulation is known as 'co-dominant'. Approximately 70% of the general population have a right-dominant system, 20% are co-dominant, and 10% are left-dominant.

Coronary collateral circulation

As coronary arteries are end vessels, collaterals provide the only alternative circulation when coronary stenoses are present. Within the myocardium, there are rich anastomoses between the right and left coronary arteries, but the vessels involved are small. Several extramural intercoronary anastomoses have been identified. These may be found at the apex between the anterior and posterior interventricular arteries, in front of the right ventricle between the anterior interventricular artery and right diagonal branches and at the back of the left ventricle between the posterior interventricular artery and the circumflex branches. These anastomoses are genetically determined and can enlarge in the event of a gradual coronary artery narrowing, providing collateral circulation to the affected area of muscle. However, if occlusion is sudden, necrosis of a segment of cardiac muscle will result as these vessels cannot enlarge acutely.

Coronary artery anomalies

The term 'coronary artery anomaly' is used for variations of the coronary arteries that occur in less than 1% of the general population. A frequency over 1% is referred to as a *variation*, such as the origin of the atrio-ventricular nodal artery that usually arises from the right coronary artery, but can be derived from the left circumflex artery. While coronary artery anomalies are less common, they may be found in up to 5% of patients undergoing coronary angiography. Most will not have caused symptoms directly, but may have contributed towards symptoms even in the absence of coronary atherosclerosis. The combination of a coronary anomaly with coronary atherosclerosis may have serious consequences. For example, a single coronary artery may be found in around 1 in 1000 individuals, with origin in the right or left coronary sinus or from the proximal segment of the RCA or LAD. Proximal occlusion of this vessel by thrombus would be fatal, as the heart would lose all its blood supply. These single vessels are also at risk of mechanical compression if they pass between the aorta and the pulmonary artery. Abnormalities in the origin, course and distribution of the coronary arteries are a common cause of sudden death in young people (Basso et al, 2001).

The nerve supply to the heart

Because of 'intrinsic rhythmicity', the heart can beat even if completely removed from the body. However, the heart is well supplied with both sympathetic and parasympathetic nerve fibres, which can modify cardiac function by changing the heart rate and the strength of myocardial contraction. Control of the autonomic nerves is via the *cardiac centre*, which is located in the medulla oblongata of the brain.

Sympathetic nerve fibres supply the SA node, atrial muscle, AV node, specialised conduction tissue and ventricular muscle. These sympathetic fibres derive from the cervical and upper thoracic sympathetic ganglia, via the superficial and deep cardiac plexuses.

Parasympathetic nerve fibres are derived from the vagus nerve, and mainly supply the sinus node and AV node and, to a lesser extent, the atrial and ventricular muscle. It is thought that most of the cardiac fibres of the right vagus terminate in the sinus node, while the majority of the fibres of the left vagus terminate in the AV node. The main action on the AV node is to slow conduction and lengthen the refractory period.

Vagal stimulation to the heart is mediated by acetylcholine, which decreases heart rate and the strength of ventricular contraction. In contrast, stimulation of the sympathetic fibres leads to the release of noradrenaline (norepinephrine), which acts specifically on beta-1 adrenergic receptors in cardiac muscle. Circulating adrenaline from the adrenal medulla may also elicit cardiac responses. Adrenergic stimulation increases both heart rate and force of contraction. Conduction velocity increases, and there is shortening of the refractory period in the AV node.

The vagal and sympathetic nerves are distributed to the heart by the cardiac plexus, which lies between the concavity of the aortic arch and the tracheal bifurcation. Pressure changes in the aorta and carotid arteries can affect cardiac performance. Sensory receptors (*baroreceptors*) can detect increased pressure in the aorta and carotid arteries. Sensory impulses travel via the vagus and glosso-pharyngeal nerves and pass to the vasomotor centre in the medulla, causing slowing of the heart rate (Marey's reflex). These baroreceptors can be artificially stimulated by carotid sinus massage.

Histology

The heart comprises two major types of cell:

- myocardial cells specialised for contraction;
- automatic cells specialised for impulse formation.

Myocardial cells

Cylindrical striated myocardial cells provide the mechanical pumping action of the heart by contracting in response to electrical stimulation. Each cell is about 100 μm long and 15 μm wide, containing a central nucleus and numerous (about 150) myofibrils aligned along the cell's axis. Each fibril runs the length of the cell and is made up of repeating functional subunits, or *sarcomeres*, containing actin and myosin arranged hexagonally. The thin *actin* filaments are attached to a limiting membrane (Z *line*) and interdigitate with the thicker central *myosin* fibres. The sarcomeres of adjacent myofibrils are aligned at the Z line. During contraction, the actin filaments slide together, bringing the Z-lines closer together. The forces that generate sliding (i.e. contraction) occur at bridges between the actin and myosin (Fig. 2.5). It is the heads of the myosin molecules that form these bridges and contain the enzyme ATPase responsible for breaking down ATP (adenosine triphosphate) to provide the energy for contraction. It is likely that the greater the number of bridges, the more forceful the contraction.

The thicker myosin filaments (seen as the A band on microscopy) are 1.5 μm in length and have a central portion (0.2 μm) that is devoid of bridges. The thin actin filaments (seen as lateral I bands) are shorter (1 μm), so it can be seen that

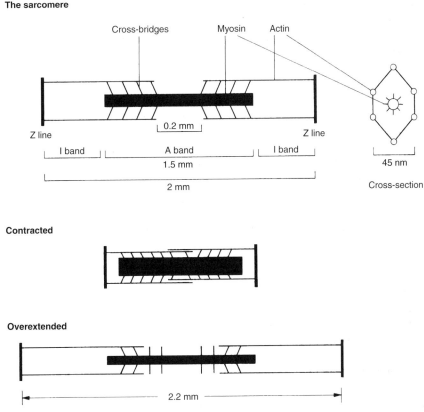

The sarcomere

Cross-bridges   Myosin   Actin

Z line

Z line

I band

A band

I band

0.2 mm

1.5 mm

2 mm

45 nm

Cross-section

Contracted

Overextended

2.2 mm

Figure 2.5   The sarcomere.

maximum bridging takes place when the overall sarcomere length is between 2.0 and 2.2 μm. If the sarcomere is stretched beyond these limits, some bridges become disengaged, which will limit the force of contraction. Starling's law of the heart (Starling, 1918) states that, within physiological limits, the greater the diastolic volume of the heart, the greater the energy of contraction. This is why the graphs demonstrating Starling's law fall off at the upper limits of myocardial stretching (Fig. 2.6).

This simplified concept is modified by the action of another contractile protein, *troponin C*. This is attached to the actin filaments and has an inhibitory effect that must be counteracted before actin and myosin can produce contraction. This is mediated by free calcium ions liberated by the sarcoplasmic reticulum in response to myocyte stimulation. There is a direct relationship between the intracellular concentration of calcium and the strength of contraction, as more binding sites are made available to the myosin heads. Projections on the myocin molecules (S1 heads) interact with actin filaments forming cross-bridges. Calcium amplifies this reaction to provide more cross-bridges, and hence the strength of contraction.

The adjacent myocardial cells are held together by the intercalated discs. Electrical resistance through these discs is about 1/400th of the resistance through the outside membrane of the myocardial fibre, allowing virtually free passage of electrical currents from one myocardial cell to the next, without encountering significant resistance. The myocardial cells are so tightly bound together that stimulation of any single cell causes the action potential to spread to all adjacent cells, eventually spreading throughout the entire myocardial network.

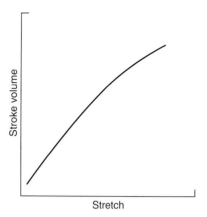

Figure 2.6 Ventricular function (Starling's) curve.

Automatic cells

Automaticity describes the ability of specialised cardiac tissue to initiate electrical impulses. The cells responsible are known as *pacemaker* or *automatic* cells. In the sinus node, these will discharge spontaneously about 80 times per minute, although automatic cells elsewhere will have a slower discharge rate. In the AV node, for example, this may be 60 times per minute, and in the ventricles, 40 times per minute. This system of 'escape rhythms' exists to prevent rhythm failure should the sinus node fail to discharge. Sometimes, the rate of discharge will increase in places other than the sinus node, and these regions then take over the pacemaker function of the heart. This is often seen following acute myocardial infarction (e.g. accelerated idio-nodal or idio-ventricular rhythms).

Both myocardial cells and automatic cells can transmit impulses, but the specialised conducting tissues are used preferentially as they allow a more rapid and ordered carriage of impulses through the heart.

Generation of the action potential

In the normal resting state, the potential across the myocardial cell membrane is about −90 mV. An active 'sodium pump' maintains the relative concentration of sodium (Na⁺) and potassium (K⁺) ions, and thus the electrical difference across the cell membrane. The pump transfers K⁺ ions into the cell up to five times more rapidly than it extrudes

Na⁺ ions and, within the cell, the concentrations of potassium and sodium are 140 and 10 mmol/L, respectively, whereas outside the concentrations are 4 and 140 mmol/L. This ionic imbalance helps to maintain the resting membrane potential at −90 mV, and the cells are then said to be 'polarised'. Should an electrical stimulus reach the cell membrane, permeability is altered, allowing a change in ionic concentrations and depolarisation of the cell.

There are distinct phases of electrical activity in myocardial cells during the generation of an action potential (Fig. 2.7).

Polarisation (phase 4)   This is the resting (inactive) state, where the cell has a membrane potential of −90 mV; the cell is said to be polarised. The cell interior is negatively charged with respect to the exterior.

Depolarisation (phase 0)   When electrical activation of the cell occurs, changes in the cell membrane permeability result, and there is an initial rapid influx of positively charged Na⁺ (the fast sodium current) followed by a more sustained influx of Ca²⁺ ions. Depolarisation is represented by the upstroke or spike on the action potential curve.

After electrical activation, the polarity of the membrane has been reversed, with the membrane potential changing from −90 mV to a slightly positive value of +20 mV (Fig. 2.8). This is the reverse pattern to that of the surrounding cells, creating a potential difference and allowing the electrical current to flow from one cell to the next, in a chain reaction. Once depolarisation has started, it is inevitably transmitted along the length of the cell to the adjacent cells. In this manner, a single electrical stimulus can depolarise the whole heart.

Repolarisation (phases 1–3)   Repolarisation is the process whereby the cell is returned to its normal resting state. This has three phases, the first of which is the 'overshoot' when chloride ions re-enter the cell and there is a slow fall in intracellular charge to +10 mV (phase 1 of the action potential). After the initial spike, the membrane remains depolarised (for 0.15 seconds in atrial muscle and 0.3 seconds in ventricular muscle), exhibiting a

Figure 2.7   The action potential in (A) myocardial and (B) pacemaker cells.

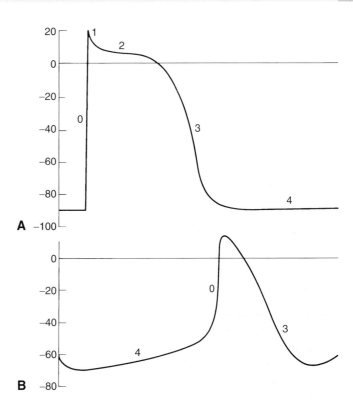

plateau, followed by the abrupt descent that represents repolarisation. The plateau phase (phase 2) of the action potential reflects a moderate and sustained slow influx of Ca^{2+}, which accompanies the more marked but less sustained influx of Na^+. The calcium entry into the cell is essential for excitation–contraction coupling (see below). An efflux of K^+ balances the calcium and sodium influx. Thus, the net effect is a relative balance of positive charges, which gives rise to the plateau. The downstroke of phase 3 represents the rapid efflux of K^+ from the cell, when membrane permeability to K^+ increases markedly.

Following repolarisation, phase 4 recovery ensues, whereby sodium is actively pumped out again and potassium in so that the cell becomes repolarised. The transmembrane potential returns to its resting level of –90 mV, and the action potential ends.

Resting state

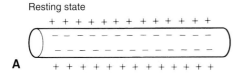

Stimulus

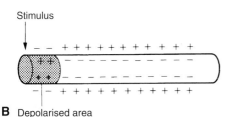

B Depolarised area

Impulse

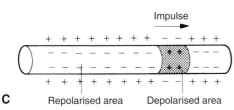

C   Repolarised area   Depolarised area

Figure 2.8   Myocardial cell transmembrane potential: (A) at rest, (B) during depolarisation and (C) during repolarisation.

The action potential in automatic cells

The action potential in automatic cells differs from that in myocardial cells. The specialised fibres of the conduction system have the inherent ability to initiate an electrical impulse spontaneously without external influence. Because these cells are responsible for initiating the electrical impulse, phase 4 of the action potential does not properly exist, and the cells have an unstable resting phase, with slow spontaneous phase 4 (diastolic) depolarisation (Fig. 2.7). A slow continuous movement of sodium ions into the cells produces this slow depolarisation during diastole, which reduces the intracellular negative charge until a threshold potential is reached and full depolarisation takes place.

The refractory period

The myocardium is normally refractory to re-stimulation for about 0.25–0.3 seconds at the start of systole. Certain antidysrhythmic agents act by lengthening or shortening this refractory period. Following this, the myocardium is relatively refractory to further stimulation for about 0.05 seconds, and this is followed by a vulnerable period, when even a very weak stimulus can evoke a response.

The normal refractory period of the atrium is about half that of the ventricles, and the relative refractory period is an additional 0.03 seconds. As a result, the atria can beat much faster than the ventricles.

Myocardial contraction

The mechanism by which the action potential causes the myofibrils to contract is known as *excitation–contraction coupling*:

Electrical excitation → mechanical activation → myocardial contraction

Electrical excitation

The function of the automatic cells is to regulate the contraction of the myocardial cells by providing the initial electrical stimulation. Their contractile elements are sparse and do not contribute significantly to the cardiac contraction.

Normally, the activating impulse spreads from the sinus node in all directions at a rate of about 1 m/second, thus reaching the most distant parts of the atrium in only 0.08 seconds. A delay of approximately 0.04 seconds in AV transmission occurs during passage through the AV node, which allows atrial systole to be completed. The wave of electrical excitement passes rapidly along the specialised muscle fibres of the AV bundle, bundle branches and peripheral ramifications of these branches in the ventricular myocardium.

Mechanical activation and myocardial contraction

The contractile process is initiated when the nerve impulse reaches the cardiac cell and travels from the limiting cell membrane (*sarcolemma*) to the inner contractile elements. Depolarisation of the sarcolemma generates an electrical impulse that travels in the sarcoplasmic reticulum along transverse tubules (T tubules) to the interior part of the cell. Depolarisation causes a dramatic transient release of calcium ions from pouches (*cisternae*) in the T tubules, producing a 'calcium transient' that is responsible for the initiation of contraction. Calcium diffuses into the myofibrils to activate myocin to split ATP and enable sliding of the actin and myosin filaments along each other, and effect contraction. The strength of myocardial contraction is dependent upon the concentration of the calcium ions. At the end of contraction, the calcium ions in the sarcoplasm are rapidly pumped back into the cisternae, and the muscle returns to its relaxed state.

Alterations in the properties of the calcium release channels in heart failure make them 'leaky' and thus impair the force of contraction.

CARDIAC PHYSIOLOGY

The heart is a double pump that maintains two circulations: the pulmonary circulation and the systemic circulation. These serve to transport oxygen and other nutrients to the body cells, remove metabolic waste products from them and convey substances (e.g. hormones) from one part of the body to another. At rest, the heart beats at about 70–80 beats/minute and pumps about 5 L of blood. During exercise, the rate may approach 200 beats/minute, and the cardiac output may increase to as much as 20 L.

The cardiac cycle

The function of the heart is to maintain a constant circulation of blood through the body. It acts as a pump whose cyclical contraction (*systole*) and relaxation (*diastole*) is known as the *cardiac cycle*. This cyclical activity is normally initiated by the spontaneous generation of an action potential at the sinus node. The impulse travels at about 1 m/second through the atrial muscle to produce atrial systole. Tissues at the AV groove prevent transmission from atrial to ventricular muscle, and conduction can take place only through specialised tissues in the AV junction. The duration of the cardiac cycle is about 0.8 seconds, producing an average heart rate of 75 beats/minute. Provided the heart receives excitation along the normal pathways, the heart rate remains constant; each successive cardiac cycle follows the same pattern of systole and diastole.

The duration of atrial systole is about 0.1 seconds and that of ventricular systole 0.3 seconds. Thus, the combined duration of atrial and ventricular systole is approximately 0.4 seconds. The timing remains fairly constant at fast heart rates, so that any increase in heart rate decreases diastolic timing. Complete cardiac diastole normally lasts 0.4 seconds but, as the pulse rate increases, the diastolic interval decreases. As coronary perfusion takes place in diastole, fast heart rates may critically impair the myocardial blood supply.

Atrial function

Atrial diastole lasts for 0.3 seconds, during which venous blood drains into the atria, which act as a reservoir, storing the blood. The AV ring moves upwards at the end of ventricular systole, causing a rise in atrial pressure and producing a '*v*' *wave* in the internal jugular vein. The AV valves then open, and the ventricles rapidly begin to fill, allowing the valve cusps to float upwards into opposition. The atria then contract (the right usually very slightly before the left), a process taking about 0.1 seconds. Blood is forced through the AV valves into the ventricles, increasing ventricular filling by about 10–20% and priming the ventricles for contraction.

As there are no valves between the right atrium and the venae cavae, some blood is also expelled backwards during atrial contraction, causing a transient rise in the central venous pressure, the '*a*' *wave* (Fig. 2.9). The delay in electrical transmission at the AV node allows the atria to empty completely before ventricular contraction starts.

Ventricular function

The pressure of blood in the ventricles begins to rise while that in the relaxing atria is falling. The cusps of the AV valves snap shut (causing the first heart sound, *S1*) and are held in opposition by the pull of the papillary muscles on the chordae tendineae. After closure of the AV valves, the intraventricular pressure rises because of isometric contraction of the ventricular muscle. During this phase, the ventricles alter their shape (becoming shorter and fatter), although not their volume (isovolumetric contraction). This momentarily causes a backward bulging of the AV valve cusps into the atria and produces a transient increase in atrial pressure (the '*c*' *wave*).

Figure 2.9 The venous pulse waveform.

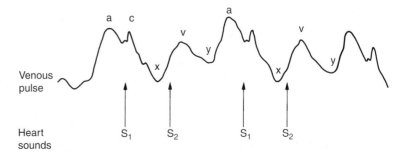

When the rising ventricular pressure exceeds the pressure in the aorta and pulmonary artery, the semi-lunar aortic and pulmonary valves open. The isotonic phase of contraction then begins, and the ventricular contents are ejected. Descent of the AV ring during ventricular systole causes a fall in right atrial pressure (the '*x*' *descent*).

As the ventricular muscle relaxes and the pressure falls below that in the aorta and pulmonary artery, the semi-lunar valves close (the second heart sound, S2), producing the dicrotic notch on arterial pressure traces. The aortic valve closes slightly before the pulmonary valve. Simultaneously, blood enters the atria and the intra-atrial pressure gradually rises, so that, when the AV valves open, blood flows rapidly from the atria to the ventricles, producing the third heart sound (S3) heard in some children and young adults.

Haemodynamics

The circulation is a continuous circuit, although it is often conveniently subdivided into the systemic and pulmonary circuits.

The pulmonary circulation

The pulmonary circuit is a low-pressure system with short, wide, thin-walled vessels and a small capacity (500–900 mL). The mean pressure in the circuit in the adult is approximately 15 mmHg – less than one-sixth of that in the systemic circulation. It circulates all the blood from the right ventricle to the left atrium. As blood is carried through the pulmonary vascular bed, carbon dioxide diffuses outwards into the lungs and oxygen is absorbed.

The pulmonary trunk carrying deoxygenated blood passes upwards from the right ventricle and divides into two main *pulmonary arteries*, one passing to each lung. Within the lungs, the arteries divide and subdivide to form the pulmonary capillary bed where gaseous exchange takes place. Eventually, these capillaries join up to form the *pulmonary veins* carrying oxygenated blood to the left atrium.

The systemic circulation

The systemic circulation is a high-pressure system that supplies all the tissues of the body (except the lungs) with blood. The aorta is elastic in nature, which helps it to function both as a reservoir for blood during the rapid ejection phase from the left ventricle and as a compression chamber to help propel the blood forward. As the branches arising from the aorta divide, the total cross-sectional area of the arteries, arterioles and capillaries increases, and the average velocity of blood flow decreases. The arterioles offer the largest resistance to flow. In the capillary bed, there is often stasis of flow in some capillaries and active flow in others. The normal systemic capillary pressure is about 24–25 mmHg, and the normal systemic capillary blood volume at rest is about 5% of the total volume (250 mL).

Coronary blood flow

The primary function of the coronary circulation is to provide an adequate supply of oxygen to support the metabolic demands of the heart. The heart extracts most of the oxygen carried in the coronary circulation (70%), and the rate of oxygen consumption is the major factor that determines coronary blood flow. Myocardial oxygen consumption is related to myocardial work in response to exercise or other stimuli, including drugs such as adrenaline, noradrenaline, calcium, thyroxine and digoxin. Coronary flow may increase by a factor of five during strenuous activity, mostly directed to the left ventricle.

About 5% of the cardiac output passes into the coronary vessels (about 250 mL/min), which fill in diastole. During systole, the coronary vessels are compressed so that the resistance to flow at that time is sharply increased. The subendocardium is more vulnerable to perfusion deficits as more tension is generated here.

Coronary blood flow is largely determined by the calibre of the coronary arteries themselves and is governed by a pressure gradient and by resistance of the vessels. Flow may be reduced because of a fixed stenosis (atheromatous plaque) or by vasospasm, which is more common in diseased coronary vessels.

Regulation of myocardial function

The normal adult blood volume is about 5 L. About 1.5 L are in the heart and lungs (central circulation) and the remaining 3.5 L are in the systemic (predominantly venous) circulation. The volume in the heart is about 0.6 L, but not all of this is expelled from the left ventricle at the end of systole. The residual volume, the *left ventricular end-diastolic volume* (LVEDV), is about 140 mL. The quantity of blood ejected during ventricular systole (the *stroke volume*) is only about 90 mL, and hence the *ejection fraction* (EF) is approximately $90/140 = 70\%$. If the heart rate is 70 beats/minute, then:

$$\begin{aligned} \text{Cardiac output} &= \text{heart rate (beats/minute)} \\ &\quad \times \text{stroke volume (mL/beat)} \\ &= \text{about 6 L/minute} \end{aligned}$$

Because the cardiac output is related to body size, it is more usually expressed as the cardiac index (L/minute/m^2 body surface area). The mean cardiac index at rest is normally 2–5 L/minute/m^2.

The ejection fraction (EF) is most commonly estimated using echocardiography, and is normally over 55%. During exercise in highly conditioned individuals, the increased stroke volume (caused primarily by increased force of contraction) can result in the EF exceeding 90%, and the cardiac output may increase up to 20 L. To alter cardiac output to meet changing bodily demands for tissue perfusion, the heart rate or stroke volume (or both) must be altered. These mechanisms normally operate together to increase the cardiac output as required.

The main determinants of cardiac output are stroke volume and heart rate. Stroke volume is determined by:

- preload (filling of the heart during diastole – venous return);
- afterload (resistance against which the heart must pump);
- contractility of the heart muscle.

Preload   Preload is the tension exerted on cardiac muscle at the end of diastole, usually expressed as the LVEDV, and is determined by the volume of blood in the left ventricle at the end of diastole. The Frank–Starling law of 1918 states that, within physiological limits, increases in LVEDV are accompanied by an increase in stroke work. In other words, the greater the volume of blood in the heart, the harder it will squeeze. This intrinsic

ability of the heart to adapt to changing loads of inflowing blood may be shown graphically (Fig. 2.6) and is approximately linear. Unfortunately, once the load increases beyond physiological limits, the heart begins to fail.

Preload can be estimated by measurement of left and right atrial pressures. The central venous pressure (CVP) is measured by a line in the right atrium, and measuring the pulmonary capillary wedge pressure approximates the pressure in the left atrium (Stokes & Jowett, 1985).

Afterload   Afterload is the force opposing ventricular emptying, and is a function of both arterial blood pressure (systemic vascular resistance) and resistance in the aortic outflow. Factors affecting afterload include aortic stenosis and hypertension.

Contractility   Contractility is an intrinsic property of the heart and exists independently of loading. Sympathetic nervous stimulation or drugs such as adrenaline, noradrenaline or dopamine can increase the speed and force of contraction (i.e. they have positive inotropic and chronotropic effects). Myocardial hypoxia, ischaemia and beta-blocking agents have the reverse effect and decrease cardiac contractility (negative inotropic and chronotropic effects). The contractile state can be gauged by the ejection fraction (normal EF is over 55%). Using the Frank–Starling graphs, contractility can be represented by different curves; higher degrees of contractility displace the curve upwards and to the left (Fig. 2.10). The greater the ventricular volume, the greater the wall tension needed to expel blood from the heart.

Blood pressure

Blood pressure may be defined as the force or pressure that the blood exerts upon the vessel walls. When the ventricle contracts, blood is forced into an already full aorta, and the pressure wave produces a systolic blood pressure of about 120 mmHg. During diastole, the arterial pressure falls to about 80 mmHg.

Blood pressure is maintained through many variables, including:

- cardiac output;
- blood volume;

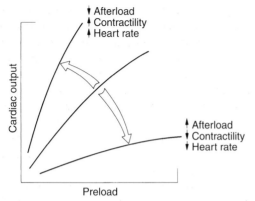

Figure 2.10 Ventricular function (Starling's) curves showing the effects of preload, afterload, contractility and heart rate.

- peripheral resistance;
- elasticity of the vessel walls;
- venous return.

Cardiac output is controlled by pulse rate and stroke volume. An increase in cardiac output raises both systolic and diastolic blood pressure, but an increase in stroke volume increases the systolic pressure to a greater degree. Blood volume is obviously important, as can be seen by the fact that blood pressure falls in shock. This may be due to an absolute loss of blood volume (e.g. haemorrhage) or a relative loss of circulating volume when there is widespread vasodilatation (e.g. septicaemic shock).

Peripheral resistance is controlled via sympathetic vasoconstrictor nerves originating in the vasomotor centre of the medulla oblongata. Normally, the artery walls are in a state of mild constriction, giving rise to 'resting tone'. Selective vasoconstriction and vasodilatation can take place around the body to ensure a constant blood supply to the vital organs, especially the heart and brain.

Venous return via the superior and inferior venae cavae also plays an important role in the maintenance of blood pressure. The force of the left ventricle is not sufficient on its own to force blood round the body. It is therefore assisted by muscular contraction and respiration. Contraction of skeletal muscle puts pressure on the veins and

squeezes blood forwards. Valves prevent backward flow. The negative intrathoracic pressure caused by inspiration also helps, by sucking blood into the heart. In addition, diaphragmatic movement raises the intra-abdominal pressure, squeezing blood out of the abdominal vessels.

The elasticity of the arterial walls is important to propel the blood forwards. During diastole, arterial recoil maintains the diastolic blood pressure. As the arterial tree ages, atheromatous deposits cause 'hardening of the arteries'. Elasticity is lost and the systolic blood pressure rises, as the arterial walls are unable to buffer the effect of the ventricular systolic shock wave.

ATHEROSCLEROSIS

In 1852, Sir Richard Quain, physician to Queen Victoria, recorded his observations on the deposition of fatty material in the blood vessels, which he attributed to poor diet. He said the 'fatty heart' was responsible for 'a languid and feeble circulation, a sense of uneasiness and oppression in the chest, embarrassment and distress in breathing, coma, syncope, angina pectoris, sudden death ...'.

The deposition of fatty material in the blood vessels that he described was atherosclerosis, a complex disorder, characterised by progressive accumulation of cholesterol within the intima of large and medium arteries, with subsequent infiltration and proliferation of vascular smooth muscle cells that causes narrowing of arteries. Coronary atherosclerosis causes *coronary heart disease*, a general term used to describe the effects of impaired or an absent blood supply on the myocardium.

Until recently, atherosclerosis was considered to be a degenerative disease, but it is clear that the development and progression of atherosclerosis is a dynamic, inflammatory process that is readily modifiable (Goldschmidt-Clermont et al, 2005). Central to its development is the passage of atherogenic lipoproteins into the arterial wall where they undergo biochemical alteration. These modified lipoproteins initiate a chronic inflammatory response that culminates in the development of atherosclerotic plaques. At least some of the cardiovascular benefits of drugs such as the statins and angiotensin-converting enzyme

(ACE) inhibitors are achieved by the reduction of these inflammatory processes (Call et al, 2004).

Endothelial function

Normal arteries have three layers:

- *the endothelium*: a single layer of endothelial cells with a basement membrane that lines the arterial lumen;
- *the media*: formed from concentric layers of smooth muscle with elastin fibres and extracellular matrix;
- *the adventitia*: the tough connective tissue coating.

The endothelium provides a link between blood within the artery and the vessel wall, and the cells play a vital role in maintaining vascular homeostasis. Crucial to this is the production of nitric oxide (NO). Nitric oxide is a labile molecule, synthesised from the amino acid L-arginine by endothelial nitric oxide synthase (eNOS), an enzyme present in endothelial cells. In turn, this is switched on by various stimuli such as wall shear stress and chemicals such as acetylcholine, estrogen and bradykinin. NO diffuses into the arterial media and the vessel lumen. The smooth muscle relaxes producing vasodilatation, and platelets are inhibited, making them less likely to aggregate. NO has many other signalling effects but, overall, it inhibits many of the processes that lead to early atherosclerosis. Such effects may be countered by high blood fats, smoking and hypertension, leading to endothelial dysfunction and abnormalities in NO-mediated vascular responses.

Endothelial dysfunction allows macrophage adhesion and initiation of inflammation, with accumulation of oxidised lipid in the vessel wall that marks the initiation of atherosclerosis. The normally quiescent vascular smooth muscle cells in the arterial media change to an 'activated repair' subtype that begin to proliferate, migrate and secrete matrix that starts the process of vessel narrowing.

Atherosclerosis evolves over decades, appearing as discrete plaques that have a soft lipid-rich core (*athere* – Greek for gruel or porridge) walled off by a hard fibrous capsule (*skleros* – Greek for hard) that keeps the prothrombotic contents away from the circulation. There is a predilection for these plaques to develop around branching vessels, or areas of arterial curvature, suggesting that haemodynamic stresses may be important in their development. In the histological classification, lesions are designated by Roman numerals I–VI, which are used to indicate plaque composition, progression and complexity (Stary et al, 1995). Each stage may stabilise temporarily or permanently, and evolution may require an additional stimulus. The role of repeated endothelial injury from local inflammation, toxins (e.g. from smoking), vasospasm and dyslipidaemia is generally assumed to be central to the initiation and evolution of these lesions.

In the early stages of atherosclerosis, progression is predictable and uniform, but lesions may subsequently evolve erratically, resulting in several lesion types in the same patient, and the development of different clinical syndromes. In general, the plaques appear as:

- *Fatty streaks (type I and II lesions)*. These are the first signs of atherosclerosis, and occur where the endothelium has been damaged. They are flat or slightly elevated pale yellow lesions of variable size and shape. They are found throughout the arterial system in patients of all ages, and are often present from early childhood in countries with high rates of coronary heart disease. Fatty streaks have been observed in the aorta and coronary arteries in children as young as 2 years (Berensen et al, 1998). The lesions are benign in themselves, causing little or no obstruction to the affected artery, but size and complexity increase as lipoprotein accumulation escalates.
- *Fibrous plaques (type III and IV lesions)*. Fatty streaks become more fibrous with time to produce raised white plaques within the intima that may protrude into the arterial lumen. The plaque becomes more fibrotic because of proliferation of the vascular smooth muscle cells (VSMCs), which synthesise and deposit matrix and connective tissue to form a tough fibrous cap, keeping the prothrombotic 'lipid pool' away from the circulating blood. This lipid pool consists of cell debris and extracellular lipids released when lipid-laden macrophages (foam cells) die, and the larger it becomes, the more

dangerous it may be. The number of fibrous plaques increases rapidly between the ages of 15 and 35 years, particularly in those with cardiovascular risk factors (Strong et al, 1999). Fibrous plaques in coronary vessels were found in 69% of those aged 26–39 years, and in 8% of those aged 2–15 years of 204 trauma death patients (Berenson et al, 1998). As the fibrous plaque enlarges, it may cause narrowing of the blood vessel, but many plaques degenerate. Some plaques do not grow into the vessel lumen at all, because expansion of the arterial media and external elastic membranes allows the atheroma to expand away from the lumen in a process called 'positive arterial remodelling'. Hence, for much of its life, the plaque grows outwards rather than inwards, and substantial atherosclerosis can accumulate without producing arterial narrowing. Large atherosclerotic loads may develop silently in both young adults and adolescents, and may be hidden at angiography (Tuzcu et al, 2001).

- *Advanced (complicated) lesions (type V and VI lesions).* These are degenerative lesions composed of fibrous tissue, fibrin and intracellular and extracellular lipid and, often, extravasated blood. The necrotic, lipid-rich core continues to increase in size, and often becomes calcified ('hardening of the arteries'). This reduces compliance of the arteries and, combined with vessel narrowing, has dramatic effects on blood pressure and blood flow, often leading to myocardial ischaemia.

Plaque rupture

Atherosclerosis is a disease that has phases of stability and instability. Mature plaques do not develop in a smooth and predictable fashion, but in sudden growth spurts. These periods of accelerated growth appear to be related to plaque erosion or rupture, dynamic processes that may occur over a period of hours or days (Davies, 1992). Plaque rupture is a common event throughout life. These events are usually asymptomatic, but may be the initiator of an acute coronary syndrome or sudden cardiac death (Fig. 2.11).

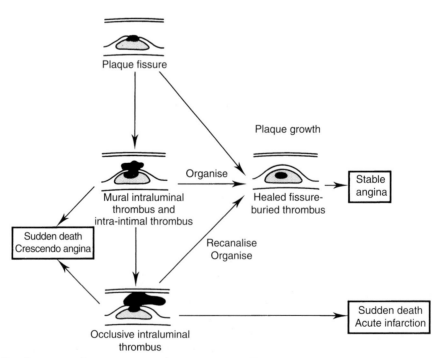

Plaque fissure

Plaque growth

Organise

Mural intraluminal thrombus and intra-intimal thrombus

Healed fissure-buried thrombus

Stable angina

Sudden death
Crescendo angina

Recanalise
Organise

Occlusive intraluminal thrombus

Sudden death
Acute infarction

Figure 2.11   Development and consequences of coronary artery disease.

Following the autopsy of Bertel Thorvaldsen, the Danish artist and sculptor who died without warning at the Royal Theatre in Copenhagen in 1844, the pathologist reported that the coronary vessel wall contained 'several atheromatous plaques, one of which quite clearly had ulcerated, pouring the atheromatous mass into the arterial lumen'. It was more than 150 years later that it was realised that patients with unstable angina and myocardial infarction almost always have a fissured or ulcerated atherosclerotic plaque that initiates the acute coronary syndrome (Davies, 2000).

Most adults in the western world have advanced atherosclerotic plaques in their coronary arteries and, although some will eventually suffer an acute coronary event, most will not, and why this is the case is not known. Plaque rupture is a random and unpredictable event, occurring in response to inflammation, mechanical stresses, coronary artery spasm and other factors acting on the coronary vasculature. Rupture exposes the highly thrombogenic collagenous matrix and lipid pool to the circulation, which inevitably triggers fibrin deposition and the formation of thrombus with partial or total vessel occlusion. The thrombus tracks down into the plaque itself, and then expands and distorts the plaque from within causing rapid changes in the severity of stenosis, and often produces total occlusion (Fig. 2.12). Platelets release vasoconstrictor agents such as serotonin and thromboxane A_2, which may induce vasospasm, either at the site of the thrombosis or within the distal microcirculation. Spontaneous thrombolysis may produce intermittent symptoms and transient electrocardiogram (ECG) changes and, as the thrombus fragments, embolisation into the small distal vessels may cause microinfarcts.

The intermittent attacks of myocardial ischaemia that occur in the unstable coronary syndromes are thus caused by:

- the thrombus waxing and waning with intermittent occlusion;
- intense vasoconstriction;
- platelet embolisation to the microvasculature.

Depending upon the duration of vessel occlusion, and the degree of repeated embolisation from the unstable plaque upstream, there may be varying effects on the myocardium, which may

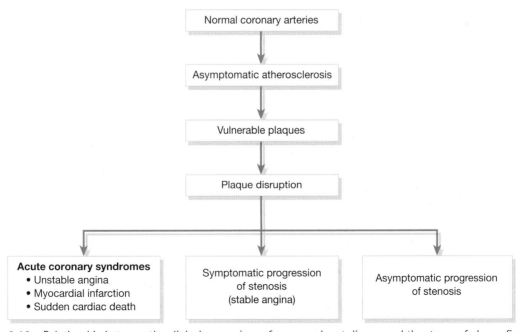

Figure 2.12   Relationship between the clinical expressions of coronary heart disease and the stages of plaque fissuring.

escape undamaged or show small focal areas of necrosis. In the past, such areas were often not detected by routine cardiac enzyme estimation. With the development of sensitive cardiac markers such as troponin, it is possible to detect as little as 1 g of myocardial necrosis, which allows a diagnosis of myocardial infarction that would previously have been missed.

Plaque vulnerability

The risk of plaque rupture does not depend on plaque numbers, plaque size or the severity of the associated stenosis, but primarily on the plaque vulnerability to fissuring (Falk et al, 1995). *Vulnerable plaques* have a large lipid pool (more than 40% of overall plaque volume) and a thin fibrous cap. Extensive macrophage accumulation indicates active inflammation. The integrity of the fibrous cap is critical in determining plaque stability, and it is the function of the vascular smooth muscle cells (VSMCs) to protect against plaque rupture. There is normally a balance between inflammation leading to breakdown of the fibrous cap and VSMC proliferation and collagen synthesis maintaining fibrosis and the integrity of the cap. Increasing accumulation of subendothelial lipid increases foam cell numbers. These secrete collagenases and produce a local inflammatory reaction with erosion of the shoulder region where the fibrous cap meets the normal arterial wall. If the healing response of VMSCs is overcome, the plaque breaks down and initiates thrombosis. Hypercholesterolaemia increases foam cell activity and the size of the lipid pool, making plaques more likely to rupture. Other risk factors such as diabetes and cigarette smoking are prothrombotic, increasing the likelihood of occlusive thrombus formation should plaque rupture occur.

While most episodes of plaque disruption are clinically silent, they can still contribute to the progression of vessel stenosis. Following plaque disruption, endogenous fibrinolysis disperses the thrombus, and VSMCs migrate into the area to 'smooth out' and repair the fibrous cap. The final result becomes a stable lesion that may cause anything from a minor irregularity in the vessel wall to a chronic occlusion. Up to 60% of patients with stable angina and 85% of those with previous myocardial infarction and angina have segments within the coronary artery where the original channel is replaced by several small channels, suggesting recanalisation through a previously occlusive thrombus. Lesions that do not 'smooth out' remain vulnerable to further disruption as shear forces from blood flow across the plaque make it more likely to fissure. Alternatively, positive vessel remodelling can expand the external diameter of the artery without impinging significantly on the lumen.

Between two-thirds and three-quarters of fatal coronary thrombi are precipitated by sudden rupture of a vulnerable plaque, 75% of which were previously causing only mild to moderate coronary obstruction. The *culprit lesion* is the plaque considered to be responsible for the clinical event, either at angiography or at post mortem. In unstable angina, myocardial infarction and sudden coronary death, the culprit lesion is usually a plaque complicated by thrombosis extending into the lumen. Although most acute coronary syndromes involve a single culprit lesion, arterial inflammation is much more diffuse, and patients may have more than one ulcerated plaque.

Plaque erosion

While rupture of a thin fibrous plaque cap is responsible for the vast majority of coronary thrombi, other mechanisms include plaque erosion and, much less frequently, erosion of calcified nodules that protrude into the artery lumen from a heavily calcified plaque. Autopsy studies show that plaque erosion may be detected in 25–40% of patients with sudden coronary death in the absence of plaque rupture. Plaque erosion is more common in younger people, smokers and women.

Plaque erosion associates with loss of the luminal endothelial cells, predisposing to thrombosis. It often occurs at the site of a pre-existing severe stenosis, although the underlying plaque is usually stable, being rich in smooth muscle cells and containing few foam cells. As such, the plaque is not classically 'vulnerable'. The reasons for plaque erosion are not clear. Unlike plaque rupture, inflammation does not appear to play a major role, but mechanical processes, such as repeated vasospasm at the same site, might be important.

Acute coronary syndromes initiated by plaque erosion result in smaller areas of myocardial infarction than those with ruptured plaque lesions, suggesting that an eroded plaque is less thrombogenic than a ruptured plaque (Hayashi et al, 2005).

Myocardial ischaemia

Myocardial ischaemia results from an imbalance between myocardial oxygen demand and supply.

Oxygen demand depends mainly upon heart rate, the strength of myocardial contraction and left ventricular wall tension. When the heart rate increases, systolic timing does not alter by very much, and the increased heart rate occurs at the expense of diastolic timing. As a result, there is a reduction in coronary perfusion time (which takes place in diastole), despite the higher demands placed upon it by the increased heart rate. Additionally, sympathetic stimulation (e.g. thyrotoxicosis) leads to an increase in the force of contraction, which increases myocardial oxygen demand. Increased wall tension will also increase myocardial work and is determined by intracardiac pressures and volumes secondary to changes in preload and afterload.

Oxygen supply varies with coronary blood flow, which is in turn determined by abnormalities of the vessel wall, abnormalities in blood flow or abnormalities in the blood itself.

Abnormalities of the coronary vessel wall

Fixed or reversible lesions may impair coronary blood supply. Atheroma is the most common cause of coronary arterial narrowing, although congenital lesions, such as coronary ectasia, may be responsible. Clinically important restriction to ordinary flow occurs when there is over 50–70% narrowing of the lumen of the artery seen at angiography, although the severity of lesions and size of distal vessels may be underestimated. An abrupt diminution or total loss of coronary blood supply will ultimately result in acute myocardial infarction.

Coronary artery spasm gives rise to an intermittent, reversible obstruction and is the underlying abnormality in 'variant angina', described by Prinzmetal et al (1959). Both spasm and atheroma are usually present in patients with symptomatic coronary heart disease, although their precise contribution to impairing myocardial perfusion at any given time will differ. Coronary artery spasm is a major component in many patients with unstable angina, and may also follow the sudden withdrawal of nitrate therapy. The usual situation is for spasm and fixed stenosis to act in combination, causing a critical reduction in flow, which leads to regional ischaemia. However, temporary occlusion of coronary flow by spasm, even in the absence of atheroma, can lead to angina or even myocardial infarction. This is a feature of cocaine abuse, although many users may have atheromatous lesions as well.

Rarely, the coronary vessel wall may be involved in inflammatory diseases, such as systemic lupus erythematosus (SLE) and polyarteritis nodosa, which may cause symptomatic occlusion.

Abnormalities in blood flow

The major determinant of blood flow is blood pressure (the perfusion pressure). Valvular heart disease, especially aortic stenosis, will impede blood flow from the left ventricle and reduce perfusion of the coronary arteries. This may provoke angina, even in the absence of coronary atheroma.

Abnormalities in the blood

Anaemia will prevent adequate oxygen carriage and may provoke angina. Hyperviscosity syndromes, such as polycythaemia and myeloma, may also result in myocardial ischaemia by slowing blood flow.

Acute coronary syndromes often occur at rest or during minimal exertion when there is little or no demand placed upon the heart. The precipitating cause would, therefore, seem to be decreased oxygen supply to the heart, rather than increased oxygen demand, where atherosclerosis, platelet adhesion, coronary thrombosis and coronary artery spasm interact to produce the clinical manifestations of acute coronary disease.

UNSTABLE CORONARY DISEASE

The main clinical manifestations of unstable coronary disease are unstable angina, myocardial infarction and sudden death. These clinical syndromes are dependent on several underlying factors including the degree, duration and abruptness of obstruction of coronary blood flow and the oxygen demand at the time of coronary obstruction.

Sudden death

A sudden death is one occurring from natural causes, in which the patient dies within 1 hour of developing symptoms and often immediately. Sudden death due to coronary disease (sudden cardiac death) is the most important cause of death in the adult population of the western world, and is responsible for about 70% of all suddenly occurring deaths. About half will have had no previously recognised heart disease. It is common, representing an estimated 25–30% of all cardiovascular deaths, and is thus responsible for up to 100 000 deaths in the UK each year.

Sudden cardiac death has two major underlying causes: vascular (thromboembolic) and dysrhythmic (electrical). These may occur alone or, more commonly, together. Ambulatory electrocardiography in patients dying suddenly suggests that ventricular tachycardia (VT) or ventricular fibrillation (VF) is the usual cause of collapse (Milner et al, 1985). Most cases are probably initiated by an acute ischaemic event, such as coronary artery spasm, acute coronary thrombosis or perhaps coronary emboli arising from ulcerated plaques, producing distal 'microinfarcts'. Histological changes of myocardial infarction do not occur for 4–6 hours, and there may be no firm morphological, enzyme or electrocardiographic evidence to make the diagnosis. About a quarter of sudden cardiac deaths cannot be confirmed as being due to myocardial infarction, and the cause is assumed to be primarily electrical, precipitated by left ventricular dysfunction secondary to myocardial ischaemia. Many of these have coronary disease, but there are other cardiac conditions that are associated with sudden 'electrical' death including cardiomyopathy, aortic stenosis, the long QT syndrome and anomalous origins of the coronary arteries.

Myocardial infarction and unstable angina

Unstable angina, non-Q wave and Q wave myocardial infarction represent a continuum of the same disease process, presenting clinically as *unstable coronary syndromes*. They are usually caused by plaque rupture, with a stuttering or abrupt reduction in coronary arterial blood flow. In unstable angina, occlusion tends to be subtotal, transient and episodic, but distal embolisation of platelets and thrombus into small intramyocardial vessels may cause myocardial infarction.

Myocardial infarction refers to the destruction of heart tissue resulting from obstruction of the blood supply to the heart muscle. This is usually associated with an occlusive thrombus in one or more of the coronary arteries, superimposed on an advanced and disrupted atherosclerotic plaque. This is the finding in up to 90% of patients immediately following myocardial infarction but, as time passes, the thrombus may disappear because of spontaneous thrombolysis. The speed with which some arteries reopen suggests that spasm may play an important role. About 1% of patients with acute myocardial infarction have normal coronary arteriograms, and the cause of the infarction remains speculative. It is possible that a small atheromatous plaque has ruptured and resolved without any residual obstruction (Da Costa et al, 2001). Patients are typically young, heavy smokers or older women.

Muscle necrosis following coronary occlusion

Abrupt coronary occlusion quickly leads to transmural myocardial ischaemia, and myocardial contraction in the area affected is compromised within seconds. The ECG may show changes within 30 seconds, and pain is usually experienced within 1 minute. Myocardial necrosis begins after about 20–30 minutes, starting in the subendocardium and progressing outwards as a 'wave front'. Ischaemic damage is greatest in the subendocardium because wall tension is greatest here, increasing oxygen requirements, and the evolving infarct will have a large area of endocardial necrosis and a smaller area of epicardial damage. About 80–90% of the ischaemic zone will be affected after 4–6 hours, If more than two-thirds of the ventricular wall thickness is involved, the infarction is termed 'transmural', usually marked by Q waves on the ECG. If it involves less than this, it is termed a non-transmural infarction, and there will be no

Q wave formation on the ECG ('non-Q wave infarct'). Smaller areas of infarction limited to the subendocardium usually give rise to symmetrical T wave inversion on the ECG ('subendocardial infarction').

The infarcted area is at first red because of 'stuffing in' of the red cells (*infarct = stuffed in*). The area later becomes pale as the necrotic muscle swells and squeezes out the extravasated blood. Finally, the infarcted area is replaced by fibrous scar tissue over the course of 1 week to 3 months.

The size of the affected area increases with the duration of coronary occlusion, plateauing at around 6 hours, after which reopening the vessel usually has no discernible effect. Prevention of cardiac damage by revascularisation procedures is therefore time dependent. As muscle necrosis mainly occurs in the first 30–90 minutes following coronary occlusion, reperfusion within 1–2 hours may allow most of the affected myocardium to be salvaged, preserving left ventricular function and therefore increasing survival (GUSTO Angiographic Investigators, 1993). Beyond 6 hours, there may be little viable tissue, but the time course of myocardial necrosis is not easily predictable, being extended in the presence of a functional coronary collateral circulation (Smith & Ilsley, 2004). Collaterals developing *after* the infarction cannot function quickly enough to affect infarct size, but may later help to modify left ventricular remodelling and reduce the risk of cardiac failure.

Another situation that may extend the window of myocardial viability is 'ischaemic preconditioning', a situation that seems to make the myocardium more resistant to the effects of ischaemia. Patients with a prior history of angina tend to suffer less myocardial damage, less cardiac failure, fewer dysrhythmias and, therefore, lower mortality (Rezkalla & Kloner, 2005), which suggests that repeated periods of myocardial ischaemia without infarction may be protective to the heart.

It must also be remembered that coronary thrombosis is a dynamic process, with spontaneous thrombolysis and restoration of some coronary flow followed by periods of reocclusion over a period of hours. Coronary occlusion may be intermittent despite the presence of continuous pain, and intermittent reperfusion may prevent or limit myocardial damage and prolong the interventional window. On the other hand, symptoms of myocardial ischaemia are variable, mild and often subjective, leading to an underestimation of occlusion time. There may also be an increased susceptibility to myocardial injury, being most pronounced in those over the age of 75 years (Lesnefsky et al, 1996).

LEFT VENTRICULAR REMODELLING

The term *left ventricular remodelling* refers to the complex structural changes in the left ventricle following myocardial infarction in response to alterations in loading. Both the infarcted and the non-infarcted myocardium are involved in this remodelling process, which has an important effect on subsequent left ventricular function and prognosis (Opie et al, 2006).

Early remodelling starts within the first 24 hours of coronary occlusion, and the infarcted area progressively stretches and thins, predisposing to cardiac rupture. The left ventricle starts to dilate and, with progressive lengthening and hypertrophy of the viable myocardium, the left ventricle alters in shape and volume, becoming more globular. The early effects of left ventricular remodelling are haemodynamically beneficial because ventricular dilatation reduces filling pressures, enabling the heart to generate larger stroke volumes, but remodelling can continue over months or even years, leading to progressive dilatation. Global ventricular dilatation increases the left ventricular volume and defines the overall prognosis – the bigger the volume, the greater the mortality.

Not all areas of myocardial infarction undergo significant remodelling, and smaller infarcts usually heal without any dilatation. Patients with extensive myocardial infarction and persistent occlusion of the infarct-related artery are most at risk of ventricular remodelling, and the site of the infarct does not seem to be important. Early reperfusion treatment improves survival by limiting infarct size, and thus preserving left ventricular function. Even late perfusion beyond the stage where there is much change for myocardial salvage seems to protect against dilatation, presumably because small islands of viable epicardium are preserved that may be sufficient to attenuate infarct expansion. The 'open artery hypothesis' suggests that myocardial reperfusion, even if too late for myocardial salvage, can prevent adverse cardiac remodelling (Abbate et al, 2003). Late reperfusion by percutaneous coronary intervention days to weeks after myocardial infarction to limit ischaemic left ventricular dilatation and myopathy is currently being evaluated in the 'occluded artery trial' (Hochman et al, 2005).

Progressive dilatation is more likely to occur where the initial left ventricular ejection fraction is less than 40%, so early use of ACE inhibitors following myocardial infarction helps to attenuate ventricular remodelling and its sequelae by limiting ventricular expansion. ACE inhibitors started within 36 hours of myocardial infarction reduce mortality and other serious cardiovascular events, particularly in the first 4 weeks (ACE Inhibitor Myocardial Infarction Collaborative Group, 1998).

Myocardial hibernation and stunning

Myocardial hibernation refers to a situation caused by chronic low-flow ischaemia, with coronary blood flow that is too feeble to fuel contraction, but just sufficient to prevent necrosis. The myocytes 'sleep', but remain viable. The longer hypoperfusion remains, the greater the likelihood of functional and structural abnormalities. Left ventricular remodelling may be initiated by hibernation, and strategies to identify viable but non-contractile myocardium that may benefit from reperfusional strategies could affect remodelling and prognosis (Futterman & Lemberg, 2000).

Myocardial stunning refers to the situation where, following reperfusion of the ischaemic myocardium, blood flow is restored but myocardial contractility does not return, even though the myocytes appear viable. Typically, this can follow thrombolysis for myocardial infarction, but it may sometimes complicate other acute coronary syndromes, angioplasty or cardiac surgery (Kluner et al, 2001). Normal contractile function may return hours, days or even weeks later, and this explains why left ventricular function takes time to recover after successful reperfusion. Repeated episodes of stunning may lead to a condition known as *chronic contractile dysfunction*, which may be difficult to differentiate from hibernation.

It can be seen that impaired left ventricular function following myocardial infarction is not always irreversible, and may recover in time or with revascularisation. Inert myocardium seen at angiography is not necessarily dead. ECG-gated myocardial perfusion scintigraphy allows data on myocardial perfusion and function to be acquired at the same time. Thallium scanning is a sensitive method for evaluating myocardial viability, where uptake of over 50% of normal in the territory of the infarct indicates that revascularisation should improve myocardial performance. Cardiac magnetic resonance imaging (MRI) and positron emission tomography (PET) are also very useful for detecting hibernating myocardium, but are not widely available.

References

Abbate A, Biondi-Zoccai GG, Baldi A et al (2003) The 'Open-Artery Hypothesis': new clinical and pathophysiologic insights. *Cardiology* 100: 196–206.

ACE Inhibitor Myocardial Infarction Collaborative Group (1998) Indications for ACE inhibitors in the early treatment of acute myocardial infarction: systematic overview of individual data from 100,000 patients in randomized trials. *Circulation* 97: 2202–2212.

Basso C, Corrado D, Thiene G (2001) Congenital coronary artery anomalies as an important cause of sudden death in the young. *Cardiology Reviews* 9: 312–317.

Berenson GS, Srinivasan SR, Bao W et al (1998) Association between multiple cardiovascular risk factors and atherosclerosis in children and young adults. *New England Journal of Medicine* 338: 1650–1656.

Call JT, Deliargyris EN, Newby LK (2004) Focusing on inflammation in the treatment of atherosclerosis. *Cardiology in Review* 12: 194–200.

Da Costa A, Isaak K, Faure E et al (2001) Clinical characteristics, aetiological factors and long-term prognosis of myocardial infarction with an absolutely normal coronary angiogram: a 3-year follow up study of 91 patients. *European Heart Journal* 22: 1459–1465.

Davies MJ (1992) Anatomic features in victims of sudden coronary death. *Circulation* 85(suppl 1): 19–24.

Davies MJ (2000) The pathophysiology of acute coronary syndromes. *Heart* 83: 361–366.

Falk E, Shah PK, Fuster V (1995) Coronary plaque disruption. *Circulation* 92: 657–671.

Futterman LG Lemberg L (2000) Hibernating myocardium, stunning, ischemic preconditioning: clinical relevance. *American Journal of Critical Care* 9: 430–436.

Goldschmidt-Clermont PJ, Creager MA, Lorsordo DW et al (2005) Atherosclerosis 2005: recent discoveries and novel hypotheses. *Circulation* 112: 3348–3353.

GUSTO Angiographic Investigators (1993) The effects of tPA, streptokinase or both on coronary artery patency, ventricular function and survival after acute myocardial infarction. *New England Journal of Medicine* 329: 1615–1622.

Hayashi T, Kiyoshima T, Matsuura M et al (2005) Plaque erosion in the culprit lesion is prone to develop a smaller myocardial infarction size compared with plaque rupture. *American Heart Journal* 149: 284–290.

Hochman JS, Lamas GA, Knatterud GL et al (2005) Occluded Artery Trial Research Group. Design and methodology of the Occluded Artery Trial (OAT). *American Heart Journal* 150: 627–642.

Kluner RA, Arimie B, Kay GL et al (2001) Evidence for stunned myocardium in humans: a 2001 update. *Coronary Artery Disease* 12: 349–356.

Lesnefsky EJ, Lundergan CF, Hodgson JM et al (1996) Increased left ventricular dysfunction in elderly patients despite successful thrombolysis: the GUSTO-I angiographic experience. *Journal of the American College of Cardiology* 28: 331–337.

Milner PG, Platia EV, Reid PR et al (1985) Ambulatory electrocardiographic recordings at the time of fatal cardiac arrest. *American Journal of Cardiology* 56: 588–592.

Opie LH, Commerford PJ, Gersh BJ et al (2006) Controversies in ventricular remodelling. *Lancet* 367: 356–367.

Prasad K, Atherton J, Smith GC et al (1999) Echocardiographic pitfalls in the diagnosis of hyper-trophic cardiomyopathy. *Heart* 82(suppl 3): III8–III15.

Prinzmetal M, Kennamer R, Merliss R et al (1959) Angina pectoris. I. A variant form of angina pectoris: preliminary report. *American Journal of Medicine* 27: 375–388.

Quain R (1852). On fatty diseases of the heart. *Edinburgh Medical and Surgical Journal* 77: 120–152.

Rezkalla SH, Kloner RA (2005) Preconditioning and the human heart. *Panminerva Medica* 47: 69–73.

Smith RD, Ilsley CD (2004) Clinical contribution of the collateral circulation to myocardial protection. *Coronary Artery Disease* 15: 393–398.

Starling EH (1918) *The Linacre Lecture on the Law of the Heart.* London: Longmans Green.

Stary HC, Chandler AB, Dinsmore RE et al (1995) A definition of advanced types of atherosclerotic lesions and a histo-logical classification of atherosclerosis: a report from the Committee on vascular lesions of the council on arteriosclerosis, American Heart Association. *Circulation* 92: 1355–1374.

Stokes PH, Jowett NI (1985) Haemodynamic monitoring with the Swan–Ganz catheter. *Intensive Care Nursing* 1: 9–17.

Strong JP, Malcom GT, McMahan CA et al (1999) Prevalence and extent of atherosclerosis in adolescents and young adults: implication for prevention from the Patho-biological Determinants of Atherosclerosis in Youth Study (PDAY). *Journal of the American Medical Association* 281: 727–735.

Tuzcu EM, Kapadia SR, Tutar E et al (2001) High prevalence of coronary atherosclerosis in asymptomatic teenagers and young adults. *Circulation* 103: 2705–2715.

Chapter 3

Prevention of cardiovascular disease

Cardiovascular disease (CVD) remains the single most common cause of morbidity and mortality in both men and women in the UK (Allender et al, 2006), the majority of which are due to coronary heart disease (CHD). Of the 216 000 cardiovascular deaths in 2004, 137 500 were from heart disease (Fig. 3.1).

CVD prevention aims to reduce the risk of atherosclerotic events, and to improve both quality and quantity of life through lifestyle and risk factor intervention. The traditional separation of 'primary' and 'secondary' prevention is artificial, as not all patients with cardiovascular disease are symptomatic, yet they have the same disease already declared by those who have had an atherosclerotic event. Modern CVD prevention now focuses on those at most risk. They are:

- people with established atherosclerotic CVD;
- people with diabetes;
- apparently healthy individuals who, following screening, are considered at high risk of developing symptomatic atherosclerotic disease.

Identifying this last group is particularly important because about half the cases of CHD present without warning with acute myocardial infarction or sudden cardiac death. Convincing asymptomatic individuals of the importance of risk factor intervention is, however, often difficult. Fewer than half of 5000 random members of the public around Europe knew that heart disease was the leading cause of death in their country (Erhardt & Hobbs, 2002). Most thought they were more likely to die from cancer.

In response to the epidemic of CVD that emerged in the first half of the twentieth century, the US public health service decided to undertake a large-scale study to explore why heart disease had become the major cause of death. Framingham, a small town in Massachusetts, was chosen for a long-term research project into the causes of atherosclerotic disease that started in 1948. Over 5000 local residents, ranging in age from 30 to 62 years, were enrolled into the study and are still under medical surveillance. In 1971, the study recruited 5124 children (and their spouses) of the original cohort for a second study (the 'Offspring study') and, in 1995, 500 members of Framingham's ethnic minority community were recruited to participate in the 'Omni' study.

Within the first 10 years of the project, the Framingham investigators established that there are many factors that predispose an individual to the development of atherosclerosis, which Dr Bill Kannel, the first director of the Framingham Heart study, termed 'risk factors'. These included those that could not be changed, such as the male gender, increasing age, ethnic origin, a low birthweight

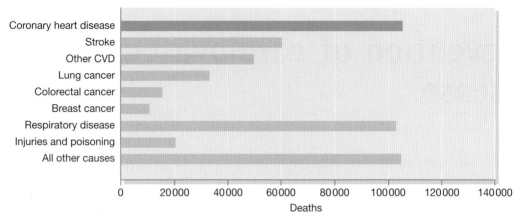

Figure 3.1   Mortality by cause in the UK, 2004 (data from Allender et al, 2006).

and a family history of premature CHD, which were termed *non-modifiable* risk factors. Of greater importance was the identification of factors that were amenable to change such as hypercholesterolaemia, cigarette smoking and hypertension. These are the *modifiable risk factors* that are very common in the adult population (Table 3.1). Because of their frequency, they tend to 'cluster' in individuals. This is important because cumulative risk is not just additive but synergistic (Kannel &

Wilson, 1995), with one factor multiplying the risk of another (Fig. 3.2). Until the late twentieth century, prevention of CVD focused on managing individual risk factors, rather than considering the effect of risk factor combinations. Emphasis was placed on the relative risk reduction for each risk factor, rather than considering how intervention would reduce absolute (i.e. overall) risk. Individuals are usually at greater risk of CVD if they have multiple mild risk factors, rather than only one severe

Table 3.1   Estimated prevalence of different risk factors in adults – England (data from Allender et al, 2006).

Risk factor	Men	Women
Total cholesterol (average)	5.5 mmol/L	5.6 mmol/L
HDL cholesterol (average)	1.4 mmol/L	1.6 mmol/L
Total cholesterol > 5.0 mmol/L	46%	43%
HDL cholesterol < 1.0 mmol/L	6%	2%
Smoking	26%	23%
Obesity (BMI > 30 kg/m²)	23%	24%
Overweight (BMI 25–30 kg/m²)	44%	35%
Central obesity (WHR > 0.95 in men or > 0.85 in women)	33%	30%
Blood pressure – mean systolic BP	135 mmHg	130 mmHg
Hypertension (BP over 140/90 mmHg)	34%	30%
Diabetes (diagnosed)	4%	3%
Diabetes (undiagnosed estimate)	3%	0.7%
Physical activity (taking less than recommended levels for health)	63%	75%

BMI, body mass index; WHR, waist–hip ratio; BP, blood pressure.

Figure 3.2   The synergistic effect of risk factors on the chances of a first major coronary episode, where blood cholesterol level is greater than 6.5 mmol/L and blood pressure is greater than 160/95 mmHg.

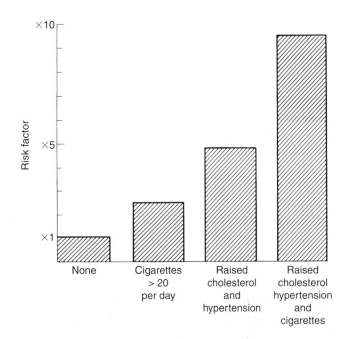

risk factor. The value of any given intervention greatly depends on how it will affect the absolute rather than the relative risk (Smith et al, 2004).

RELATIVE AND ABSOLUTE CARDIOVASCULAR RISK

Cardiovascular risk is defined as the probability of developing cardiovascular symptoms or a vascular event. Appropriate intervention requires knowledge of the level of risk, quoted as the absolute risk, attributable risk or relative risk.

- *Absolute cardiovascular risk* is the risk of developing cardiovascular disease over a time period. It is calculated from cohort or longitudinal studies and randomised controlled trials, where risk is simply the incidence of the event in a particular group. Comparing the absolute risk in two or more groups having different exposures to the risk factor may be expressed as attributable risk (risk difference) and relative risk (risk ratio).
- *Attributable risk* measures the excess risk accounted for by exposure to a particular risk factor (e.g. smoking), and is simply the difference between the absolute risks in the two groups.
- *Relative cardiovascular risk* compares the risk in two different groups of people, and expresses it

as a ratio (%). For example, patients with hypercholesterolaemia have a higher risk of CVD compared with (relative to) those with low blood cholesterol levels. Relative risk is the ratio of two absolute risks for these two groups of patients.

The importance of absolute risk

Guidelines for the prevention of CVD are designed to give a quantitative prediction of absolute risk, which is of particular value when assessing asymptomatic individuals who may have a number of slightly abnormal risk factors that may not attract medical attention. Many such people may be at a much higher level of absolute cardiovascular risk than those with just one high risk factor that brings them under medical care. Individuals in the top 10% of levels of systolic blood pressure, cholesterol and body mass index (BMI) account for only 20–30% of the total number of cases of stroke, ischaemic heart disease and diabetes. Absolute risk equations acknowledge the multifactorial causation of CVD, and can estimate the likelihood of developing an event(s) over a particular time period. Interventions based on elevated levels of a single risk factor may allocate treatment to individuals with little chance of gain because of low absolute risk. When intervening to reduce risk in clinical practice, the *relative* risk reduction associated with treatment of serum cholesterol or high blood pressure is the same at different levels of absolute risk. The *absolute* risk reduction associated with treatment is therefore proportional to the initial absolute risk, i.e. the benefit will be greater in those at higher overall risk.

Calculating risk

Using absolute risk to inform clinical decision-making allows prioritisation of medical resources to those with the highest probability of developing CVD, and risk assessment tables or computer programs have been included in many clinical guidelines to help both clinicians (and patients) to assess overall risk and the need for intervention. Many of these have been derived from the original observations in Framingham. The *Framingham risk equations* were developed to predict coronary disease, heart failure or stroke, and estimate the 10-year risk of each event compared with the average risk in control subjects matched for age and sex. Although the data used to construct this tool were based on a predominantly white, American, middle-class population, the risk equations have been found to be reasonably accurate when applied to North European populations. However, caution is required in extrapolating these results elsewhere, as they overestimate risk in populations with a lower baseline risk, such as those in France, Italy and Spain. The European Systematic Coronary Risk Estimation (SCORE) uses a large data set from several European cohorts and has separate risk charts for low- and high-risk regions of Europe (Conroy et al, 2003). This avoids overestimation of CHD rates in low-risk populations that can occur when using risk equations developed using data from high-risk populations, such as the Framingham cohort. However, because SCORE only predicts fatal CVD, it underestimates the total cardiovascular risk based on non-fatal and fatal cardiovascular events together. As a result, the Joint British Societies (JBS) representing the British Cardiac Society, the British Hypertension Society, Diabetes UK, HEART UK, the Primary Care Cardiovascular Society and the Stroke Association in the UK still use the Framingham data for

calculating risk, despite the known limitations. The JBS have now published revised guidelines for the prevention of atherosclerotic disease and, importantly, like the European SCORE charts, they have replaced estimation of CHD with the prevention of CVD (de Backer et al, 2003). This takes the emphasis away from just cardiac disease, and combines the risk of coronary disease (fatal and non-fatal myocardial infarction and new angina) plus stroke (fatal and non-fatal stroke and cerebral haemorrhage) and transient cerebral ischaemia. Their guidance for preventing CVD in clinical practice uses charts for estimating CVD risk in asymptomatic individuals from major risk factors, expressing risk as the probability (percentage chance) of developing CVD over 10 years (JBS-2, 2005). This aids decisions on risk factor intervention, but should not replace clinical judgement when considering the individual patient.

Using the JBS guidelines

Calculation of cardiovascular risk using the JBS tables requires knowledge of the individual's age, sex, blood pressure, total cholesterol to high-density lipoprotein (HDL) cholesterol ratio and past and present smoking status (Box 3.1). Smoking status is based upon lifetime exposure to tobacco and not tobacco use at the time of assessment. Those who have only recently given up smoking should be regarded as current smokers for risk assessment, as it may take up to 10 years to reach the risk level of those people who have never smoked. The initial blood pressure and the first random (non-fasting) total cholesterol and HDL cholesterol can be used to estimate an individual's risk but, if drug treatment is being contemplated, evidence should be based on a series of pretreatment measurements to allow for biological variability in these readings. If the HDL is not available, it may be assumed to be 1 mmol/L. Random blood glucose testing is helpful to exclude diabetes.

To estimate an individual's total 10-year risk of developing CVD, the JBS guidelines provide individual tables appropriate to age and sex. Level of risk is defined according to the point at which the co-ordinates for systolic blood pressure and the ratio of total cholesterol to HDL cholesterol meet.

> **Box 3.1** Assessing cardiovascular risk in asymptomatic patients.
>
> **Who should be screened?**
>
> All adults 40–80 years
> Younger adults with strong family histories of premature CVD
>
> **Who should not be screened?**
>
> People with known CVD
> Patients with diabetes
> Patients with renal dysfunction
> Patients with inherited dyslipidaemias
> Patients with BP > 160/100 (or end-organ disease)
> Patients with total/HDL cholesterol ratio > 6
>
> **What is needed to assess risk?**
>
> Age
> Sex
> Smoking history
> Random total cholesterol (+ HDL if possible)
> Random blood glucose
> Blood pressure
> Joint British Societies Risk Charts (JBS-2, 2005)
>
> **What other risk factors should be considered?**
>
> Ethnic group
> Family history (first-degree male < 55 years; female < 65 years)
> Premature menopause/polycystic ovary syndrome
> Obesity (especially abdominal)
> Low HDL-C and hypertriglyceridaemia

CVD, cardiovascular disease; BP, blood pressure; HDL, high-density lipoprotein.

There are some additional factors that can increase the risk of CVD above that calculated from the simple risk factors mentioned above, and these should be taken into account in reaching a final decision about the need for lifestyle intervention and, more particularly, drug therapy. These additional factors are:

- family history of premature CVD (men under 55 years and women under 65 years);
- obesity (BMI > 30 kg/m^2) and especially central obesity (waist circumference in white Caucasians over 102 cm in men and over 88 cm in women and, in Asians, over 90 cm in men and over 80 cm in women);
- low HDL cholesterol (< 1.0 mmol/L in men and < 1.2 mmol/L in women);
- raised triglycerides (> 1.7 mmol/L);
- impaired fasting glucose (fasting blood glucose > 6.1 mmol/L but < 7.0 mmol/L) or impaired glucose tolerance (2-hour glucose > 7.8 mmol/L and < 11.1 mmol/L during an oral glucose tolerance test);
- women with premature menopause or polycystic ovaries.

Patients with established atherosclerotic disease have already declared themselves to be at high risk for recurrent events and do not need to have their risk assessed. These individuals require aggressive risk factor modification, as discussed in Chapter 15. Similarly, patients with familial hypercholesterolaemia (or certain other inherited dyslipidaemias), diabetes, raised total cholesterol to HDL cholesterol ratio of > 6 or severe hypertension (systolic blood pressure > 160 mmHg and/or diastolic blood pressure > 100 mmHg) are already at high risk, and the assessment charts do not apply. To identify other high-risk individuals in the population requires either formal or opportunistic screening. It is recommended that all adults from 40 years onwards should be considered for screening at least every 5 years.

The threshold of total CVD risk at which drug treatments are suggested is arbitrary based on the evidence of benefits, as well as financial considerations in relation to the ability of the health services to provide care. Whatever threshold is chosen, it must target those at highest risk, where the absolute benefits of treatment will be greatest. Lesser degrees of risk remain important, but a progressive staged approach to CVD prevention will ensure that delivery of care is balanced with the ability of the medical services to identify, investigate and treat patients in the long term. While certain pharmacological interventions have been shown to reduce absolute risk at levels of less than 1% per year, managing everyone at this low level of risk, particularly with expensive therapies, would be hugely demanding on medical resources. There is little point in turning people into patients if we cannot offer appropriate care.

If a decision is made not to intervene pharmacologically, this must be reviewed at regular intervals. With advancing age, an individual's risk will increase and may rise to levels that warrant intervention.

THE MAJOR CARDIOVASCULAR RISK FACTORS

Five independent risk factors have a major and direct role in promoting atherosclerosis. These are:

- cigarette smoking;
- hypertension;
- elevated total cholesterol and low-density lipoprotein (LDL) cholesterol;
- diabetes;
- low HDL cholesterol.

In addition, there are predisposing risk factors that interact with these causal risk factors to increase overall risk (Grundy, 1999). These are:

- age;
- obesity;
- physical inactivity;
- family history of premature CVD;
- male sex;
- race;
- metabolic syndrome.

The INTERHEART study has shown that the risk factors associated with CHD are essentially the same all over the world, and CVD is mostly preventable by cessation of smoking, taking more exercise and eating a healthy diet (Yusuf et al, 2004).

Age

Mortality from CHD rises steeply with increasing age, approximately doubling every 5 years. The incidence of new and recurrent heart attacks also increases with age, and most coronary events occur in the elderly. While it is assumed that the increase in frequency of heart disease in the elderly is part of the ageing process, it is probably due to a cumulative effect of exposure to known modifiable risk factors such as smoking, hyperlipidaemia and hypertension, rather than simple degeneration. Many people over the age of 70 years are at a 10-year CVD risk of over 20%,

and decision to intervene requires individual clinical judgement with research evidence where available. For example, hypertension trials consistently confirm the benefits of lowering blood pressure in patients up to 80 years of age, and the Medical Research Council/British Heart Foundation heart protection study (Heart Protection Study Collaborative Group, 2002) has now shown the benefits of cholesterol lowering with simvastatin in patients up to 80 years of age. Because the absolute risk of CVD is higher in the elderly, risk factor modification should have a greater effect than the same interventions in younger age groups. On the other hand, although the short-term total CVD risk of younger people may not be great, their total lifetime risk exposure may be exceptionally high. In addition, as blood pressure, cholesterol and glucose all rise, and HDL cholesterol falls with age, their risk can only worsen unless there is some intervention.

Sex

Coronary heart disease has been thought to be primarily a problem that affects men and, while most women worry about breast cancer, only 4% will die from this, but over half will die as a result of heart attack or stroke. Risk factors for CHD are the same in women as they are in men, but their relative weighting is different, and this has important implications for prevention.

Female issues

The absolute risk of CHD is lower at all ages in women until old age when the level of risk converges with that of males. At the time of presentation with heart disease, women tend to be 10 years older than men and, at the time of their first myocardial infarction, they are usually 20 years older. The menopause marks an approximate threefold increase in the risk of CHD, when it has been assumed that it is the lack of the protective effects of estrogens that is mostly responsible. However, hormone replacement therapy does not seem to be protective (Hulley et al, 1998), and what is more relevant is that, after the age of 55 years, many women become obese and have higher blood cholesterol and glucose concentrations

> **Box 3.2** Cardiovascular risk factors in women.
>
> **Higher risk in women**
> Smoking
> High triglyceride levels
>
> **Higher prevalence in women**
> Diabetes
> Obesity
> Depression
>
> **Other risk factors**
> Oral contraceptive use
> Hormone replacement therapy
> Polycystic ovary syndrome

than men. Women with diabetes have 2.6 times the risk of dying from CHD than women without diabetes compared with a 1.8-fold risk among men with diabetes. In addition, smoking, hypertension and hypertriglyceridaemia appear to be more dangerous in women (Box 3.2). Levels of physical activity in girls show a sharp decline after the age of 8 or 9 years, and few women in the UK take regular physical activity.

Women are poorly represented in risk factor modification trials, but current recommendations on risk factor intervention make no distinction between men and women.

Male issues

Endothelial dysfunction underlies both atherosclerosis and erectile dysfunction (ED), and the incidence of coronary disease is increased in patients with impotence (Jackson et al, 2006). Approximately 50% of men aged over 40 years experience some degree of ED, and it is more common in those with hypertension, diabetes and coronary artery disease. A patient with ED and coronary artery disease is more likely to have multivessel than single-vessel coronary disease (Solomon et al, 2003). If there are no cardiac symptoms, ED should be considered as a marker for occult vascular disease, and individuals should be screened for cardiac risk factors and evidence of established CVD (Thompson et al, 2005).

Race

Atherosclerosis affects all races, but there are marked international differences in the occurrence of CHD, even allowing for the differences made in disease classification by various countries. The rates of CHD are very high in those of South Asian origin (India, Bangladesh, Pakistan and Sri Lanka), intermediate in those of European origin (Northern rates higher than Southern European rates), with the lowest rates in those from Africa and China. However, at any given time, different countries are at varying stages of epidemiological transition, with adverse lifestyle changes that accompany industrialisation and urbanisation. Further, as life expectancy increases, the duration of exposure to risk factors increases. Certain risk factors are more common among South Asians. These vary between communities, but include high levels of smoking (particularly among Bangladeshi men), low rates of exercise and diets high in fat and low in fruit and vegetables. In general, migrants who move from low-risk to high-risk areas change their risk of CVD to that of the host country, although with prolonged exposure to the environment, disease rates tend to return to the incidence of their country of origin.

It is thus unclear whether the variation in CHD in different races is due to environmental or genetic factors, but one review suggested that the apparent increased risk in Asians disappears when the higher incidence of diabetes has been accounted for (Bhopal, 2000). Diabetes is up to six times more common in South Asians and, while cardiovascular risk factors are the same in all nationalities, the metabolic response to various risk factors may differ in different populations (Yusuf et al, 2004).

Risk assessment tables should be used with caution when assessing patients from ethnic minorities, as they have not been validated in these populations and may grossly underestimate risk (Bhopal et al, 2005). Adding 10 years to the age of South Asian people is a simple way of calculating CHD risk using current risk charts (Aarabi & Jackson, 2005), or multiplying the CVD risk by 1.4. Lifestyle advice appropriate to the individual's culture is required, but all risk factors should be managed as for other nationalities.

Genetic predisposition and a family history of premature CVD

Mortality from CHD in the UK fell by 42% in the decade 1987–1997. This large decline can only be explained by improvements in prevention and treatment, as alterations in the genetic structure of the population cannot have taken place sufficiently fast to account for such dramatic changes. Nevertheless, it is clear that genetic influences are of importance in the aetiology of coronary heart disease (Jowett, 1984). Genetic factors affecting susceptibility to CHD may operate through known modifiable risk factors that run in families, such as dyslipidaemia, diabetes and hypertension, or through as yet undefined genetic mechanisms. Modern recombinant DNA technology has already ascertained the risks of some genetic diseases that increase the risk of CHD, such as familial hypercholesterolaemia, homocysteinaemia, type III and familial combined hyperlipidaemia. Other suggested 'candidate genes' include those affecting coagulation factors, growth factors, vessel wall proteins, the insulin receptor gene, the angiotensin-converting enzyme (ACE) gene and apolipoprotein genes (Jowett et al, 1984; Rees et al, 1985). Variants of certain haemostatic genes, including that encoding the factor V Leiden and the 20210A variant of the prothrombin gene, both of which increase circulating thrombin generation, might each be moderately associated with the risk of coronary disease (Ye et al, 2006). Several regions in the human genome have been shown to be associated with either hypertension or CHD (Broeckel et al, 2002).

Genetic testing is likely to become an established component of preventing coronary artery disease, with identification of genetic variants that have a predictive value. This will allow a more cost-effective method of risk factor intervention, by directing preventive therapy and counselling to those who will benefit most.

When considering risk from a positive family history, this does not just mean having a family member with heart disease. Given the prevalence of CHD, most people have an affected relative. The family history risk for CHD increases:

1 when a first-degree relative (parent, sibling or offspring) has CHD;

2 as the number of family members with CHD increases;

3 when a family member develops CHD at a young age.

In the Framingham Offspring study, the risk of CVD was greater if a sibling rather than a parent was already affected (Murabito et al, 2005). Families of patients with early onset CHD are a priority group for risk identification and monitoring. Family history information of an individual is not static and, over time, other young family members may develop premature CVD. It is important that the family history is updated at regular intervals.

Current cardiovascular risk assessment tables do not consider family history. If there is a first-degree relative with CVD in a male before the age of 55 years or in a female before the age of 65 years, the calculated absolute risk should be multiplied by a factor of 1.3.

Lipids, lipoproteins and dyslipidaemia

The major lipids are triglycerides and cholesterol. Cholesterol forms an integral cell membrane component. Triglycerides are stored energy reserves found predominantly in adipose tissue, and are the main vehicles for the transport of fatty acids. Fatty acids are carried from the liver and intestine to the tissues (including the myocardium) for energy, and to the endothelium for prostaglandin synthesis.

Lipids are insoluble in water and, in order for them to be transported in the blood, they are converted to water-soluble complexes called lipoproteins. The main lipoproteins are:

- *Chylomicrons*: the largest lipoprotein. They consist mainly of dietary triglyceride absorbed by the small intestine.
- *Low-density lipoprotein (LDL)*: the main transport vehicle for cholesterol.
- *Very low-density lipoprotein (VLDL)*: small, triglyceride-rich lipoproteins. They transport lipids synthesised mainly in the liver.
- *High-density lipoprotein (HDL)*: the smallest lipoproteins. They contain cholesterol transported away from cells to the liver.

The typical high-fat diet of most western populations in the twentieth century has proved to be one of the main underlying factors in the cardiovascular epidemic. The INTERHEART case–control study estimated that around 40% of heart attacks in Europe are associated with abnormal blood lipids (Yusuf et al, 2004).

There is a clear correlation between raised serum cholesterol levels and the risk of CHD (Law et al, 1994), the relationship being virtually linear with no threshold value (Fig. 3.3). The average level of serum cholesterol in different countries roughly predicts the risk of CHD – the higher the national average cholesterol, the higher the risk – so there is really no such thing as a 'normal' serum cholesterol level. For every 1% increase in the level of total cholesterol, there is a 2–3% increase in the incidence of coronary artery disease. The UK population has among the highest serum cholesterol concentrations in the world. The mean blood cholesterol level for men aged 16 years and above in England is 5.5 mmol/L and for women 5.6 mmol/L. About 45% of the adult population have blood total cholesterol concentrations of over 5.0 mmol/L.

While high total plasma cholesterol concentrations are a very strong risk factor for CVD, risk is principally determined by the concentrations of LDL cholesterol (LDL-C). LDL-C concentrations can be measured directly in the laboratory, but are usually estimated indirectly by the Friedewald formula:

$$LDL–C \, (mmol/L) = (total \; cholesterol–HDL-C) \\ – (triglyceride \times 0.45)$$

The Friedewald formula only gives an estimation of LDL concentrations, and cannot be used if the triglyceride concentrations are more than 4.5 mmol/L or in some patients with diabetes. Measuring lipids in the non-fasting state will underestimate LDL cholesterol concentrations, particularly if there is hypertriglyceridaemia. Measuring the levels of apolipoprotein B, a structural protein present in all atherogenic particles, may be particularly useful for estimating risk in individuals with hypertriglyceridaemia, because it reflects the total atherogenic load. Apolipoprotein B is a better estimator of cardiovascular risk than LDL-C alone (Sniderman et al, 2003).

Dyslipidaemia

The term *hyperlipidaemia* has previously been used to identify those with particularly high blood lipid concentrations, but the term *dyslipidaemia* is now preferred because blood lipid abnormalities that predispose to CHD are not always present in high concentrations. For example, it is *decreased* concentrations of HDL-C that predispose to CVD (particularly the HDL$_2$ subfraction). Low HDL-C and high LDL-C levels are the major associates of atherosclerotic disease, and a ratio of these two lipoproteins of less than 0.2 appears to be an important predictor of CHD. There is also a small dense type of LDL-C (the type 'B' phenotype) that particularly associates with atheromatous disease. This type B LDL-C particle is more common in those with the metabolic syndrome, and high concentrations associate with low HDL-C levels and hypertriglyceridaemia.

The role of high triglycerides in the aetiology of CHD is a little harder to interpret. Raised triglyceride levels appear to be more strongly correlated with CVD risk in women but, while raised levels associate with the risk of ischaemic heart disease,

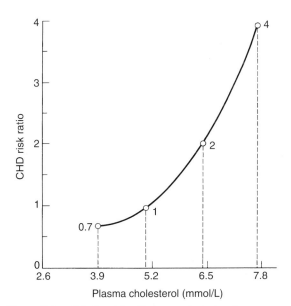

Figure 3.3 Relationship of plasma cholesterol concentrations to mortality, based on a 7.5-year follow-up of 17 718 men in the Whitehall study (data from Rose and Shipley, 1980).

it is not an independent risk factor, as hypertriglyceridaemia normally associates with raised LDL-C and reduced HDL-C concentrations (Jackson, 1996). Interestingly, patients with genetic hypertriglyceridaemia (e.g. familial lipoprotein lipase deficiency) are not at increased risk of CVD, but it is important to detect severe hypertriglyceridaemia, as it may cause acute pancreatitis and peripheral neuropathy.

The mean HDL-C level in the UK is 1.5 mmol/L, and relatively few individuals have concentrations low enough to affect health. However, low HDL-C levels often associate with other risk factors, such as lack of exercise, diabetes, obesity and cigarette smoking. Overall, about 6% of men and 2% of women have HDL-C levels of < 1.0 mmol/L.

Raised HDL levels are often found in premenopausal women, joggers and moderate, regular drinkers of alcohol. Although as many women as men die of CHD per year, the mean age at death is substantially higher. The reason for this sex gap may be the substantially higher concentrations of HDL cholesterol in women.

Screening for dyslipidaemia Lipid abnormalities are usually asymptomatic and are ordinarily detected by screening. Opportunistic screening should be offered to all adults from 40 years of age onwards, but selective screening will be required in those with strong family histories of premature CVD and familial dyslipidaemias.

Family screening Measurement of serum lipids should be offered to first-degree relatives of patients with marked dyslipidaemia, particularly younger males, in whom early therapy will be of most value. This is especially important in monogenic familial hypercholesterolaemia (FH), an autosomal dominant disorder that carries a high risk of early cardiovascular morbidity and death. FH affects 1 in 500 of the UK population, and is caused by one of many mutations of the LDL receptor gene on chromosome 19 (Humphries et al, 1985). Typically, the patient has a cholesterol concentration over 7.5 mmol/L, together with cutaneous signs such as early corneal arcus, xantholasma and tendon xanthomata. The last are very suggestive of heterozygous FH, and are found in three-quarters of sufferers over the age of 20 years. Early diagnosis and therapy offer the best hope of improving cardiovascular prognosis, and tracing of family members is very important for case finding (Marks et al, 2002). Diagnostic criteria for FH in adults are defined by the Simon Broome register (Box 3.3).

There are two other monogenic disorders that associate with hypercholesterolaemia and premature vascular disease:

- *familial defective apolipoprotein-B* (FDP) is caused by mutations in apo-B100 (the protein constituent of LDL);
- *autosomal recessive hypercholesterolaemia* (ARH), that associates with mutations in an adapter protein that prevents cellular uptake of LDL-C from the blood.

Familial combined hyperlipidaemia is found in up to 20% of survivors of myocardial infarction. Both cholesterol and triglycerides are moderately raised.

Box 3.3   Diagnostic criteria for familial hypercholesterolaemia in adults (Simon Broome Register Group, 1999).

Definite familial hypercholesterolaemia

Total cholesterol > 7.5 mmol/L (or LDL-C > 4.9 mmol/L), PLUS
Tendon xanthomata in the patient or a first- or second-degree relative

Possible familial hypercholesterolaemia

Total cholesterol >7.5 mmol/L (or LDL-C > 4.9 mmol/L), PLUS either:
Premature myocardial infarction (< 60 years in first-degree relative or < 50 years in a second-degree relative), OR
Total cholesterol > 7.5 mmol/L (or LDL-C > 4.9 mmol/L) in a first- or second-degree relative

It is probably dominantly inherited, but no single gene defect has yet been identified.

Familial dysbetalipoproteinaemia (often known as type III hyperlipidaemia) patients are at increased risk of vascular disease, despite low LDL levels. There is a defect in the clearance of remnant particles that are thought to be atherogenic. Palmar crease and tuberous xanthomata are common.

Laboratory requests   The most commonly employed screening test is random serum cholesterol estimation, although both total and HDL-C concentrations are needed to calculate the 10-year CVD risk. This is particularly important in women, who frequently have high HDL-C levels. A low HDL-C is often found in the presence of other risk factors, particularly diabetes, and relying on total cholesterol alone may be misleading. If the total cholesterol is less than 4 mmol/L, there is usually no need for further analysis, unless there is suspicion of another abnormality. If the random cholesterol is greater than 4 mmol/L, or if there is likely to be another lipid abnormality, total cholesterol, HDL-C and triglyceride levels should be measured in a sample of venous blood taken, preferably without venous stasis, after an overnight (12-hour) fast. Because of the biological and laboratory variability in assessing cholesterol concentrations, a reliable estimate requires at least three separate fasting estimations. Some centres would further explore the index of risk by measuring *apolipoprotein* levels. There are at least 10 of these structural parts of the lipoprotein particle. Each is involved with a specific lipoprotein and is concerned with its transport, activation or receptor recognition. ApoA-1 and ApoB are the major apolipoproteins of HDL and LDL, respectively, and measurement may permit more accurate prediction of coronary disease than HDL-C or LDL-C levels alone (Sniderman et al, 2003). Lipoprotein 'little a' (Lpa) is an LDL-like lipoprotein that has structural similarities to plasminogen, and may be associated with increased cardiovascular risk. Supportive evidence has been conflicting, and no trial has yet looked at the effects of reducing Lpa concentrations (Harjai, 1999).

It should be noted that acute illness such as infection, trauma (including surgery) and myocardial infarction might alter serum lipoprotein concentrations so that they are not representative of the patient's baseline values. For example, for about 3 months after acute myocardial infarction, plasma triglycerides may be higher and total cholesterol lower than preinfarction levels (Brugada et al, 1996).

There are sometimes underlying causes of dyslipidaemia ('secondary dyslipidaemias') such as diabetes, thyroid disease, renal disease, cholestasis, alcohol and drugs (Jowett & Galton, 1987). These must be excluded and addressed before assessing cardiovascular risk. Appropriate routine laboratory tests are urea and electrolytes, liver and thyroid function tests and random blood glucose.

Management of dyslipidaemia   Management of blood cholesterol according to risk in asymptomatic people without CVD is shown in Figure 3.4. Any measure that reduces serum cholesterol is effective in the prevention of CVD, whether dietary, pharmacological or surgical (Downs et al, 1998). All people should receive lifestyle advice to modify their lipoproteins favourably (to reduce total and LDL cholesterol, raise HDL cholesterol and lower triglycerides). Drug therapy is recommended for those at high total risk (CVD risk > 20% over 10 years), and for those with diabetes over the age of 40 years. Younger patients with diabetes should also be considered for statins if there is evidence of microvascular disease, poor glycaemic control, hypertension or an adverse family history. The aim is to reduce total cholesterol concentrations to below 4 mmol/L, or LDL-C of 2 mmol/L, marking the level above which there is a marked rise in atherosclerotic cardiovascular events, notably CHD (Fig. 3.3).

Having reduced the total and LDL cholesterol to target, some patients may still have harmful blood lipid concentrations (e.g. diabetes, metabolic syndrome, genetic dyslipidaemia), and a full lipid profile may be helpful in this group of patients. Non-HDL-C (i.e. total cholesterol minus HDL-C) is a measure of atherogenic triglyceride-rich lipoproteins. Desirable concentrations are < 3 mmol/L. The HDL-C should preferably be > 1 mmol/L in men and > 1.2 mmol/L in women. Individuals with hypertriglyceridaemia (> 1.7 mmol/L) usually have a slightly higher CVD risk than that shown in the charts, and it is appropriate to increase that risk by a factor of 1.3.

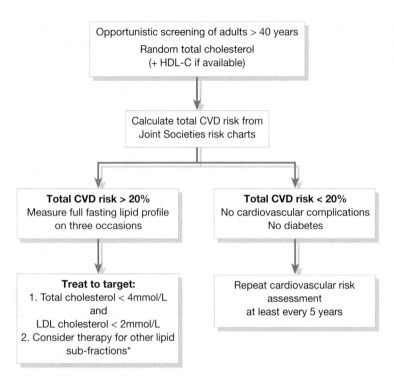

Figure 3.4 Assessing blood lipids according to risk in asymptomatic people without CVD (adapted from JBS-2, 2005).

Risk charts should not be used to decide whether to introduce lipid-lowering medication when the ratio of serum total to HDL cholesterol exceeds six, as treatment is usually indicated regardless of estimated CVD risk.

Smoking

Smoking increases the risk of coronary, cerebral and peripheral arterial disease and depends upon both the amount of tobacco smoked daily and the duration of smoking. Smoking remains the single most important public health issue in the UK, and has been for over 400 years, since 1604 when King James I of England (James VI of Scotland)

produced a paper entitled 'Counterblaste to Tobacco'. He noted that smoking was a 'custome loathsome to the eye, hateful to the nose, harmful to the brain and dangerous to the lungs'. Little did the monarch realise that, four centuries later, this loathsome habit was killing more than 100 000 subjects in the UK every year, most dying from cancer, chronic obstructive pulmonary disease and coronary heart disease. About half of all regular smokers will eventually be killed by their habit (Doll et al, 2004) and, currently, 23% of all male deaths and 12% of all female deaths are attributable to smoking (Twigg et al, 2004). Smoking 20 cigarettes/day doubles the risk of coronary death, and smoking caused around 30 600 deaths from

CVD alone in 2000 in the UK (Allender et al, 2006). The risk of dying increases proportionally with the number of cigarettes smoked, and appears to be greater for women (Prescott et al, 1998).

Tobacco smoke is a complex aerosol containing two implicated cardiovascular toxins, nicotine and carbon monoxide.

1 *Nicotine.* Nicotine absorption during smoking varies from about 5% to 100%, depending upon smoking patterns, and a heavy smoker may absorb about 100 mg of nicotine per day. Nicotine stimulates catecholamine release, and increases myocardial work by raising heart rate, blood pressure and force of myocardial contraction. Additionally, there is a thrombogenic action caused by inhibition of fibrinolysis and an increase in platelet aggregation.

2 *Carbon monoxide.* Carbon monoxide is a cellular poison and makes up about 3–6% of inhaled cigarette smoke. This is eight times the maximum air pollution allowed in industry! It binds 200 times more readily with haemoglobin than does oxygen, which it displaces to form carboxyhaemoglobin. Typically, the haemoglobin of a heavy smoker will be 20% carboxylated, which shifts the oxygen dissociation curve to the left, thereby impairing oxygen release in tissues. Oxygenation is therefore reduced, despite increased myocardial requirements due to nicotinic stimulation. Carbon monoxide may additionally cause endothelial dysfunction, increasing permeability to foam cells and predisposing to atheroma.

The number of packs smoked per day multiplied by the number of years gives the *pack–years*, a widely accepted method for smoking quantification. Pipe, cigar and chewing tobacco use should also be noted. The cardiovascular risk from pipe and cigar smoke is more variable but, if inhaled, is probably not very different from the risk produced by cigarette smoke. The hazards to pipe and cigar smokers who have never smoked cigarettes is thought to be less, because smoking patterns usually differ, with reduced intake of smoke into the lungs. Former cigarette smokers who switch to cigars or a pipe do not reduce their risk of cardiovascular events, presumably because of the tendency to inhale the smoke more like

a cigarette. It is also worth noting that self-reports on the depth of inhalation of smoke are extremely inaccurate.

Smoking often associates with other unhealthy behaviours such as a high-fat, high-calorie diet, and tobacco exposure is associated with the development of glucose intolerance. In the CARDIA study, a strong association was found between both active and passive tobacco smoke exposure and subsequent development of impaired fasting glucose or diabetes over 15 years. Increasing total pack–years smoked associates with increasing risks of diabetes (Houston et al, 2006).

The proportion of male smokers declined from 28% in 1993 to 26% in 2004 and, in women, the proportion fell from 26% to 23%. The UK now has the second lowest proportion of male smokers in the European Union, whereas women are among the highest. Just over one-third of adults in England are ex-smokers.

Smoking remains particularly prevalent in the young. By the age of 15 years, 1 in 10 children in the UK are regular smokers, and most smokers are now found in the 20- to 24-year age group. Those who start smoking before the age of 20 years increase their cardiovascular risk by three to five times. The highest rates of smoking are found among men aged 25–34 years, in whom prevalence is estimated to be as high as 40% (Twigg et al, 2004).

Smokers and former smokers are at twice the risk of a heart attack as those who have never smoked. Stopping smoking will reduce cardiovascular risk, although it may take 10 years to reach the risk level of those people who have never smoked. However, in those with coronary disease, excess risk falls much faster, so that, within 2–3 years, it is similar to those people with coronary disease who have never smoked.

Environmental tobacco smoke

Second-hand (environmental) smoke consists of *side-stream smoke* (from the burning tip of a cigarette between puffs) and the *mainstream smoke* (exhaled by the smoker). Second-hand smoke is a mixture of more than 4000 chemical compounds including at least 40 known carcinogens. Higher levels of many of these carcinogens are found in side-stream smoke, which makes up 85% of second-hand smoke and is at least four times more toxic than mainstream smoke (Wallace-Bell, 2003). Side-stream smoke from filtered (or light) cigarettes is considerably more toxic than that from full flavour cigarettes.

Passive smoking is the term applied to breathing second-hand smoke, and it is recognised as a significant public health issue, increasing the risk of both lung cancer and CVD by about 20–30% (Law et al, 1997; Scientific Committee on Tobacco Health, 1998). Passive smoking in the workplace is a major health issue, being responsible for more than 600 deaths per year, as well as major effects on lost productivity through sickness-related absences (Jamrozik, 2005). Those who work in the hospitality industry (pubs, hotels and restaurants) are at particular risk. Exposure within the home may contribute to over 10 000 adult deaths, and children living in smoking households may 'smoke' up to 150 cigarettes each year. This predisposes them to childhood asthma, chronic chest and middle ear infections, and probably provides a stimulus for accelerated atherosclerosis. Treatment of these children costs the NHS an estimated £410 million in England and Wales alone.

In 2004, the Health Development Agency provided a summary of evidence-based strategies to reduce smoking initiation and increase smoking cessation for all population groups, with particular reference to the young (Naidoo et al, 2004). This has been supplemented by the Government's *Choosing Health* white paper (Department of Health, 2004a), which recognises that exposure to second-hand smoke in both the workplace and public areas can be significantly reduced by interventions that seek to ban or restrict smoking. By restricting smoking in public places, tobacco use can be 'denormalised', rendering it less acceptable as a social behaviour, and smoking prevalence should fall as a result (Chapman et al, 1999). Legislation that bans smoking in all enclosed (or substantially enclosed) public places and places of work was passed by the UK government in February 2006. Prohibition is already in place on trains and buses and in schools and shops. From summer 2007, this will be extended to include all bars, clubs, cinemas, restaurants and offices. On 29 March 2004, a similar ban was implemented in Ireland. Despite concerns about unemployment with falling numbers in pubs,

a survey at 12 months found that the number of smokers going to pubs remained the same, but more non-smokers were now visiting. Carbon monoxide levels in non-smoking bar workers dropped by 45%. Almost 1 in 5 Irish smokers now choose not to smoke at all when out socialising, and the vast majority of workers now find their workplace a more pleasant place to work in.

Blood pressure

Individuals with blood pressure levels at the upper limits of the population distribution have an increased incidence of atherosclerotic vascular disease and an increased morbidity and mortality resulting from stroke, myocardial infarction and peripheral vascular disease. High blood pressure also associates with a decline in renal and cognitive function, and is one of the most important preventable causes of premature death worldwide (Ezzati et al, 2002). The risk of CHD is directly related to both systolic and diastolic blood pressure levels and, in adults aged 40–69 years, each 20-mmHg increase in usual systolic blood pressure, or 10-mmHg increase in usual diastolic blood pressure, approximately doubles the risk. At older ages, the increase in the risk of death from CHD is smaller. The INTERHEART study estimated that about a quarter of heart attacks in Europe are associated with high blood pressure, and a history of hypertension places individuals at just under twice the risk of a heart attack compared with those with no history of hypertension (Yusuf et al, 2004).

Blood pressure levels in the UK are generally high, rise with age and do so more rapidly after the age of 45 years. As a result, all adults from 40 years onwards should have their blood pressure measured as part of an opportunistic CVD risk assessment. This should be repeated at least 5-yearly. Currently, the mean systolic blood pressure in English adult males is 135 mmHg, and in adult females 130 mmHg.

The distribution of blood pressure values in the population is a continuum, and the cut-off point above which patients are considered hypertensive is arbitrary. Hypertension in adults (> 18 years) is currently graded as shown in Table 3.2.

Hypertension (more than 140/90 mmHg) affects about a billion people worldwide. In the UK,

Table 3.2 Grading of hypertension in adults.

	Systolic BP (mmHg)	Diastolic BP (mmHg)
Normal	< 120	< 80
High-normal	135–139	85–89
Hypertension		
Mild hypertension (grade 1)	140–159	90–99
Moderate hypertension (grade 2)	160–179	100–109
Severe hypertension (grade 3)	> 180	> 110

the prevalence of hypertension has been estimated to be 42% in people aged 35–64 years (Wolf-Maier et al, 2003).

While rising levels of both systolic and diastolic blood pressure increase the risk of death, the systolic blood pressure is the better predictor of subsequent CVD. Isolated systolic hypertension (ISH) is a particular problem in the elderly that remains poorly recognised and poorly treated. The evaluation of blood pressure levels in older people is often difficult, because there is a higher prevalence of postural hypotension and greater blood pressure variability through the day. Multiple measurements are required, with both sitting and standing values to exclude any significant postural drop. Standing blood pressure levels are often a better basis for initiating and assessing response to treatment.

In people over the age of 80 years, treatment of hypertension reduces stroke and heart attacks, but total mortality may be unaffected (Gueyffier et al, 1999), so treatment decisions should balance potential benefits with other co-morbidities. It is probably unwise to stop longstanding therapy when patients get older.

The risks of hypertension are not uniform, but are higher in those with other risk factors, and the British Hypertension Society guidelines (Williams et al, 2004) support initiation of treatment on both the mean blood pressure measurement and the level of overall cardiovascular risk (10-year risk of CVD ≥ 20%). The exception to this applies to those with average sustained systolic blood pressures > 160 mmHg and diastolic pressures > 100 mmHg

(90 mmHg in the elderly), who usually require intervention, regardless of absolute CHD risk.

Clinical trials consistently provide compelling evidence of the effectiveness of antihypertensive therapy in reducing the risk of CVD (Blood Pressure Lowering Treatment Trialists' Collaboration, 2003). The absolute risk reduction will be greatest in those at highest risk, so lower intervention thresholds and lower optimal treatment targets are recommended for people with target organ disease or diabetes. Markers of target organ damage include:

- cerebrovascular disease (stroke/transient ischaemic attack);
- peripheral vascular disease;
- coronary artery disease;
- heart failure;
- hypertensive (or diabetic) retinopathy;
- abnormal renal function tests (proteinuria or eGFR);
- left ventricular hypertrophy.

Managing blood pressure according to risk in asymptomatic people without CVD is shown in Figure 3.5. Ambulatory blood pressure monitoring (ABPM) or home blood pressure readings are usually lower than clinic readings, and so 10/5 mmHg should be added for both thresholds and targets. For ambulatory readings, the mean daytime figure is preferable for decision-making rather than the average for the 24-hour period.

In hypertensive patients younger than 55 years, the first choice of initial therapy is usually an angiotensin-converting enzyme (ACE) inhibitor (or an angiotensin-II receptor antagonist if an ACE inhibitor is not tolerated). For patients over 55 years or black patients (African or Caribbean descent, not mixed race, Asian or Chinese) of any age, the first choice of initial therapy should be either a calcium channel blocker or a thiazide diuretic (NICE, 2006).

For most patients, a treatment target of < 140 mmHg systolic and < 85 mmHg diastolic pressure is recommended. A lower target of less than 130/80 is used for patients with diabetes, renal impairment or established CVD (Table 3.3).

The benefits of blood pressure reduction depend upon how well the blood pressure is controlled. National surveys continue to show substantial underdiagnosis, undertreatment and poor rates of

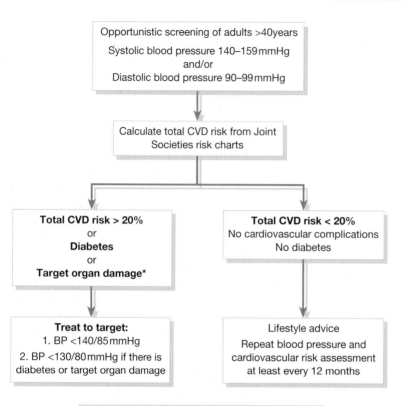

Figure 3.5 Managing blood pressure according to risk in asymptomatic people without CVD (adapted from JBS-02, 2005). TIA, transient ischaemic attack.

Table 3.3 Target blood pressure during antihypertensive treatment (Williams et al, 2004).

	Measurement in clinic		Mean daytime ambulatory measurement or home measurement	
	No diabetes	With diabetes	No diabetes	With diabetes
Blood pressure (mmHg)	< 140/85	< 130/80	< 120/75	< 120/70
Optimal Audit Standard[a]	< 150/90	< 140/80	< 130/80	< 130/75

aThe audit standard reflects the minimum recommended target for blood pressure control.

blood pressure control (Primatesta et al, 2001). Target blood pressures may only be achieved in 10% of the hypertensive population (Wolf-Maier et al, 2004).

All people with high normal blood pressures or a family history of hypertension should receive lifestyle advice to help reduce their blood pressure and CVD risk. Following salt restriction and weight reduction, the need for drug therapy may be reduced.

Hypertension and aspirin

Aspirin is recommended for primary prevention in well-controlled hypertensive patients (with blood pressure < 150/90 mmHg) aged 50 years and above with any of:

- evidence of target organ damage;
- a 10-year cardiovascular disease risk > 20%;
- type 2 diabetes mellitus.

Diabetes and glucose intolerance

Like blood cholesterol concentrations, it appears that the blood glucose level is a continuous cardiovascular risk factor – the higher the mean blood glucose, the greater the risk. This risk extends from a blood glucose concentration of 4.2 mmol/L upwards, a level well below the threshold for the diagnosis of diabetes and glucose intolerance (Coutinho et al, 1999). The term 'dysglycaemia' has been used to indicate that the blood glucose is higher than it should be, without defining a threshold (Gerstein & Yusuf, 1996). Reflecting the concern that the risk of CVD exists in people with even slightly elevated blood glucose levels, the American Diabetes Association have suggested that the cut-off for 'normality' is a fasting blood glucose of 5.6 mmol/L (American Diabetes Association, 2003). The concept of dysglycaemia and its consequences is poorly appreciated in primary care (Wylie et al, 2002).

Diagnosing glucose intolerance

All people who develop diabetes go through stages of rising blood sugars, although the length of these phases may vary depending on the extent of the underlying disease process. The term 'prediabetes' is a practical and convenient term to describe this period of dysglycaemia, which places individuals at risk of developing diabetes and CVD (American Diabetes Association, 2002). The term 'impaired glucose regulation' is sometimes used as an alternative.

In the past, the diagnostic criteria for diabetes have been based on predisposition to microvascular complications (e.g. retinopathy, renal disease). However, over 70% of patients with diabetes die from macrovascular disease (mainly CHD), and modern diagnostic criteria attempt to capture all those with prediabetes because of their increased risk of future diabetes (American Diabetes Association, 2003). In the Hoorn study, the risk of conversion to diabetes in patients with prediabetes during 6.5 years of follow up was more than 10 times higher than in people with normal glucose tolerance (Vegt et al, 2001).

Patients with hyperglycaemia may be broadly classified as having:

- type 1 diabetes (previously known as insulin-dependent diabetes or IDD);
- type 2 diabetes (previously known as non-insulin-dependent or maturity onset diabetes – NIDDM or MOD);
- impaired glucose tolerance (IGT);
- impaired fasting glucose (IFG).

The diagnosis of glucose intolerance is based on fasting or random blood glucose measurement but may need a formal 75-g oral glucose tolerance test (OGTT) (Table 3.4).

In patients with symptoms (polyuria, polydipsia, weight loss, etc.), diabetes is confirmed with:

- a random plasma glucose > 11.1 mmol/L; or
- a fasting plasma glucose > 7.0 mmol/L; or
- a 2-hour plasma glucose > 11.1 mmol/L following a formal OGTT.

In patients without symptoms, the tests should be repeated at least once at another time. A random glucose of < 6 mmol/L usually excludes glucose intolerance.

Prediabetes may be subdivided into IGT or IFG.

1 Patients with IGT have a 1.5 times increased risk of developing CVD compared with those with normal glucose tolerance (DECODE Study

Table 3.4 Plasma glucose levels for the diagnosis of IFG, IGT and diabetes.

	Fasting plasma glucose (mmol/L)[a]		2-h plasma glucose (mmol/L) following OGTT
IFG	6.1–7.0		N/A
IFG (isolated)	6.1–7.0	and	< 7.8
IGT (isolated)	< 6.1	and	7.8–11.0
IFG and IGT	6.1–6.9	and	7.8–11.0
Diabetes	> 7.0	or	> 11.1

IFG, impaired fasting glucose; IGT, impaired glucose tolerance; OGTT, oral glucose tolerance test.

aThe cut-off value of 6.1 mmol/L is currently advised by UK authorities (JBS-2, 2005). The American Diabetes Association (2003) recommends that this threshold should be reduced to 5.6 mmol/L. The next World Health Organization technical report on 'Definition, diagnosis and classification of diabetes mellitus and its complications' will hopefully clarify this.

Group, 2001). They are also at risk of developing diabetes. Patients are identified by having a fasting plasma glucose of > 6.1 mmol/L (but under 7 mmol/L) or a 2-hour post-OGTT of > 7.8 mmol/L (but < 11.1 mmol/L).

2 Patients with IFG do not seem to be at increased risk of cardiovascular events, but are at high risk of developing type 2 diabetes. Insulin resistance is common. This patient group is defined as having fasting plasma glucose over 6.1 mmol/L but less than 7 mmol/L. Such patients need an OGTT to exclude diabetes and, if negative, should be followed up with annual fasting blood glucose estimation.

Identification of patients with dysglycaemia is of major importance, as effective delivery of appropriate lifestyle intervention should reduce the number of patients with both diabetes and related cardiovascular complications. Most patients with dysglycaemia are overweight, and the rise in the incidence of type 2 diabetes in the young is largely due to increasing obesity (World Health Organization, 1999). Worldwide, the number of adults with diabetes is predicted to increase to 300 million by 2025 (King et al, 1998). As weight reduction improves glucose tolerance, hyperglycaemia remains one of the strongest modifiable risk factors for CVD.

Three major randomised controlled trials have shown that that effective lifestyle intervention, with increased physical activity and weight loss, can prevent or delay the progression to type 2 diabetes in patients with prediabetes (Pan et al, 1997; Tuomilehto et al, 2001; Diabetes Prevention Program

Research Group, 2005). Intensive lifestyle intervention also reduces blood pressure, increases HDL cholesterol levels and lowers triglyceride levels.

Patients with established diabetes

Around 3–4% of the adult population in England is known to have diabetes, but numbers are increasing, and not all diabetes is diagnosed. The Health Survey for England (2004) estimates that 3% of men and 0.7% of women aged 35 years and over have undiagnosed diabetes. This means there are around 2.5 million adults in the UK with diabetes today, plus at least another half a million cases undiagnosed.

Type 2 diabetes is up to six times more common in people of South Asian decent, compared with the white UK population, and usually has an earlier onset. As such, it should no longer be regarded as 'maturity onset' diabetes. In some parts of the USA, it already accounts for one-third of newly diagnosed patients with diabetes under 20 years of age (Fagot-Campagna et al, 2000).

Patients with diabetes mellitus, particularly type 2 diabetes, are at a substantially increased risk of CHD, with the risk being perhaps two to four times greater in men and three to five times greater in women. Risk is particularly high if there is diabetic retinopathy, autonomic neuropathy, erectile dysfunction, microalbuminuria and proteinuria. The reason for the greater risk in women is not known, but it has been suggested that the excess risk of coronary death may be because they do not always receive standard treatment or attain therapeutic targets (Huxley et al, 2005).

Patients with type 1 diabetes are also at increased risk of CVD, although this may not declare itself until 20–30 years after diagnosis. In contrast, many patients with type 2 diabetes have obvious CVD at diagnosis, or may have already had a cardiovascular event.

Multifactorial intervention in diabetes

A multifactorial lifestyle and evidence-based polypharmacy approach has been suggested in the Steno-2 study (Gaede et al, 2003). Most people with diabetes will need aspirin, a statin and anti-hypertensive drugs because of the high preva-lence of cardiovascular co-morbidities.

- *Hypertension* (blood pressure > 140/90 mmHg) is twice as common in patients with diabetes as in those without, and may be present at diagno-sis in nearly 40% of patients. It is highly predic-tive of cardiovascular complications. Trials such as the United Kingdom Prospective Diabetes Study (UKPDS, 1998) and the HOT trial (Hansson et al, 1998) support reducing blood pressure in patients with diabetes to under 130/80 mmHg.
- *Dyslipidaemia* requires treatment in most patients with diabetes. The CARDS trial (Colhoun et al, 2004) showed that reducing cholesterol with atorvastatin in patients with type 2 diabetes and LDL-C concentrations under 4.14 mmol/L was associated with a reduction in cardiovascular events. Statin therapy is therefore recommended for all adults with diabetes (both type 1 and type 2) over the age of 40 years, regardless of the cholesterol level. It is also recommended in those aged 18–39 years who have other adverse risk factors such as microvascular complications (e.g. retinopathy, nephropathy), hypertension, hypercholesterolaemia (> 6.0 mmol/L), poor glycaemic control (HbA1c > 9%), a strong family history of CVD or the metabolic syndrome.
- *Aspirin* is recommended for all type 2 diabetics over 50 years, those with hypertension and those with microvascular disease. It is probably of value in all adults who have had diabetes for over 10 years.

Screening for dysglycaemia

All adults from 40 years onwards should have a random (non-fasting) blood glucose measured as part of an opportunistic CVD risk assessment (Fig. 3.6). If the random glucose is potentially abnormal (> 6.1 mmol/L) but not indicative of dia-betes (< 11.1 mmol/L), then a fasting blood glucose should be taken, followed by an OGTT if indicated.

Apparently healthy individuals with a 10-year CVD risk > 20% who have IFG or IGT should receive appropriate lifestyle and risk factor inter-vention, including the use of cardiovascular pro-tective drug therapies, to achieve the risk factor targets and therapy to obtain glycaemic control.

Obesity

Obesity occurs when a person's calorie intake repeatedly exceeds the amount of energy expended. This relationship may be influenced by genetic, social, cultural, psychological, environ-mental and economic factors.

Obesity is an independent risk factor for high blood pressure, raised blood cholesterol, diabetes and impaired glucose regulation, and associates with CVD. Around a third of patients with CHD and ischaemic stroke, and almost 60% of hyperten-sive disease in developed countries, are due to increasing obesity (World Health Organization, 1998). Even if there are no other cardiovascular risk factors, individuals who are obese in middle age have a higher risk of hospitalisation and mortality from cardiovascular disease and diabetes than those who are normal weight (Yan et al, 2006).

The numbers of overweight and obese individ-uals are increasing rapidly. Obesity is progressive, taking years, and sometimes decades, to develop. The prevalence will therefore always lag behind any aetiological factors, virtually all of which are environmental. In England alone, adult obesity has increased by over 50% in the last decade.

Obesity is often familial, suggesting an element of individual susceptibility, but the excuse of 'low metabolism' or 'hormones' to explain why partic-ular individuals are unable to regulate energy balance has not been demonstrated. Endocrine disorders such as hypothyroidism and Cushing syndrome usually present with other symptoms.

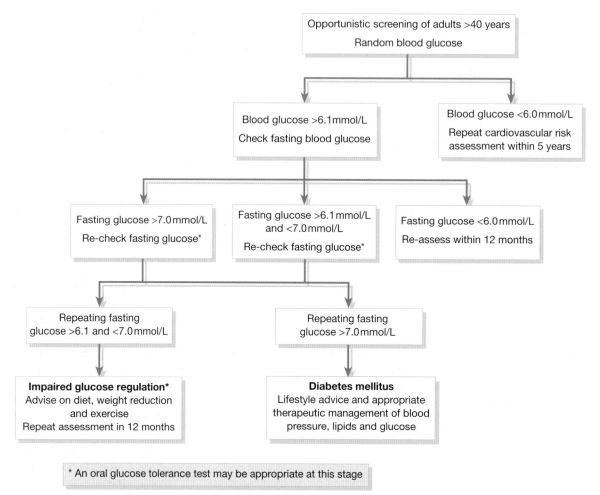

Figure 3.6 Assessing plasma blood glucose in asymptomatic people without CVD (adapted from JBS–2, 2005).

The rising trends in obesity indicate that the primary causes of the problem must lie in environmental or behavioural changes affecting large sections of the population, as the escalating rates of obesity are occurring in a relatively constant gene pool. Affluence, familial obesity due to role modelling and eating habits with the western sedentary lifestyle all contribute. Big serving bowls at home, supersized fast food and buckets rather than packets of popcorn at the cinema encourage overeating (Wansink & Cheney, 2005). It is also clear that obese people tend to provide biased diet records and habitually eat far more than they claim (Lichtman et al, 1992).

The diet in industrialised countries has changed dramatically since the nineteenth century when most dietary energy was derived from carbohydrate in cereals and potatoes. Over the past 50 years, fat consumption has increased markedly, mostly from increased ingestion of meat and dairy produce. In the 1940s, half as much energy was derived from fat as from carbohydrate, but now fat and carbohydrate provide the same amount.

Despite the drift towards high-fat diets, the British are consuming less energy than in the 1970s. Even after adjustments for meals eaten outside the home, and for consumption of alcohol, soft drinks and confectionery, average per capita energy intake seems to have declined by 20% since 1970. The paradox of increasing obesity in the face of decreasing food intake can only be explained if levels of energy expenditure have declined faster than energy intake. Thus, despite our diets being of lower energy value, we have reduced our energy expenditure even further, and the low levels of physical activity now prevalent in Britain play a dominant role in the development of obesity. Only 20% of men and 10% of women are employed in active occupations (Allied Dunbar National Fitness Survey, 1992), and motorised transport, mechanised equipment and energy-saving domestic appliances have displaced previously physically arduous tasks. Leisure pursuits are dominated by television viewing and other inactive pastimes, such as computer games. Central heating also reduces the need to expend energy for thermoregulation and probably encourages lethargy.

There are periods of life when weight gain seems more likely. For men, this is between the ages of 35 and 40 years, after marriage and after retirement. For women, the greatest increases in weight are between the ages of 15 and 19 years, after pregnancy and after the menopause. Asian and African populations are more prone to obesity, and particularly the accumulation of abdominal fat. Once weight has been gained, it is difficult to lose, and obese children are twice as likely to become obese adults.

Assessing obesity

A distinction should be made between 'average' weights and 'ideal' weights. Average weights are always higher in the west, where we overeat relative to energy expenditure. Ideal weights are based on the pooled experience of life assurance companies, who have calculated desirable weight, based on excess mortality figures. Subjective assessments of obesity, including the presence of central obesity, are often inaccurate, and the body mass index (BMI), which adjusts weight for height, has been widely adopted.

$$BMI = [weight\ (kg)/(height\ (m)^2]$$

Internationally accepted ranges of BMI used to define degrees of obesity in Caucasians are shown in Table 3.5.

The term *morbid obesity* is applied to people with a BMI of 40 or more, or a BMI of between 35 and 40 and other significant disease (e.g. diabetes, hypertension) that may be improved if they lose weight. In 1998, an estimated 0.6% of men and 1.9% of women in England and Wales had a BMI of over 40.

There is a progressive increase in the incidence of chronic diseases such as hypertension, diabetes and CHD with an increasing BMI (World Health Organization, 1998). Other risks of obesity are obstructive sleep apnoea, osteoarthritis of weight-bearing joints, accidental injury and a number of different cancers (e.g. breast, prostatic and colorectal). Respiratory symptoms, varicose veins, depression, hernias and gallstones are also more frequent. On average, life expectancy is decreased by 15% for every 10% excess of ideal body weight, and obesity must therefore be viewed as a serious medical condition rather than as a concern surrounding current fashion. Obesity is also associated with decreased quality of life. Those affected

Table 3.5 Internationally accepted ranges of BMI used to define degrees of obesity in Caucasians.

WHO classification (1998)	BMI (kg/m²)	Health risks[a]
Underweight	< 18.5	Low (but may indicate other health problems)
Normal	18.5–24.9	Average ('ideal' weight)
Overweight (pre-obese)	25.0–29.9	Mild increase
Obese	> 30.0	
Class I	30.0–34.9	Moderate
Class II	35.0–39.9	Severe
Class III	> 40.0	Very severe

a Risk of diabetes, hypertension and cardiovascular diseases.

often face prejudice and discrimination. Obesity has a negative impact on mobility, productiveness, employment and psychosocial functioning, with many obese people left feeling depressed, defensive and unable to live life to the full.

Using the BMI, the prevalence of obesity among adults in Britain has more than trebled in the last 20 years, and only 27.2% of men and 35.8% of women are at normal weight. The Heath Survey for England (2004) found that, between 1993 and 2004, the proportion of adults with a BMI > 30 (i.e. obese) had increased from 13.2% to 23.6% in men and from 16.4% to 23.8% in women. The UK has the second highest proportion of obese adults in the European Union (Greece has the most). Only 6.4% of Norwegian adults are obese.

The percentage of children in England aged 2–10 years with a BMI > 25 rose from 22.7% in 1995 to 27.7% in 2003, and obesity prevalence in children has been increasing faster in more recent years (Stamatakis et al, 2005). The combination of low birthweight coupled with excessive weight gain after 12 months of age is especially hazardous and may account for the increased rates of CHD and type 2 diabetes in people of South Asian origin. For this group, health risks start at a BMI of 23, with severe health risks associating with a BMI > 30 (Inoue & Zimmet, 2000).

Using other definitions of obesity

While the BMI provides a guide to obesity, it is a poor indicator of body fat in many individuals. It does not differentiate between muscle and fat mass; many athletes will have a BMI > 30 because of increased muscle bulk. There are also sex differences in body fat composition. Women have less visceral fat than men, but more fat in total (about 20% of body weight).

The cardiovascular risk associated with excess weight is particularly marked if the fat is concentrated mainly in the abdomen rather than on the hips and limbs, and people with central obesity are at over twice the risk of a heart attack compared with those without. The INTERHEART case–control study estimated that 63% of heart attacks in western Europe and 28% of heart attacks in central and eastern Europe were associated with abdominal obesity.

Around 33% of men and 30% of women in England have central obesity (Yusuf et al, 2004). An abdominal girth of over 94 cm (37 in) in men and over 80 cm (32 in) in women should alert the clinician that intervention is required. Levels of risk relating to abdominal circumference have been suggested by the World Health Organization (1998) (Table 3.6).

Correct measurement of waist circumference is between the lower border of the ribs and the iliac crest in a horizontal plane. The trouser waist size measurement is highly inaccurate, as most men wear the trousers with the waistband under the iliac spines or under a very large gut! Studies support the benefits of reducing waist circumference to improve metabolic parameters and cardiovascular risk (Wang et al, 2005).

Waist–hip ratio (WHR)

Measurement of hip circumference at the widest point over the buttocks in addition to measuring the waist allows the waist–hip ratio to be calculated. WHR is obtained by dividing the waist circumference by the hip circumference.

- Men with a WHR of 0.90–0.99 and women with a WHR of 0.80–0.84 are classified as overweight.
- Men with a WHR > 1.00 and women with a WHR > 0.85 are classified as obese.

A study of more than 27 000 people from diverse ethnic groups across the world showed that, of the common measures of obesity (BMI, waist circumference, WHR), WHR is the best for assessing coronary risk and BMI is the worst (Yusuf et al, 2005). Even at low BMI levels, an increased WHR increases risk, while those who have a high BMI but normal WHR are not at excess risk. Redefining obesity

Table 3.6 Levels of risk relating to abdominal circumference.

Men	Women	Risk
< 94 cm	< 80 cm	Low
94–102 cm	80–88 cm	Moderate
> 102 cm	> 88 cm	High

using WHR instead of BMI increases the estimate of myocardial infarction attributable to obesity in most ethnic groups, so the contribution that obesity makes to public health may be higher than currently quoted estimates (Merchant et al, 2006).

Central obesity and the metabolic syndrome

Abdominal obesity is associated with dyslipidaemia, hypertension, impaired glucose tolerance and CVD, all features of the metabolic syndrome. Visceral fat originates from brown fat that is metabolically very active, unlike subcutaneous fat that is a fat store for excess triglycerides. Visceral fat cells are smaller with more lipolytic activity and expose the liver to high concentrations of fatty acids. While brown fat provides a rapid access reservoir of fatty acids for energy, as abdominal adiposity increases, these fatty acids are released in such high concentrations that they swamp the liver and interfere with insulin release. As a result, blood glucose levels rise, with elevated triglyceride concentrations and reduced HDL-C levels. The metabolic syndrome (syndrome X or Reaven syndrome) links this clustering of cardiovascular risk factors that complicates central obesity. A large waist circumference is the main diagnostic clue. The International Diabetes Federation (IDF, 2005) have proposed that the diagnosis of the metabolic syndrome should be based on a waist measurement of > 94 cm in men or > 80 cm in women with any two features of:

- glucose intolerance (fasting blood glucose > 5.6 mmol/L);
- hypertension (> 130/85 mmHg);
- hypertriglyceridaemia (> 1.7 mmol/L);
- low HDL-C levels (< 1 mmol/L in men and < 1.3 mmol/L in women).

These are more stringent than previous definitions, but have been revised because associated insulin resistance may predate the development of diabetes by as much as 10 years. Patients with the metabolic syndrome, but free from CVD, are also five times more likely to develop a cardiovascular event than those without the syndrome (Bonora et al, 2004). Early management of obesity may prevent diabetes and CVD, and drugs that target the endocannabinoid system (e.g. rimonabant) may help to reduce the multiple risk factors that make up the syndrome (Finer & Pagotto, 2005).

Exercise

Lack of physical activity is a major underlying cause of death, disease and disability, and a sedentary lifestyle is associated with an increased risk of CVD (Thompson et al, 2003). Inactivity is one of the 10 leading global causes of death and disability, with over 2 million attributed deaths per year (World Health Organization, 2002). Physical activity levels are low in the UK, and 60% of men and 70% of women can be classed as sedentary. Whereas the manual worker in the past was protected from the adverse effects of a sedentary occupation, the advent of mechanical aids, including the car, conveyor belts, lifts and other devices, has minimised the amount of exercise taken, even by manual workers. Over the last 25 years, there has been a significant decrease in physical activity as part of daily routines, but there has been a small increase in the proportion of people taking physical activity for leisure in the UK. Physical activity declines rapidly with increasing age for both men and women, although for women this decline does not begin until the mid-forties.

Between 1975 and 2002, the average number of miles per year travelled by foot fell by around a quarter and by cycle by around a third. Over the same period, the average number of miles per year travelled by car increased by just under 70%.

The White Paper *Saving Lives: Our Healthier Nation* (Department of Health, 1999) emphasises the importance of physical activity as one of the key determinants of good health. Those who engage in vigorous sports and keep-fit exercises have half the incidence of fatal and non-fatal coronary events, compared with those who do not. This remains the case regardless of age or the presence of other risk factors. In addition, physical activity can prevent or delay the onset of hypertension, increases HDL-C concentration and lowers the risk of developing diabetes.

Numerous studies have demonstrated a reduced rate of initial CHD events in physically active people, and provide strong evidence that regular physical activity of at least moderate intensity reduces the risk of coronary events. An even greater impact is seen when the endurance exercise programme is of sufficient intensity and duration to improve aerobic capacity. Vigorous intensity exercise has been shown to increase aerobic fitness more effectively than moderate intensity exercise and may thus be more cardioprotective (Swain & Franklin, 2006). However, it is sedentary individuals becoming moderately active who gain the largest reduction in risk, with a more modest reduction in those who are already moderately active increasing to vigorous activity. Cardiovascular benefits are lost when physical activity is reduced.

The UK Department of Health recommends that adults should undertake at least 30 minutes of physical activity on five or more days of the week for general health benefits (Britton & McPherson, 2000). This can be achieved either by doing all the daily activity in one session or through several shorter bouts of activity of 10 min or more. The activity can be simple walking, structured exercise programmes, sport or a combination of these. As little as 30 minutes per week of strength training may reduce the risk of an initial coronary event (Tanasescu et al, 2002).

In April 2004, the Chief Medical Officer restated this recommendation in his report *At Least Five a Week* for the prevention of CHD, diabetes and obesity (Department of Health, 2004b). There has been a small increase in the overall proportion of adults meeting the recommended level of physical activity between 1997 and 2003, but over one-third still exercise for less than 30 minutes a week (Health Survey for England, 2004). The target proposed in 2004 by the Government's Strategy Unit – to increase the proportion of the adult population who participate in 30 minutes of moderate physical activity five or more times a week to 70% by 2020 – seems a forlorn hope.

Psychosocial well-being

The influence of personality factors on the incidence of CHD has become a subject of increasing interest (Hemingway et al, 2003). Four different types of psychosocial factors have been found to associate with an increased risk of CHD:

- stress – especially work related;
- anxiety and depression;
- lack of social support;
- personality – especially hostility.

Acute mental stress, anger or excitement can precipitate angina, and it is likely that recurrent episodes could lead to transient elevation of blood pressure, which provides the stimulus for plaque rupture and, hence, myocardial infarction, heart failure or sudden death. Psychosocial stressors such as pressure at work or at home, financial stress and major life events (marriage, divorce, moving job or house) associate with an increased risk of acute myocardial infarction (Rosengren et al, 2004). Occupations that make very high demands on individuals, or in which they have little or no control, increase the risk of CHD and premature death (Department of Health, 1999). In contrast to the usually perceived image of a stressed individual being a young male executive working in the city, the effect of stress on the heart in the INTER-HEART study was shown to be independent of sex, social group, economic status or geographical location.

Among the personality traits long thought to be related to heart disease are hostility and so-called 'type A' behaviour. Type A characteristics include abrupt gestures, hurried speech, impatience, with overcommitment to vocation or profession and excessive drive. However, trial data do not support a connection. Furthermore, randomised trial data of psychosocial interventions for hostility, anxiety and depression following myocardial infarction have produced conflicting results in terms of improvements in mortality.

Diet

It is recognised that a diet that is high in fat, salt and free sugars, and low in complex carbohydrates, fruit and vegetables increases the risk of CVD (World Health Organization, 2002).

Poor diet plays a fundamental role in the development of CHD, and is a key modifiable risk factor. Eating adequate amounts of essential nutrients, coupled with energy intake in balance with energy expenditure, is vital to maintain health and to prevent or delay the development of CVD, stroke, hypertension and obesity.

Individual foods as well as foods within the same food group vary in their nutrient content. No one food contains all the known essential nutrients, and eating a variety of foods helps to ensure that all nutritional needs are met. Portion number and size should be monitored to ensure adequate nutrient intake without exceeding energy needs. Excessive food intake, especially of energy-dense foods high in saturated fat and sugar, should be avoided. Vitamin and mineral supplements are not a substitute for a balanced and nutritious diet.

In 1992, *The Health of the Nation* initiative set targets for reductions in the incidence of CHD and stroke. This was the first time since the Second World War that there had been an explicit nutrition policy in the UK, and it signalled a shift to a greater emphasis on disease prevention and health promotion. The nutrition targets were:

- to reduce intake of total fat to no more than 35% of food energy;
- to reduce intake of saturated fatty acids to no more than 11% of food energy;
- to reduce the number of obese adults to no more than 6% (men) and 8% (women);
- to reduce the proportion of men drinking more than 21 units of alcohol per week and women drinking more than 14 units of alcohol per week to 18% of men and 7% of women.

In 1994, the committee on medical aspects of food and nutrition policy (COMA) published a report on diet and CVD (Department of Health, 1994).

Recommendations for fats and other nutrients are shown in Table 3.7.

Cardiovascular health is strongly influenced not only by the quantity, but also by the quality of dietary fat, as well as the quantity of fruit, vegetables and salt consumed. Dietary advice should emphasise a varied diet, rich in vegetables, legumes, fruits, cereals and fish. This 'Mediterranean diet', with a modest intake of wine, may reduce mortality by 7% (EPIC, 2005).

Fat intake

Dietary fats and cholesterol play a major role in CHD development, mostly by their effect on plasma lipoprotein concentrations. The average British diet contains 37% of energy as total fat, and this has fallen slightly from around 41% in the last 25 years. This has largely been due to reductions in milk and butter intake, which have been replaced by 'low-fat' equivalents. The major dietary sources of fats are spreading fats (butter and margarine), cooking fats, meat and dairy produce. Much of the fat intake is hidden in foods such as cakes and biscuits. Offal (liver, kidney and pâté), shellfish and eggs all contain large amounts of cholesterol, although these foods only have a small effect on serum cholesterol concentrations.

Table 3.7   Recommendations from the COMA report on diet and cardiovascular disease (Department of Health, 1994).

Food type	Total recommended intake
Total fat	Less than 35% (saturated fats < 11%, but more monounsaturated and polyunsaturated fats)
Carbohydrate	Over 50% (mostly complex carbohydrates and sugar in fruit and vegetables)
Protein	10–20%
Fibre	Over 35 mg/day
Cholesterol	Under 300 mg/day
At least five portions of fruit and vegetables per day	
Less salt (under 6 g/day)	
More potassium (over 3.5 g/day)	
Less alcohol (under 21 units for men, and under 14 units for women per week)	

The two main categories of fat in the diet are saturated fats (which tend to raise serum cholesterol levels) and unsaturated fats (which tend to lower blood cholesterol). The intake of saturated fats has fallen quite markedly since the 1980s from nearly 20% to just under 15% of total energy intake. Simple low-fat diets do not significantly reduce serum cholesterol unless combined with an increase in polyunsaturated fats (Oliver, 1996), so total fat intake should be reduced to less than 35% of the total food energy intake, with two-thirds of this as vegetable fat. Not all vegetable fats are acceptable; palm and coconut oil, for example, are high in saturated fat, and olive oil (a monounsaturated fat) is a better source of vegetable fat. Unlike polyunsaturated fat, olive oil does not reduce HDL-C levels, which may explain the negative correlation between olive oil consumption and coronary deaths.

Fish oils have notable antithrombotic activity, and high intake reduces blood fibrinogen levels, as well as blood pressure, and eating oily fish has therefore been emphasised in cardioprotective diets. Omega-3 fatty acids are essential fatty acids that cannot be manufactured by the body and must be obtained from food. The omega-3 essential fatty acids in oily fish are called eicosapentaenoic acid (EPA) and docosahexaenoic acid (DHA).

The richest sources of EPA and DHA are in cold-water fish such as salmon, sardines, mackerel, herring, trout and pilchards. Wild fish are superior to those from fish farms, because commercial fish foods contain less vitamin A and C and less of the omega-3 fatty acids than ocean foods. Fresh fish is also superior in omega-3 fat content to frozen or canned varieties.

In the Diet And Re-infarction Trial (DART) of 2033 men recovering from myocardial infarction, advice on eating oily fish on a daily basis reduced all-cause mortality by 29% in the first 2 years, compared with those who were not advised (Burr et al, 1989). Interestingly, there was no significant effect on serum cholesterol in those eating oily fish. Regular consumption of fish and marine foods is recommended to provide over 200 mg daily of essential fatty acids (World Health Organization, 2002).

The 'Mediterranean' type of diet is also rich in omega-3 fatty acids and has these characteristics:

- high in fruits, vegetables, bread and other cereals, potatoes, beans and nuts;
- dairy products, fish and poultry consumed in low to moderate amounts, little red meat;
- includes regular olive oil as a source of monounsaturated fat;
- eggs consumed less than four times weekly;
- wine consumed in low to moderate amounts.

In the Lyon trial (de Lorgeril et al, 1994), there was a 70% reduction in cardiac events in post-infarct patients adopting such a diet, independent of changes in cholesterol concentrations. This suggests that the beneficial effects of omega-3 fatty acids are possibly due to a direct antithrombotic effect, rather than mediated through changes in serum cholesterol. Omega-3 fats provide little if any benefit if there are excessive dietary omega-6 fats, because they compete for the same rate-limiting enzymes. A high ratio of omega-6 to omega-3 fat is implicated in many chronic diseases, including atherosclerosis, arthritis and cancer (Simopoulus & Cleland, 2003). Omega-6 and omega-3 essential fatty acids (also known as polyunsaturated fatty acids or PUFAs) are best consumed in a ratio of about 3:1. Most western diets range between 10 and 20 to 1 in favour of omega-6, mostly as a result of the large amounts of plant oils used for cooking or in prepared foods.

For primary prevention, adults should eat a variety of (preferably oily) fish at least twice a week, and include oils and foods rich in alpha-linolenic acid (flaxseed, canola and soybean oils, walnuts), which are converted to omega-3 essential fatty acids.

Fruit and vegetables

Eating at least five 100-g portions of a variety of fruit and vegetables a day could lead to an estimated reduction of up to 20% in overall deaths from chronic diseases, such as heart disease, stroke and cancer. An adequate intake of potassium from fruit and vegetables (> 90 mmol) will also benefit the blood pressure (Whelton et al, 1997). Each increase of one portion of fruit and vegetables per day lowers the risk of CHD by 4% and the risk of stroke by 6%.

The average consumption of fruit and vegetables among adults in England is less than 300 g a day and, while more fruit is being eaten, fresh vegetable consumption is declining. Only 13% of men and 15% of women consume five or more portions of fruit and vegetables a day (Department for Environment, Food and Rural Affairs, 2002).

There are wide differences in fruit and vegetable consumption between social classes, with those in lower social class groups consuming about 50% less than those in professional groups. Children's consumption of fruit and vegetables is particularly low. One in five children aged 4–18 years eat no fruit at all.

There is also considerable variation in eating habits by ethnic group. Bangladeshi adults have the lowest levels of fruit consumption, with only 15% of men and 16% of women consuming fruit six or more times a week. The lowest levels of vegetable consumption are in the Pakistani community, with just 7% of men and 11% of women eating vegetables on six or more days a week.

Salt intake

Salt intake is directly correlated with mean blood pressure across all populations, and limiting salt consumption will reduce blood pressure (Elliott et al, 1996). Three-quarters of consumed salt is hidden in processed food, and this makes if very difficult for individuals to influence their intake. Public health attempts to influence the amount of salt in food have been directed at the food industry, but there is continued resistance to changing the contents of their foods (DeCrane, 2004). Common salt is the main source of flavour in processed foods, and low-salt foods are often unappetising and do not sell so well. It is argued that improving flavour by adding more natural ingredients (such as fruit and vegetables) would be too expensive.

The average salt consumption at the population level is too high (9.5 g/day in the UK), and may be as much as 60 g daily in some western populations. A reduction to no more than 6 g/day (100 mmol of sodium) is desirable and not harmful, even in the very hot summer months. Sodium homeostasis will regulate sodium excretion in sweat and urine to maintain physiological amounts. Only 15% of men and 31% of women in the UK consume < 6 g of salt per day.

Alcohol

There is an inverse or 'U-shaped' relationship between alcohol intake and the risk of CHD (Rimm et al, 1996). A consistent beneficial effect on mortality has been observed for consumption of 1–3 units of alcohol per day (one unit equates to about 80 mL of wine, 250 mL of normal strength beer and 30–50 mL of spirits), largely due to fewer heart attacks (Thun et al, 1997). Moderate drinking of alcohol, particularly of wine, is associated with a 20% reduction in coronary events, which is lower than in those who do not drink alcohol (Department of Health, 1995). Optimum consumption of alcohol is less for women.

Alcohol may exert benefits by raising HDL-C levels, inhibiting platelets and ameliorating stress, but these potential health benefits must be evaluated against the adverse effects of too much alcohol, which include cardiomyopathy, hypertension, haemorrhagic stroke, cardiac dysrhythmias and sudden death. The World Health Organization (2004) has estimated that 2% of CHD and 5% of stroke in men in developed countries is caused by excess alcohol and that, overall, alcohol contributes to 9% of all disease burden. Most of these adverse effects are associated with long-term alcohol consumption of over three drinks per day, which fits with the current guidelines that men should not drink more than 21 units a week and women no more than 14 units a week.

From the late 1950s, alcohol consumption has been steadily increasing, and intake has virtually doubled over the last 50 years. Overall, 27% of men and 17% of women in the UK consume more alcohol than the weekly recommended limits and, while this has remained a stable over the last few years in men, the numbers have more than doubled in women. Binge drinking has also become more common, and is associated with a higher risk of sudden death and stroke, possibly due to an acute hypertensive effect. The relation between blood pressure and alcohol intake is virtually linear beyond 2–3 units/day. Binge drinking (> 6 units in one session) is particularly common in the 16- to 24-year age group with 32% of young men and 24% of young women binge drinking at least once a week.

Adults from all minority ethnic groups in the UK, with the exception of the Irish, are less likely to drink alcohol than the general population. Levels of alcohol consumption in the UK are below the average in the European Union but, while levels are declining in other European countries, this has not been seen in the UK.

'Emerging' risk factors

Despite the power of current knowledge to explain the occurrence of CVD in populations, the search for new risk factors, often termed 'emerging' risk factors, continues. These include thrombotic factors (such as Lpa, fibrinogen), serum homocysteine levels, infectious agents (e.g. chlamydia), prenatal factors (low birthweight), genetic influences and estrogen deficiency. None of these factors will add substantially to CVD risk prediction above that of the major classical risk factors. Individuals who do not smoke, whose diet is good and who remain physically active (primarily reflected by favourable lipid concentrations, low BMI and low blood pressure) rarely develop CVD (Beaglehole & Magnus 2002). Routine assessment of these emerging risk factors is usually unhelpful, and is not presently indicated outside the sphere of research.

References

Aarabi M, Jackson PR (2005) Predicting coronary risk in UK South Asians: an adjustment method for Framingham-based tools. *European Journal of Cardiovascular Prevention and Rehabilitation* 12: 46–51.

Allender S, Peto V, Scarborough P et al (2006) *Coronary Heart Disease Statistics*. London: British Heart Foundation. Statistics database: www.heartstats.org.

Allied Dunbar National Fitness Survey (1992) *A Report on Activity Patterns and Fitness Levels*. London: Sports Council and Health Education Authority.

American Diabetes Association (2002) The prevention or delay of type 2 diabetes. *Diabetes Care* 25: 742–749.

American Diabetes Association (2003) Follow-up report on the diagnosis of diabetes mellitus. *Diabetes Care* 26: 3160–3167.

de Backer G, Ambrosioni E, Borch-Johnsen K et al (2003) Third Joint Task Force of European and Other Societies on Cardiovascular Disease Prevention in Clinical Practice. European guidelines on cardiovascular disease prevention in clinical practice. *European Heart Journal* 24: 1601–1610.

Beaglehole R, Magnus P (2002) The search for new risk factors for coronary heart disease: occupational therapy for epidemiologists? *International Journal of Epidemiology* 31: 1117–1122.

Bhopal R (2000) What is the risk of coronary heart disease in South Asians? A review of UK research. *Journal of Public Health Medicine* 22: 375–385.

Bhopal R, Fischbacher C, Vartiainen E et al (2005) Predicted and observed cardiovascular disease in South Asians: application of FINRISK, Framingham and SCORE models to Newcastle Heart Project data. *Journal of Public Health Medicine* 27: 93–100.

Blood Pressure Lowering Treatment Trialists' Collaboration (2003) Effects of different blood-pressure-lowering regimens on major cardiovascular events: results of prospectively designed overviews of randomised trials. *Lancet* 362: 1527–1545.

Bonora E, Targher G, Formentini G et al (2004) The metabolic syndrome is an independent predictor of cardiovascular disease in type 2 diabetic subjects. Prospective data from the Verona Diabetes Complications study. *Diabetic Medicine* 21: 52–58.

Britton A, McPherson K (2000) *Monitoring the Progress of the 2010 Target for Coronary Heart Disease Mortality: Estimated Consequences on CHD Incidence and Mortality from changing Prevalence of Risk Factors*. London: National Heart Forum.

Broeckel U, Hengstenberg C, Mayer B et al (2002) A comprehensive linkage analysis for myocardial infarction and its related risk factors. *Nature Genetics* 30: 210–214.

Brugada R, Wenger NK, Jacobson TA et al (1996) Changes in plasma cholesterol levels after hospitalization for acute coronary events. *Cardiology* 87: 194–199.

Burr ML, Fehily AM, Holliday RM et al (1989) Effects of changes in fat, fish and fibre intakes on death and myocardial re-infarction: diet and re-infarction trial (DART) *Lancet* 343: 1454–1459.

Chapman S, Borland R, Scollo M et al (1999) The impact of smoke free workplaces on declining cigarette consumption in Australia and the United States. *American Journal of Public Health* 89: 1018–1022.

Colhoun HM, Betteridge DJ, Durrington PN for the CARDS investigators (2004) Primary prevention of cardiovascular disease with atorvastatin in type 2 diabetes in the Collaborative Atorvastatin Diabetes Study (CARDS): multicentre randomised placebo-controlled trial. *Lancet* 364: 685–696.

Conroy RM, Pyorala K, Fitzgerald AP et al (2003) Estimation of 10-year risk of fatal cardiovascular disease in Europe: the SCORE project. *European Heart Journal* 24: 987–1003.

Coutinho M, Gerstein HC, Wang Y et al (1999) The relationship between glucose and incident cardiovascular events. A meta-regression analysis of published data from 20 studies of 95 783 individuals followed for 12.4 years. *Diabetes Care* 22: 233–240.

DECODE Study Group (2001) Glucose tolerance and cardiovascular mortality: comparison of fasting and 2-hour diagnostic criteria. *Archives of Internal Medicine* 161: 397–405.

DeCrane SK (2004) Have we underestimated the effects of sodium excess on the health of the public? *Policy Politics and Nursing Practice* 5: 25–33.

Department for Environment, Food and Rural Affairs (2002) *The National Food Survey Annual Report on Food Expenditure, Consumption and Nutrient Intakes*. London: The Stationery Office.

Department of Health (1994) *Nutritional Aspects of Cardiovascular Disease*. Report of the Cardiovascular Review Group of the Committee on Medical Aspects of Food Policy. Report on Health and Social Subjects 46. London: The Stationery Office.

Department of Health (1995) *Sensible Drinking*. The report of an Inter-Departmental Working Group. London: The Stationery Office.

Department of Health (1999) *Saving Lives: Our Healthier Nation*. London: The Stationery Office.

Department of Health (2004a) *Choosing Health: Making Healthy Choices Easier*. London: The Stationery Office.

Department of Health (2004b) *At Least Five a Week: Evidence on the Impact of Physical Activity and its Relationship to Health*. London: The Stationery Office.

Diabetes Prevention Program Research Group (2005) Impact of intensive lifestyle and metformin therapy on cardiovascular disease risk factors in the Diabetes Prevention Program. *Diabetes Care* 28: 888–894.

Doll R, Peto R, Boreham J et al (2004) Mortality in relation to smoking: 50 years' observations on male British doctors. *British Medical Journal* 328: 1519–1527.

Downs JR, Clearfield M, Weis S et al (1998) Primary prevention of acute coronary events with lovastatin in men and women with average cholesterol levels: results of the AFCAPS/TexCAPS. Air Force/Texas coronary atherosclerosis prevention study. *Journal of the American Medical Association* 279: 1615–1622.

Elliott P, Stamler J, Nicholas R for the INTERSALT Cooperative research Group (1996) Intersalt revisited: further analysis of 24hr sodium excretion and blood pressure within and between populations. *British Medical Journal* 312: 1249–1255.

EPIC (2005) Elderly prospective cohort study Modified Mediterranean diet and survival. *British Medical Journal* 330: 991–995.

Erhardt L, Hobbs FD (2002) Public perceptions of cardiovascular risk in five European countries: the react survey. *International Journal of Clinical Practice* 56: 638–644.

Ezzati M, Lopez AD, Rodgers A et al (2002) Selected major risk factors and global and regional burden of disease. *Lancet* 360: 1347–1360.

Fagot-Campagna A, Petit DJ, Engelgan MM et al (2000) Type 2 diabetes among North American children and adolescents: an epidemiological review and a public health perspective. *Journal of Pediatrics* 136: 664–672.

Finer N, Pagotto U (2005) The endocannabinoid system: a new therapeutic target for cardiovascular risk factor management. *British Journal of Diabetes and Vascular Disease* 5: 121–124.

Gaede P, Vedel P, Larsen N et al (2003) Multifactorial intervention and cardiovascular disease in people with type 2 diabetes. *New England Journal of Medicine* 348: 383–393.

Gerstein HC, Yusuf S (1996) Dysglycaemia and the risk of cardiovascular disease. *Lancet* 347: 949–950.

Grundy SM (1999) Primary prevention of coronary heart disease: integrating risk assessment with intervention. *Circulation* 100: 988–998

Gueyffier F, Bulpitt C, Boissel JP et al (1999) Antihypertensive drugs in very old people: a subgroup meta-analysis of randomised controlled trials. *Lancet* 353: 793–796.

Hansson L, Zanchetti A, Carruthers SG et al (1998) Effects of intensive blood pressure lowering and low-dose aspirin in patients with hypertension: principal results of the hypertension optimal (HOT) randomised trial. *Lancet* 351: 1755–1762.

Harjai KJ (1999) Potential new cardiovascular risk factors: left ventricular hypertrophy, homocysteine, lipoprotein (a), triglycerides, oxidative stress and fibrinogen. *Annals of Internal Medicine* 131: 376–386.

Health Survey for England (2004) www.ic.nhs.uk/pubs/hlthsvyeng2004upd.

Heart Protection Study Collaborative Group (2002) MRC/BHF Heart Protection Study of cholesterol lowering with simvastatin in 20 536 high-risk individuals: a randomised placebo controlled trial. *Lancet* 360: 7–22.

Hemingway H, Kuper H, Marmot M (2003) Psychosocial factors in the primary and secondary prevention of coronary heart disease: an updated systematic review of prospective cohort studies. In: Yusuf S, Cairns JA, Fallen E et al (eds) *Evidence Based Cardiology*, Vol. 2. London: British Medical Journal Publishing.

Houston TK, Person SD, Pletcher MJ et al (2006) Active and passive smoking and development of glucose intolerance among young adults in a prospective cohort: CARDIA study. *British Medical Journal* 332: 1064–1069.

Hulley SB, Grady D, Bush T et al (1998) Randomised trial of estrogen plus progestin for secondary prevention of coronary heart disease in post-menopausal women. *Journal of the American Medical Association* 280: 605–613.

Humphries SE, Kessling AM, Horsthemke B et al (1985) A common DNA polymorphism of the low-density lipoprotein receptor gene and its use in diagnosis. *Lancet* 1: 1003–1005.

Huxley R, Barzi F, Woodward M (2005) Excess risk of fatal coronary heart disease associated with diabetes in men and women: meta-analysis of 37 prospective cohort studies. *British Medical Journal* 332: 73–76.

IDF (2005) Consensus worldwide definition of the metabolic syndrome. www.idf.org/webdata/docs/DF_Metasyndrome_definition.pdf.

Inoue S, Zimmet P (2000) *The Asia-Pacific Perspective: Redefining Obesity and its Treatment*. International Diabetes Institute Health Commission, Australia. http://www.diabetes.com.au/pdf/obesity_report.pdf.

Jamrozik K (2005) Estimate of deaths attributable to passive smoking among UK adults: database analysis. *British Medical Journal* 330: 812–815.

Jackson G, Kloner R, Kostis J (2006) The second Princeton consensus on sexual dysfunction and cardiac risk: new guidelines for sexual medicine. *Journal of Sexual Medicine* 3: 28–36.

Jackson R (1996) Models of absolute risk assessment. In: *The Lipid Guidelines*. National Heart Foundation, Australia. www.heartfoundation.com.au.

JBS-2 (2005) Joint British Societies' guidelines on prevention of cardiovascular disease in clinical practice. Prepared by: British Cardiac Society, British Hypertension Society, Diabetes UK, HEART UK, Primary Care Cardiovascular Society, The Stroke Association. *Heart* 91: 1–52.

Jowett NI (1984) *Recombinant DNA Gene-specific Probes and the Genetic Analysis of Diabetes, Hyperlipidaemia and Coronary Heart Disease*. London: University of London.

Jowett NI, Galton DJ (1987) The management of the hyperlipidaemias. In: Hamer J (ed.) *Drugs for Heart Disease*, 2nd edn. London: Chapman and Hall.

Jowett NI, Rees A, Caplin J et al (1984) DNA polymorphisms flanking the insulin gene and atherosclerosis. *Lancet* 2: 348.

Kannel WB, Wilson PW (1995) An update on coronary risk factors. *Medical Clinics of North America* 79: 951–971.

King H, Aubert RE, Herman WH (1998) Global burden of diabetes, 1995–2025: prevalence, numerical estimates and projections. *Diabetes Care* 21: 1414–1431.

Law MR, Wald NJ, Wu T et al (1994) Systematic underestimation of association between serum cholesterol and ischaemic heart disease in observational studies: data from the BUPA study. *British Medical Journal* 308: 363–366.

Law MR, Morris JK, Wald N (1997) Environmental tobacco smoke exposure and ischaemic heart disease: an evaluation of the evidence. *British Medical Journal* 315: 937–980.

Lichtman SW, Pisarska K, Berman ER et al (1992) Discrepancy between self-reported and actual caloric intake and exercise in obese subjects. *New England Journal of Medicine* 327: 1893–1898.

de Lorgeril M, Renaud S, Mamelle N et al (1994) Mediterranean alpha-linoleic acid-rich diet in the secondary prevention of coronary heart disease. *Lancet* 343: 1454.

Marks D, Wonderling D, Thorogood M et al (2002) Cost effective analysis of different approaches to screening for familial hypercholesterolaemia. *British Medical Journal* 324: 1303–1308.

Merchant A, Yusuf S, Sharma AM (2006) A cardiologist's guide to waist management. *Heart* 92: 865–866.

Murabito JM, Pencina MJ, Nam BH et al (2005) Sibling cardiovascular disease as a risk factor for cardiovascular disease in middle-aged adults. *Journal of the American Medical Association* 294: 3117–3123.

Naidoo B, Warm D, Quigley R et al (2004) *Smoking and Public Health: A Review of Reviews of Interventions to Increase Smoking Cessation, Reduce Smoking Initiation and Prevent Further Uptake of Smoking*. London: Health Development Agency.

NICE (2006) *Management of Hypertension in Adults in Primary Care*. Clinical guideline 34. London: NICE. www.nice.org.uk.

Oliver MF (1996) Which changes in diet prevent coronary heart disease? *Acta Cardiologica* 51: 467.

Pan XR, Li GW, Hu YH et al (1997) Effects of diet and exercise in preventing NIDDM in people with impaired glucose tolerance: the Da Qing IGT and diabetes study. *Diabetes Care* 20: 537–544.

Prescott E, Hippe M, Schnohr P et al (1998) Smoking and risk of myocardial infarction in women and men: longitudinal population study. *British Medical Journal* 316: 1043–1047.

Primatesta P, Brookes M, Poulter NR (2001) Improved hypertension management and control: results from the Health Survey of England, 1998. *Hypertension* 38: 827–832.

Rees A, Stocks J, Williams LG et al (1985) DNA polymorphism in the apolipoprotein C-III and insulin genes and atherosclerosis. *Atherosclerosis* 58: 269–275.

Rimm EB, Klatsky A, Grobbee D et al (1996) Review of moderate alcohol consumption and reduced risk of coronary heart disease: is the effect due to beer, wine or spirits? *British Medical Journal* 312: 731–736.

Rose G, Shipley MJ (1980) Plasma lipids and mortality: a source of error. *Lancet* i: 523–526.

Rosengren A, Hawken S, Ôunpuu S (2004) Association of psychosocial risk factors with risk of acute myocardial infarction in 11 119 cases and 13 648 controls from 52 countries (the INTERHEART study): case–control study. *Lancet* 364: 953–962.

Scientific Committee on Tobacco and Health (1998) *Report of the Scientific Committee on Tobacco and Health*. www.archive.officialdocuments.co.uk/document/doh/tobacco/contents.htm.

Simon Broome Register Group (1999) Mortality in treated heterozygous familial hypercholesterolaemia: implications for clinical management. *Atherosclerosis* 142: 105–112.

Simopoulus AP, Cleland LG (2003) Omega-6/omega-3 essential fatty acid ratio: the scientific evidence. *World Review of Nutrition and Dietetics* 92: 1–174.

Smith SC Jr, Jackson R, Pearson T et al (2004) Principles for national and regional guidelines on cardiovascular disease prevention. A scientific statement from the World Heart and Stroke Forum. *Circulation* 109: 3112–3121.

Sniderman AD, Furberg CD, Keech A et al (2003) Apolipoproteins versus lipids as indices of coronary risk and as targets for statin treatment. *Lancet* 361: 777–780.

Solomon H, Man JW, Wierzbicki AS et al (2003) Relation of erectile dysfunction to angiographic coronary artery disease. *American Journal of Cardiology* 91: 230–231.

Stamatakis E, Primatesta P, Chinn S et al (2005) Overweight and obesity trends from 1974 to 2003 in English children: what is the role of socioeconomic factors? *Archives of Disease in Childhood* 90: 999–1004.

Swain DP, Franklin BA (2006) Comparison of cardioprotective benefits of vigorous versus moderate intensity aerobic exercise. *American Journal of Cardiology* 97: 141–147.

Tanasescu M, Leitzmann MF, Rimm EB et al (2002) Exercise type and intensity in relation to coronary heart disease in men. *Journal of the American Medical Association* 288: 1994–2000.

Thompson IM, Tangen CM, Goodman PJ et al (2005) Erectile dysfunction and subsequent cardiovascular disease. *Journal of the American Medical Association* 294: 2996–3002.

Thompson PD, Buchner D, Pina IL (2003) Exercise and physical activity in the prevention and treatment of atherosclerotic cardiovascular disease. A statement from the Council on Clinical Cardiology (subcommittee on exercise, rehabilitation and prevention) and the Council on Nutrition, Physical Activity and Metabolism (subcommittee on physical activity) *Circulation* 107: 3109–3116.

Thun MJ, Peto R, Lopez AD et al (1997) Alcohol consumption and mortality amongst middle aged and elderly US adults. *New England Journal of Medicine* 337: 1705–1714.

Tuomilehto J, Lindstorm J, Eriksson JG et al for the Finnish Diabetes Prevention Study Group (2001) Prevention of type 2 diabetes mellitus by changes in lifestyle among subjects with impaired glucose tolerance. *New England Journal of Medicine* 333: 1343–1350.

Twigg L, Moon G, Walker S (2004) *The Smoking Epidemic in England*. London: NICE. www.publichealth.nice.org.uk.

UKPDS (1998) The United Kingdom Prospective Diabetes Study Group 38. Tight blood pressure control and risk of macrovascular and microvascular complications in type 2 diabetes. *British Medical Journal* 317: 703–713.

Vegt F, Dekker JM, Jager A et al (2001) Relation of impaired fasting and postload glucose with incident type 2 diabetes in a Dutch population: the Hoorn study. *Journal of the American Medical Association* 285: 2109–2113

Wallace-Bell M (2003) The effects of passive smoking on adult and child health. *Professional Nurse* 19: 217–219.

Wang Y, Rimm EB, Stampfer MJ et al (2005) Comparison of abdominal adiposity and overall obesity in predicting risk of type 2 diabetes among men. *American Journal of Clinical Nutrition* 81: 555–563.

Wansink B, Cheney MM (2005) Super Bowls: serving bowl size and food consumption. *Journal of the American Medical Association* 293: 1727–1728.

Whelton PK, He J, Cutler JA et al (1997) Effects of oral potassium on blood pressure: meta-analysis of randomised controlled clinical trials. *Journal of the American Medical Association* 275: 1016–22.

Williams B, Poulter NR, Brown MY (2004) Guidelines for management of hypertension: report of the fourth working party of the British Hypertension Society, 2004 – BHS IV. *Journal of Human Hypertension* 18: 139–185.

Wolf-Maier K, Cooper RS, Banegas JR et al (2003) Hypertension prevalence and blood pressure levels in 6 European countries, Canada, and the United States. *Journal of the American Medical Association* 289: 2363–2369.

Wolf-Maier K, Cooper RS, Kramer H et al (2004) Hypertension treatment and control in five European countries, Canada, and the United States. *Hypertension* 43: 10–17.

World Health Organization (1998) *Obesity: Preventing and Managing the Global Epidemic*. Geneva: WHO.

World Health Organization (1999) *Expert Committee on Diabetes Mellitus: Diagnosis and Classification of Diabetes Mellitus and its Complications*. WHO Department of Non-communicable Disease Surveillance. Geneva: WHO.

World Health Organization (2002) *Reducing Risks, Promoting Healthy Life*. Geneva: WHO.

World Health Organization (2004) *Global Status Report on Alcohol*. Geneva: WHO.

Wylie G, Hungin APS, Neely J (2002) Impaired glucose tolerance: qualitative and quantitative study of general practitioner's knowledge and perceptions. *British Medical Journal* 324: 1190–1195.

Yan LL, Daviglus ML, Liu K et al (2006) Midlife body mass index and hospitalization and mortality in older age. *Journal of the American Medical Association* 295: 190–198.

Ye Z, Liu EHC, Higgins JPT et al (2006) Seven haemostatic gene polymorphisms in coronary disease: meta-analysis of 66,155 cases and 91,307 controls. *Lancet* 367: 651–658.

Yusuf S, Hawken S, Ôunpuu S on behalf of the INTER-HEART Study Investigators (2004) Effect of potentially modifiable risk factors associated with myocardial infarction in 52 countries (the INTERHEART study): case–control study. *Lancet* 364: 937–952.

Yusuf S, Hawken S, Ôunpuu S on behalf of the INTER-HEART Study Investigators (2005) Obesity and the risk of myocardial infarction in 27 000 participants from 52 countries: a case–control study *Lancet* 366: 1640–1649.

Chapter 4

Assessing patients with coronary heart disease

Initial contact with patients suspected of having coronary heart disease (CHD) may be in primary care, the cardiology clinic or following an acute admission to hospital. Patient assessment may be divided into:

- defining symptoms;
- demonstrating clinical signs;
- organising appropriate investigations.

The initial assessment usually gives significant clues to the diagnosis and, in patients presenting with acute chest pain, rapid triage is essential to ensure that those qualifying for reperfusion receive it as quickly as possible. Initial details of the presenting history need to be succinct, but can be supplemented later with information from the family, the referral letter or previous medical and nursing notes.

While coronary care units (CCUs) manage many cardiac problems other than acute coronary syndromes, admission data from our unit suggest that approximately one in five patients admitted to coronary care do not have a cardiological problem (Table 4.1). Paradoxically, the CCU may be a dangerous place for patients who do not have a cardiovascular disease (CVD). All too often it is assumed that ill patients attached to a cardiac monitor must have something wrong with their heart, and it is important to consider both alternative and concomitant diagnoses. So, for patients admitted directly to the CCU without triage, the immediate decision is whether or not the patient has a CVD illness.

SYMPTOMS OF CORONARY HEART DISEASE

Chest pain and breathlessness are two of the most common complaints that lead to a patient seeking medical advice. Patients suspected of having an acute coronary syndrome should be referred to hospital urgently, so that prognosis may be improved by early intensive care. Patients admitted to medical wards are often not considered soon enough for thrombolytic therapy, or for secondary interventions later on (Lawson-Matthew et al, 1994). Symptom evaluation is of utmost importance and, while the natural focus is on confirming an acute coronary syndrome, there may be other dangerous diagnoses, including aortic dissection, pulmonary embolism or pneumothorax.

Chest pain

The frequency with which non-cardiac pain appears on CCUs demonstrates how difficult it is to determine the origin of chest pain. Many people in the community suffer episodes of chest pain,

Table 4.1   Primary discharge diagnosis for all patients admitted to our coronary care unit in 1 year (Withybush General Hospital, 2005).

Cardiac (81%)	
Myocardial infarction (STEMI/NSTEMI)	35.0%
Dysrhythmias	24.6%
Left ventricular failure	8.8%
Unstable angina	5.8%
DC cardioversion	3.0%
Stable angina	2.1%
Other cardiac	1.0%
(e.g. post cardiac arrest, pericarditis)	
Non-cardiac (19%)	
Chest pain of uncertain origin	6.3%
Gastrointestinal causes	4.0%
Respiratory tract infection	4.0%
Syncope	1.0%
Cerebrovascular accident	1.0%
Anxiety/hyperventilation	0.6%
Aortic dissection	0.3%
Musculoskeletal	0.1%
Pulmonary embolus	0.1%
Others (carcinoma of lung, anaemia, gastrointestinal haemorrhage, constipation, diabetic ketosis, renal failure, hypothermia)	0.1%

STEMI, ST elevation myocardial infarction; NSTEMI, non-ST elevation myocardial infarction; DC, direct current.

Box 4.1   Some causes of chest pain.

Cardiovascular causes

Myocardial ischaemia
Coronary artery spasm
Myocardial infarction
Pericarditis
Dissecting aortic aneurysm
Pulmonary embolism
Mitral valve prolapse

Non-cardiac causes

Herpes zoster
Oesophageal reflux
Oesophageal spasm
Hiatus hernia
Pneumonia
Pneumothorax
Pleurisy
Peptic ulceration
Gallbladder disease
Musculoskeletal pain
Da Costa syndrome (cardioneurosis)

and the cause is usually benign. Such patients have a lower prevalence of cardiovascular risk factors, apart from smoking, and those who repeatedly attend the GP surgery often have a history of psychiatric problems such as anxiety, depression or alcohol abuse.

Chest pain can originate from most tissues in the chest (Box 4.1), and an accurate diagnosis is often difficult because the pain may be coming from more than one site. For example, many patients presenting with angina may also have gastro-oesophageal reflux or chest wall tenderness. Even those with CVD may present with atypical symptoms, particularly the elderly (Then et al, 2001). Obtaining the history may also be difficult if the patient is in pain, distressed or simply frightened. Although certain elements of the chest pain history are associated with an increased or decreased probability of coronary disease, none can be relied on alone or in combination to accurately identify cardiac patients (Swap & Nagurney, 2005). The severity of symptoms and the final outcome in patients with acute coronary syndromes are not directly related either. One helpful guide is clinical evidence of autonomic nervous system activation, which often accompanies acute cardiac conditions. Sweating and pallor (mostly in men) and nausea and vomiting (mostly in women) are important clues when present.

Myocardial ischaemia

New onset exertional angina is the most common presentation of CHD (Fox, 2005), but many people with significant coronary disease do not have angina, either because the atheroma is not causing significant obstruction or because gradual obstruction has been compensated for by a collateral circulation. Anginal symptoms are not always due to coronary disease either, and can occur in patients with anaemia, aortic or pulmonary valve stenosis, hypertrophic cardiomyopathy or pulmonary hypertension. Patients with diabetes often have atypical symptoms of myocardial ischaemia, and some people do not get chest pain at all (Airaksinen, 2001). About half the patients presenting with an acute coronary syndrome will have had a previous heart attack or suffer from angina, so the diagnosis is often made easier.

The discomfort of myocardial ischaemia is generally described as tightness, heaviness, pressure or constriction, rather than pain. The origin of the pain is probably the myocardium itself. Pain impulses travel via sympathetic fibres to the thoracic sympathetic ganglia and the nerve roots of T1–T5. For that reason, the pain is felt in the anterior chest wall and the ulnar aspect of the arms and hands. Even in atypical presentations, ischaemic pain rarely extends beyond the region bordered by the lower jaw and the epigastrium. Usually, the pain is felt in the central chest, with other common sites including the throat, jaw, back, epigastrium, left chest and arms. The location is never so sharply localised that it may be identified with a pointing finger. It is much more usual for patients to indicate the nature and location of the pain with a squeezed fist held over the sternum (Levine's sign) or the flat of both hands placed on either side of the upper chest (Edmonstone, 1995). Pain that is stabbing, pleuritic, positional or reproducible by palpation is unlikely to be cardiac. Ischaemic pain usually comes on gradually over a minute or two, lasts minutes rather than seconds or hours and is usually not affected by respiration or changes in position. It is typically precipitated by exercise, particularly after meals, or in the wind and cold, and is usually predictable. Associated symptoms include sweating, dyspnoea, nausea, vomiting, lightheadedness, weakness and malaise. Common precipitants include:

- exertion, particularly hills or stairs;
- cold, windy weather;
- anger and anxiety;
- heavy meals;
- exciting television ('Match of the Day' angina);
- vivid dreams;
- sexual intercourse.

Middle-aged people with longstanding partners engage in sex approximately twice a week, with intercourse lasting about 10–15 minutes. The energy demand varies between 2 and 6 metabolic equivalents (METs) depending upon enthusiasm, a level similar to climbing two flights of stairs. With a usual partner, sexual activity is usually pleasurable and stress free, but with a new partner, or an extramarital encounter, stress levels and energy expenditure are likely to be much higher.

Chest pain is a particularly common symptom in women, but nearly half do not have CHD. The clinical, investigative and prognostic features in men with chest pain are not necessarily applicable to women (Sullivan et al, 1994). Women presenting with acute myocardial infarction report pain more frequently in the back, neck and jaw.

The four-level Canadian Cardiovascular Society (CCS) classification (Campeau, 1976) is the most commonly used measure of angina severity, ranging from class I, denoting effort-induced chest pain, to class IV, denoting profound limitation in undertaking ordinary physical activities (Table 4.2). The higher the CCS class, the greater the number of diseased vessels and the worse the all-cause mortality (Hemingway et al, 2004).

- *Stable angina* refers to a predictable pattern of episodic pain (and sometimes breathlessness), usually exercise or stress related and relieved by rest. This usually associates with stable fixed coronary occlusions.

Table 4.2 The Canadian Cardiovascular Society (CCS) classification of angina.

CCS class	Description
I	No angina with normal physical activity. Angina with strenuous or prolonged activity
II	Slight limitation of ordinary activity, such as climbing stairs fast, emotional stress or walking in cold wind or after meals
III	Marked limitation of ordinary activity
IV	Angina with minimal physical activity. Occasional rest pain

- *Unstable angina* is much more serious, associating with myocardial infarction and sudden death (see Chapter 8).
- *Decubitus angina* describes chest pain that is induced by lying down or during sleep. It may be caused by increased wall stress produced by increased cardiac preload or by coronary spasm induced by dreaming.
- *Prinzmetal (or variant) angina* develops spontaneously and is associated with increased coronary arterial tone giving rise to vasospasm. Smokers appear to be at particular risk. Although originally described as coronary spasm at the site of an atheromatous stenosis, about 10% of patients have normal coronary angiograms.
- *Microvascular angina* (syndrome X) describes the triad of angina, a positive exercise stress test and angiographically normal epicardial coronary arteries. It has a benign course, but is frequently associated with debilitating symptoms, psychological problems and a poor quality of life (Asbury & Collins, 2005). The exact pathogenesis of the condition is not known, but may be due to microvascular dysfunction that is either idiopathic or secondary to hypertension, cardiomyopathy or valvular disease. It is more common in women.
- *Cocaine abuse* frequently causes angina, and occasionally myocardial infarction, even in the young. The aetiology is complex but appears to be the result of coronary artery vasoconstriction, intracoronary thrombosis and accelerated atherosclerosis (Benzaquen et al, 2001). Drug abuse is a frequently overlooked cause of chest pain, but should be considered in any young patient with minimal cardiovascular risk factors presenting with symptoms of myocardial ischaemia or heart failure.

'Silent' myocardial ischaemia

Silent myocardial ischaemia (SMI) describes anginal pain that appears late (or not at all) with exertion, even in the presence of ischaemic changes on the electrocardiogram (Stern & Tzivoni, 1974). The exact mechanism is not clear, but may include cardiac autonomic neuropathy (as in patients with diabetes), a high pain threshold (in patients who produce high levels of endorphins) or perhaps because the symptoms are not recognised by the patient as being related to the heart.

Two types of silent ischaemia have been described:

- Type 1 SMI occurs in patients who never experience anginal pain and probably have a defective warning system. The presence of asymptomatic ischaemia may be detected on exercise testing or Holter monitoring, and identifies a high-risk group of patients. Frequently, the presence of occlusive coronary disease may not be discovered until the patient has a myocardial infarction or dies.
- Type 2 SMI patients experience periods of both silent and symptomatic ischaemia. Asymptomatic episodes of ST segment depression may be found in about 50% of patients with stable angina during ambulatory monitoring, and seem to be more common in the morning.

Most patients with silent ischaemia have single vessel disease, particularly in the left anterior descending artery. If silent ischaemia occurs during sleep, advanced coronary disease is usually present. In general, the prognosis of coronary ischaemia is not determined by the presence or absence of anginal pain, but by the total ischaemic burden, taking into account the total number, duration and extent of ischaemic episodes over 24 hours, whether symptomatic or not (Lichtlen, 1996).

Painless heart attacks

During the 30-year follow-up of 5127 participants in the Framingham study, 708 myocardial infarctions were detected on routine biennial electrocardiograms (ECGs) rather than from the medical history (Kannel & Abbott, 1984). Of these unrecognised infarctions, almost half were truly 'silent'. The others caused symptoms that were not appreciated as being significant at the time. About a third had shortness of breath, a third had other cardiac symptoms, such as vague chest pains, sweating or presyncope, but a third had seemingly non-cardiac complaints. The proportion of all unrecognised infarcts was higher in women and in older men. Silent infarcts were uncommon in persons with known angina, suggesting most cases of silent myocardial infarction associate with type 1 silent myocardial ischaemia.

In the UK, a 3-month hospital audit found that a fifth of patients with myocardial infarction had presented without chest pain (Dorsch et al, 2001). Again, patients were older, female and, in this study, more likely to have a history of heart failure. They also had worse baseline haemodynamics and more severe left ventricular impairment than those who presented with chest pain. Because of the delayed diagnosis, they tended to receive suboptimal care. For example, only 39% spent time in a CCU, compared with 77% of patients who presented with chest pain. They were also less likely to be discharged on aspirin or a beta-blocker, were less likely to attend rehabilitation programmes and had fewer follow-up outpatient appointments. The mortality rates at 30 days were higher in this group, and the increased risk of death persisted for up to 2 years. Overall, presentation without chest pain associated with a 60% increase in mortality. Hence, painless myocardial infarction is more common than many of us realise, and these patients are at high risk of further serious adverse cardiac events (Wong & White, 2002).

Pericardial pain

Pain is the usual presenting feature of pericarditis. The visceral pericardium is insensitive, and the pain arises from the parietal pericardium. The pain is sharp, aching and usually made worse by lying back or swallowing. Diaphragmatic pericarditis associates with pain that radiates to the left shoulder (trapezius ridge) or the neck. The diagnosis is sometimes confirmed by the presence of a pericardial friction rub. Apart from following acute myocardial infarction, the most frequent cause of pericarditis is a viral infection. The patient is usually young and fit, and there is often a history of a recent flu-like illness. Other causes of pericarditis include connective tissue disorders (e.g. systemic lupus erythematosus, rheumatoid arthritis or sarcoidosis), tuberculosis and renal failure. The ECG classically shows widespread concave ST segment elevation, as well as PR segment depression, but may show T wave changes or even be normal.

Aortic dissection

The chest pain of aortic dissection is described as tearing, and classically radiates through to the back, particularly between the shoulder blades. The condition associates with shock and loss of peripheral pulses. In type A dissection, obstruction of the right coronary ostium may produce inferior or posterior myocardial infarction by dissection rather than by thrombosis. Dissection of the left coronary artery is rapidly fatal. A haemopericardium is common and may associate with pericardial pain or tamponade. The mixture of pains coming from these different tissues can make diagnosis difficult. A history of trauma, hypertension, a bicuspid aortic valve or a family history of Marfan syndrome or aortic dissection makes the diagnosis more likely, and the diagnosis of aortic dissection should always be considered prior to thrombolysis.

Pain from the lungs

Pleurisy is caused by inflammation or irritation of the parietal pleura, which is innervated by branches of the intercostal nerves and by the phrenic nerve over the diaphragm. The visceral pleura does not have pain fibres. Most lung disorders are localised on one side, so pleuritic pain is usually restricted to one side of the chest and characteristically relates to breathing. The pain may be variously described as sharp, dull, burning or simply a 'catch'. Coughing or sneezing may cause intense distress, and many patients adopt a body position that restricts movement of the affected region. An audible pleural rub helps to confirm the diagnosis.

Pulmonary embolism usually causes chest pain (60%), sometimes accompanied by dyspnoea and haemoptysis. Peripheral emboli associate with pleuritic pain, but larger central emboli may mimic myocardial infarction, presenting with shock and central chest pain. Symptoms of deep vein thrombosis may only be present in a quarter of cases.

A left-sided *pneumothorax* can be confused with myocardial pain, particularly if there is a tension pneumothorax when shock may be present.

Table 4.3 Site of chest pain and radiation in 200 consecutive medical patients with cardiac and oesophageal pain (Withybush General Hospital, 1991).

Radiation	Primary source of pain	
	Cardiac (%)	Oesophageal (%)
Chest	100	100
Left arm		
All	55	20
To elbow	60	25
Right arm		
All	33	4
To elbow	40	12
Throat/jaw	33	8
Epigastrium	7	35

Oesophageal pain

Oesophageal pain (heartburn) is a very common cause of chest discomfort in the general population but, because it is so frequent, a confident diagnosis does not rule out the presence of other pathologies, particularly myocardial ischaemia. Differentiating cardiac from oesophageal pain can be difficult, and both sources of pain may co-exist (Table 4.3). Oesophageal pain may be described as burning, gripping, boring or stabbing. The pain is usually in the anterior chest and tends to be felt mainly in the throat or epigastrium. Like cardiac pain, it may radiate to the arms, back or neck. Many patients have a long history of oesophageal reflux and heartburn. An association with eating, dysphagia or relief by antacids may be helpful clues.

Altered oesophageal motility (sometimes referred to as oesophageal spasm) may associate with gastro-oesophageal reflux and can produce severe and distressing substernal pain. It is responsive to sublingual glyceryl trinitrate (GTN). Mucosal (Mallory–Weiss) tears can occur after bouts of vomiting, as may oesophageal rupture. Both present with chest pain, and the latter with shock. Other gastrointestinal disorders, such as peptic ulceration and gallbladder disease, often cause difficulty with differential diagnosis. An upper gastrointestinal bleed may present with lower chest/epigastric pain and shock.

Musculoskeletal pain

The most common cause of chest wall pain is trauma, including fractures of the ribs, vertebral collapse and other muscular strains. The original injury may have been unrecognised or forgotten, or may relate to a bout of coughing or sneezing. Because the muscles and bones move during breathing, there may be a 'pleuritic' element to the resulting pain, but chest wall pain is more limited in its distribution and is nearly always associated with localised tenderness.

Bornholm's disease (intercostal myalgia) is chest pain associated with a flu-like illness in the younger patient. The onset may be sudden or insidious and is often severe. *Costochondral pain* (usually of the third/fourth costal cartilage) and *Tietze syndrome* (sternal costochondritis) are very common. Costochondritis associates with inflammation of the costochondral joints, but there may be swollen tender lumps palpable in patients with Tietze syndrome. The lumps may persist for years. *Texidor's twinge* (precordial catch) is a benign cause of acute recurrent chest pain at the cardiac apex in younger women (Miller & Texidor, 1959). The cause is unknown, but may relate to posture.

Skin

Herpes zoster often presents with pain or parasthesia a day or two before the rash appears. If this affects a thoracic nerve root, chest pain may be so severe that it may be indistinguishable from the pain of myocardial infarction.

Chest pain of unknown origin

This is a proper diagnosis, which may be applied to patients presenting with chest pain in whom myocardial ischaemia seems unlikely and no other cause can be found. The typical patient is a middle-aged male presenting with chronic, intermittent stabbing pain in the left breast, lasting for a few seconds, often radiating down the left arm. GTN has usually been tried and, although claimed to be useful, only works after 30 minutes. Most patients have multiple, normal tests, sometimes including coronary angiography carried out for purposes of reassurance. Unfortunately, a large number have psychological problems and are not reassured by normal investigation. About a half of sufferers remain on cardiac medication, most continue to experience pain, and 50% become unemployed (Chambers & Bass, 1998). Providing a diagnosis can be difficult, but addressing the patient's concerns may be more important than offering a precise medical label. Effective management of non-cardiac chest pain releases time and resources for those individuals who have CHD.

Dyspnoea

Dyspnoea means difficulty with breathing, and it is entirely subjective. Many patients who are obviously short of breath at rest will not complain of respiratory difficulties, yet others claim to be short of breath on exertion but are able to complete exercise stress tests with apparent ease. Breathlessness is usually due to a cardiorespiratory disorder, obesity, physical deconditioning or anaemia. Cardiologically, the main causes of breathlessness are:

- pulmonary oedema;
- dysrhythmias;
- low cardiac output states;
- angina.

Left ventricular failure is the classical cardiac cause of acute breathlessness, with pulmonary oedema causing increased lung rigidity and decreased oxygen transfer. Respiration will, therefore, require greater effort, which is not helped by oedematous narrowing of the larger airways. Dyspnoea may also be caused by a raised left atrial pressure alone, which causes pulmonary venous congestion with few physical signs. Venous congestion reduces vital capacity and stimulates pulmonary stretch receptors, which cause the shortness of breath.

Symptoms and exercise capacity have been used by the New York Heart Association Criteria Committee (NYHA, 1964) to classify patients with heart failure according to *functional* ability (not severity of the condition) (Table 4.4).

Orthopnoea is difficulty with breathing when lying flat. It is often an early symptom of left ventricular failure, but may not be volunteered by the patient who learns to sleep propped up with three

Table 4.4 New York Heart Association (NYHA) classification of patients with heart failure (NYHA, 1964).

NYHA I	Heart disease with no limitation on ordinary physical activity
NYHA II	Slight limitation. Ordinary physical activity produces symptoms (e.g. fatigue, palpitations, angina, dyspnoea)
NYHA III	Marked limitation. Unable to walk on the level without disability. Less than ordinary activity produces symptoms
NYHA IV	Dyspnoea at rest. Inability to carry out any physical activity

or four pillows. The increase in venous return in the recumbent patient reduces vital capacity and lung compliance. In patients with right ventricular failure, an enlarged liver and ascites may contribute to orthopnoea, by diaphragmatic splinting. Orthopnoea does not always indicate heart failure. Patients with chronic obstructive airways disease often complain of waking with dyspnoea and wheezing, which is due to the loss of the diaphragmatic component of their respiratory pattern, corrected by sitting up. Periods of sleep apnoea may also cause obese patients to wake with breathlessness.

Paroxysmal nocturnal dyspnoea (PND) may be viewed as a delayed form of orthopnoea, when breathlessness develops if the patient slides down the bed into a horizontal position. The increase in pulmonary congestion leads to dyspnoea, which is reversed by the patient sitting up or standing. Typically, the patient jumps out of bed to an open window, gasping for breath.

Patients with chronic heart failure do not usually have pulmonary oedema, and exertional breathlessness is caused by a mismatch between oxygen demand and delivery. It is tissue hypoxia and acidosis that produce the symptoms.

Cheyne–Stokes breathing was described independently by John Cheyne in 1818 and William Stokes in 1846. It describes a respiratory pattern that begins with a hardly perceptible respiratory effort that gradually increases in depth until very much exaggerated. The effort then dies away, until breathing ceases for a period of about 20–30 seconds.

The whole cycle is then repeated, each cycle lasting for between 1 and 3 minutes. The mechanism is complex, but essentially the pauses in respiration allow the levels of arterial carbon dioxide to rise, which stimulates the respiratory centre to set off a fresh cycle of breathing. Cheyne–Stokes breathing is common in the elderly, especially during sleep. It is also found in those with chronic chest disease or following a stroke. In cardiac patients, it is frequent in heart failure, and patients are often aware of breathlessness in the fast phase of respiration. Cheyne–Stokes breathing may also be associated with heart rhythm disturbances, such as junctional rhythms and heart block.

Syncope

Dizziness is a common and non-specific symptom, affecting about a third of patients over the age of 65 years. The cause is often multifactorial with a combination of drugs, CVD and impaired circulatory reflexes. In cardiac patients, it is important to define whether or not such episodes describe presyncope. Syncope is a transient loss of consciousness resulting from inadequate cerebral blood flow.

Cardiac syncope can reflect serious underlying disease, and associates with a high mortality. Exclusion of structural or conduction system disease is a priority.

Vasovagal attacks are the most common cause of syncope caused by a combination of vasodilatation and vagally induced bradycardia. Attacks may occur following prolonged standing or in response to emotion or pain.

Postural (orthostatic) hypotension describes presyncope on standing. This is more common in the elderly and often induced by drugs. The face is pale, the pupils are dilated, and the pulse and respiration are slow. Peripheral pulses are often impalpable, leading to the frequent diagnosis of cardiac arrest.

Carotid sinus syncope may result from stimulation of the carotid sinus, usually when the head is rotated, particularly if the patient's neckwear is too tight.

Micturition syncope typically occurs in older men with enlarged prostate glands who lose consciousness while voiding urine. This is either because straining reduces venous return and cardiac output (Valsalva manoeuvre) or because sudden decompression of an overfull bladder causes reflex vasodilatation. Elderly men should be encouraged to sit when emptying their bladder at night.

Exertion syncope is a characteristic feature of aortic stenosis, when the cardiac output through the narrow valve cannot meet the demands of increased activity. Similar obstructive lesions occur in pulmonary stenosis and hypertrophic obstructive cardiomyopathy (HOCM).

Rhythm-induced syncope may result from heart rates that are too slow or too fast to maintain cerebral blood flow. Paroxysmal tachycardias often lead to a marked fall in cardiac output, with resulting syncope. Stokes–Adams attacks may be missed as the ECG is usually normal between attacks. The usual underlying problem is complete heart block or sinus arrest. Attacks may terminate in a convulsion, leading to an erroneous diagnosis of epilepsy. However, in dysrhythmia-associated collapse, there is no aura, and recovery is prompt, often accompanied by flushing, as blood flows again through vessels dilated by hypoxia. The desire to sleep does not occur, and headache is not as common.

Oedema

Oedema is an abnormal accumulation of fluid in the interstitial tissues that is usually preceded by weight gain of 3–5 kg of extracellular fluid. It is a relatively late manifestation of heart failure. Normally, fluid is exuded into the tissues because arterial capillary pressure (30 mmHg) exceeds plasma oncotic pressure (25 mmHg). However, the fluid is forced back into circulation at the venous end of the capillaries because pressure here (12 mmHg) is exceeded by the oncotic pressure. If the venous pressure rises, as in heart failure, the resorption of fluid is impaired and oedema results (Fig. 4.1).

Oedema will preferentially collect in loose tissues, so the distribution of fluid is determined by both gravity and the degree of ambulation. In most patients, the legs and feet are affected but, in those who are confined to bed, the fluid accumulates over the sacrum. The oedema characteristically pits when pressure is applied (*pitting oedema*). Greater degrees of oedema will gradually affect the whole of the lower extremities, extending to the torso and eventually the face (*anasarca*). Unilateral or bilateral pleural effusions and abdomen (*ascites*) may occur in advanced heart failure.

Figure 4.1   Changing pressures within a capillary.

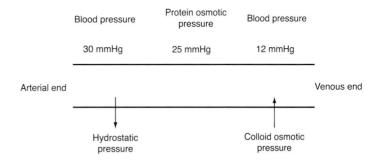

Haemoptysis

Coughing up blood is an unusual indicator of cardiac disease. When related to circulatory rather than lung pathology, the volume of blood is small, and the sputum is usually only streaked. Haemoptysis related to exercise might indicate mitral stenosis, with pulmonary veins rupturing under high pressure. Following thrombolysis, patients with left ventricular failure often cough up moderate amounts of fresh blood, but severe haemoptysis usually indicates important pulmonary disease such as bronchial carcinoma, tuberculosis or pulmonary infarction.

Palpitations

Palpitation is an awareness of the heartbeat, familiar to those awaiting examinations! However, it is used by patients to describe various sensations in the chest, only some of which have a cardiac basis. Most people are aware of their heartbeat at some time in their lives, especially at night when lying on the left side. Anxiety is a very common underlying cause, with unusual awareness of their own heartbeat, sometimes accompanied by 'flutters' or missed beats.

Palpitations are a very common referral to cardiology clinics (about 30% of referrals). In the vast majority, the symptoms are benign and are not associated with significant cardiac disease. Features that may indicate a more serious form of dysrhythmia include:

- the presence of pre-existing cardiovascular disease;
- a family history of syncope, dysrhythmia or sudden death;
- an association with falls and/or syncope.

Palpitations may be felt and described in many different ways. Some complain of a racing heart, others of thumping or feeling a missed beat, but the description does not always help with diagnosis. A thumping or pounding heart is the most common complaint and is usually the awareness of normal beats, sometimes exaggerated in strength and speed by sympathetic overactivity (e.g. stress and anxiety). This frequently occurs for prolonged periods and on a daily basis. Dropped beats are probably the next most common complaint, and these are more frequent if basic sinus rhythm is slow. Patients report that their heart keeps stopping.

Important points to establish include:

- precipitants including smoking, caffeine or alcohol consumption, bronchodilators and nasal decongestant sprays, slimming preparations and recreational drugs;
- the onset, duration and frequency of episodes;
- the effects of vagal manoeuvres, such as stooping, breath-holding, gagging;
- accompanying symptoms including dyspnoea, sweating, chest pain and polyuria.

Racing of the heart is usually abnormal if the pulse rate exceeds 130 beats/minute. The history may go back for many years if attacks are infrequent. Sustained palpitations that begin and end abruptly suggest an abnormal tachycardia. If the heart is giving irregular flutters, it is usually due to paroxysmal atrial fibrillation. Frequent ectopic beats may produce the same feeling, and both are common in the elderly. A slow heart rate may be due to sinus node disease or heart block.

Psychological problems

Patients with chronic cardiac disease are prone to anxiety and depression, with fear of death, recurrent hospital admission or becoming dependent.

IMPORTANT CARDIAC SIGNS

Clinical examination of the patient remains an important skill, although with modern developments in echocardiography, the time-honoured stethoscope could soon be replaced by handheld ultrasound machines.

Cyanosis

Cyanosis describes the blue discoloration (cyan) of the skin and mucous membranes when there is more than 5 g of oxygen-depleted haemoglobin in the blood. Cyanosis is described as either peripheral or central.

Peripheral cyanosis occurs in the fingers and toes. It usually indicates a slowing of peripheral circulation, allowing more oxygen to be extracted as the blood passes through the constricted capillaries. It occurs most commonly in cold weather. In hospital practice, it may be seen in patients with low cardiac output or shock.

Central cyanosis is observed in the lips and tongue, and becomes apparent at arterial oxygen saturations of less than 85%. Central cyanosis is produced by inadequate oxygenation of the blood as it passes through the lungs (as in pulmonary disease) or sometimes when the lungs are bypassed all together (as in right-to-left intracardiac shunts). Pulmonary cyanosis should respond to increased inspired oxygen concentrations (FiO_2), but there will be little effect if there is an intracardiac right-to-left shunt.

The arterial pulse

Arterial pulses should be examined for rate, rhythm and character of the waveform. Although the rate and rhythm are usually assessed by palpation of the radial artery, an artery closer to the heart is usually better for appreciating pulse waveform. In clinical practice, all features may be best assessed by palpation of the right brachial artery.

Rate

The normal adult pulse rate varies between 60 and 100 beats/minute. Slower rates are found in athletes and patients taking beta-adrenergic blocking agents, but otherwise may indicate a brady-dysrhythmia. Pulse rates in excess of 100 are often associated with anxiety or pain, and those above 130 beats/minute at rest usually indicate an abnormal tachycardia.

Rhythm

The normal pulse is regular, or very slightly irregular if there is a *sinus arrhythmia*, when the heart quickens on inspiration. An occasional irregularity indicates an ectopic beat, and an irregularly irregular pulse indicates either multifocal ectopic beats or atrial fibrillation. Gently exercising the patient will produce a regular pulse in the former cases, when the resulting rise in heart rate will abolish the ectopics. This will have no effect on the irregularity produced by atrial fibrillation.

Waveform character

The character of the pulse waveform is not often easily appreciated but can help with diagnosis. Examples include:

- *Pulsus alternans*: alternate high- and low-volume beats as found in left ventricular failure. It indicates poor left ventricular function.
- *Pulsus paradoxus*: an excessive reduction in pulse pressure (over 10 mmHg) on inspiration. It may be found in severe asthma, pericardial tamponade or pericardial constriction.
- *Collapsing pulse*: a large-volume pulse, with rapid rise and fall as may occur in thyrotoxicosis or aortic incompetence. This is often best appreciated with the arm elevated and the palm of the hand place across the wrist.
- *Plateau pulse*: low volume, slow rise and slow fall, as found in aortic stenosis.
- *Absent pulse*: due to atherosclerosis, aortic dissection or peripheral embolisation.

Jugular venous pressure (JVP)

The filling of the internal jugular vein is used to assess the central venous pressure (CVP), may be observed in front of the sterno-mastoid muscle and may give important information about right heart function. With a normal CVP, pulsation of the internal jugular vein is usually only visible when the patient lies flat. When observing for elevation, the height above the sternal angle should be measured with the patient lying at 45°. If the light is poor, a bedside lamp directed obliquely across the neck can help. Confirmation of the level may be made by pressing on the liver, which transiently increases the CVP by increasing venous return to the heart (*hepato-jugular reflux*). Tender liver enlargement may occur in chronic heart failure, and pulsation may be felt in severe tricuspid incompetence. An elevated JVP indicates high right-sided cardiac pressures, as in heart failure, pulmonary embolism or cor pulmonale. An elevated JVP early after acute myocardial infarction may signify involvement of the right ventricle, but may be seen if there was cardiac failure preceding the infarct.

Much has been written about the pulsation in the jugular vein, but clinical interpretation is often difficult. Sometimes 'a' and 'v' waves may be seen, which correspond to right atrial and right ventricular contractions. The 'a' wave occurs just before the carotid arterial pulse, and very large 'a' waves (cannon waves) may be seen when the right atrium contracts against a closed tricuspid valve, as may occur in complete heart block when atrial and ventricular contraction are not synchronised. There will be no 'a' waves if the heart is in atrial fibrillation, as the atria do not contract.

Blood pressure

The first recorded measurement of blood pressure was in 1730, by the Reverend Stephen Hales, who measured the height of a column of blood in a glass tube inserted into the neck veins of a horse. The tube had to be more than 8 feet long! Fortunately, Scipione Riva-Rocci devised the sphygmomanometer in 1896, which greatly cleaned up and simplified blood pressure estimation. The 'Riva-Rocci' or 'auscultatory' method of blood pressure estimation employs a sphygmomanometer to occlude the brachial artery and a stethoscope to detect sounds of turbulent blood flow within the artery following the release of arterial compression. These sounds are known as the Korotkoff sounds, named after Nicholi Korotkoff, a Russian army surgeon who described them in 1905. The auscultatory method using the mercury sphygmomanometer has been the mainstay of clinical blood pressure measurement for many years but, with the withdrawal of mercury for health and safety reasons, there has been a move in favour of well-validated, accurate and reasonably priced semi-automated monitors. An enormous number of different electronic oscillometric monitors are now available, but they vary considerably in their accuracy, size, weight and noise level, as well as ease of use. The European Society of Hypertension (ESH) has published standards for the evaluation of blood pressure measuring devices (O'Brien et al, 2002), and those not certified by ESH or the American National Standards for electronic or automated sphygmomanometers (ANSI/AAMI) should not be used (Jowett, 1997). Aneroid sphygmomanometers are still widely used, but are notoriously difficult to maintain in an accurate state over time and cannot be recommended for routine use (Williams et al, 2004). Most wrist and finger devices are unvalidated.

Self-measurement of blood pressure

Despite improvements in blood pressure monitors suitable for patient use, management of hypertension based exclusively on self-measurement at home is not recommended at the moment (Celis et al, 2005). The Treatment of Hypertension based on Home or office Blood Pressure (THOP) trial (Den Hond et al, 2004) showed that antihypertensive treatment based on home instead of clinic blood pressure measurements led to less intensive drug treatment, but also to less hypertensive control. A home blood pressure of < 135 mmHg systolic and 85 mmHg diastolic is usually considered normal. The use of accurate and validated measuring devices is obviously important, and measurements should preferentially be storable.

Ambulatory blood pressure monitoring (ABPM)

ABPM permits non-invasive measurement of blood pressure over prolonged periods, provides a more reproducible estimate of the blood pressure

Table 4.5 Recommended blood pressure levels (mmHg) for ABPM.

	Normal	Abnormal
Daytime	< 135/85	> 140/90
Night-time	< 120/70	> 125/75
24 hour	< 130/80	> 135/85

than either clinic or home measurements (O'Brien et al, 2000; O'Brien 2001) and is a much stronger predictor of cardiovascular morbidity and mortality than conventional blood pressure estimation (Verdecchia, 2001). Measurements are usually made at half-hourly intervals so as not to interfere with activity during the day and with sleep at night, but can be made more frequently if necessary. Recommended blood pressure levels (mmHg) for ABPM are given in Table 4.5.

For diagnostic and monitoring purposes, the average daytime readings are used, where an ABPM of < 135 mmHg systolic and 85 mmHg diastolic is generally considered normal. Lower blood pressure targets are suggested in high-risk groups, such as following myocardial infarction, or in diabetic patients, where levels < 130/80 mmHg are considered optimal.

Ambulatory measurement of blood pressure is not currently recommended by the British Hypertension Society for assessment of all hypertensive patients, but may be useful in:

- excluding white coat hypertension;
- deciding on treatment in elderly patients;
- accurate diagnosis in patients with borderline hypertension;
- assessing patients with resistant hypertension;
- diagnosing hypotension.

White coat hypertension describes a blood pressure of over 140/90 mmHg when measured in the clinic by conventional methods, but found to be less than 135/85 mmHg by ABPM. It may be seen in up to 30% of the general population, particularly the elderly. Conventional measurement of systolic pressure in elderly people may produce results that are on average 20 mmHg higher than daytime ambulatory pressure, leading to an overestimation of the occurrence of isolated systolic hypertension among elderly patients and probably excessive treatment.

Resistant hypertension is defined as a blood pressure that remains consistently above 150/90 mmHg in spite of treatment with three antihypertensive drugs. ABPM may either confirm this or indicate that the apparent lack of response is caused by the white coat phenomenon. Poor compliance with antihypertensive treatment remains the commonest cause of poor blood pressure control.

Measuring the blood pressure

There is considerable variability in blood pressure through the day, and readings may be affected by such factors as emotion, pain, a full bladder or circadian rhythm. For example, anxiety may raise the blood pressure by as much as 30 mmHg. As far as is practicable, it is important for the patient to be both relaxed and rested, preferably with the patient sitting still for at least 5 minutes, not moving or speaking. The arm must be supported at the level of the heart, and no tight clothing should constrict the arm. Atrial fibrillation can make the measurement of blood pressure particularly difficult due to marked beat-to-beat variability. This is a particularly important consideration when using automated devices, when multiple readings may be needed.

Most devices for measuring blood pressure are dependent on occlusion of an artery with a constricting cuff, and by detection of the Korotkov sounds on release of the pressure by auscultation or oscillometry. The correct selection and application of the pressure cuff is important, especially in small women and obese patients. The choice of cuff size should be based upon the arm circumference, which should be measured at the midpoint between the shoulder and elbow. The width of the cuff bladder should be not less than 40% of the midarm circumference (range 40–50%), and it should encircle at least 80% of the circumference of the arm (but not over 100%). Terms such as 'paediatric' or 'small adult' are misleading – the correct size is solely dependent upon arm circumference. A simple guide can be employed to show the best available cuff width based upon arm size (Fig. 4.2). The cuff size selected should be recorded, and the same size should always be used for serial measurements in the same patient.

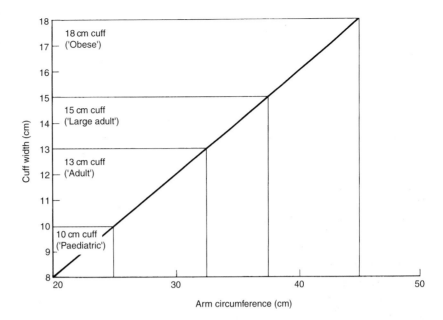

Figure 4.2 Selecting the correct blood pressure cuff. The ratio of cuff to arm should be greater than 40%.

The cuff should be applied firmly so that the lower edge is 2.5 cm above the antecubital fossa, with the bladder overlying the brachial artery. It must not be twisted or in contact with the patient's clothing. The patient should be comfortable and the forearm supported, slightly extended and externally rotated. The midpoint of the cuff is often marked and should rest over the artery. If the arm is small, it may be easier to put the cuff on upside down so that the tubing is well away from the artery and pointing towards the patient's shoulder.

Correct positioning of the arm is required for accurate blood pressure measurement. The blood pressure rises as the arm is lowered below the level of the heart, and vice versa. Additionally, if the arm is unsupported, isometric muscle contraction needed to hold the arm up against gravity will raise the blood pressure. Hence, the arm should be supported horizontally on a level with the heart. Automatic machines will determine pulse rate, systolic and diastolic blood pressure, although there are some patients in whom oscillometric methods are difficult.

Estimation of blood pressure (non-electronic)

- Palpate the brachial pulse in the antecubital fossa.
- Rapidly inflate the cuff to 20 mmHg above the point where the brachial pulse disappears.
- Deflate the cuff and note the pressure at which the pulse reappears: the approximate systolic pressure.
- Reinflate the cuff to 20 mmHg above the point at which the brachial pulse disappears.
- Using one hand, place the stethoscope over the brachial artery ensuring complete skin contact with no clothing in between.
- Slowly deflate the cuff at 2–3 mmHg/second listening for Korotkoff sounds:

  1 *Phase I*: systolic blood pressure is indicated by the first appearance of faint tapping sounds that gradually become louder.
  2 *Phase II*: the sounds become soft and may disappear altogether (auscultatory gap).
  3 *Phase III*: sharp heart sounds return.
  4 *Phase IV*: abrupt muffling then occurs.
  5 *Phase V*: the point at which the sounds disappear marks the diastolic blood pressure.

Both phase IV and phase V have been used in the past as an indication of diastolic blood pressure. Phase IV usually differs by less than 5 mmHg from phase V, but the latter correlates best with intra-arterial pressure. In certain patient groups (children, pregnant women, elderly, anaemic), there may be a large discrepancy between phase IV and phase V, but phase V should still be used to indicate diastolic blood pressure, unless sounds are heard down to zero. In this instance, both phase IV and phase V blood pressure should be recorded (e.g. 140/80/0).

Normally, the diastolic blood pressure rises a little on standing, with a slight fall in the systolic blood pressure. In patients with autonomic failure (such as diabetics and the elderly), taking vasodilator medication or in shock, this fall may be very marked (postural or orthostatic hypotension). There is little difference between sitting and lying blood pressure. It is usual to record the blood pressure twice, recording the average at each of a number of visits. The arm used for recording should be noted and, initially, the pressure in both arms should be recorded, so that a subclavian arterial stenosis is not missed. Subsequent measurements should be in the arm with the higher blood pressure.

When using an electronic device, most will allow manual blood pressure setting selection. Other monitors will automatically inflate and reinflate to the next setting if required. Measurements should be repeated three times and the results recorded as displayed.

There may be several occasions on which blood pressure estimation is difficult (Table 4.6). This is particularly so in hypotensive patients or in those with unstable blood pressure when invasive blood pressure monitoring may be required (see Chapter 5).

Blood pressure continues to be measured in the original units introduced by Poiseuille for the mercury manometer – millimetres of mercury (mmHg), despite the International System of Units being adopted by many countries (including the UK). While the kilopascal is used in reporting blood gases (1 mmHg = 0.13 kPa, or 1 kPa = 7.52 mmHg), replacing the millimetre of mercury with the kilopascal for estimating blood pressure has been postponed.

The apex beat and cardiac impulse

The apex beat marks the maximal thrust of the left ventricle, and is normally seen and felt just inside the mid-clavicular line in the fifth left intercostal space with the patient lying at 45°. If the apex beat is seen towards the left, there is usually cardiac enlargement, but it may also be displaced by abnormalities of the lungs or rib cage. Collapse of

Table 4.6 Problems in measuring blood pressure.

Problem	Cause	Reasons
False high reading	Cuff too small	Small cuff does not adequately disperse the pressure over the arterial surface
	Bladder not centred over the brachial artery	More external pressure is needed to compress the artery
	Cuff not applied snugly	Uneven and slow inflation results in varying tissue compression
	Arm positioned below heart level	Hydrostatic pressure imposed by weight of blood column above site of auscultation additive to arterial pressure: reposition arm to appropriate level
	Very obese arm	Cuff too small for a large arm will cause too little compression of the artery at the suitable pressure level: apply a large thigh cuff to the upper arm if necessary
False low reading	Cuff too large	Pressure is spread over too large an area and produces a damping effect on the korotkoff sounds
	Arm positioned above heart level	Hydrostatic pressure in the elevated arm causes resistance to pressure generated by the heart

the right lung, for example, will pull the heart to the right, and a thoracic scoliosis may displace the mediastinum either way.

When felt, the apex may feel normal, hyperdynamic (thrusting) or sustained (heaving). Sustained impulses are usually due to pressure overload, as in aortic stenosis or hypertension. Hyperdynamic impulses occur in volume overload as in aortic or mitral regurgitation or after exercise. The left ventricle produces a sustained heaving or thrusting apex beat if hypertrophied but, when enlargement is due to dilatation, it is weak and diffuse. It has a tapping quality in mitral stenosis. If there is a left ventricular aneurysm, there may be a double or rocking apical beat. The right ventricular impulse is usually not palpable in health. In pulmonary hypertension or right-sided valve disease, the right ventricle gives rise to a parasternal heave. More usually, this is due to mitral incompetence.

Seeing, or even feeling, the apex beat is probably only possible in 50% of cases, and it is particularly difficult in the obese or in those with hyperinflated chests.

The heart sounds

The heart sounds are produced by closure of the valves. Mitral and aortic valve closure precedes that of the tricuspid and pulmonary valves and is louder.

The first sound

The first sound (S_1) is related to closure of the mitral and tricuspid valves at the onset of systole, and is best heard at the apex. The mitral component is louder, and occurs fractionally before closure of the tricuspid valve. At the onset of ventricular systole, the valve cusps have been forced downwards into the ventricle by atrial contraction, and the sound relates to them snapping back up again, the movement being checked by the chordae tendineae. The position of the cusps is determined by the volume and pressure of blood on either side of the valve, so the more the valve is forced down, the louder S_1.

Loud first heart sounds will occur if the left atrial pressure is abnormally high (as in mitral stenosis), during fast heart rates or if the atrium contracts very close to ventricular systole (marked by a short PR interval on the ECG). A soft first heart sound

occurs if the mitral valve is calcified, does not move well or if left ventricular contraction is poor.

When there is dissociated contraction of the atria and ventricles, as in complete heart block or ventricular tachycardia, the first sound varies in intensity depending on the position of the valve at the onset of ventricular systole.

The second sound

The second sound (S_2) is related to closure of the pulmonary and aortic valves at the end of ventricular systole, and is best heard in the second left intercostal space. The sound is normally split because the aortic valve closes before the pulmonary valve on inspiration when the right ventricle takes longer to expel the increased venous return. The aortic subcomponent (A_2) is accentuated in hypertension, when the cusps do not move well (aortic valve calcification) or in thin patients. A loud pulmonary component (P_2) may be a feature of acute pulmonary embolism or pulmonary hypertension.

Wide splitting is caused when the right ventricle is overloaded, as in pulmonary stenosis or cor pulmonale, and the valve is unable to close quickly. It also occurs in right bundle branch block, when there is delayed right ventricular activation.

Reversed splitting means that P_2 precedes A_2, and the splitting is best heard on expiration. It occurs if the ventricle is overloaded, as in left ventricular failure, or cannot empty fast enough (aortic stenosis). It may also occur in left bundle branch block, because the right ventricle is activated prematurely.

Fixed splitting means that the components of the second heart sound do not vary with respiration, and it occurs when increased venous return affects both ventricles (e.g. atrio-septal defect, right heart failure, left-to-right shunts).

A *single* S_2 usually infers a calcific aortic valve with stenosis (or rarely pulmonary stenosis), but it may be heard in obese patients or in pericardial effusion.

The third sound

The third sound (S_3) is low pitched and best heard at the apex. It may be normal in the young and in pregnancy, but is usually abnormal in patients over the age of 40 years. In the first phase of diastole, 80% of the blood stored in the atria during systole is transferred to the ventricles. If the volume transferred is abnormally large, the ventricles tense during this rapid filling and produce this added heart sound. S_3 implies heart failure or a widely open mitral valve (mitral regurgitation). A third heart sound is found in 5–10% of patients admitted with myocardial infarction and is an important indicator of left ventricular dysfunction and poor outcome.

The fourth sound

The fourth sound (S_4) is heard just before S_1, at the apex of the heart. It is probably produced by the atrial kick associated with emptying of the remaining 20% of atrial blood into a non-distending ventricle, as may exist in left ventricular hypertrophy or hypertrophic obstructive cardiomyopathy (HOCM). A prominent fourth heart sound is common in patients admitted to the coronary care unit, but probably has no prognostic significance.

Gallop rhythm is often heard in heart failure. The addition of a third heart sound with a tachycardia makes the heart sounds sound like a galloping horse. If both third and fourth heart sounds are present, it is called a *summation gallop*. Gallop rhythm may be normal in young adults and children.

Other heart sounds

Ejection clicks occur immediately after the first heart sound at the time of aortic and pulmonary valve opening, and are usually associated with stenosis of the valves. They are sometimes confused with a fourth heart sound. A mid-systolic click may be heard with mitral valve prolapse. An opening snap of the mitral valve is heard in mitral stenosis, but disappears as the valve becomes calcific. The opening snap may be confused with a third heart sound, but is much more widely conducted.

A pericardial friction rub causes a scratchy sound (like sandpaper) produced by the inflamed visceral and parietal pericardia rubbing against each other. It may be localised, generalised, longlasting or transient. It is best heard with the patient sitting forward.

Heart murmurs

Murmurs are sounds caused by turbulent blood flow. This may be either because the blood flow is more rapid or because it is running a turbulent course.

Murmurs are heard during either systole or diastole. Their intensity is sometimes classed as grades 1–6 for systolic murmurs and 1–4 for diastolic murmurs, but such practice is usually unhelpful. The intensity of the murmur does not reflect the severity of the valve defect. It is more important to determine where the murmur occurs in the cardiac cycle, where and how it is best heard and, finally, where the murmur radiates to.

Innocent or functional murmurs are due to minor turbulence unassociated with any structural abnormality. Functional murmurs are very common in children, and most disappear around puberty. Most are pulmonary flow murmurs. A continuous *venous hum* may be heard over the right clavicle, radiating into the neck. It is reduced by compressing the internal jugular vein on the same side or by lying down.

Pathological murmurs are indicative of a structural or functional cardiac abnormality. Patients on the coronary care unit may develop murmurs related to myocardial infarction, but may have pre-existing murmurs unrelated to their acute problem. It is therefore very important that murmurs are precisely documented to distinguish them from newly developed murmurs.

Systolic murmurs These are either pan-systolic (i.e. heard throughout systole) or mid-systolic (loudest in mid-systole). The latter are sometimes called ejection systolic murmurs, as they are usually associated with the ejection of blood from the ventricles through a stenosed pulmonary or aortic valve. The A_2 is then heard clearly at the apex of the heart, whereas with regurgitant murmurs, the A_2 is better heard at the base of the heart.

Innocent and physiological murmurs are virtually always systolic. An apical systolic murmur is common following acute myocardial infarction, and is usually due to papillary muscle dysfunction. The sudden development of a harsh pan-systolic murmur may indicate severe mitral regurgitation due to papillary muscle rupture or a post-infarction ventriculo-septal defect. It may be difficult to differentiate the two clinically, and echocardiography should be carried out urgently.

Diastolic murmurs   These can be early diastolic, mid-diastolic or late diastolic (presystolic). They are always low pitched. Early diastolic murmurs are common in the elderly due to mild aortic regurgitation. A loud aortic diastolic murmur in patients presenting with severe chest pain usually indicates aortic dissection.

Common murmurs heard on CCU

Pulmonary systolic murmur   This short, 'blowing' murmur is often found in younger patients, usually admitted with supraventricular tachycardia. It may be heard down the left sternal edge and apex. Some patients will be noted to have a sternal depression or an abnormally straight back ('straight back syndrome') that presumably squashes the heart from front to back, altering blood flow patterns. Echocardiography is needed, as it sometimes associates with mitral valve prolapse (Spapen et al, 1990).

Aortic ejection murmur   These are common in middle-aged and elderly patients, especially those with hypertension, in which aortic valve thickening and dilatation of the proximal aorta are usual. Differentiation from significant aortic stenosis is difficult, and patients should have an echocardiogram.

Mitral systolic murmur   Fibrosis and calcification of the mitral annulus is common in the elderly and produces a murmur identical to that of mitral incompetence. Mitral regurgitant murmurs are common following myocardial infarction, caused by either dilatation of the mitral ring or damage to the mitral apparatus.

A short, late systolic murmur may be due to prolapse of a mitral leaflet into the left atrium at the end of ventricular systole. *Mitral valve prolapse* is the most common valvular abnormality in the UK, with a prevalence of up to 17% in women and 12% in men. Most cases are asymptomatic, and the overall prognosis is excellent, although a small subset will

develop serious complications, including infective endocarditis and severe mitral regurgitation (Hayek et al, 2005). Mitral valve repair is the treatment of choice for symptomatic prolapse. Many patients are prone to atypical chest pains and palpitations.

Signs of hyperlipidaemia (Fig. 4.3)

A *corneal arcus* is a partially or completely opaque white ring seen at the periphery of the cornea. It is common among the elderly as a result of hyaline degeneration, but may indicate deposition of fatty granules in association with hypercholesterolemia and hypertriglyceridaemia (Chua et al, 2004).

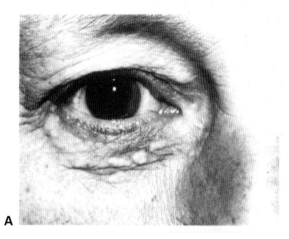

A

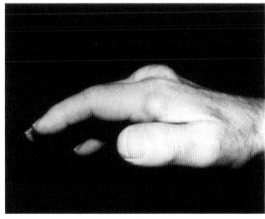

B

Figure 4.3   Cutaneous signs of high blood lipids: (A) xantholasma; (B) tendon xanthomas.

In younger patients, it should raise the suspicion of dyslipidaemia and, in those with symptoms of coronary disease, the presence of a corneal arcus usually indicates multivessel coronary atherosclerosis (Hoogerbrugge et al, 1999).

Xanthelasma are small, raised, yellow plaques on the eyelids, which contain cholesterol, but do not always associate with abnormal blood lipid concentrations. *Tendon xanthomata* are hard nodules found over the knuckles, knees and in the Achilles tendon. These are important signs of familial hypercholesterolaemia (FH), a condition associated with a very high incidence of early and severe CHD.

Eruptive xanthomata are papules with yellow centres that appear over extensor surfaces and are a clinical clue to severe hypertriglyceridaemia (Jowett, 2002). This often associates with acute pancreatitis, sometimes resulting in admission to the coronary care unit because of lower chest/upper abdominal pain and shock.

The diagonal earlobe crease

There is an association between coronary atherosclerosis and the presence of a diagonal earlobe crease that runs at a 45° downward angle towards the shoulder (Fig. 4.4). In one study, the presence of a unilateral earlobe crease was associated with a 33% increase in the risk of a heart attack, and the risk increased to 77% when the earlobe crease appeared bilaterally (Elliott & Powell, 1996).

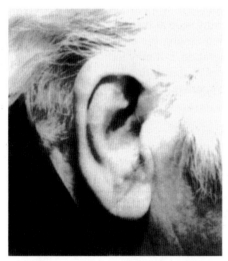

Figure 4.4　Diagonal earlobe crease.

References

Airaksinen KE (2001) Silent coronary artery disease in diabetes – a feature of autonomic neuropathy or accelerated atherosclerosis? *Diabetologia* 44: 259–266.

Asbury EA, Collins P (2005) Cardiac syndrome X. *International Journal of Clinical Practice* 59: 1063–1069.

Benzaquen BS, Cohen V, Eisenberg MJ (2001) Effects of cocaine on the coronary arteries. *American Heart Journal* 142: 402–410.

Campeau L (1976) Grading of angina pectoris. *Circulation* 54: 522–523.

Celis H, Den Hond E, Staessen JA (2005) Self-measurement of blood pressure at home in the management of hypertension. *Clinical Medicine & Research* 3: 19–26.

Chambers J, Bass C (1998) Atypical chest pain: looking beyond the heart. *Quarterly Journal of Medicine* 91: 239–244.

Chua BA, Mitchell J, Wang PP et al (2004) Corneal arcus and hyperlipidaemia: findings from an older population. *American Journal of Ophthalmology* 137: 363–365.

Den Hond E, Staessen JA, Celis H et al (2004) Treatment of Hypertension Based on Home or Office Blood Pressure (THOP) Trial Investigators. Antihypertensive treatment based on home or office blood pressure – the THOP trial. *Blood Pressure Monitoring* 9: 311–314.

Dorsch MF, Lawrance RA, Sapsford RJ et al EMMACE Study Group (2001) Poor prognosis of patients presenting with symptomatic myocardial infarction but without chest pain. *Heart* 86: 494–498.

Edmonstone WM (1995) Cardiac chest pain: does body language help the diagnosis. *British Medical Journal* 311: 1660–1661.

Elliott WJ, Powell LH (1996) Diagonal earlobe creases and prognosis in patients with suspected coronary artery disease. *American Journal of Medicine* 100: 205–211.

Fox KM (2005) Investigation and management of chest pain. *Heart* 91: 105–110.

Hayek E, Gring CN, Griffin BP (2005) Mitral valve prolapse. *Lancet* 365: 507–518.

Hemingway H, Fitzpatrick NK, Gnani S et al (2004) Prospective validity of measuring angina severity with Canadian Cardiovascular Society class: the ACRE study. *Canadian Journal of Cardiology* 20: 305–309.

Hoogerbrugge N, Happee C, van Domberg R et al (1999) Corneal arcus: indicator for severity of coronary atherosclerosis? *Netherlands Journal of Medicine* 55: 184–187.

Jowett NI (1997) Monitoring the central venous and arterial blood pressure. In: Jowett NI (ed.) *Cardiovascular Monitoring*. London: Whurr, pp. 122–144.

Jowett NI (2002) Milky serum. *Practical Diabetes International* 19: 122.

Kannel WB, Abbott RD (1984) Incidence and prognosis of unrecognized myocardial infarction. An update on the Framingham study. *New England Journal of Medicine* 311: 1144–1147.

Lawson-Matthew PJ, Wilson AT, Woodmansey PA et al (1994) Unsatisfactory management of patients with acute myocardial infarction admitted to general medical wards. *Journal of the Royal College of Physicians of London* 28: 49–51.

Lichtlen PR (1996) The concept of total ischaemic burden: clinical significance. *European Heart Journal* 17(suppl G): 38–47.

Miller AJ, Texidor TA (1959) The 'precordial catch,' a syndrome of anterior chest pain. *Annals of Internal Medicine* 51: 461–467.

New York Heart Association Criteria Committee (1964) In: *Diseases of the Heart and Blood Vessels: Nomenclature and Criteria for Diagnosis*. Boston, MA: Little Brown & Co., p. 114.

O'Brien E (2001) Blood pressure measurement is changing! *Heart* 85: 3–5.

O'Brien E, Coats A, Owens J et al (2000) Use and interpretation of ambulatory blood pressure monitoring: recommendations of the British Hypertension Society. *British Medical Journal* 320: 1128–1134.

O'Brien E, Pickering T, Asmar R et al (2002) Working Group on Blood Pressure Monitoring of the European Society of Hypertension International Protocol for validation of blood pressure measuring devices in adults. *Blood Pressure Monitoring* 7: 3–17.

Spapen HD, Reynaert H, Debeuckelaere S et al (1990) The straight back syndrome. *Netherlands Journal of Medicine* 36: 29–31.

Stern S, Tzivoni D (1974) Early detection of silent ischaemic heart disease by 24-hour electrocardiographic monitoring of active subjects. *British Heart Journal* 36(5): 481–486.

Sullivan AK, Holdright DR, Wright CA et al (1994) Chest pain in women: clinical, investigative and prognostic features. *British Medical Journal* 308: 883–886.

Swap CJ, Nagurney JT (2005) Value and limitations of chest pain history in the evaluation of patients with suspected acute coronary syndromes. *Journal of the American Medical Association* 294: 2623–2629.

Then KL, Rankin JA, Fofonoff DA (2001) Atypical presentation of acute myocardial infarction in three age groups. *Heart and Lung* 30: 285–293.

Verdecchia P (2001) Reference values for ambulatory blood pressure and self-measured blood pressure based on prospective outcome data. *Blood Pressure Monitoring* 6: 323–327.

Williams B, Poulter, NR, Brown, MJ for the British Hypertension Society (2004) British Hypertension Society guidelines for hypertension management 2004 (BHS-IV): summary. *British Medical Journal* 328: 634–640.

Wong C-K, White HD (2002) Recognising 'painless' heart attacks. *Heart* 87: 3–5.

Chapter 5

Investigation of patients with coronary heart disease

Exertional chest pain is the most common presenting symptom of coronary heart disease (CHD), and there are over 600 000 primary care consultations for angina in the UK each year (Nilsson et al, 2003). Prompt investigation of these patients is needed for diagnostic, therapeutic or prognostic reasons and, apart from the very elderly and infirm, all patients with symptoms suggestive of myocardial ischaemia should be referred to a cardiologist for confirmation of the diagnosis and objective assessment of severity. Early assessment is important, because 10% of patients with new exertional angina suffer death or myocardial infarction within 12 months, and a further 20% have to undergo revascularisation (Gandhi et al, 1995). Prognosis can be favourably influenced by intervention in most cases, as the majority of patients have an undamaged left ventricle at presentation (Sutcliffe et al, 2003).

Assessment may take place in the following settings:

Community. Patients may present to their own general practitioner (GP), walk-in centres, NHS Direct, a hospital emergency department or the emergency medical services (EMS). Walk-in centres that use protocol-based assessment have been reported to perform better than either GP surgeries or NHS Direct (Grant et al, 2002), but the role of the GP should not be underestimated, as they often have knowledge of the patient, their past medical history, the family and their home circumstances. Appraisal of cardiovascular risk factors often aids diagnosis and, while physical examination seldom adds much in confirming a diagnosis of myocardial ischaemia, it may identify other causes of the presenting symptoms. Initial investigations by the primary care team should include a resting electrocardiogram (though normal in 50% of cases), chest radiograph and blood testing for haemoglobin, erythrocyte sedimentation rate (ESR), renal function tests, fasting blood glucose and lipid profile. Priority cardiology referral is suggested for patients with:

- recent onset or rapidly progressive chest pain and/or breathlessness;
- possible aortic stenosis with symptoms;

- change in severity of symptoms (minimal exertion or nocturnal angina);
- threatened unemployment (especially vocational drivers).

Secondary care (district general hospital). Physicians accredited in cardiovascular medicine provide optimal secondary care, and all cardiology departments should be able to perform exercise stress testing, dynamic (Holter) electrocardiography, ambulatory blood pressure monitoring and echocardiography. Myocardial perfusion scintigraphy, stress echocardiography, transoesophageal echocardiography and cardiac catheterisation laboratories are now established within many district general hospitals.

Patients referred with suspected angina can be assessed through a rapid access chest pain clinic to avoid prolonged worry (doctor and patient) or hospital admission (Dougan et al, 2001). Low-risk stable angina patients seen in the emergency department can also be referred to the rapid access clinic, rather than to cardiology outpatients or back into primary care.

All acute hospitals should have provision for rapid triage of patients presenting with acute chest pain. Those with likely or confirmed acute coronary syndromes should be admitted to the coronary care unit (CCU) without delay, and the majority with more benign causes of chest pain can be referred to the chest pain clinic. Patients at indeterminate risk may benefit from assessment in a dedicated chest pain unit (CPU) to establish which have symptoms of acute myocardial ischaemia and require early therapy, and prevent the 2–4% of patients (usually women) with evolving myocardial infarction being sent home with a diagnosis of non-cardiac chest pain (Pope et al, 2000). Randomised trials support the introduction of CPUs as a safe and effective method for evaluation of low- and intermediate-risk chest pain patients, and these are cost-effective compared with usual in-hospital evaluation (McManus et al, 2002).

Tertiary care (regional cardiac centre). Specialist investigation and management facilities with appropriately skilled personnel are needed in regional cardiac centres for electrophysiological testing, complex cardiac pacing, vascular imaging techniques, percutaneous coronary intervention (PCI) and cardiac surgery. Direct referral to tertiary units from primary care often overloads these specialist units.

INVESTIGATIONAL TOOLS

The electrocardiogram

The normal cardiac electrical impulse originates in the sinus node and is conducted as a wave over the atrium to initiate atrial systole. An electrical barrier exists between the atrial and ventricular myocardium, and further activation can only take place via the atrio-ventricular (AV) node, a group of specialised cells situated on the right side of the interatrial septum, just below the entrance of the coronary sinus. The atrial depolarisation wave activates the AV node, and the impulse is then transmitted to the ventricles by the left and right divisions of the *bundle of His*. The left bundle reaches the left heart by perforating the interventricular septum, and both bundles carry the impulse onwards, the septum being activated from left to right. The impulse then spreads over the endocardial surface of the ventricles via the *Purkinje fibres* and through the ventricular myocardium, in a wave passing from the endocardium outwards to the epicardium.

The electrical forces generated by the heart travel in multiple directions simultaneously. The electrocardiogram (ECG) is designed to record these electrical impulses via electrodes placed on the body surface, and the generated waveform has been divided into P, Q, R, S, T and U waves. The *P wave* represents atrial activation, and the *QRS complex* ventricular activation. The *T wave* represents ventricular repolarisation. Repolarisation of the atria (T_a wave) is not usually seen, being buried in the QRS complex. The origins of the U wave (if seen) are not clear.

The signals are amplified and, by convention, the display is arranged so that impulses moving towards a surface electrode give rise to an upward (positive) deflection, while impulses moving away from the electrode give a downward (negative) deflection. To help to interpret the patterns of electrical movement, electrocardiography is carried out in different planes. The three major planes are recorded via electrodes on the right arm (RA), left arm (LA) and left leg (LL). A fourth electrode is traditionally placed on the right leg, but this is

Figure 5.1 The Einthoven triangle (named after Willem Einthoven, 1860–1927, Professor of Physiology, University of Leiden).

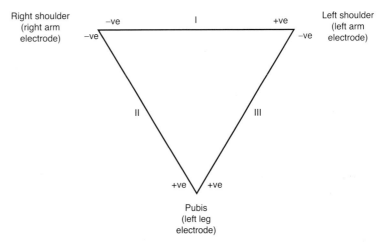

not used for recording and serves as a ground (earth) electrode. The three planes form an electrical triangle (Einthoven's triangle) that surrounds the heart (Fig. 5.1). These *bipolar* limb leads are used to record the potential difference between two specified electrodes (hence bipolar) designated standard leads I, II and III.

The normal ECG uses recordings from 12 leads. In addition to the three standard limb leads (I, II and III), there are three *unipolar* leads (VR, VL and VF), which measure the potential difference between one of the limb electrodes (the 'exploring' electrode) and a reference potential derived by joining the other two limb lead electrodes. The ECG machine records and boosts this signal automatically to produce 'augmented' unipolar leads aVR, aVL and aVF. Six additional chest (V) leads complete the standard 12-lead ECG and view the heart electrically from the front, as shown in Figure 5.2. These are also unipolar leads that record the potential difference between the set points on the chest wall and the average potential obtained from the three limb leads.

Positioning of the leads

Standard (limb) lead placement is with the electrodes attached to both arms and legs slightly above the wrists and ankles. The leads are normally labelled RA (right arm – red), LA (left arm – yellow), LL (left leg – green) and RL (right leg – black). Changes in the cardiac axis may occur if the limb lead electrodes are placed proximally on the trunk instead of on the wrists and ankles (Jowett et al, 2005). Positioning of the chest leads also needs to be precise to prevent artefactual ECG changes between serial recordings. V1 and V2 are often placed too high on the chest and the lateral leads (V5 and V6) too low down. Correct positions are:

- V1: fourth intercostal space, immediately to the right of the sternum;
- V2: fourth intercostal space, immediately to the left of the sternum;
- V3: midway between V2 and V4;
- V4: fifth intercostal space, mid-clavicular line;
- V5: left anterior axillary line, on the same horizontal line as V4;
- V6: left mid-axillary line, horizontal with V4 and V5.

In female patients, V4–V6 should be placed *under* the breast unless the breast is particularly pendulous to ensure close apposition to the chest wall. The breast tissue will otherwise attenuate the signal and may produce changes in the ECG.

Many other additional electrode placements can be used to demonstrate particular aspects of the heart (Jowett, 1997), such as V7 and V8 (further laterally) or $V3_R$ and $V4_R$ (V3 and V4 positions on the right side of the chest).

Assessing the quality of the recording

Before analysing an ECG, it is essential to ensure that the recording was obtained correctly. Errors in

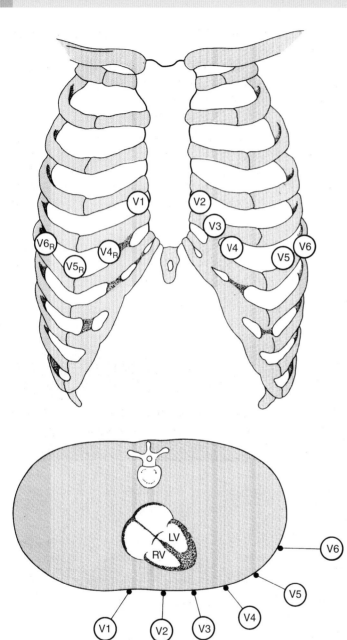

Figure 5.2 The positioning of ECG V leads on the chest.

lead placement or connection, selection of paper speed, standardisation and lead labelling are very common. Hence, the technical quality of the recording should not be assumed to be correct and should always be assessed first.

1 *Standardisation.* A potential of 1 mV should be represented by a 10-mm vertical deflection. A standard, test deflection should be recorded at the start and finish of a 12-lead recording.

2 *Speed.* Recordings are usually made with a paper speed of 25 mm/second.

3 *Clear tracings.* Mains interference may produce a fuzzy trace, as may patient movement caused by cold, shock or anxiety.

4 *Correct lead placement and labelling.* The net electrical movement in the heart is from lead

aVR towards lead II. Hence, the complexes should usually be totally positive in lead II (upright P, QRS and T waves) and totally negative in aVR. If the ECG does not show this, check the leads and/or repeat the ECG, particularly if the changes are very abnormal.

Analysing the ECG

If a standard approach is made to interpreting an ECG, important changes will not be missed. The sequence should be rate, rhythm, axis and waveform.

Rate The ECG is recorded at 25 mm/second on standard ECG paper, which has fine lines at 1-mm intervals and heavier divisions every 5 mm. Each millimetre therefore represents 0.04 seconds, and each large division is 0.2 seconds.

To calculate the rate, the number of large squares between two successive complexes should be measured and divided into 300. If the heart rhythm is irregular, a greater number of complexes should be assessed. Special ECG rulers can simplify the calculation of rate and also give anticipated values for the QT interval. A pair of dividers is also useful to measure intervals.

Rhythm Normal sinus rhythm appears as a normal P wave preceding each QRS complex, with a constant PR interval. If this is not the case, a dysrhythmia is present.

Axis The cardiac axis represents the net electrical direction that the cardiac impulse takes as it spreads through the myocardium. It does not represent the anatomical position of the heart – right axis deviation does not mean that the heart has swivelled around to point over the right shoulder! Axis is assessed in the frontal plane, with lead I designated 0°, and the 360° circle surrounding the heart divided into +180° (clockwise) and −180° (anti-clockwise). Normally, the cardiac axis lies between −30° and +90° and can be quickly approximated in the following manner:

- *Which lead has equal positive and negative QRS components?* This will be at right angles (90°) to the cardiac axis. However, the impulse could be in either direction, which leads to a further question.
- *Which lead has the predominant QRS deflection?* The net electrical movement must be in this direction, as movement towards a surface electrode gives a positive deflection.

Determining the cardiac axis may help in the diagnosis of broad complex tachycardias, pre-excitation syndromes (e.g. Wolff–Parkinson–White syndrome), pulmonary embolism, conduction defects (hemi-blocks) and congenital heart disease (Box 5.1).

Waveform The size of the different waves and the intervals between them are subject to biological variability, such as heart rate, age and sex. Values are shown in Figure 5.3.

Box 5.1 Some causes of axis deviation on the resting ECG.

A. Right axis deviation (> 90°)

Normal finding in children and tall, thin adults
Right ventricular hypertrophy
Chronic lung disease
Pulmonary embolus
Left posterior hemi-block
Antero-lateral myocardial infarction
Atrial septal defect
Ventricular septal defect
Wolff–Parkinson–White syndrome (left-sided accessory pathway)

B. Left axis deviation (< −30°)

Left anterior hemi-block
Inferior myocardial infarction
Hyperkalaemia
Artificial cardiac pacing
Emphysema
Wolff–Parkinson–White syndrome (right-sided accessory pathway)

C. Extreme left or right axis deviation

ECG leads applied incorrectly
Ventricular tachycardia

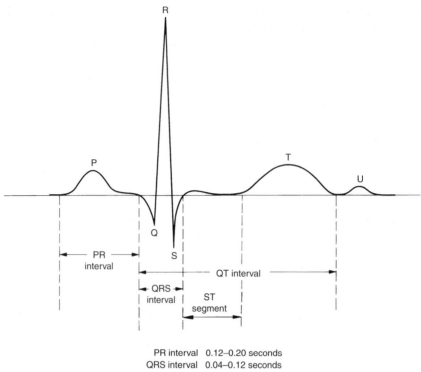

PR interval   0.12–0.20 seconds
QRS interval   0.04–0.12 seconds
QT interval   0.30–0.44 seconds (0.45 for women)

PR and QT intervals vary with heart rate

Figure 5.3   The electrocardiographic cycle showing nomenclature and time intervals.

P wave The normal P wave results from the spread of activity from the sinus node across the atria. Because the sino-atrial (SA) node is located on the right side of the interatrial septum, right atrial depolarisation occurs first, and causes the initial P wave deflection. Left atrial depolarisation occurs later and causes the terminal deflection. The net electrical movement during atrial depolarisation is from right to left, so the P wave will be upright in leads I, II and aVF and inverted in aVR. The normal P wave axis lies between +30° and +80°, so the P wave may be positive, negative or biphasic in leads III and aVL. The P wave is upright in lead II and biphasic in V1. The P wave should not be greater than 0.11 seconds in duration and should not be taller than 3 mm in the standard leads or 2.5 mm in the chest (V) leads.

Abnormalities may be:

- *Inversion*. This means that the atria are being depolarised from an unusual site, rather than the sinus node (unless there is dextrocardia).

The origin may be elsewhere in the atria, in the AV node or even below this.

- *Excessive height*. A tall, peaked P wave (> 2.5 mm) results from right atrial enlargement. Because this is often secondary to pulmonary hypertension, the wave is sometimes referred to as *P pulmonale*.
- *Excessive width*. With left atrial enlargement, the P wave becomes broad and notched, like the letter M. The bifid appearance arises because of slight asynchrony between right and left atrial depolarisation. This is normal, but a pronounced notch often results because of left atrial enlargement in mitral valve disease, and the appearance is then known as *P mitrale*.
- *Absent*. The P wave is missing during junctional rhythm or may be replaced by flutter or fibrillation waves.

PR interval This represents the total time taken for atrial activation and AV nodal delay. It is measured from the start of the P wave to the first deflection of the QRS complex. This may be a

Q wave, but the term PR interval is still used. It is normally 0.14–0.21 seconds long. A shortened PR interval is seen when the impulse originates in junctional tissue, or when there are accessory conduction pathways (e.g. Wolff–Parkinson–White syndrome). An increased PR interval indicates atrio-ventricular block and is more common in the elderly.

QRS interval   This represents the total time taken by ventricular depolarisation, and is measured from the first deflection of the QRS complex (whether a Q or R wave) to the end of the S wave. A value greater than 0.12 seconds (three little squares) is abnormal, and usually indicates an intraventricular conduction disorder (e.g. bundle branch block).

When the depolarisation wave travels through the conduction tissues to the ventricles, it depolarises the left side of the interventricular septum first, then spreads to the right side, reflected as a small initial positive R wave in lead V1. Small septal Q waves register simultaneously in leads I, aVL, V5 and V6. These are normal, and differ from pathological Q waves that may be seen in many leads and are more than two small squares deep and more than 1 small square wide. A large Q wave is normal in aVR.

The shape of the QRS complex varies and, because depolarising of the left ventricle predominates (having the largest muscle mass), the R wave gradually becomes taller from V1 to V6, while the S wave slowly diminishes. The transition point (where S = R) is usually V3. This transition point may move towards V4 in the obese. Poor R wave progression (meaning little or no R wave height change until V4) may indicate an old anterior myocardial infarction.

In general, the size of the S waves and R waves together should not be greater than 30 mm, unless there is ventricular hypertrophy.

QT interval   This represents the complete electrical activity time of ventricular stimulation and recovery (depolarisation and repolarisation). It is measured from the beginning of the QRS complex to the end of the T wave, and varies with heart rate (i.e. the QT interval shortens as the heart rate increases). The QT interval should therefore be corrected for heart rate (QT_c) by the formula:

$$QT_c = \frac{QT}{\sqrt{RR}}$$

where QT is the QT interval and RR is the RR interval. This is an approximation, and does not allow for the effect of drugs and circadian variation. Practically, the QT interval should be less than 50% of the preceding cycle length (RR) and should not exceed 0.46 seconds. A long QT interval may predispose to ventricular tachycardia (torsades-de-pointes).

The QT interval lengthens in heart failure, following myocardial infarction, with hypocalcaemia and with some drugs (antidysrhythmic agents, antibiotics, psychiatric drugs, etc.). It is shortened in hypercalcaemia and hyperkalaemia.

T wave   The T wave results from repolarisation of the ventricles and might, therefore, be assumed to produce a negative deflection. However, because repolarisation takes place in the opposite direction to depolarisation, i.e. from epicardium to endocardium, the T wave is usually positive and has the same axis as the QRS complex. The T wave may be inverted in leads V1 and V2 in healthy individuals and in V3 in healthy negroes.

T waves are normally no more than 5 mm tall in the standard leads or more than 10 mm in the chest leads. Peaked T waves may be seen in hyperkalaemia, myocardial infarction or ischaemia. Flattening or asymmetrical T wave inversion is a non-specific abnormality, but may reflect hypothyroidism or hypokalaemia. T wave inversion depends upon whether the R or S wave is dominant. The T wave is normally inverted in III, aVF, aVR and V1. T wave inversion may be found in myocardial infarction, ventricular hypertrophy or bundle branch block. T wave inversion in two or more of the right precordial leads in the young is termed *persistent juvenile pattern*.

ST interval   The ST segment is measured from the *J point* (at the junction of the S wave and the ST segment) to the start of the T wave, and should be level with the subsequent TP segment. The ST segment is very slightly curved upwards, but is isoelectric. ST displacement or changes in shape are of major importance in electrocardiographic interpretation. Horizontal displacement beyond 1–2 mm upward or 0.5 mm downwards is abnormal. ST elevation typically occurs in myocardial infarction (when the segment is convex upwards) and pericarditis (when the segment is concave upwards). ST depression is found in myocardial ischaemia and with digoxin therapy. Ventricular hypertrophy associates with ST depression over the relevant ventricle.

Benign early repolarisation is responsible for ST elevation in about 1% of the population. It appears almost exclusively in males under 40 years, and disappears as the subject becomes older. It is particularly frequent in those of African origin. There is ST elevation of up to 2 mm in leads V1 to V3 that is often maximal in V4 where the rapid ascending S wave merges with the T wave, making the J point difficult to see. A slight notch is often present on the downstroke of the preceding R wave. The ST segment remains concave, and the T wave is normal. *High ST take-off* is common in the right-sided chest leads, and is usually normal when isolated to V2 and V3, where the ST segment often slopes upwards rather than being flat.

U wave These are low-voltage, broad waves following the T wave that may be seen in healthy individuals, particularly athletes, and are often prominent in hypokalaemia and hypocalcaemia. The origins are not clear, but they are probably part of the T wave, and similarly reflect repolarisation of the ventricular myocardium (Ritsema van Eck et al, 2005). This may have implications for the measurement of the QT interval (QU).

Intraventricular conduction blocks

Intraventricular conduction blocks may be found in patients with or without cardiac disease. The term refers to block of conduction in one or more of the fascicles of the conducting tissue distal to the bundle of His or within the ventricles.

Bundle branch block The main bundle of His divides into two bundle branches (left and right) that depolarise the ventricles, the left ventricle slightly before the right. Either of these bundles may fail to convey the conduction of electrical activity, resulting in asynchronous ventricular depolarisation and contraction. This abnormal activation will alter the shape and duration of the QRS complex, which will lengthen to more than 0.12 seconds. Bundle branch block may complicate 10–20% of cases of acute myocardial infarction

and is more common with anterior myocardial infarction.

Left bundle branch block (LBBB) When the left bundle branch is blocked, septal depolarisation commences from right to left, instead of left to right as normally occurs. Hence, the initial q wave in leads I, aVL, V5 and V6 is lost and is replaced by a small, upright R wave. The right ventricle is then depolarised before the left, which produces an initial R wave in chest lead V1 and an S wave in lead V6. The left ventricle depolarises later, producing a deep wide S wave in V1–V3 and a second R wave (R^1) in V6. The delay in biventricular activation prolongs the QRS duration to more than 0.12 seconds and alters the QRS morphology, such that a W-shaped complex appears in V1 with an M-shaped complex in V6 (Fig. 5.4). There is ST elevation in V1–V3, and ST depression with T wave inversion in V4–V6, standard lead I and aVL.

Right bundle branch block (RBBB) When the right bundle branch is blocked, activation is from the left bundle, and right ventricular depolarisation is abnormally delayed. This produces a secondary R wave (R^1) in the right chest leads and a deep S wave in the left chest leads. The QRS complex is prolonged to greater than 0.12 seconds, and in V1 there is an M-shaped complex (rSR^1 or qR), and in V6 a W-shaped complex (Fig. 5.5). There is ST depression with T wave inversion in V1–V3.

RBBB complicates about 2% of myocardial infarcts and is associated with the later development of complete heart block.

Hemi-blocks The left bundle divides into two hemi-fascicles, an anterior branch running superolaterally and a posterior branch running inferomedially. Each of these may become blocked, either on its own or in addition to the main right and left bundles.

Although hemi-block associates with a slight prolongation of the QRS duration, this is usually not appreciated because the duration is still less than 0.12 seconds. Hemi-block is assumed to be present if there is a change in the frontal QRS axis that cannot be explained by any other cause. Left anterior hemi-block (LAHB) is manifest by left axis deviation to less than −30°, while left

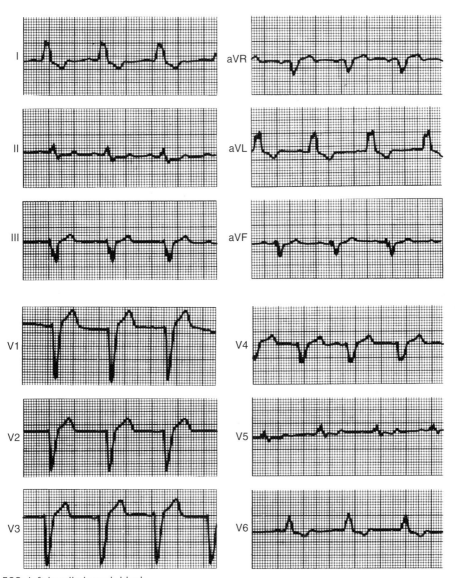

Figure 5.4 ECG: left bundle branch block.

posterior hemi-block (LPHB) produces right axis deviation in excess of +90°. Additionally, QRS morphology may alter to show an RS pattern in lead I and a QR in lead III if there is left posterior hemi-block, while the reverse is seen in left anterior hemi-block.

LAHB complicating myocardial infarction is considered benign, but LPHB is usually only seen with extensive myocardial infarction, and therefore associates with a high mortality.

Bifascicular block means block affecting any two hemi-fascicles, such as RBBB + LAHB/LPHB or LAHB + LPHB. Bifascicular block after myocardial infarction commonly leads to complete heart block, and prophylactic temporary pacing is sometimes carried out.

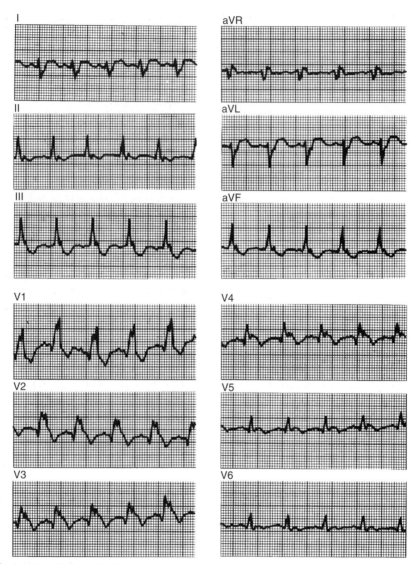

Figure 5.5   ECG: right bundle branch block.

Trifasicular block is a term applied to patients with:

- LBBB and a long PR interval;
- RBBB with alternating LAHB/LPHB;
- LBBB with alternating RBBB.

Such patients have advanced conduction tissue disease, and require permanent cardiac pacing.

Incomplete bundle branch block   This term is used when the morphology of the QRS complex is similar to that observed in established bundle branch block, but the QRS duration is within normal limits (i.e. under 0.12 seconds). The changes are not thought to be due to actual conduction block, but are indicative of delays caused by prolonged depolarisation of enlarged ventricles.

Ventricular hypertrophy   Ventricular hypertrophy increases the amplitude of the QRS complex. Hypertrophy of the left ventricle increases the height of the R waves in V4–V6, while that of the right ventricle increases the height of the R waves in leads V1–V3. Septal hypertrophy produces a large, narrow Q wave in the left-sided chest leads.

The ECG is poor at determining right ventricular hypertrophy and pulmonary hypertension.

Unfortunately, these ECG changes are very non-specific, as many factors can influence the magnitude of the QRS complex, including age, thickness of the chest wall, overexpanded chests (as in chronic obstructive airways disease), hypothyroidism and pericardial effusions. However, the following measurements are suggestive of ventricular hypertrophy ('voltage criteria').

Left ventricular hypertrophy (LVH) LVH is suggested by:

- an R wave in V5 or V6 > 27 mm;
- an S wave in V1 or V2 > 25 mm;
- when the R wave in V5 or V6 added to the S wave in V1 is > 35 mm (40 mm in the young);
- when the R wave in aVF is > 20 mm and the QRS axis is vertical.

Left axis deviation less than −30°, ST depression and T wave inversion in V4–V6 may also be seen. Left atrial abnormalities of dilatation or hypertrophy may also be present suggested by an M-shaped P wave in lead II (P mitrale) or a prominent terminal negative component to P wave in lead V1.

A normal ECG does not exclude significant left ventricular hypertrophy. Similarly, many people with LVH criteria on ECG have a normal left ventricle at echocardiography, particularly if they are young and thin.

Right ventricular hypertrophy (RVH) RVH is suggested by:

- an R wave that is bigger than the S wave in V1, and measures more than 5 mm;
- an R wave in V1 added to the S wave in V5 or V6 that is greater than 11 mm.

Confirmatory evidence is right axis deviation (more than +90°), ST depression and T wave inversion in V1–V3 and possible P pulmonale.

Atrial hypertrophy Because of conduction delay through the hypertrophied atrial muscle, the P wave duration is increased to > 120 ms, seen best in V1.

Left atrial hypertrophy The increased voltage component made by the left atrium may give rise to an M-shaped P wave, the hypertrophied left atrium making a second and delayed peak (P mitrale).

Box 5.2 Some normal resting ECG findings in healthy adults.

Sinus bradycardia or sinus tachycardia
Sinus arrhythmia
Prominent U waves
Wandering atrial pacemaker
First-degree heart block
Second-degree heart block (Mobitz type 1)
Junctional rhythm
High ST take-off/benign early repolarisation
Tall R waves in the chest leads

Right atrial hypertrophy Even when hypertrophied, depolarisation of the right atrium is usually completed before depolarisation of the left atrium, and the P wave duration does not change. However, the additional voltage makes the P wave peak (P pulmonale) to > 2.5 mm, seen best in lead II.

A summary of resting ECG abnormalities found in healthy adults is shown in Box 5.2.

STATIC ECG MONITORING

Monitoring cardiac rhythm forms a vital part of the assessment of patients in coronary care and other high-dependency units, and has had a major impact on reducing mortality from acute myocardial infarction by allowing prompt detection and treatment of dysrhythmias. The results of such monitoring vary according to whether all potentially serious dysrhythmias are recognised. Fatigue, boredom or distraction limits much 'manual' recording, but computer-linked monitors can detect almost all significant dysrhythmias. Personnel from all specialities often care for patients attached to cardiac monitors and should be familiar with electrode placement and monitor operation, as well as being able to recognise and distinguish normal and abnormal rhythms.

Electrodes

Electrodes are small sensors that can be fixed to the skin to allow the electrical activity of the heart to be detected and transmitted to the monitor for amplification and display. Great advances have been made in the design of these electrodes, and modern disposable, self-adhesive electrodes usually obtain excellent skin contact with minimal or no skin preparation. If the signal is poor, the following may be tried:

- Shaving the skin. Not only will skin contact be enhanced, but the patient will also be grateful during electrode removal.
- Rubbing the skin with dry gauze or a wooden spatula will remove loose, dry skin (the stratum corneum) and aid electrode contact.
- Wiping the skin with alcohol will remove excess tissue debris, body oil and sweat.

The electrode site should be examined daily for allergic skin reactions, but otherwise there is no need to change the electrodes routinely, unless the signal becomes poor. Non-allergenic electrodes may be used if the patient is sensitive to the adhesive, and any inflammation may be treated with a small quantity of 1% hydrocortisone cream.

The monitor wires either clip or snap on to the chest wires, although it is preferable to do this before the electrodes are placed on the chest, so that the patient is not hurt if pressure is required to push them on.

The monitor cable

The signals detected by the electrodes are transmitted to the monitor by a cable. At the distal end, this comprises thin wires about 30 cm (12 inches) in length, which connect directly to the surface electrodes. These may be of different colours or labelled 'right', 'left' and 'ground' (or 'earth'). These correspond to the right arm electrode (RA), the left arm electrode (LA) and the right leg electrode (RL) respectively. Multichannel cables may allow a full 12-lead ECGs to be recorded. The contacts with the electrodes should be clean and compatible with the surface electrodes being used. The wires should be inspected regularly for breaks in the insulation and any bends or knots. It is useful to form a 'stress loop' with this part of the cable to prevent traction on the electrodes and monitor connections, with consequent electrode separation and movement artefact.

The bedside monitor

The monitor displays the patient's ECG tracing on a continuous basis. Where there is a central monitoring system with a central console, the ECG pattern is duplicated for all monitored beds and occasionally for telemetry units too.

The monitor uses the interval between the tallest component of the complexes (usually the R wave) to calculate the heart rate. False heart rates may be registered if, for example, the T wave is of amplitude equal to that of the R wave, as this will be read as another QRS complex. The amplitude of the complexes may be adjusted by using the gain control or, if this is insufficient, another lead can be selected by the lead selector control. This control allows the ECG complexes to be recorded in different selected patterns without moving the chest electrodes. A three-electrode system allows the standard limb leads I, II and III to be selected. Five-electrode systems allow leads aVR, aVL and aVF to be obtained as well, and 12 leads will allow a full 12-lead ECG to be displayed. Alarms are set to sound when predetermined parameters are met or exceeded.

Most bedside units have a secondary trace under the actual 'real-time' trace. Depending on the degree of sophistication, this holds a memory loop of a few seconds to many minutes. It may allow specific rhythm retrieval and a 'hard copy' rhythm strip to be obtained for more detailed examination or to provide a permanent copy for the patient's records.

Monitoring

Standard electrocardiographic limb leads (I, II and III) are normally used for basic ECG monitoring. Chest electrodes are placed in the two infraclavicular spaces (right, negative; left, positive) and at the right sternal edge (earth), which are areas free from underlying muscular masses, thus minimising muscle potential artefact. In this configuration, a tracing similar to standard limb lead I is obtained, but leads II and III may be achieved by lead selection on the monitor. Dysrhythmias may be recognised in any lead, but using chest lead V1 is often the best, because it clearly demonstrates the P wave and usually

MCL$_1$ (modified CL$_1$)

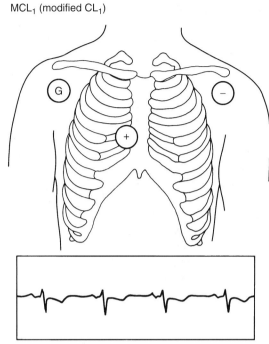

Figure 5.6 Modified chest lead 1 (MCL$_1$). +, positive electrode; −, negative electrode; G, ground electrode (from Jowett et al, 1985, reproduced by kind permission of Churchill Livingstone).

allows clear differentiation between ventricular ectopic beats and those arising from the supraventricular region but being conducted aberrantly. Recording chest lead V1 is reproduced by modifying the chest leads as shown in Figure 5.6. The positive (+) electrode is placed in the normal V1 intercostal space (fourth right), while the negative (−) and the earth (G) electrodes are located near the left shoulder and right shoulder respectively. Modern coronary care practice utilises continuous 12-lead electrocardiography, which allows both rhythm interpretation and ST segment monitoring.

Computerised monitoring

Although visual observation of the monitor by a trained observer was originally used on many units (and is still usual on general wards), many dysrhythmias were missed. The use of computers for the detection of dysrhythmias in acute care units and for the review of rhythms over an extended period is now usual. Computer technology has led to the development of monitors that are able to recognise most dysrhythmias and sound alarms appropriately. Analysis can be performed at various levels of sophistication, from simple dysrhythmia recognition to full reporting of standard 12-lead ECGs. Using a storage mode, display of premature ventricular beat counts and trend analysis is possible for a 24-hour period.

AMBULATORY ECG MONITORING

Abnormalities of cardiac rhythm are common and may affect individuals with or without cardiac disease. Such abnormalities may be detected by static monitoring but, if the dysrhythmia is infrequent or transient, extended monitoring techniques are required (Crawford et al, 1999). The standard 12-lead ECG provides little information about cardiac rhythm. The average ECG records about 50 complexes, typically taken with the patient lying down and at rest. Static monitoring techniques also have their limitations and are unsuitable for the detection of short rhythm disturbances, especially if induced by exertion or other factors in the daily life of the patient (Jowett & Thompson, 1985; Jowett et al, 1985). Documentation of abnormal electrical activity may require prolonged continuous recording during exercise. Ambulatory ECG monitoring was initially designed to document transient disturbances in heart rhythm and conduction, with the aim of establishing a relationship between symptoms and accompanying disturbances in cardiac rhythm. The role of ambulatory monitoring has now expanded to assessing antidysrhythmic therapy, detecting ischaemia and determining prognosis.

Norman 'Jeff' Holter put forward ideas for a portable ECG recorder in the late 1940s and, hence, these recording machines are often known as 'Holter recorders'. From the initial bulky, short-duration recorders, these monitors have been refined to light, small, strong machines capable of recording the heart rhythm continuously for several days, often with multiple channels of ECG data being recorded simultaneously. Improvements in digital technology have improved data acquisition, and allow electronic or telephonic transmission of ECG data.

The classic Holter monitor continuously records an electrocardiographic signal for 24–48 hours, and does not need patient activation. The recording allows capture of both symptomatic and asymptomatic dysrhythmias as well as documentation of circadian variation in pulse rate. The device is battery operated and is connected to bipolar electrodes that allow the recording of two or three different leads. The data are converted to a digital format and are analysed by software that helps to identify abnormalities in heart rhythm. A diary of timed symptoms and the referral note are of major value during tape analysis and interpretation.

Event recorders store only a brief period of ECG activity when activated by the patient in response to symptoms. These devices often miss the onset of the rhythm disturbance, or may miss the event completely if the episode is brief.

Continuous-loop event recorders record the ECG continuously, but store only a brief period of ECG recording in the memory when the patient activates the event marker at the time of symptoms. The small monitor is worn around the neck or attached to the patient's belt and uses two patch electrodes applied to the patient's chest. The duration of saved data is programmable, but will typically keep recordings of rhythm before and after the event marker.

Event and loop recorders can be loaned to the patient for prolonged periods of time to identify infrequently occurring arrhythmias or symptoms that would not be detected by conventional 24-hour continuous recorders.

Implantable loop recorders (e.g. Reveal Plus) are subcutaneously placed, leadless recorders with a battery life of approximately 18 months. The recorder is small (about the size of a pack of chewing gum), requires no electrodes and can be implanted quickly and easily under local anaesthetic. The recorder may be interrogated through the skin, and removed when no longer needed (Seidl et al, 2000). While direct patient activation of the insertable loop recorder through a small handheld activator is the primary means of capturing a symptomatic dysrhythmic event, the Reveal Plus can automatically detect significant bradycardic and tachycardic events to supplement patient activation.

High-speed electrocardioscanners are used to analyse the data. Presentation of the data depends upon the clinical circumstances. A full disclosure presentation can print all the complexes in miniature, which is particularly useful for identifying periods of interest. If the patient has experienced symptoms, these periods may be selectively recalled, with a normal-sized ECG printout, including the periods before and after the event. Precise timing is noted on the strips, to allow comparison with the patient's diary, to correlate symptoms and dysrhythmias with confirmation of a dysrhythmia-induced symptom. Asymptomatic recordings do not usually help, although evidence of asymptomatic abnormalities, such as short runs of ventricular tachycardia or ischaemic episodes, may help in further management. Up to a third of recordings will be normal despite the presence of symptoms during the recording period. On the other hand, ambulatory monitoring may disclose many dysrhythmias in apparently normal individuals. These are not necessarily pathological but, currently, there are no consistent ways of separating normality from abnormality. Most of the general population have isolated ventricular ectopic beats, two-thirds have sinus bradycardia, and about one-fifth have very brief episodes of atrial fibrillation. About 0.2% of apparently healthy adults have periods of ventricular bigeminy. Pauses of 2–3 seconds are very common in athletes, who have high vagal tone. In general, rhythm disturbances are more important (and are tolerated less well) in the elderly. The interpretation of the pathological significance of rhythm abnormalities is very much dependent on the circumstances.

Telemetric units

Telemetry is often used for extended peri-infarction cardiac monitoring. The patient is fitted with standard chest electrodes attached to a small transmitter carried in a chest harness or the pyjama pocket. The cardiac rhythm is transmitted continuously to a receiver (normally situated in the CCU), where it is displayed, observed and analysed in the same way as for patients on static monitors. The advantage of this system is that patients may be mobilised in the early period following myocardial infarction, while still having the benefits of dysrhythmia monitoring. The transmission range of these units is usually short, and thus relatively free from extrinsic radiointerference. Longer range units have been developed for use by cardiac arrest teams who may be further away from the receiver units, and by ambulance and paramedic teams outside the hospital. In both cases, the cardiac rhythm may be monitored and advice on drug therapy may be given by more experienced physicians 'back at base'.

PULSE OXIMETRY

Pulse oximetry is a simple non-invasive method of monitoring the percentage of haemoglobin that is saturated with oxygen (SaO_2). Oxygen saturation tells us how much of the oxygen-carrying capacity of the haemoglobin is being utilised. Hence:

Oxygen saturation ($SaO_2\%$) =

Amount of oxygen being carried by the haemoglobin

Amount that can be carried by the haemoglobin

The pulse oximeter consists of a probe attached to the patient's finger or ear lobe, which is linked to a computerised unit that displays the percentage of haemoglobin saturated with oxygen.

How oximetry works

The principle of oximetry was developed following the simple observation that oxygenated blood is usually red whereas deoxygenated blood appears blue. When the two are mixed, the ratio of oxygenated to deoxygenated arterial blood can be measured by the amount of red and infrared light absorbed by the different colours as a light sources shines through the capillary beds in the extremities. The oximeter probe contains the two light-emitting diodes that shine towards a detector located opposite. The diodes are rapidly switched on and off, and the detector records how much of the two types of light have been absorbed on their passage through the capillaries. To eliminate the light-absorbing effects of other tissues, the resulting signal registers only the readings from blood pulsating in the capillaries (hence 'pulse' oximetry). The corresponding arterial oxygen saturation is calculated as an average based on the previous few seconds of recording and is constantly being updated.

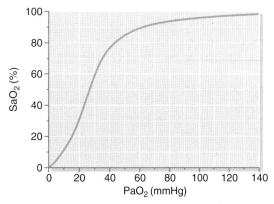

Figure 5.7 The oxyhaemoglobin dissociation curve.

When haemoglobin carries oxygen, it is converted to oxyhaemoglobin, and the amount of oxygen that can be carried is closely related to the PaO_2 of the blood. This relationship is shown by the oxyhaemoglobin dissociation curve (Fig. 5.7). Importantly, this relationship is not linear, but 'S' shaped so, while a saturation of over 97% equates with a normal PaO_2 of over 97 mmHg, an apparently minor fall in saturation to 90% actually equates to a fall in the PaO_2 to 60 mmHg. This is because of the rapid descent at the end of the plateau, where saturation falls quite quickly as the PaO_2 declines. The consequence of this is that, if the SaO_2 is found to be less than 80%, there is usually severe hypoxia (PaO_2 of under 45 mmHg), and arterial blood gases should be taken urgently. Target saturation during oxygen therapy will vary with such changes as pCO_2, pH and body temperature, which cause lateral shifts in the oxygen dissociation curve, either to the left or to the right. In general, oxygen is needed if the SaO_2 is less than 90%. Oximeters give no information about the level of $PaCO_2$, and cannot give warning of respiratory failure associated with carbon dioxide retention.

Problems with oximetry

The pulse oximeter can only function if enough pulsatile blood passes between the light source and the detector. If tissue perfusion is poor or the pulse is weak, the generated signal will be liable to error. Movement artefact is common when the probe slips across the skin whenever the hand is moved. A lopsided probe will allow light from the two light emitters to pass directly into the detector, and not through the tissues of the finger. Persistent limb tremor is an occasional problem best circumvented by application of the ear probe. Excessive ambient light from sunlight or flickering fluorescent lights may saturate the detector and cause erroneous readings.

Compounds that absorb light at the same wavelengths as haemoglobin and oxyhaemoglobin will introduce errors (e.g. nail varnish!). The microprocessor in the oximeter is programmed to parameters derived from the normal oxyhaemoglobin dissociation curve, and abnormal haemoglobins may produce errors. In most cases, the oximeter will underestimate the true saturation, but of far more concern are situations in which the oximeter may overestimate saturation, particularly in the presence of carboxyhaemoglobin, which may form 5–10% of the total haemoglobin in heavy smokers.

HAEMODYNAMIC MONITORING

The ability to recognise and assess serious circulatory changes in patients with acute coronary syndromes is of major importance, both diagnostically and for assessing therapy and prognosis. While clinical examination of the patient remains of major importance, it may be difficult to assess some patients without invasive monitoring. For example, infarction of the right ventricle may complicate one-third of inferior myocardial infarctions and is associated with a low left atrial pressure, despite elevation of the jugular venous pressure. In patients with longstanding cardiac failure, selective peripheral vasoconstriction may maintain blood pressure, while masking a low cardiac output. This group of patients may also develop thickening of the pulmonary vessel walls, allowing a substantial rise in pulmonary capillary pressures before the clinical signs of pulmonary congestion develop. So, while the patient may be judged to have mild left ventricular failure on clinical grounds, haemodynamically, there may be pulmonary hypertension, with a substantial reduction in cardiac output.

The term 'haemodynamic monitoring' describes methods of monitoring blood pressure, blood volume and circulation, usually by indwelling catheters inserted into the heart or major blood vessels.

The catheters are connected by fluid-filled tubing to pressure transducers and recording systems. The most frequently measured parameters in coronary care are the pulse, arterial blood pressure, central venous pressure (CVP), intracardiac pressures and cardiac output. In recent years, many techniques have become available that permit easy bedside analysis of the patient's haemodynamic status and cardiac function. The precise method of obtaining and recording these haemodynamic data varies from hospital to hospital and is usually dependent upon the expertise of the staff and available equipment. Typical indications for invasive monitoring are shown in Box 5.3.

Once the catheter has been inserted, it is usually the responsibility of the nursing staff to ensure the patient's comfort and safety and the maintenance of the system, and to obtain and record data. As the patient's treatment will often rely heavily on the results of monitoring, it is essential that such data are accurate. The nurse should be aware of problems inherent in data acquisition, including common technical and physiological variables that may affect the data. In addition, they should be aware of the effect that specific nursing interventions (e.g. feeding, bathing and positioning) may have on haemodynamic measurements.

Pressure transducer systems

Pressure transducers are electromechanical devices that detect energy changes (e.g. those in pressure and temperature) and convert them to electrical signals. In most forms of haemodynamic monitoring,

---

Box 5.3   Some indications for invasive haemodynamic monitoring.

Cardiogenic shock
Unexplained hypotension
Haemodynamic instability with suspicion or presence of:
- Pulmonary embolism
- Right ventricular infarction
- Aortic dissection
- Mechanical heart defects (e.g. ruptured interventricular septum or papillary muscle)

they detect intravascular pressure changes and convert them into electrical charges for amplification and digital readout. Usually, pressure changes are transmitted via fluid-filled tubing to a supple diaphragm located in a transducer dome. Pressure waves detected by the diaphragm are transmitted to a strain gauge. The more the diaphragm is moved by the pressure waves, the greater is the electrical charge generated and the higher the pressure reading on the monitor.

Measuring the central venous pressure (CVP)

Central venous pressure monitoring is used to measure the pressure of blood in the right atrium or superior vena cava. The CVP reflects right ventricular end-diastolic pressure (filling pressure or preload) and is determined by blood volume, vascular tone and cardiac performance. Elevation of the CVP is common following acute myocardial infarction, usually reflecting raised right-sided pressures secondary to left ventricular failure. Other causes are right ventricular infarction and cardiac tamponade. Low CVP readings are usually due to hypovolaemia, when infusion of fluid may improve cardiac performance.

CVP catheters are inserted percutaneously, usually into the subclavian or jugular veins, and are advanced to lie in the superior vena cava or right atrium. During central venous catheterisation, it is important that the patient is placed in the Trendelenburg position (i.e. head down). This distends the central veins, which not only reduces the risk of air embolism, but also makes cannulation easier. The right side of the patient is chosen preferentially to prevent damage to the thoracic duct. Placement of the catheter is confirmed by chest radiograph, which will also exclude a pneumothorax.

The CVP is often measured using manometry although, because of the sluggish response, an electrical pressure transducer may be preferred, particularly if continuous display of the CVP is required.

Manometry

The manometer should be placed with the baseline at the level of the right atrium. The baseline may be at zero on the scale, but it is preferable to set it at a higher value (e.g. 10 cm), so that negative pressures may be recorded. A spirit level should be used to ensure that the zero reference points on both the patient and the manometer coincide. The line should be well flushed, by opening up the intravenous fluid line. Free passage of fluid through the system should occur when the infusion rate is turned up, and blood should be freely aspirated if required. Respiratory oscillations should be visible.

Figure 5.8 Central venous pressure (CVP) monitoring, showing stopcock positioning.

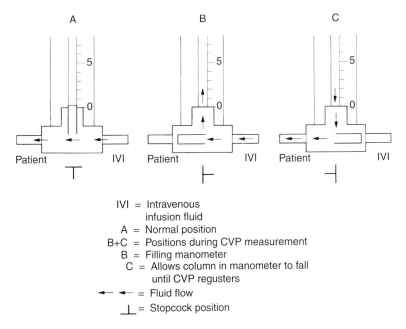

IVI = Intravenous
infusion fluid
A = Normal position
B+C = Positions during CVP measurement
B = Filling manometer
C = Allows column in manometer to fall
until CVP regusters
= Fluid flow
⊥ = Stopcock position

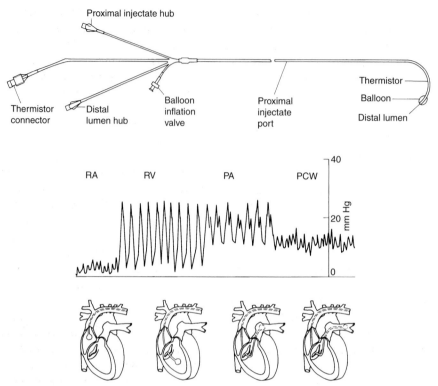

Figure 5.9   The Swan–Ganz thermodilution catheter and typical pressures recorded during its passage through the heart (from Stokes & Jowett, 1985, reproduced by kind permission of Churchill Livingstone).

Turning the stopcock from the normal position A to position B (Fig. 5.8) should fill the manometer column. The stopcock is then turned to position C, and the fluid is allowed to run down and equilibrate through the CVP line. Normally, the fluid falls freely, although it fluctuates with venous pulsation and respiration. Once the column has settled, the CVP should be measured at the end of expiration and expressed in cmH_2O (normal = 0–10 cmH_2O).

Following CVP measurement, the stopcock should be returned to position A, and the infusion rate adjusted as required.

Electrical pressure transducers

This method is most frequently used when measurements are made via the right atrial port of a four-channel Swan–Ganz catheter (Fig. 5.9). The reading recorded by the transducer is displayed in mmHg (normal = 0–8 mmHg). Correlation of CVP in mmHg and cmH_2O is shown in Table 5.1.

Positioning the patient is extremely important during measurement of the CVP. Ideally, the patient should be lying flat, without a pillow but, if the patient's condition does not permit this,

Table 5.1   Conversion of mmHg to cmH_2O (approximate).

(mmHg × 1.36 = cmH_2O)	
1 = 1	11 = 15
2 = 3	12 = 16
3 = 4	12 = 16
4 = 5	13 = 18
5 = 7	14 = 19
6 = 8	16 = 22
7 = 10	17 = 23
8 = 11	18 = 24
9 = 12	19 = 26
10 = 14	20 = 27
(cmH_2O/1.36 = mmHg)	

he can be positioned at 45° or less. During normal respiration, the intrathoracic pressure falls on inspiration. Measuring haemodynamic pressures at end expiration is considered to be the most valid, because the intrathoracic pressure is closest to zero at this point.

Intra–arterial blood pressure monitoring

In haemodynamically unstable patients, measurement of the blood pressure is often difficult, and indirect readings may differ from the actual arterial blood pressure by over 30 mmHg. The insertion of an arterial pressure line is then useful for directly and continuously measuring systolic, diastolic and mean arterial blood pressures, as well as for giving easy access for repeated blood gas sampling. Sites commonly employed are the radial, brachial and dorsalis pedis arteries. However, the closer the cannula is to the heart, the more accurate the waveform and pressure reading, and so the radial artery is the most commonly utilised site.

Cannulation is performed under local anaesthetic, using a 20-gauge Teflon catheter, which is attached to a T-connector and a pressurised heparin/saline flushing system. This runs continuously at 3–5 mL/hour to minimise clotting, vasospasm and intimal damage. A transducer converts the pressures into a digital readout and displays the arterial waveform. The readings displayed are systolic blood pressure, diastolic blood pressure and mean blood pressure. It should be noted that the mean arterial pressure (MAP) is not half the sum of the systolic and the diastolic pressures, but is a measurement that integrates the area under the arterial waveform curve to obtain a true mean.

Complications of intra-arterial monitoring are not common but include arterial spasm and occlusion, bleeding and air embolism. When the line is removed, pressure over the insertion site should be maintained for at least 5 minute, or longer if thrombolytic agents or anticoagulants have been used.

Pulmonary artery and pulmonary artery wedge pressures

Pulmonary artery (Swan–Ganz) balloon flotation catheters are sometimes helpful in assessing patients with low cardiac output, hypotension, severe pulmonary oedema and cardiogenic shock (Stokes & Jowett, 1985). They allow quick and easy differentiation of inadequate intravascular volume with a resultant low left-sided filling pressure, and adequate intravascular volume and a high left-sided filling pressure due to extensive left ventricular dysfunction.

Insertion requires central venous cannulation, which may be particularly hazardous in patients who have recently been thrombolysed. Inappropriate use or use by the inexperienced may associate with increased mortality and morbidity (Manikon et al, 2002). A meta-analysis of trials in which patients were randomly assigned to monitoring by Swan–Ganz catheterisation or not found that the catheter had no effect on mortality and hospital stay (Shah et al, 2005).

THE CHEST RADIOGRAPH (CXR)

In patients presenting to hospital with chest pain, about 25% of chest radiographs will be abnormal, showing such abnormalities as cardiomegaly, pulmonary oedema or consolidation, making it a worthwhile routine investigation. However, it should be remembered that radiation exposure requires justification under the European Union ionising radiation (medical exposure) regulations, 2000. This is a legal requirement.

The standard postero-anterior (PA) chest radiograph is taken at full inspiration, with the patient standing facing the film, which is 1.5 m away from the X-ray tube focus. In the standard PA view, the right border of the heart consists (from top to bottom) of the superior vena cava, the ascending aorta and the right atrium. The left border is formed by the aortic arch, the descending aorta, the pulmonary artery and the left ventricle (Fig. 5.10). A standard PA chest film should always be requested where possible because:

- the diaphragm is flattened and allows the bases of the lungs to be seen;
- the erect position lowers hydrostatic pressure in the low-pressure pulmonary vascular tree;
- the scapulae are slid away from the lung fields;
- the PA projection reduces magnification of the heart shadow.

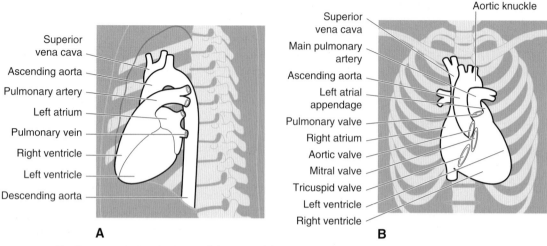

Figure 5.10   Cardiac anatomy on the lateral (A) and PA (B) chest radiograph.

The radiograph should be assessed by a routine method so that nothing is missed.

Technical quality

Conventional chest radiographs still use films, but modern picture archiving communication systems (PACS) now use digital technology that stores the image on a reusable photostimulation plate. This is usually stored within a computer database, but can allow printing on to film. All images should be correctly identified and dated. Right and left markers will avoid a misdiagnosis of dextrocardia. If the film is taken straight, the medial ends of the clavicles should be equidistant from the midline, marked by the spinous processes of the vertebrae. If the patient is rotated, the CXR may suggest cardiomegaly or hilar tumours. An underpenetrated film will enhance lung markings, often leading to an erroneous diagnosis of pulmonary congestion, and is particularly common in the obese patient. The images generated on PACS can be manipulated electronically, allowing contrast changes and magnification if required. A previous radiograph image can easily be recalled for comparison.

The heart

The cardiac size is assessed radiologically by determining the cardiothoracic ratio (CTR). This is the ratio of the widest part of the heart shadow to the widest transverse thoracic diameter, measured from the inner surface of the ribs. The CTR should be less than 50% in adults, but assessing cardiac size radiologically may be misleading. Cardiomegaly is common in athletes and does not necessarily indicate dilatation or hypertrophy. Apparent cardiomegaly may be a feature of those who are obese when fat pad is sometimes seen adjacent to the cardiac border. If the patient has not fully expanded their lungs, the heart shadow may also suggest cardiomegaly. The diaphragm should expand to the level of the fifth rib anteriorly on full inspiration.

The heart may appear enlarged because of individual chamber enlargement or an overall increase in size. The most frequent causes of significant cardiac enlargement are dilatation due to volume overload (heart failure) or pericardial effusion. Large effusions make the heart outline globular, but small effusions are hard to detect radiologically and are best detected by echocardiography. Hypertrophy normally leads to a volume reduction within the heart chambers, so that the overall cardiac diameters are only very slightly increased.

The lung fields

The normal divisions of the pulmonary artery can be traced to within about a centimetre of the lung edge. The pulmonary veins are larger, and horizontal in the lower lung fields, but are seen as smaller linear opacities draining towards the left atrium in the upper lung fields. As pressure in the pulmonary veins rises (as in heart failure), there is increasing congestion seen in the pulmonary vessels until a critical pressure of about 30 mmHg is reached, which marks the onset of frank pulmonary oedema. Pulmonary congestion occurs first in the lower pulmonary veins, where perivascular interstitial oedema develops, resulting in local hypoxia and reflex vasoconstriction in the affected vessels. The blood is then shunted to the upper lung vessels (upper lobe diversion), producing a characteristic radiological picture. The interstitial oedema collects around hilar vessels to produce the 'bat wing' sign, and perivascular cuffing may be seen as thickened and blurred walls of end-on bronchi near the hilum. Oedema in and around the pulmonary lymphatics gives rise to thin linear opacities called Kerley lines. The *Kerley A lines* (engorged intralobular lymphatics) run from the periphery to the hilum, and the more common *Kerley B lines* (septal lines) of interstitial oedema are short parallel lines that run horizontally at the lung peripheries, particularly in the costophrenic angles. As the pulmonary oedema worsens, fluid collects in the alveoli of the lower zones, producing opacities, and later outside the lung to produce pleural effusions.

In patients with longstanding pulmonary hypertension and heart failure, there may be thickening of the pulmonary vessel walls, allowing substantial elevation of pulmonary capillary pressures without clinical congestion.

There may be a lag of up to 48 hours between haemodynamic stabilisation and resolution of radiological signs, so frequent chest radiographs are not helpful. The presence of any of the signs of acute pulmonary congestion reliably indicates acute congestive heart failure (CHF), but absence does not exclude it (Mueller-Lenke et al, 2006).

The mediastinum

The position and size of the aorta should be noted. Unfolding of the aorta is common in the elderly and hypertensive patient, and calcification of the aortic knuckle may be seen. An increase in the size of the aortic outline with widening of the mediastinal shadow may indicate aortic dissection, particularly in the presence of a small left pleural effusion.

Bones

Sternal depression (pectus excavatum) may displace the heart and is the cause of a systolic murmur with apparent cardiac enlargement (the 'straight back' syndrome). This may only be visible with a lateral chest film. The heart shadow will also be displaced if there is a thoracic scoliosis. Rib lesions such as fractures or metastases may be a cause of the presenting chest pain.

The neck and upper abdomen

A retrosternal goitre may be misdiagnosed as an aortic aneurysm. The presence of intraperitoneal air (air under the diaphragm) should be excluded, as peritonitis may present with chest and shoulder tip pain.

ECHOCARDIOGRAPHY

Echocardiography allows the heart to be studied non-invasively, and is a powerful tool for assessing cardiac anatomy, pathology and function. The echocardiogram uses a transducer that generates high-frequency pulses of short duration, which travel through the body at differing velocities, depending upon the tissues encountered, and are echoed back, to be recorded by the same transducer. Cardiac ultrasound uses frequencies of 1.9–10.0 MHz, and the higher the frequency, the better the resolution (although the worse the tissue penetration).

The two main techniques used are M-mode and cross-sectional (real-time or two-dimensional) echocardiography. The Doppler shift effect during ultrasound can be combined with these techniques to provide information on the velocity and direction of blood flow. Colour flow mapping uses a multigated, pulsed Doppler technique to estimate the mean velocity of blood cells within the heart and can identify patterns of blood flow and abnormal jets.

Transthoracic echocardiography is the usual method of obtaining cardiac images by ultrasound. The transducer is placed on the chest wall to obtain different views of the heart through anatomical 'windows'. The technique is limited by the size of these windows found between the ribs and the lungs, as ultrasound does not travel through bone or air. Technical difficulties may be encountered in up to one-quarter of recordings.

Transoesophageal echocardiography (TOE) uses a miniature transducer mounted on a modified endoscope, which may be swallowed and positioned directly behind the heart. The image quality is much better because of the proximity of the structures as well as the absence of bone. Biplane probes incorporate two transducers at right angles to each other, and multiplane probes can permit a 180° view of the heart. The probe uses very high frequencies as depth is not so important, which allows very high resolution. The investigation is invasive, and requires adequate facilities and staff. There is a risk of both morbidity (inhalation, bleeding, oesophageal perforation) and even death. The study including preliminary transthoracic imaging takes about 1 hour. Patients should be prepared as for a minor operative intervention with fasting for 4–6 hours, intravenous access, a consent form and nurse escort.

Indications for TOE include assessment and diagnosis of infective endocarditis and aortic dissection, assessment of prosthetic heart valves and the detection of left atrial thrombus in patients with atrial fibrillation prior to cardioversion.

Cross–sectional echocardiography

Two-dimensional images are built up by the ultrasound beam being swept through a 90° sector of the heart, producing up to 50 cross-sections per second, and generating a recognisable 'real-time' moving image of the heart. Lung tissue impedes the passage of ultrasound, so the two most commonly used 'windows' for ultrasound imaging are between the ribs, over the cardiac apex and at the left sternal edge. The most easily understood projection is the apical four-chamber view, in which both ventricles are visualised from base to apex, along with both atrio-ventricular valves and both atria. Rotation of the transducer along its axis images the left ventricular outflow tract and the two chambers of the left heart (apical long-axis and two-chamber views). The parasternal views provide images of the mitral and aortic valves, left ventricle, left atrium, right heart and proximal aorta. Most modern machines use second harmonic imaging

where reception is at twice the frequency of the transmitted wave, which improves image quality.

The images are usually recorded on super-VHS videotape or digitally on optical discs. Photographs can be obtained as a hard copy to file with the notes. Online computers can be used to measure cardiac dimensions and calculate various parameters, such as ejection fraction and cardiac output.

M–mode echocardiography

The 'motion' or M-mode echocardiogram uses ultrasound transmitted and received along a specific line of interest and produces a graph of depth of tissues against time. A single 1-cm ultrasound beam is directed through the heart using a scan line selected from the two-dimensional image. Cardiac motion is sampled approximately 1000 times/second, thereby increasing temporal resolution and enabling greater appreciation of the movement of cardiac structures. The graph is recorded on rapidly moving paper, which allows the measurement of intracardiac structures (such as wall thickness and cavity dimensions) with timing of events. The M-mode trace does not demonstrate cardiac anatomy and probably should not be interpreted without reference to the cross-sectional image. It is principally used to measure chamber size and wall thickness, but is also helpful in precisely timing cardiac events such as systolic anterior motion of the mitral valve (SAM) in patients with hypertrophic cardiomyopathy (HOCM).

Doppler echocardiography

Doppler can be used to assess the direction and velocity of moving blood by measuring the change in frequency of an ultrasound impulse reflected from red blood cells. If they are moving towards the ultrasound transducer, they will shorten the wavelength of the returning signal; if they are moving away, the wavelength lengthen. The greater the velocity of red blood cells, the larger the frequency shift. The returning signals are displayed graphically, with velocity on the vertical axis plotted against time horizontally. By convention, velocities obtained from blood moving towards the transducer are displayed above the baseline, and those moving away below. In addition, the density of the signal reflects the number of red cells moving at the indicated velocity. Blood velocity can be measured by either pulsed or continuous wave ultrasound.

Pulsed wave (PW) Doppler assesses the velocity of blood at one site, selected by a cursor superimposed on the two-dimensional image. Signals are transmitted intermittently and received after a set delay. This enables the velocity of blood within a defined area to be examined, but limits the maximum velocity that can be measured. PW Doppler is mainly used to determine the pattern of ventricular filling through the mitral valve in diastole, to assess flow patterns in the pulmonary and hepatic veins and to measure the blood velocity in the left ventricular outflow tract. Doppler tissue imaging, using low-frequency ultrasound, can be used to measure the slower velocities of myocardial tissue. This is particularly useful in measuring the velocity of the mitral valve annulus during diastole – an indicator of myocardial relaxation that is relatively unaffected by loading conditions and is thus helpful in defining diastolic function.

Continuous wave (CW) Doppler signals are transmitted and received constantly. They measure frequency shifts along the entire length of the ultrasound beam and are most useful for measuring high velocities (such as those that occur across a stenotic aortic valve). The beam can be steered within the two-dimensional image so that specific areas of the heart can be interrogated. The signal can, however, originate from any point along the length of the beam.

Colour flow echocardiography

Colour Doppler flow mapping has been one of the most important developments in cardiac ultrasound since cross-sectional echocardiography, and has allowed a better understanding of flow physiology in health and disease. As red blood cells move through the heart at relative high velocities, the Doppler shift can be detected and assigned a colour depending upon the direction and velocity of blood flow. The blood flow information is displayed over the two-dimensional or M-mode image and, by convention, flow towards the transducer is displayed in red, flow away from the transducer is coloured blue, and turbulence produces a mosaic of different colours. Different colour maps can be applied depending upon operator preferences. The technique is very sensitive and can detect the trivial regurgitation that occurs through normal valves when they close, so overinterpretation of the images is possible. For example, around 90% of the normal population have tricuspid and pulmonary regurgitation and one-third have mitral regurgitation.

Colour flow imaging is invaluable in the detection of abnormal flows within the heart and great arteries. It may be combined with M-mode echocardiography for timing flow events and distinguishing between systolic and diastolic abnormalities.

USES OF ECHOCARDIOGRAPHY

Assessment of left ventricular function

Although it often possible to identify patients with significant left ventricular systolic dysfunction clinically, echocardiography can quantify the severity and may help to determine the underlying cause. In addition, many patients with heart failure have concomitant or predominant diastolic dysfunction, which may be more difficult to detect clinically. Because regional wall abnormalities can corrupt estimates of global function, left ventricular systolic function is often assessed subjectively and graded as normal or mildly, moderately or severely impaired. Many requesting echo assessment of the left ventricle want to know the ejection fraction, but echocardiographic estimation is notoriously inaccurate, particularly if there is regional ischaemic dysfunction.

Murmurs

Cardiac murmurs are caused by turbulence of blood, which may be due to valvular heart disease, increased flow across a normal valve or shunts related to congenital or acquired defects. Echocardiography is the investigation of choice to define the aetiology and assess the severity of the underlying abnormality. Many heart murmurs are benign, and are not always accompanied by an echocardiographic abnormality.

Atrial fibrillation

Atrial fibrillation is common, often related to valvular or coronary heart disease, hypertension or cardiomyopathy, and an echo should be carried out in all patients. In those under 50 years, there may be no associated abnormalities of cardiac structure or perfusion (lone atrial fibrillation). Although echocardiographic findings are not the sole determinants of a patient's suitability for cardioversion, those with major structural abnormalities, left ventricular systolic dysfunction or a left atrial diameter of over 4.5 cm are unlikely to maintain sinus rhythm, even if an initial attempt works.

Stroke

Up to a fifth of ischaemic neurological events may be caused by a cardioembolic source, particularly in younger patients who have a lower prevalence of significant atherosclerosis. Neurological events in multiple cerebrovascular territories make a cardiac source more likely. Echocardiography rarely shows intracardiac thrombus (unless contrast is used), but often reveals abnormalities that could predispose to embolisation, such as mitral valve disease or a left ventricular aneurysm. Rarely, stroke may be secondary to infective endocarditis.

Echocardiography and coronary care

A modern, two-dimensional ultrasound machine is an essential piece of equipment for the coronary care unit, because it is non-invasive, has rapid acquisition time and can be brought to the bedside. In patients with cardiovascular collapse of unknown cause, echocardiography can quickly differentiate between hypovolaemia, severe left ventricular dysfunction, pulmonary embolism and pericardial effusion with tamponade. The intimal flap of an aortic dissection can be seen in many cases of aortic dissection, and critical aortic stenosis can also be demonstrated and quantified.

Other frequent applications of echocardiography in patients on coronary care include:

- *Defining the aetiology of cardiomegaly.* Clinical and radiological cardiomegaly may be due to ventricular dilatation, ventricular hypertrophy or pericardial effusion. Echocardiography allows the correct interpretation.
- *Supporting the diagnosis of ischaemic chest pain.* Healthy myocardium thickens and contracts inwards in systole. In ischaemic myocardium, contraction may be diminished (hypokinesis) or, in extreme cases, absent (akinesis). Akinesis usually indicates infarcted tissue, which may also show disco-ordinate contraction and cause the myocardial wall to bulge outwards in systole (dyskinesis). Regional left ventricular wall dyskinesia is a feature of myocardial ischaemia and may occur before there are any ECG changes. Stress echocardiography, using exercise or pharmacological stress, may be used to detect regional wall motion abnormalities (see below).
- *Assessing complications of myocardial infarction.* Echocardiography is essential for the prompt diagnosis of the mechanical complications of acute myocardial infarction. It can quickly distinguish between acute mitral incompetence and an acquired ventriculo-septal defect, and is an essential investigation in patients with cardiogenic shock, to distinguish severe left ventricular damage from right ventricular infarction or cardiac rupture with tamponade.
- *Assessment of cardiac failure.* Echocardiography should be carried out in all patients presenting with heart failure to establish the aetiology and severity (Cheesman et al, 1998).
- *Assessing prognosis.* Stress echocardiography has been used to assess residual ischaemia and define prognosis following acute myocardial infarction, although standard treadmill testing is appropriate for most patients. Intravenous myocardial contrast echocardiography may be a useful tool to assess reperfusion following thrombolysis or angioplasty (Kaul, 1999).
- *Miscellaneous problems*
  1 *Vegetations* over 3 mm in size may be demonstrable in over half the patients with infective endocarditis. They are seen as rapidly moving masses attached to, or replacing, normal cardiac tissue. TOE is usually required for confirmation of the diagnosis and to show complications such as mycotic abscesses.
  2 *Mitral valve prolapse* is common (depending upon precise definitions) and is easily identifiable with echocardiography. Patients may

present with dysrhythmias or atypical chest pain.

3   *Hypertrophic cardiomyopathy (HOCM)* may present with chest pain and dysrhythmias. The ECG is usually abnormal, but the diagnosis may be confirmed with echocardiography.

4   *Prosthetic valve function* may need to be assessed in coronary care admissions to ascertain whether valvular dysfunction is the source of symptoms. TOE is the best way to assess valve dysfunction because of artefactual signals from the prosthesis that are a particular problem with transthoracic echocardiography.

STRESS ECHOCARDIOGRAPHY

Acute myocardial ischaemia is accompanied by the development of regional left ventricular wall motion abnormalities initiated by the 'ischaemic cascade' (Fig. 5.11). These wall motion abnormalities serve as a marker of the presence and location of flow-limiting coronary arterial stenoses and may be determined by stress echocardiography (Marwick, 2003). Stress echocardiography uses exercise or pharmacological stress to diagnose coronary artery disease, detect myocardial viability or assess prognosis.

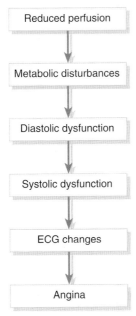

Figure 5.11   The ischaemic cascade.

A dobutamine infusion is the most commonly used pharmacological stressor, and it increases myocardial oxygen consumption through increments in heart rate and blood pressure. Vasodilator agents such as adenosine and dipyridamole are an alternative, and work by diverting blood away from diseased coronary vessels (coronary steal), which occurs in the setting of severe or extensive coronary disease. For diagnostic indications, the sensitivity of dobutamine echo is somewhat greater, especially in patients with single vessel disease. Serious complications occur in about 3 in 1000.

The left ventricle is viewed in parasternal and apical views, often using *acoustic quantification*, an automatic online computerised technique that helps to detect the interface between the left ventricular endocardial surface and the blood displayed on the two-dimensional image. It enables beat-to-beat estimation of the ejection fraction, and using colour enables regional wall abnormalities to be highlighted. Myocardial thickening is assessed before, during and after stress, and global and regional function is evaluated using a scoring system for regional wall motion abnormalities. Digital imaging allows side-by-side comparison of regional function at rest and during stress. Motion abnormalities are recorded in different segments of the left ventricle, allowing correlation with the expected coronary anatomy.

The sensitivity and specificity of stress echocardiography are much better than exercise stress testing, especially in women, and comparable with nuclear stress testing. It is, however, very operator dependent, as well as being time-consuming. Not all patients are good echo subjects, which may also limit its application.

Contrast echocardiography uses microbubbles to produce a cloud of echoes as they pass through the heart, which is easily detectable by echocardiography. The technique has been used to detect right-to-left shunts, for example through septal defects, and may be used to define the endocardial border of the left ventricle, to better assess intracardiac thrombus and wall motion artefacts.

Tissue Doppler imaging (TDI) uses Doppler pulses on the valves and myocardium. Colour assignment helps to determine both the velocity and the direction of tissue movement, and is thus a powerful technique for assessing regional wall abnormalities and determining global left ventricular function. Another potential use of tissue Doppler is the localisation of accessory conduction pathways prior to radiofrequency ablation (e.g. in the Wolff–Parkinson–White syndrome). Premature ventricular activation through the accessory pathway is accompanied by earlier contraction in that area.

Real-time three-dimensional (RT3D) echocardiography imaging provides a more accurate estimation of left ventricular mass, quantification of intracavity volumes, mitral valve structure and congenital anomalies.

Portable echocardiography is now possible to take to the patient who is critically ill, or even at home. It may complement clinical examination in the CCU, and can carry out most basic echo functions, with excellent images. Portable echocardiography is likely to extend to non-cardiologists in many different clinical areas (e.g. GP surgeries, emergency departments). Adequate training is vital.

Intravascular ultrasound (IVUS) provides a cross-sectional, three-dimensional image of the full circumference of a coronary artery, and allows precise measurements of plaque length, thickness and lumen diameter. It may therefore be used to clarify ambiguous angiographic findings and to identify wall dissections or thrombus. It is most useful during percutaneous coronary intervention, when target lesions can be assessed before, during and after the procedure and at follow-up. Stents that seem to be well deployed on angiography may actually be suboptimally expanded. Unfortunately, the procedure is expensive and requires experience. As such, it is not a routine procedure.

EXERCISE STRESS TESTING

Many patients with cardiac disease have no signs, symptoms or abnormal investigations at rest, and exercise stress testing may reveal hitherto

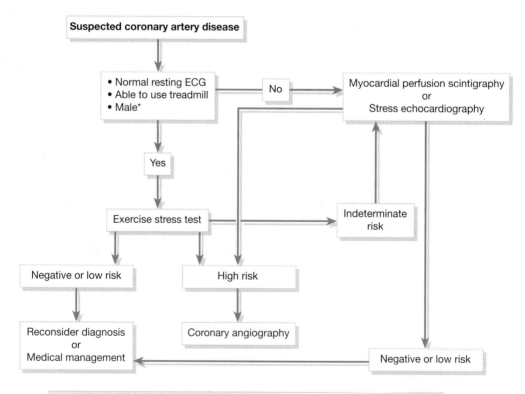

Figure 5.12 Investigation of suspected angina.

undocumented abnormalities. Exercise tolerance testing with continuous 12-lead ECG monitoring is the first non-invasive test for the evaluation of suspected ischaemic chest pain (Fig. 5.12). The main aims of stress testing are:

- to provoke symptoms, such as chest pain and dyspnoea;
- to demonstrate ECG changes with progressive workload;
- to determine maximum workload;
- to assess prognosis.

The procedure has a low complication rate, although any investigation of patients with myocardial disease carries a risk. If patients are carefully selected for exercise testing, the rate of serious complications (death or acute myocardial infarction) is about 1 in 10 000 tests. The incidence of ventricular tachycardia or fibrillation is about 1 in 5000 tests. Full cardiopulmonary resuscitation facilities must be available, and test supervisors must be trained in cardiopulmonary resuscitation. The British Cardiac Society (1993) has drawn up guidelines for performing exercise tests in the absence of direct medical supervision.

Despite a wealth of experience and a great deal of published work on the investigation, controversy still surrounds the interpretation of the test. Exercise testing has a sensitivity of 78% and a specificity of 70% for detecting coronary artery disease. It cannot therefore be used to rule in or rule out ischaemic heart disease unless the probability of coronary artery disease is taken into account. For example, in a low-risk population (e.g. young women), a positive test result is more likely to be a false positive than true, and negative results add little new information. In a high-risk population, a negative result cannot rule out ischaemic heart disease, although the results may be of some prognostic value. Exercise testing is therefore of greatest value in patients with a moderate probability of coronary artery disease, rather than in those with low or high probability. Despite its limitations, it remains an extremely useful tool.

While ECG changes are important, it is important to interpret these in the context of symptoms, pulse and blood pressure response and recovery time following exercise. The specificity of ST segment depression as the main indicator of myocardial

ischaemia is limited, and may be seen in 20% of normal individuals on ambulatory electrocardiographic monitoring. In general, early onset of angina, marked and widespread ST depression, slow recovery and a poor blood pressure response are indicative of severe ischaemic heart disease.

If the resting electrocardiogram is abnormal, the usefulness of an exercise test is reduced or may even be precluded. Repolarisation and conduction abnormalities (e.g. left ventricular hypertrophy, left bundle branch block) or patients taking digoxin make accurate interpretation of the electrocardiogram during exercise very difficult, and other forms of exercise test (for example nuclear scans) or angiography are required for evaluation.

Methods of stress testing

Stress testing is usually performed with a treadmill or bicycle, the choice being largely determined by the available space. There are several contraindications to stress testing, which are shown in Box 5.4.

Box 5.4   Contraindications to ECG stress testing.

Cardiac (absolute)

Within 2 days of acute myocardial infarction
Unstable angina (not stabilised)
Uncontrolled symptomatic heart failure
Acute myocarditis or pericarditis
Severe aortic stenosis
Serious uncontrolled dysrhythmias

Cardiac (relative)

Moderate stenotic valve disease
Severe hypertension
Hypertrophic cardiomyopathy
Heart block (advanced)

Non-cardiac considerations

Anaemia
Elderly or infirm patient
Gross obesity
Severe respiratory disease
Digoxin toxicity
Electrolyte imbalance

Table 5.2 Bruce protocol for exercise (treadmill) ECG test.

Stage	Speed (mph)	Gradient (%)	Duration (min)	METs (units)	Total time (min)
1	1.7	10	3	4.6	3
2	2.5	12	3	7.0	6
3	3.4	14	3	10.1	9
4	4.2	16	3	12.9	12
5	5.0	18	3	15.0	15
6	5.5	20	3	16.9	18
7	6.0	22	3	19.1	21

Exercise testing for patients on coronary care is best performed close to the CCU for safety reasons.

The patient is first connected to the exercise ECG machine. Resting electrocardiograms, both sitting and standing, are recorded as electrocardiographic changes, particularly T wave inversion, may occur as the patient stands up to start walking on the treadmill. A short period of recording during hyperventilation is also valuable for identifying changes resulting from hyperventilation rather than from coronary ischaemia.

Recommended lead systems for detecting regional myocardial ischaemia may employ 2–20 electrodes. The simplest and most useful lead for recording is MCL5 (the positive lead in the V5 interspace and the negative on the manubrium), which will demonstrate up to 90% of detectable abnormalities. However, the most common lead system uses the normal 12-lead recording positions using the torso rather than the limbs for the limb leads, to prevent entanglement and to reduce movement artefact.

There are many different protocols designed for different circumstances and available equipment (ACC/AHA, 1997). The protocol should offer:

- an appropriate workload for the patient, which will not cause excessive stress;
- A gradually increasing workload, with enough time at each level to attain steady state;
- continuous ECG, heart rate and blood pressure recording;
- resuscitation facilities.

The most common test in the UK uses the Bruce protocol (Bruce et al, 1963), which produces a fast increase in progressive workload (Table 5.2). The protocol has seven stages, each lasting 3 minute, with the speed and incline of the treadmill increasing with each stage. Automatic ECG recorders will usually record a full 12-lead ECG at predetermined time intervals, and the test is continued until completion or another endpoint has been reached (Box 5.5). At the end of testing, the level of the test achieved [with timing and metabolic equivalent (MET)] should be recorded, with the reason for stopping. All symptoms and blood pressure readings should be recorded.

The modified Bruce protocol is much slower, taking 21 minute to reach the 12-minute equivalent

---

Box 5.5   Endpoints of the exercise stress test.

Absolute

Fall in systolic blood pressure > 10 mmHg
  with ischaemia
Signs of poor perfusion (pallor, cyanosis)
Patient request
Sustained ventricular tachycardia
ST elevation in leads without Q waves
Moderate or severe angina

Relative indications

Attainment of target heart rate (220 – age in
  men; 210 – age in women)
Fall in systolic blood pressure > 10 mmHg
Increasing chest pains
Exaggerated hypertensive response
Marked ST–T wave changes
Dysrhythmias

Table 5.3   Modified Bruce protocol for exercise (treadmill) ECG test.

Stage	Speed (mph)	Gradient (%)	Duration (min)	METs (units)	Total time (min)
1	1.2	0	3	1.9	3
2	1.7	0	3	2.3	6
3	1.7	5	3	3.5	9
4	1.7	12	3	4.6	12
5	2.5	14	3	7.0	15
6	3.4	16	3	12.9	18
7	4.2	18	3	15.0	21
8	5.0	20	3	16.9	24
9	5.5	22	3	19.1	27

of the Bruce protocol (Table 5.3), but it is more suited to older patients or those with recent myocardial infarction or stabilised acute coronary syndrome.

Oxygen uptake (VO$_2$) and metabolic equivalents (METs)

The rate of oxygen uptake by the body relates to the ability to achieve a given workload. At rest, oxygen uptake (VO$_2$) is about 3.5 mL/kg/minute, and is described as 1 MET (1 metabolic equivalent). Average peak VO$_2$ in cardiac patients is about 21 mL/kg/minute (6 METs). As exercise protocols differ, effort capacity should be expressed in METs. Those who can achieve around 10 METs (9 minute of the Bruce protocol) have a prognosis with medical therapy as good as those with operative intervention, and those who can achieve 13 METs (stage 4 of the Bruce protocol) have an excellent prognosis regardless of other exercise responses. The patient should be encouraged to exercise for as long as possible, but signs of fatigue, pain and dyspnoea should be noted, especially in the stoic patient.

Results

There are various parameters that can be observed and assessed during an exercise test, such as:

1 *Symptomatic*: onset of symptoms and relationship to exercise. Angina during exercise is predictive of coronary disease, particularly if accompanied by ECG changes.

2 *Haemodynamic*: changes in blood pressure and heart rate. Blood pressure may fall or remain static during the initial stage of exercise as the patient relaxes. Thereafter, the systolic blood pressure should rise as exercise increases, sometimes to levels up to 225 mmHg. Diastolic blood pressure tends to fall slightly. The maximum predicted heart rate is calculated as 220 (210 for women) minus the patient's age. A satisfactory heart rate response is achieved on reaching 85% of the maximum predicted heart rate. A fall in systolic blood pressure associates with poor prognosis in patients with coronary heart disease.

3 *Electrocardiographic*: changes in the ST segment and cardiac rhythm.

During exercise, the P wave increases in height and the R wave decreases in height. The QT interval shortens and the T wave decreases in height. J point depression is normal (the junction of the S wave and ST segment), so that the ST segment slopes sharply upwards. Abnormalities include:

• *ST depression* that worsens with increasing exercise, returning to normal on stopping, is very suggestive of myocardial ischaemia. The greater the ST depression, and the longer it persists into recovery, the greater the likelihood of coronary disease. The absence of such changes does not exclude coronary disease. The standard criterion for an abnormal ST segment response is horizontal (planar) or downsloping depression of more than 1 mm over at least three consecutive complexes. If 0.5 mm of depression is taken, the sensitivity of the test increases and the specificity decreases (vice versa if 2 mm of depression is selected). By convention, ST segment depression is measured relative to the isoelectric baseline (between the T and P waves) at a point 60–80 ms after the J point. There is intraobserver variation in the measurement of this ST segment depression and, therefore, computerised analysis can assist, but not replace, the clinical evaluation of the test. Up to 50% of patients will demonstrate ST depression without pain, but the absence of pain probably indicates a better prognosis (except in diabetes). ST depression *after* exercise often indicates coronary disease, but ST depression on the pre-exercise ECG, which normalises with exercise to return after exercise, usually indicates a normal heart. Some patients depress the ST segment during hyperventilation or changes in body position. Beta-blockade and exercise may abolish these changes.

- *ST elevation* usually represents left ventricular dyskinesia in leads over an old infarct or aneurysm. In the absence of a previous history, or Q waves, ST elevation suggests severe transmural ischaemia, and is thus a sign of poor prognosis.
- *T wave changes* such as inversion and pseudo-normalisation (an inverted T wave that becomes upright) are non-specific changes.
- *U wave inversion* is a highly specific sign for ischaemia but, as U waves are often difficult to identify, especially at high heart rates, this finding is not sensitive.
- *Rhythm abnormalities* may be provoked or suppressed. The presence of extrasystoles that have been induced by exercise is neither sensitive nor specific for coronary artery disease. Supraventricular ectopic beats will be provoked in a third of normal people. *Ventricular dysrhythmias* usually associate with coronary artery disease. The more complex these are, the more likely there is coronary disease or poor left ventricular function.
- *Bradycardia and hypotension* post exercise are usually benign.
- *Bundle branch block* may develop during exercise in some patients. It is usually rate dependent (over 125 beats/minute) and benign but, at lower heart rates, may suggest coronary or conduction disease.

Misleading results

False-positive tests

Many normal people may develop ST depression on exercise (10% of men and 25% of women), usually related to hyperventilation or increased sympathetic tone. Some young women without heart disease may be found to have widespread ST/T wave changes on the resting ECG, which worsen (often dramatically) on exercise. Treadmill stress testing is therefore of limited value in women (Sullivan et al, 1994) and in those with pre-existing repolarisation abnormalities such as bundle branch block, ventricular hypertrophy, digoxin therapy or hypokalaemia.

False-negative tests

These may occur because:

- Coronary disease is mild.
- The patient has good collateral coronary arteries.
- The ECG leads do not cover the affected myocardium.
- Drug therapy may delay the onset of ECG changes (e.g. beta-blockers).
- The test has been submaximal. Tests should be reported as inadequate rather than negative if the heart rate is under 85% of the predicted maximum.

The Duke treadmill score

This scoring system has been used to improve the sensitivity of treadmill stress testing. It combines exercise time, symptoms and ST segment shift to divide patients into high-, low- and intermediate-risk groups (Shaw et al, 1998). The score also correlates with the angiographic severity of coronary disease, and high-risk patients usually require coronary artery bypass surgery.

Indications for exercise stress testing

There are three main reasons for exercise stress testing:

- assessing patients with chest pain;
- assessing prognosis;
- assessing other exercise-related symptoms.

Assessing patients with chest pain

The major indication for exercise stress testing is for diagnosis of the cause of chest pain. Unfortunately, ST changes are not always present during exercise in patients with angiographically defined coronary artery disease, especially if lesions are limited to the circumflex and distal right coronary arteries. Typical pain during stress testing usually indicates coronary disease, even if there are no ECG changes.

Assessing prognosis

Stress testing may be used for:

- risk stratification after myocardial infarction;
- risk stratification in patients with hypertrophic cardiomyopathy;
- evaluation of revascularisation or drug treatment;
- evaluation of exercise tolerance and cardiac function (e.g. dilated cardiomyopathy or heart failure);
- assessment of treatment for dysrhythmias.

Exercise testing has become routine in most hospitals to determine prognosis in patients with ischaemic heart disease. The greater the degree of ST segment shift on exercise, the greater the chance of significant multivessel disease. The exercise time is very important and is often used for risk stratification and to determine mortality (Table 5.4).

The prognosis of patients following myocardial infarction is mostly dependent on left ventricular function, which may be reflected by workload and blood pressure response to formal exercise, as well as circulation to the unaffected myocardium. Patients with low exercise capacity and hypotension induced by exercise have a poor prognosis. Asymptomatic ST segment depression is associated with a more than 10-fold increase in mortality compared with a normal exercise test. Conversely, patients who reach stage 3 of a modified Bruce protocol with a blood pressure response of over 30 mmHg have an annual mortality of under 2%. Inability to perform the test and/or a rise of less than 30 mmHg in the systolic blood pressure seem to identify the high-risk patients and are predictive of future cardiac events.

Symptom-limited exercise stress testing may be carried out safely before discharge in selected patients following myocardial infarction. Typically, these are patients under 65 years of age, without dysrhythmias, recurrent ischaemic pain or cardiac failure. Information on functional capacity is not only useful for prognostic reasons, but may also help in advising on future activities and the appropriateness of rehabilitation. The usual recommendation is that predischarge tests should be limited to 5 METs (about 12 minute of the modified Bruce protocol). For logistical reasons, exercise testing often has to be carried out following discharge from hospital. Those patients who were unable to have a predischarge stress test should have a symptom-limited test performed prior to their first outpatient appointment. Patients without post-infarct angina and without ST changes during exercise stress testing do not need coronary angiography. Those with abnormal tests should be assessed further, usually by coronary angiography.

Assessing other exercise-related symptoms

The aetiology of atypical anginal pain, dyspnoea, palpitations and dizziness may all be clarified by

Table 5.4 Mortality for patients with coronary heart disease assessed by the Bruce exercise test (Coronary Artery Surgery Study, 1983).

Stage completed	Mortality at 12 months	24 months	Risk
Stage III	1%	5%	Low
Stage II	2%	11%	Intermediate
Stage I	5%	19%	High

an exercise test. Functional capacity can be gauged by an objective assessment of the severity of symptoms and the degree of limitation imposed by cardiac or other disease. Occasionally, intermittent dysrhythmias may be recorded, and an exercise test may form part of the evaluation of patients with suspected cardiac rhythm abnormalities.

In patients with cardiac failure, an exercise capacity of less than 6 METs associates with decreased survival.

CARDIAC CATHETERISATION AND CORONARY ANGIOGRAPHY

Selective coronary angiography was introduced in 1958 and, despite advances in imaging techniques, it is still considered the gold standard for defining the anatomy of the main epicardial coronary arteries. In non-urgent cases, routine angiography without prior non-invasive testing is not advisable, because of the high cost and associated mortality and morbidity.

In addition to coronary angiography, cardiac catheterisation may need to be carried out:

- to record intracardiac pressures and demonstrate pressure gradients;
- to measure cardiac output and detect shunting (by measuring blood gases) at different levels;
- to identify anatomical and functional anomalies, such as ventricular aneurysms and valvular disease.

Providing the catheter laboratory is handling between 1500 and 2000 diagnostic cases per year to ensure efficient use of the facility, and the competence of the staff, there is no reason why these cannot be located in district general hospitals.

Coronary angiography

Before the procedure, patients usually fast and may be given a sedative. Insertion of an arterial sheath with a haemostatic valve minimises blood loss and allows catheter exchange. Despite local anaesthesia, arterial access may be uncomfortable, although patients do not usually feel catheter manipulation. The catheter is engaged in the opening of the relevant coronary artery (ostium), and 5–10 mL of contrast medium is injected into the

coronary artery through the lumen of the catheter. Moving radiograph images are obtained and recorded using digital image storing techniques to provide a dynamic record of ventricular wall movement, blood flow and intravascular anatomy. Typically, six to eight views are taken of the left coronary artery and three of the right coronary artery.

A pigtail catheter that has additional side-holes may be passed across the aortic valve into the left ventricle for left ventricular angiography. About 30–40 mL of contrast medium is injected by a motorised pump, and provides visualisation of left ventricular contraction over two to four cardiac cycles. Pressures within the ventricle and across the aortic valve in the aorta are also recorded as the catheter is withdrawn ('pull-back' pressures) in cases of aortic stenosis. A gradient of 50 mmHg or more usually indicates that surgery is required. Echo gradients measure instantaneous gradients that normally differ by more than 10 mmHg and may overestimate the severity of aortic stenosis. Pull-back gradients are underestimated if there is poor left ventricular function.

Modern contrast agents only rarely cause nausea and vomiting, but may cause a transient hot flush and a strange hallucination of urinary incontinence. Transient angina may occur during injection of contrast, especially if there is diffuse or severe arterial disease.

After completion of the procedure, the catheter and sheath are removed, and haemostasis is achieved by manual compression, an arterial closure device (AngioSeal, VasoSeal) or direct repair (Perclose). The femoral artery has traditionally been the preferred access site for angiography, but it is relatively contraindicated in the presence of severe peripheral vascular disease, and is sometimes difficult in patients with hip pain. The rate of complications at the femoral access site is 2–8%. The radial artery has become the access route of choice for many coronary procedures. It virtually eliminates access site complications, and allows rapid mobilisation and discharge (Archibald et al, 2004).

A significant coronary arterial stenosis is usually defined as one that occludes 70% or more of the internal diameter of the coronary vessel (50% for the left main stem artery). Involvement of the

Table 5.5 Survival and coronary artery stenosis (Coronary Artery Surgery Study, 1983).

Number of vessels stenosed > 70%	1-year survival	5-year survival
One	98%	89%
Two	96%	88%
Three	89%	67%
Left main stem stenosis > 50%	71%	57%

right coronary artery is generally less serious than involvement of the left coronary artery. Left main stem stenosis, or stenosis of the left anterior descending artery proximal to the first septal branch, is particularly unfavourable. The number and distribution of coronary vessels stenosed affects prognosis (Table 5.5).

Indications for coronary angiography

Angiography is usually recommended for:

- class I or II stable angina with an early positive exercise stress test;
- class III or IV angina;
- angina not controlled by drug treatment;
- where coronary artery disease cannot be excluded by non-invasive testing;
- patients at high risk following an acute coronary syndrome;
- post-infarction angina (or positive stress test);
- angina after revascularisation.

Following acute transmural myocardial infarction, the need for angiography is usually not urgent, and it is probably better to await healing of the infarct with endogenous remodelling of the coronary vasculature before assessment. Most do not have multivessel coronary disease, and will not need surgery to improve their prognosis. At-risk groups can be identified non-invasively (Cross et al, 1993). Up to 10% of patients will have a significant left main stem stenosis, and 30% will have triple artery disease requiring surgical intervention.

Early angiography (immediately or within a few hours of admission) may be performed following failed thrombolysis ('rescue angioplasty'), or re-infarction, but is made more difficult because of the cumulative anticoagulant effects of aspirin, clopidogrel, heparin and thrombolytic agents. In the GUSTO angiographic study (1993), in which patients underwent angiography within 24 hours of thrombolysis, 6% had major bleeds requiring transfusion, and 1.4% required vascular repair.

Patients with cardiogenic shock and those who develop mechanical complications of myocardial infarction (ruptured papillary muscle or acquired ventricular septal defect) usually undergo angiography with a view to revascularisation and surgical repair. Prior stabilisation with an intra-aortic balloon pump is usual.

Risks of coronary angiography

While coronary angiography is usually a quick and easy investigation, it is invasive and there are associated morbidities and even occasional mortality. The overall complication rate is around 8 in 1000 (West et al, 2006). The commonest complications are transient and minor, including arterial access bleeding and haematoma, pseudoaneurysm, dysrhythmias, reactions to the contrast medium and vagal reactions (during sheath insertion or removal). Athero-embolism to the kidneys is particularly frequent in the elderly, sometimes leading to renal failure (Cuddy et al, 2005). Major complications, although rare in experienced hands, include death (1 in 1400), stroke or myocardial infarction (1 in 1000), coronary artery dissection (1 in 1000) and arterial access complications (1 in 500).

Contrast nephropathy may complicate angiography in some patients, particularly those with prior renal impairment or diabetes. This is hypoxic tubular injury caused by vasoconstriction induced by the contrast, resulting in renal failure, with serum creatinine peaking at 3–5 days after exposure. High-risk patients should be identified prior to investigation (e.g. the elderly and those with hypoxia, hypotension and using non-steroidal anti-inflammatory drugs). Dehydration should be avoided.

Improvements in catheter design and technique have helped to reduce some of these complications but, because more older and sicker patients are now undergoing angiography, overall complication rates have not changed in recent years.

NUCLEAR SCANS AND NUCLEAR ANGIOGRAPHY

In recent years, there has been a rapid development of radioisotope techniques for the assessment of myocardial disease (Hesse et al, 2005). Nuclear scanning can be used to assess:

- myocardial perfusion;
- ventricular function;
- myocardial viability;
- prognosis.

Myocardial perfusion scintigraphy (MPS)

MPS involves the intravenous injection of a radioactive tracer at peak stress to evaluate coronary perfusion of living cardiac muscle. After injection, the tracer is taken up by cardiac muscle cells, is distributed throughout the myocardium in proportion to regional blood flow and may be imaged with a gamma camera. There are three tracers commonly used. *Thallium-201* is a potassium analogue, which concentrates in normal myocardial cells. Overall image quality is not good with thallium, and image interpretation is often hampered by tissue attenuation artefacts from the breasts and diaphragm. Attenuation correction is available on some scanners, which helps to eradicate soft tissue artefact, and *technetium-labelled* sestamibi or tetrofosmin ('Myoview') often produces superior imaging.

Comparison of the myocardial distribution of the tracer after stress and at rest provides information on myocardial viability, inducible perfusion abnormalities and, when ECG gated imaging is used, global and regional myocardial function. Cardiovascular stress can be induced by exercise, but is most commonly induced by pharmacological agents, such as vasodilators (adenosine or dipyridamole) or positive inotropic agents (dobutamine).

Images are obtained after stress and again when the heart is rested 3–4 hours later. Total scanning time is about 20 minute.

Homogeneous uptake of tracer throughout the myocardium indicates the absence of clinically significant infarction or coronary stenosis. A defect in the stress images that normalises in the rest images usually corresponds to a significant coronary stenosis. A defect in both stress and rest images indicates an area of non-viable myocardium, such as myocardial infarction. The distribution of perfusion defects roughly corresponds with the affected coronary artery or arteries. Antero-septal defects indicate disease in the left anterior descending artery, lateral defects correspond with the circumflex artery, and inferior wall defects usually indicate right coronary artery or left circumflex lesions depending upon dominance.

Myocardial perfusion imaging is also of value in defining prognosis. A normal stress perfusion study predicts a risk of cardiac death or myocardial infarction at less than 1% per year, even where there is angiographically proven coronary artery disease. This is the same event rate for the general population without coronary disease. In contrast, those patients with markedly abnormal tests have an event rate approaching 6% per year. Abnormal perfusion tests predict acute coronary syndromes, and left ventricular dysfunction predicts sudden death. Patients with more than 10% of the left ventricle appearing ischaemic derive prognostic benefit from revascularisation. Some indications for MPS are shown in Box 5.6.

MPS was originally developed as a planar (two-dimensional) imaging technique, but SPECT (single photon emission computerised tomography) uses a three-dimensional imaging technique to accurately localise perfusion defects, and is of particular value in identifying the coronary vessel involved. The National Institute for Health and Clinical Excellence (NICE, 2003) recommends SPECT for the diagnosis of suspected coronary artery disease as the preferred investigation when stress electrocardiography causes difficulties in interpretation (e.g. in women and in those with left bundle branch block or diabetes) and for those unable to exercise on a treadmill.

SPECT can provide information additional to that from conventional stress tests or coronary

Box 5.6 Some indications for myocardial perfusion scintigraphy.

As an alternative to exercise stress testing where:

The resting ECG prevents interpretation (e.g. bundle branch block)
Patients are unable to use a treadmill (e.g. amputees)
The patient is female

Where significant coronary disease may still exist following exercise stress testing:

Symptomatic treadmill test without ECG changes
Abnormal ECG changes, but asymptomatic treadmill test

angiography, which may help to risk stratify patients with suspected or known coronary disease or following myocardial infarction, and may avoid the need for percutaneous intervention (Mowatt et al, 2005).

Gated MPS SPECT imaging allows regional and global estimation of left ventricular function. Radioactivity is measured within the heart as it beats and is recorded frame-by-frame by the gamma camera, which is activated by the ECG (8–16 frames per ECG R–R interval). Multiple cardiac cycles are averaged, and this enables regional wall motion to be visualised (for defining dyskinetic segments and ventricular aneurysms) and provides information on ventricular volumes, ejection fraction and cardiac output.

Magnetic resonance imaging (MRI)

MRI is a safe, non-invasive imaging technique that utilises a strong magnetic field to generate a three-dimensional image. *Cardiac MRI* is an evolving technology, providing information on cardiac morphology, perfusion and left ventricular function.

MRI can demonstrate the complications of acute myocardial infarction, including left ventricular aneurysm, intraventricular clot and ventriculo-septal defects. Using ECG gated cine-MRI, left ventricular

function may also be assessed. Perfusion imaging using intravenous gadolinium leads to a better diagnosis and treatment of patients with angina and normal coronary angiograms. The procedure takes less than 20 minute, involves no ionising radiation and has much higher resolution than SPECT scanning. It can also demonstrate transmural perfusion.

Because it uses a strong magnetic field, some patients are not suitable for MRI, such as those with cardiac pacemakers or defibrillators. Scanning should also be avoided in patients with metallic fragments near a vital structure, such as the retina, or with brain aneurysm clips.

MULTIDETECTOR COMPUTERISED TOMOGRAPHIC ANGIOGRAPHY

While angiography remains the gold standard for the investigation of suspected coronary disease, it can only detect advanced atheroma causing obstruction of the coronary lumen. It is also invasive, with a small associated morbidity and mortality. Although there are still some technical difficulties, multidetector (or multislice) computerised tomography (MDCT) could soon replace conventional coronary angiography (Mollet et al, 2005). MDCT is able to confirm the presence or absence of significant coronary stenoses and can also provide an indication of plaque morphology.

MDCT imaging needs to 'freeze' the coronary arteries in the diastolic phase of the cardiac cycle when coronary flow takes place. Hence, drugs are often given to reduce heart rate, prolong diastole and reduce heart rate variability. Early four-detector channel models have been replaced with 64-detector scanners with shorter scan times and improved resolution. As traditional CT scanners are upgraded, the MDCT will be of special value in those hospitals where there is no 'on-site' catheter laboratory (Donnelly et al, 2005).

Electron beam computerised tomography (EBCT)

EBCT is used to detect coronary arterial calcification, and the calcium score derived by scanning may predict the risk from obstructive coronary disease (Nallamothu et al, 2001). Coronary vessel wall calcium is a reliable marker of the total atherosclerotic plaque burden, and includes lesions that may not be seen on angiography.

Positron emission tomography (PET) scanning

Many patients with poor left ventricular function can benefit from revascularisation if non-functional cardiac muscle can be shown to be affected by hibernating or stunning, rather than fibrosis. *Positron emission tomography (PET)* is the most accurate non-invasive imaging technique for detecting myocardial viability, and it employs short-lived tracers of blood flow and metabolism, commonly N-13 ammonia and F-18 fluorodeoxyglucose (FDG). Normally functioning myocardium takes up this FDG, which is a glucose analogue, and PET scanning can differentiate between normal myocardium (preserved contractility and positive FDG uptake), infarcted myocardium (impaired contractility and no FDG uptake) and hibernating myocardium (impaired contractility and positive FDG uptake). Patients with a PET mismatch have been shown to have improvements in mortality and functional capacity following revascularisation (Di Carli, 1998). Unfortunately PET scanners are a very limited resource.

References

ACC/AHA (1997) American College of Cardiology/American Heart Association guidelines for exercise stress testing. *Circulation* 96: 345–354.

Archibald RA, Robinson NM, Schilling RJ (2004) Radial artery access for coronary angiography and percutaneous coronary intervention. *British Medical Journal* 329: 443–446.

British Cardiac Society (1993) Guidelines on exercise testing when there is not a doctor present. *British Heart Journal* 70: 488.

Bruce RA, Blackman J R, Jones JW et al (1963) Exercise tests in adult normal subjects and cardiac patients. *Pediatrics* 32: 742–756.

Cheesman MG, Leech G, Chambers J et al for the British Society of Echocardiography (1998) Central role of echocardiography in the diagnosis and assessment of heart failure. *Heart* 80 (suppl 1): S1–S5.

Coronary Artery Surgery Study (CASS) (1983) A randomised trial of coronary artery bypass surgery: survival data. *Circulation* 68: 939–950.

Crawford MH, Bernstein SJ, Deedwania PC et al (1999) ACC/AHA guidelines for ambulatory electrocardiography: executive summary and recommendations: a report of the American College of Cardiology/American Heart Association Task Force on Practice Guidelines (Committee to Revise the Guidelines for Ambulatory Electrocardiography) *Circulation* 100: 886–893.

Cross SJ, Lee H S, Kenmure A et al (1993) First myocardial infarction in patients under 60 years old: the role of exercise tests and symptoms in deciding who to catheterise. *British Heart Journal* 70: 428–432.

Cuddy E, Robertson S, Cross S et al (2005) Risks of coronary angiography. *Lancet* 366: 1825.

Di Carli MF (1998) Positron emission tomography for assessment of myocardial perfusion and viability. *Cardiology Reviews* 6: 290–301.

Donnelly PM, Higginson JDS, Hanley PD (2005) Multidetector CT coronary angiography: have we found the holy grail of non-invasive coronary imaging? *Heart* 91: 1385–1388.

Dougan JP, Mathew TP, Riddell JW et al (2001) Suspected angina pectoris: a rapid-access chest pain clinic. *Quarterly Journal of Medicine* 94: 679–686.

Gandhi MM, Lampe F, Wood DA (1995) Incidence, clinical characteristics and short-term prognosis of angina pectoris. *Heart* 73: 193–198.

Grant C, Nicholas R, Moore L et al (2002) An observational study comparing quality of care in walk-in centres with general practice and NHS Direct using standardised patients. *British Medical Journal* 324: 1556–1559.

GUSTO Angiographic Investigators (1993) The effect of tissue plasminogen activator, streptokinase, or both on coronary artery patency, ventricular function and survival after acute myocardial infarction. *New England Journal of Medicine* 329: 1615–1622.

Hesse B, Tagil K, Cuocolo A et al (2005) EANM/ESC procedural guidelines for myocardial perfusion imaging in nuclear cardiology. *European Journal of Nuclear Medicine & Molecular Imaging* 32: 855–897.

Jowett NI (1997) *Cardiovascular monitoring*. London: Whurr.

Jowett NI, Thompson DR (1985) Electrocardiographic monitoring. II. Ambulatory monitoring. *Intensive Care Nursing* 1: 123–129.

Jowett NI, Thompson DR, Bailey SW (1985) Electrocardiographic monitoring. I. Static monitoring. *Intensive Care Nursing* 1: 71–76.

Jowett NI, Turner AM, Cole A et al (2005) Modified electrode placement must be recorded when performing 12-lead electrocardiograms. *Postgraduate Medical Journal* 81: 122–125.

Kaul S (1999) Myocardial contrast echocardiography in acute myocardial infarction: time to test for routine clinical use? *Heart* 81: 2–5.

McManus RJ, Mant J, Davies MK et al (2002) A systematic review of the evidence for rapid access chest clinics. *International Journal of Clinical Practice* 56: 4–5.

Manikon M, Grounds, Rhodes A (2002) The pulmonary artery catheter. *Clinical Medicine* 2: 101–104.

Marwick T (2003) Stress echocardiography. *Heart* 89: 113–118.

Mollett NR, Cademartiri F, de Feyter PJ (2005) Non-invasive multi-slice CT coronary imaging. *Heart* 91: 401–407.

Mowatt G, Brazzelli M, Gemmell H et al (2005) Systematic review of the prognostic effectiveness of SPECT myocardial perfusion scintigraphy in patients with suspected or known coronary artery disease and following myocardial infarction. *Nuclear Medicine Communications* 26: 217–229.

Mueller-Lenke N, Rudez J, Staub D et al (2006) Use of chest radiography in the emergency diagnosis of acute congestive heart failure. *Heart* 92: 695–696.

Nallamothu BK, Saint S, Bielak L et al (2001) Electron-beam computed tomography in the diagnosis of coronary artery disease: a meta-analysis. *Archives of Internal Medicine* 161: 833–838.

NICE (2003) *Myocardial Perfusion Scintigraphy for the Diagnosis and Management of Angina and Myocardial Infarction*. Technology Appraisal No. 73. www.nice.org.uk.

Nilsson S, Scheike M, Engblom D et al (2003) Chest pain and ischaemic disease in primary care. *British Journal of General Practice* 53: 378–382.

Pope JH, Aufderheide TP, Ruthazer R et al (2000) Missed diagnosis of acute cardiac ischaemia in the emergency department. *New England Journal of Medicine* 342: 1163–1170.

Ritsema van Eck HJ, Kors JA, van Herpen G (2005) The U wave in the electrocardiogram: a solution for a 100-year-old riddle. *Cardiovascular Research* 67: 256–262.

Seidl K, Rameken M, Breunung S et al (2000) Diagnostic assessment of recurrent unexplained syncope with a new subcutaneously implantable loop recorder. Reveal Investigators. *Europace* 2: 256–262.

Shah MR, Hasselblad V, Stevenson LW et al (2005) Impact of the pulmonary artery catheter in critically ill patients. *Journal of the American Medical Association* 294: 1664–1670.

Shaw LJ, Peterson ED, Shaw LK et al (1998) Use of a prognostic treadmill score in identifying diagnostic coronary disease sub-groups. *Circulation* 98: 1622–1630.

Stokes PH, Jowett NI (1985) Haemodynamic monitoring with the Swan–Ganz catheter. *Intensive Care Nursing* 1: 9–17.

Sullivan AK, Holdright DR, Wright CA et al (1994) Chest pain in women: clinical, investigative and prognostic features. *British Medical Journal* 308: 883–886.

Sutcliffe SJ, Fox KF, Wood DA et al (2003) Incidence of coronary heart disease in a health authority in London: review of a community register. *British Medical Journal* 326: 20.

West R, Ellis G, Brooks N on behalf of the Joint Audit Committee of the British Cardiac Society and Royal College of Physicians of London (2006) Complications of diagnostic cardiac catheterisation: results from a confidential inquiry into cardiac catheter complications. *Heart* 92: 810–814.

Chapter 6

An introduction to the acute coronary syndromes

The term 'acute coronary syndromes' defines clinical expressions of acute coronary artery disease classified by the appearance of the presenting 12-lead electrocardiogram (ECG) and concentrations of cardiac biomarkers detected in the blood. It includes all cases of acute myocardial infarction and unstable angina, whether accompanied by ST elevation or ST depression, or resulting in Q wave or non-Q wave patterns on the ECG.

Acute coronary syndromes result from the abrupt, total or subtotal obstruction of a coronary artery. Occlusion may be transient (and typically recurrent) or permanent and, in most cases, is initiated by rupture or erosion of an atheromatous plaque, with later contributions from thrombus, platelet emboli and coronary arterial spasm.

Clinical presentation of the syndromes depends upon:

- the site of the occlusion (left coronary artery is worse than the right coronary artery; proximal occlusion is worse than distal occlusion);
- whether the obstruction is abrupt or stuttering;
- whether the coronary occlusion is total or subtotal;
- whether a coronary collateral circulation is present.

In the absence of an effective collateral blood supply, persistence of an occlusive thrombus in a major epicardial coronary artery results in transmural myocardial infarction, which later associates with pathological Q waves on the ECG. The presence and degree of myocardial damage following prolonged ischaemia can be assessed in different ways including electrocardiography, concentration of biochemical cardiac markers ('cardiac enzymes'), echocardiography or myocardial perfusion scintigraphy. Individually, and collectively, these methods will give an indication of the extent of myocardial necrosis, residual left ventricular function and, hence, prognosis.

Spontaneous thrombolysis or the relief of coronary arterial spasm sometimes allows reperfusion of the myocardium and relief from the effects of myocardial ischaemia. However, repetitive embolisation of platelets and other debris from the unstable plaque may result in focal myocardial necrosis, often too small to be identified by electrocardiography or traditional cardiac enzymes, but now detectable by sensitive cardiac biomarkers. The presence and magnitude of intracoronary thrombus is directly related to the concentration of serum troponin. The resulting myocardial infarction may be classed as:

- microscopic (microinfarction);
- small (less than 10% of the left ventricle);
- medium (10–30% of the left ventricle);
- large (over 30% of the left ventricle).

In the past, myocardial infarction (MI) has been defined by a combination of two from the three classical characteristics – chest pain, elevation of cardiac enzymes or ECG changes (World Health Organization, 1979). These diagnostic criteria usually meant that a large enough area of myocardium had to infarct, sufficient to produce elevations in non-specific cardiac enzymes [lactate dehydrogenase (LDH), aspartate aminotransferase (AST), creatine kinase (CK)] and/or characteristic ECG changes. Minor infarcts were often not detected, and these at-risk patients were frequently discharged with benign diagnoses such as 'chest pain – MI ruled out' or 'anginal attack'. Where the ECG showed more definite changes, other diagnostic labels such as crescendo angina and subendocardial infarction were applied, made on the basis of negative enzymes and often implying little or no risk. We now know that all acute coronary syndromes (ACS) associate with an adverse prognosis that is amenable to modification if diagnosed correctly and promptly. The risk is not small, and ACS patients presenting without ST elevation on the ECG have a 6-month mortality of between 8% and 13%, and a further 20% will be readmitted to hospital with another episode of unstable coronary disease (Fox et al, 2002). Fortunately, current technology can now quantify as little as 1 g of myocardial necrosis, so about a quarter of patients formerly diagnosed as having unstable angina are now being correctly diagnosed as suffering myocardial infarction (McKenna & Forfar, 2002). This should reduce future morbidity and mortality, although the increased number of patients now diagnosed with acute myocardial infarction may still cause spurious changes in epidemiological data over the next few years. This information should allow healthcare systems to expand to ensure appropriate investigation, treatment and rehabilitation for the increased number of patients who are likely to come to medical attention.

Given the sensitivity of these new biomarkers, the modern definition of acute myocardial infarction is thus based primarily on their typical rise and fall in the blood, which confirms myocardial necrosis. Supportive evidence of an acute ischaemic event is still required in the form of typical symptoms of myocardial ischaemia, acute ST–T wave changes on the ECG or the late development of pathological Q waves (ESC/ACC, 2000).

As diagnosis of acute myocardial infarction is now based upon troponin (or other biomarker) concentrations, there is no threshold below which troponin positivity is without implication. There is continuity from minor cardiac damage detected by minimal troponin concentrations (but negativity of traditional cardiac enzymes) to the classical transmural infarct associated with Q waves on the ECG, large rises in cardiac enzyme concentrations and subsequent complications such as heart failure and dysrhythmias. Troponin elevation also indicates an increased risk of myocardial complications, and helps to identify patients who may derive benefit from early medical or surgical intervention (Morrow et al, 2001).

Although troponin elevation is a true indication of myocardial damage, it does not indicate the *cause* of the damage. A positive result indicates the presence of, but not the underlying reason for, myocardial injury. A variety of conditions may associate with myocyte necrosis (reflected accurately by troponin release) in patients who may not have acute coronary disease (Box 6.1). Even those presenting with an acute cardiological illness, such as tachycardias, pericarditis or heart failure, may have increased troponin concentrations, but no suggestion of an acute coronary syndrome and, while troponin positivity may indicate some myocyte injury, antiplatelet and antithrombotic therapies are unlikely to help. The term *false-positive troponin* should be restricted to problems with biochemical analysis (assay interference).

As many as 40% of acutely ill medical patients may have elevated troponin levels, but no clinical evidence of myocardial ischaemia, and the relevance of a raised troponin level must be made in a

> **Box 6.1** Conditions associated with elevation of cardiac troponin in the blood.
>
> **Ischaemic injury**
>
> *Primary*
>
> Coronary thrombosis (myocardial infarction)
>
> *Secondary*
>
> Distal embolisation of thrombus/atheroma following percutaneous coronary intervention
> Global ischaemia (especially following coronary artery bypass graft)
> Heart failure
> Dysrhythmias
> Renal failure
> Pulmonary embolism
> Severe infections (especially pneumonia)
> Stroke
> Coronary artery spasm (spontaneous or induced by drugs, especially cocaine and amphetamines)
> Extreme endurance sports/marathons
>
> **Non-ischaemic injury**
>
> Cardiac trauma (stabbing, crush injuries)
> Myocarditis
> Hypertrophic cardiomyopathy/hypertension (left ventricular hypertrophy)
> Metabolic (sepsis, multiorgan failure)
> Cardiotoxic drugs (adriamycin, doxorubicin)
> Following laser ablation of electrical pathways
>
> **Assay interference**
>
> Heterophilic antibodies
> Rheumatoid factor
> Fibrin clots
> Skeletal muscle injury

clinical context (Watt et al, 2005). The usefulness of troponin largely depends on the quality of the clinical judgement and the level of clinical probability. A label of myocardial infarction will have many implications for the individual patient in terms of work, life insurance, vocational driving and psychological status, so patients should not be told they have had a heart attack based on a positive troponin alone (Turner, 2003).

CLASSIFICATION OF THE ACUTE CORONARY SYNDROMES

The acute coronary syndromes may be divided into two main groups.

ST elevation myocardial infarction (STEMI)

This is an acute myocardial infarction presenting with ST elevation or new bundle branch block on the ECG, and it defines those patients who require urgent myocardial reperfusion by thrombolysis or primary angioplasty. Diagnosis is based on the clinical history and the standard resting 12-lead ECG alone, although confirmatory evidence may be obtained later by measurement of troponin or other cardiac biomarker concentrations. Acute coronary syndrome patients presenting with ST elevation are likely to be younger and to have fewer diseased coronary arteries than those who present with other acute coronary syndromes.

Unstable angina (UA) and non–ST elevation myocardial infarction (NSTEMI)

Patients with UA/NSTEMI present with symptoms of myocardial ischaemia, but have an admission 12-lead ECG that does *not* show ST segment elevation or bundle branch block. If there is subsequently no elevation in the concentration of cardiac biomarkers, the patient is said to have unstable angina (UA) but, if there is positivity of the markers, the patient will have sustained myocardial damage as a result of the ischaemic event and is said to have a non-ST elevation myocardial infarction (NSTEMI). UA and NSTEMI are referred to as the *unstable coronary syndromes* and are serious, having a 10-year mortality of 70% (Herlitz et al, 2001).

Differentiation of the acute coronary syndromes based on the presenting 12-lead ECG and biomarker concentrations is shown in Table 6.1.

The British Cardiac Society (BCS) has suggested that precise cut-off levels of troponin concentrations should be used to refine the diagnosis, as short-term mortality in patients presenting with an acute coronary syndrome is reflected by the degree of troponin elevation (Fox et al, 2004). The BCS first suggests separation of high-risk

Table 6.1 Differentiation of the acute coronary syndromes.

Clinical syndrome	ECG features	Cardiac biomarkers
Acute myocardial infarction (STEMI – eligible for thrombolysis)	ST elevation (± Q waves) New bundle branch block Posterior infarction	Positive
Non-ST elevation myocardial infarction (NSTEMI)	ST depression T wave inversion Transient or aborted ST elevation Non-specific changes	Positive
Unstable angina (UA)	Any of the above or a normal ECG	Negative

NB Troponin positivity depends upon local assay values, and details should be obtained from the biochemistry laboratory. Blood samples should be assayed within 2 h for maximum reliability.

patients (troponin positive) from low-risk patients (troponin negative), and then dividing those with troponin positivity into those patients with high troponin concentrations from those with lower levels. This latter subdivision is important because those with smaller troponin increases will typically develop any adverse cardiac events (e.g. further infarction or hospitalisation) in days and weeks rather than immediately. High troponin patients will need immediate intervention, but those with lesser degrees of elevation may be dealt with electively. The three BCS classes are termed:

- ACS with unstable angina (undetectable troponin or CK-MB markers, but supporting evidence of coronary disease, e.g. an abnormal ECG or prior documented coronary disease);

- ACS with myocyte necrosis [troponin T < 1.0 ng/mL or AccuTnI < 0.05 ng/mL (or equivalent threshold with other troponin I methods)];
- ACS with clinical myocardial infarction [typical clinical syndrome and troponin T > 1.0 ng/mL or AccuTnI > 0.05 ng/mL (or equivalent threshold with other troponin I methods)].

The different definitions of acute myocardial infarction according to troponin T concentrations are shown in Table 6.2. A troponin T concentration of > 1.0 ng/mL implies a level of risk equivalent to the World Health Organization definition of myocardial infarction.

ACS TRENDS

The relative proportion of patients presenting with unstable angina and myocardial infarction

Table 6.2 Contemporary definitions of acute coronary syndromes (ACS) based on troponin T concentrations.

	Troponin T concentration		
	≤ 0.01 ng/mL	0.01–1.0 ng/mL	≥ 1.0 ng/mL
WHO definition	Unstable angina	Unstable angina	Myocardial infarction
ESC/ACC definition	Unstable angina	Myocardial infarction	Myocardial infarction
BCS definition	ACS with unstable angina	ACS with myocyte necrosis	ACS with clinical myocardial infarction

WHO, World Health Organization (1979); ESC/ACC, European Society of Cardiology/American College of Cardiology (2000); BCS, British Cardiac Society (Fox et al, 2004).

has increased since the widespread use of sensitive biomarkers of myonecrosis that has allowed improved diagnostic accuracy. Extensive application of primary and secondary cardiovascular prevention measures (including revascularisation) is also reducing the severity of acute cardiac presentations. We are no longer seeing the predominance of patients presenting with ST elevation myocardial infarction and left ventricular damage (Dauerman et al, 2000). In our hospital, between 2003 and 2005, STEMI patients represented only 28.7% of all troponin-positive ACS cases admitted. Future coronary care design and organisation will need to change to manage the increasing volume of patients with non-ST elevation acute coronary syndromes, to allow early diagnosis, risk stratification and prompt medical and percutaneous intervention. While virtually all our STEMI patients passed through the coronary care unit (CCU), most NSTEMI patients did not, in part because of the high numbers. This is important, as patients are more likely to receive evidence-based therapies when treated by cardiology specialists in dedicated units (Dorsch et al, 2004).

PREHOSPITAL CARE

Most patients who die as a result of coronary thrombosis do so before reaching the hospital. Ventricular fibrillation or pulseless ventricular tachycardia is the precipitating rhythm of cardiac arrest in most of these deaths, and such dysrhythmias are most likely to develop early following the onset of symptoms. The risk of myocardial infarction and sudden cardiac death are increased during bouts of sudden high-intensity activity, particularly in those who are usually sedentary (Burke et al, 1999).

Treatment of the acute coronary syndromes aims to prevent, or rapidly treat, these acute rhythm disturbances, and preserve left ventricular function by minimising the extent of any myocardial damage. Hence, patients presenting with symptoms consistent with an acute coronary syndrome should be referred to hospital urgently for further assessment, as effective interventions are extremely time-sensitive, particularly for those presenting with ST elevation on the initial ECG. Out-of-hospital electrocardiography, with advanced notification to the receiving facility, speeds the diagnosis, shortens the time to treatment and helps to reduce mortality rates (Canto et al, 1997). Prehospital administration of fibrinolytic agents should be considered for patients with a transport time to hospital of over an hour (Morrison et al, 2001).

TRIAGE

Chest pain is described and experienced very differently by different patients. The severity of the pain is a poor predictor of diagnosis and complications, including cardiac arrest. The initial diagnostic steps should serve two purposes:

- to quickly identify high-risk cardiac patients who need reperfusion ('fast tracking');
- to delineate patients in whom there is little or no suspicion of a life-threatening disorder (e.g. aortic aneurysm, pulmonary embolism).

Separating patients with acute coronary ischaemia from the larger number of individuals who present with non-cardiac pain is a major challenge. Chest pain is one of the most common symptoms presenting to emergency departments, yet only 10–15% of these patients will have an acute coronary syndrome. Three symptom patterns suggest an acute coronary syndrome:

- new onset of severe chest pain suggestive of myocardial ischaemia (less than 2 months);
- abrupt worsening of previous anginal symptoms [symptoms becoming more frequent, more severe, more prolonged and less responsive to glyceryl trinitrate (GTN)];
- chest pain suggestive of ischaemia occurring at rest (often lasting more than 15 minutes).

Patients presenting with acute coronary ischaemia usually indicate pain over a wide area of the anterior chest wall rather than localised pain. The pain might radiate to the arms, as well as to the neck and back. Women more often describe pain radiating to the neck and jaw, or through to the back. When such symptoms develop within the first 2 weeks following acute myocardial infarction, there is a high risk of reinfarction, and these patients should be sent directly to the CCU without delay.

The 12-lead ECG and cardiac biomarkers are the main tools for risk stratification in the emergency setting. A rapid physical examination is helpful to rule out other causes of chest pain, and will detect any immediate complications related to acute myocardial ischaemia. Emergency physicians must be expert in identifying ACS patients and initiate first steps in management (Fig. 6.1). Patients with high-risk features should be admitted to the CCU without delay, but those at intermediate risk may be better evaluated in chest pain units than in the emergency department (Bahr, 2000). These units have been shown to be a safe, effective and cost-saving means of ensuring

appropriate care to patients with unstable coronary syndromes and at intermediate risk of future adverse cardiovascular events (Farkouh et al, 1998).

THE ECG AS A TOOL FOR TRIAGE

The most important investigation is the 12-lead ECG, preferably carried out during an episode of pain. While the main role is to identify those with myocardial ischaemia, the ECG may also reveal important clues such as dysrhythmias, signs of left ventricular hypertrophy, bundle branch block or right ventricular strain (suggesting pulmonary embolism). ECG changes compatible with ischaemia usually confirm the diagnosis of an acute coronary syndrome, but the initial ECG in patients with acute myocardial infarction can

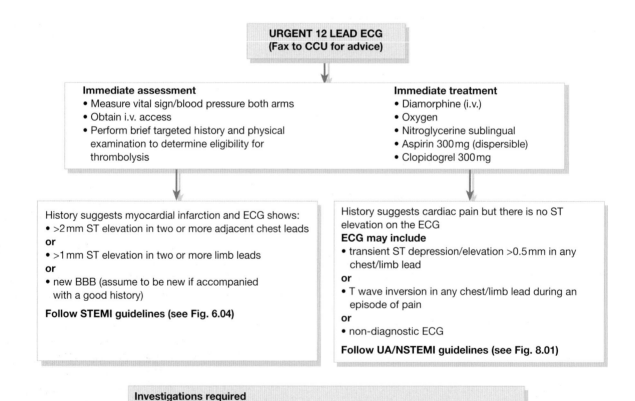

Figure 6.1   Triage of suspected cardiac chest pain.

be normal or non-diagnostic in up to 50% of cases. ST segment depression or elevation is frequently transient in the early stages, so a single ECG represents a 'snapshot' of what is actually a dynamic process. Repeat ECGs can help to identify injury or ischaemia when compared with the baseline ECG. Automated serial 12-lead ECG monitoring is an alternative (Jowett, 1997).

- *ST segment elevation* is the most sensitive and specific ECG marker for acute myocardial infarction, and usually appears minutes after the onset of symptoms. Patients with ST segment elevation or new bundle branch block need immediate consideration for reperfusional therapy (thrombolysis or primary angioplasty).
- *ST depression* signifies severe transmural myocardial ischaemia, and is a significant risk for myocardial infarction and death. These patients usually have triple artery disease.
- *T wave inversion* is a non-specific sign that might indicate various disorders including myocardial ischaemia, myocarditis and pulmonary embolism. Patients often have normal coronary angiograms. However, *deep symmetrical T wave inversion* across the precordial leads may indicate a critical stenosis of the left anterior descending coronary artery (Wellen's phenomenon).

One-month mortality is lowest in patients with simple T wave inversion, intermediate in those with ST elevation or ST depression, and highest in those with ST elevation and depression. The benefit of early revascularisation is proportional to the degree of ST deviation on the presenting ECG in patients with UA/NSTEMI. The risk of death and myocardial infarction may be reduced by 50% by early percutaneous coronary intervention (PCI)/coronary artery bypass graft (CABG) in those with the most extensive ST changes, independent of age, sex or troponin status (Mueller et al, 2004).

SERUM CARDIAC BIOMARKERS

When myocytes are damaged, their cell membrane integrity is lost, and large intracellular proteins leak out and may be detected in the blood. While measuring 'cardiac enzymes' has been routine on CCUs for many years, modern biochemical tests are not for enzymes, so the preferred term is *serum cardiac biomarkers*. The cardiac troponins are currently the best markers for the detection of myocardial damage, and are proving highly effective in the risk stratification of patients with chest pain, reducing unnecessary admissions and allowing targeted drug therapy in high-risk patients. Where troponin estimation is not available, other markers may be used such as total creatine kinase, CK-MB and myoglobin, and these can also be helpful because of their different release profiles (Fig. 6.2). Point-of-care ('near-patient') testing in the emergency department or chest pain unit can accelerate decision-making by providing CK-MB and troponin levels within 15–20 minutes after presentation (Novis et al, 2004).

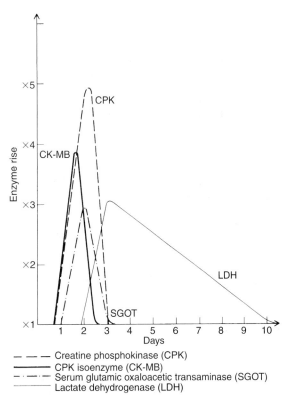

Figure 6.2 Serum cardiac marker release following acute myocardial infarction.

Cardiac troponins

The troponin complex consists of three subunits – troponin C, troponin I and troponin T – and is located on the myofibrillar thin (actin) filament of striated skeletal and cardiac muscle. Troponin T and I are only expressed in cardiac muscle, and assays are available for both that are equivalent in diagnostic and prognostic efficacy.

Troponin is released into the blood within 3 hours of injury to the heart, peaking at 12–24 hours and remaining elevated for up to 14 days. The profile of troponin release is initially similar to that of creatine kinase (see below), but protein-bound troponin is released slowly for many days after the myocardial infarction. Troponin is therefore very useful for making a late diagnosis of myocardial infarction. Restoration of coronary blood flow by thrombolysis is associated with a rapid 'washout' of troponin, so the peak occurs earlier, and levels may be undetectable at 5–7 days (Fig. 6.3). About 50% of patients with acute myocardial infarction will have a positive troponin 6 hours after the onset of chest pain, but it takes 12 hours to become reliably positive in 99% of cases. Hence, if the troponin is not elevated on presentation, it should be repeated 12 hours after the onset of symptoms.

If this is then positive, the diagnosis of an acute coronary syndrome is confirmed. If the troponin remains negative, patients have an *unconfirmed acute coronary syndrome*, and an alternative diagnosis should be considered and managed appropriately. Further investigations to confirm or refute myocardial ischaemia are often appropriate, as even troponin-negative patients do not have a benign prognosis if they have coronary disease; around 5% will die within 6 months (Fox et al, 2002). While troponin or other cardiac biomarkers give an indication of myocardial damage, they fail to provide information on the underlying cause (plaque disruption and platelet activation). The CD-40 ligand and its receptor are important contributors to the inflammatory process associated with acute coronary thrombosis. In patients presenting with chest pain who are troponin negative, soluble CD-40 identifies those who have coronary disease and are at risk of a subsequent major adverse cardiac event (Heeschen et al, 2003).

Creatine kinase (CK)

CK is found in high concentrations in both skeletal and cardiac muscle, as well as the brain, but the

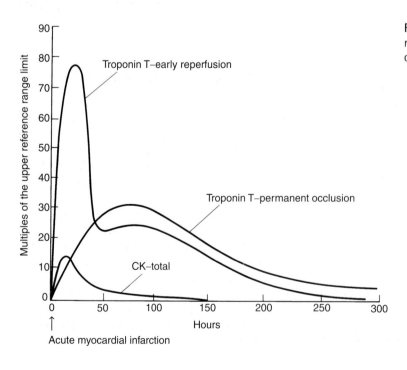

Figure 6.3 Pattern of troponin T release following early perfusion of the myocardium.

MB subfraction (CK-MB) is almost exclusively found in the human heart. CK-MB activity rises within 4–8 hours of myocardial infarction to reach a peak between 12 and 24 hours and disappear again by about 72 hours. Detecting raised levels of myocardial CK-MB (CK-MB$_2$) improves sensitivity and specificity for detecting myocardial damage within 6 hours of myocardial infarction. Levels are first detectable in the blood at 2–4 hours and peak at 6–12 hours.

Myoglobin

Myoglobin is a small haem protein found in skeletal and cardiac muscle. It is released 1–3 hours following myocardial infarction, peaking at 4–8 hours and returning to normal within 24 hours. It has been found to be more sensitive than CK-MB, but is not specific for cardiac damage. Results can be obtained in < 2 minutes, and bedside estimation in the emergency room or on the CCU may allow early exclusion of myocardial infarction.

Fatty acid–binding proteins

Fatty acid-binding proteins (FABPs) are involved in the intracellular transport of long-chain fatty acids. Three main types of FABPs were initially discovered in the heart, liver and gut, and many other isoforms have now been identified. Heart-type FABP is readily released into the circulation after myocardial injury. Concentrations peak earlier than myoglobin, returning to normal within 24 hours, and may thus become a useful biomarker for early detection of myocardial damage.

Practical use of biochemical markers

The different cardiac markers may be of value in different clinical situations, but using multiple tests both together and at different times may enhance diagnosis. For example, nearly all cases of myocardial infarction may be identified within 90 minutes by measuring troponin I, CK-MB and myoglobin (Ng et al, 2001). Positivity of any of these three indicates myocardial infarction, so negativity of all three will exclude the diagnosis. These combination tests may help with early triage of patients presenting with chest pain, but are more expensive. The diagnostic value of total CK-MB, CK-MB isoforms, myoglobin and troponin was compared in patients presenting to the emergency department with chest pain (Fromm et al, 2001). The CK-MB isoforms were the most useful marker for triage. Troponin estimation was best for late diagnosis, and they all provided similar prognostic information.

Peak CK and CK-MB levels are sometimes used to assess infarct size, and the plateau stage of troponin at 72 hours shows an inverse relationship to the left ventricular ejection fraction at 3 months (Panteghini et al, 2002).

Reinfarction after initially successful reperfusion often passes unrecognised because of the reduced sensitivity of the ECG, which remains abnormal following acute infarction, and the possibility that cardiac markers may have not returned to baseline values. Within the first 12–24 hours of an infarction the detection of reinfarction relies on clinical symptoms plus re-elevation of the ST segments in the affected territory of the ECG, with a rise in cardiac markers to more than 50% above a previous peak concentration. The long half-life of the troponins reduces their sensitivity for the detection of reinfarction, and biomarkers with shorter half-life markers (CK-MB, myoglobin, fatty acid-binding protein) may be helpful.

ASSESSING RISK IN PATIENTS PRESENTING WITH ACUTE CORONARY SYNDROMES

The hazards of acute coronary syndromes have been underestimated in the past, and all ACS patients should be risk stratified before discharge from hospital. Patients presenting with unstable coronary syndromes will be at differing levels of risk for progression to myocardial infarction or death. Risk is highest in the first few days following presentation, and decreases slowly over the next few weeks. Two-thirds of adverse events will occur in the first month following presentation, so risk assessment cannot wait for the usual 6-week follow-up visit in outpatients. Acute myocardial infarction or death will affect more than 12% of patients within 6 months (Collinson et al, 2000).

Table 6.3   Some clinical features that define risk in acute coronary syndromes.

High risk	Medium risk	Low risk
Age over 70 years	History of MI/LVF	No high-risk features
ST depression on first ECG	Diabetes	Normal ECG
Refractory angina	Recurrent ischaemia	Clinically stable
Haemodynamic instability	Already on aspirin	No known CAD
Markedly raised troponin	Mildly raised troponin	Troponin not raised

MI, myocardial infarction; LVF, left ventricular failure; CAD, coronary artery disease.

Risk stratification is not only needed to define prognosis, but may also determine the treatment strategy. The process is complex, and several risk scores, based on clinical, ECG and laboratory variables, have been developed for evaluating the short-tem risk of adverse outcomes (de Araujo Goncalves et al, 2005). In general, risk is defined by the haemodynamic severity of the presentation and prior risk factors, which may indicate extensive underlying cardiac disease (age, diabetes, hypertension, smoking, heart failure or previous myocardial infarction).

Acute risk is signalled by recurrent episodes of chest pain with ST segment changes on the ECG and positivity of cardiac markers (Table 6.3), but risk may change with time (Table 6.4). Elevated cardiac troponin concentrations identify patients at high risk of complications and, in general, the higher the cardiac troponin concentration, the greater the risk of further events (including death), and the sooner they will occur. However, troponin elevation should not be viewed in isolation and should be interpreted in perspective, with knowledge of the patient, the ECG appearances and assessment of left ventricular function. A rise in troponin could simply reflect a sustained episode of ischaemia to a small area of myocardium and, as such, probably represents low risk. However, a similar concentration of troponin might be produced by a brief episode of ischaemia to a large (but perhaps vulnerable) area of myocardium, or perhaps episodes of recurrent ischaemia. These latter situations are more likely to associate with adverse cardiovascular events. Minor ischaemic events may have serious consequences in those with prior extensive coronary disease.

INITIAL MANAGEMENT

Patients should be managed by cardiac specialist services on a dedicated unit. Evidence-based therapy for the acute coronary syndromes has been established, and associates with improved outcomes. Effective therapy of acute coronary syndromes should target both the acute lesion and other potential culprit lesions. The three initial steps are relief of pain, ensuring adequate oxygenation and relief of ischaemia.

Sublingual nitrates are an effective and easily administered treatment for ischaemic chest pain,

Table 6.4   Methods of risk stratification for patients with unstable coronary syndromes.

Time of assessment	Method of assessment		
At presentation	Clinical history	Baseline ECG	Cardiac markers
At 6 h	Recurrent pain	ST instability	Cardiac markers
At 24 h	Recurrent pain	Response to therapy	Cardiac markers
Predischarge	Echocardiography	Stress test	Angiographic findings

and have some beneficial haemodynamic effects (e.g. dilatation of the coronary arteries and the venous capacitance vessels). These pharmacological effects associate with reduced myocardial oxygen consumption, but no trial has shown survival benefits. Care is required in those with hypotension.

Diamorphine is the analgesic of choice for nitrate-refractory pain and, like nitrates, it will dilate venous capacitance vessels. It also relieves anxiety, and the associated fall in catecholamine levels inhibits thrombus propagation and makes dysrhythmic episodes less frequent.

Oxygen should be started in those with arterial oxygen saturation of under 90% and/or pulmonary congestion, particularly if there are continuing symptoms of ischaemia. The combination of diamorphine, oxygen and nitrates is extremely efficient in pain relief.

Antiplatelet therapy should be given as soon as possible (aspirin 300 mg and clopidogrel 300 mg). Aspirin on its own reduces absolute mortality at 35 days by 2.4% (ISIS-2, 1988) but, in combination with clopidogrel, there is improved patency in the culprit artery and further reductions in mortality.

Low molecular weight heparin should be started immediately and continued for at least 48 hours.

Patients with STEMI usually have complete occlusion of an epicardial coronary vessel and require urgent reperfusion therapy through the administration of fibrinolytic agents or primary angioplasty. Intravenous thrombolytic therapy is the standard care for patients with acute myocardial infarction, based upon its widespread availability and efficacy, although it has limitations. Many patients are ineligible for treatment and, of those treated, some have persistent occlusion or late reocclusion of the infarct-related artery. The evidence for switching to primary angioplasty for all cases of acute myocardial infarction appears to be overwhelming. Randomised trials comparing primary PCI with intravenous thrombolytic treatment (Keely et al, 2003) have shown that primary PCI:

- leads to better thrombolysis in myocardial infarction (TIMI) grade 3 flow in the infarct-related artery;
- leads to a shorter hospital stay;

- prevents more cases of reinfarction;
- associates with less heart failure;
- results in less post-infarct angina;
- associates with fewer strokes;
- has less hospital readmission;
- improves short- and long-term mortality.

However, trial evidence often differs from real-world cardiology and, while angioplasty provides a short-term clinical advantage over thrombolysis, this may not be significant, nor sustained in the long term (Cucherat et al, 2003). The benefits for primary angioplasty over thrombolysis probably equate to fewer than one or two lives saved per 100 patients treated, but much depends on the choice of thrombolytic agent, time to treatment, place of treatment and adjunctive therapy (Brophy & Bogaty, 2004). Current arguments over whether we should use mechanical or pharmacological reperfusion should be replaced by strategies in which both interventions are integrated to provide the greatest benefits to individual patients, and the two treatments should be viewed as complementary rather than competitive. It is evident that one strategy will not be universal, and that there may be many different solutions that are applicable and optimal under different geographical and organisational situations. Thrombolysis remains a clinically and economically attractive option for the treatment of acute myocardial infarction, and does not require the radical restructuring of healthcare systems. Even in developed countries, the majority of patients do not have access to primary PCI, and almost a third of patients presenting with STEMI still receive no reperfusion therapy at all. A reperfusion plan for patients presenting to hospital with an acute ST elevation myocardial infarction is shown in Figure 6.4.

In the absence of ST segment elevation, patients with ischaemic-type chest pain do not benefit from thrombolytic therapy, which may actually be harmful. These ACS patients usually have a partially or intermittently occluding thrombus, and clinical features often correlate with the dynamic nature of the thrombus as it waxes and wanes. Antiplatelet and anticoagulant therapy with beta-blockade and nitrates is appropriate with risk assessment. Early revascularisation by

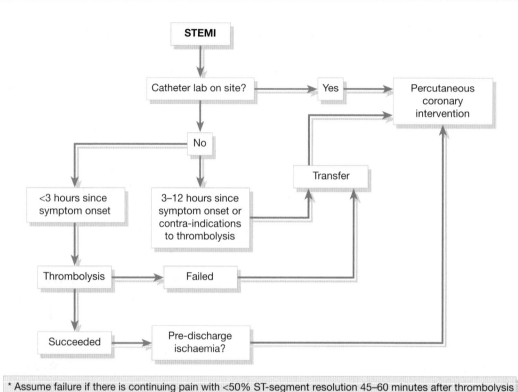

Figure 6.4   Reperfusion plan for patients presenting to hospital with an acute ST elevation myocardial infarction (STEMI).

CABG surgery or PCI is usually considered for the following groups of patients:

- those identified as being at high risk;
- those with refractory symptoms;
- those identified not to be at immediate high risk, but thought to have significant residual ischaemia;
- patients already awaiting CABG surgery.

There is wide variation in the number and type of patients presenting with acute coronary syndromes who are referred for revascularisation, but those hospitals with high revascularisation rates do not necessarily have better outcomes compared with those with lower rates (Fox et al, 2002). Routine rather than selective invasive strategies may reduce myocardial infarction, severe angina and rehospitalisation, but associate with a higher mortality and are not appropriate for all (de Winter et al, 2005; Mehta et al, 2005). Local guidelines between secondary and tertiary centres

are desirable to optimise the timing of intervention. An overview of management of the acute coronary syndromes is shown in Figure 6.5.

CARE OF PATIENTS AFTER LEAVING HOSPITAL

The risk of an unstable coronary syndrome progressing to myocardial infarction or death is highest within the first 8 weeks, after which patients resume a clinical course similar to those who have chronic stable angina. Hospital evaluation should not just concentrate on short-term intervention, but should be used to assess long-term care and preparing the patient for return to normal activities. All people who have recovered from an acute coronary syndrome should have access to a comprehensive cardiovascular prevention and rehabilitation programme. Care should be integrated between hospital and primary care using agreed protocols designed to ensure optimal long-term

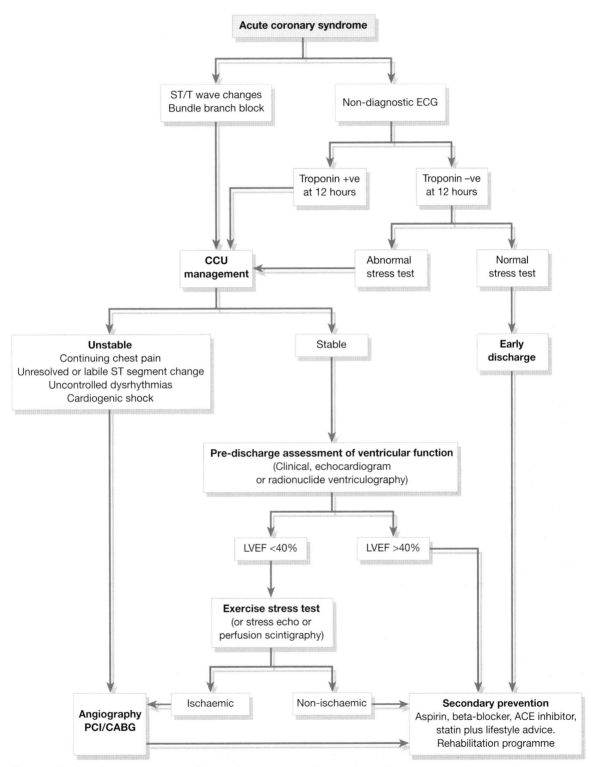

Figure 6.5   Overview management of the acute coronary syndromes.

lifestyle, risk factor and therapeutic management (JBS-2, 2005).

Aggressive management of established risk factors is the most practical and cost-effective intervention (Carbajal & Deedwania, 2005). Lifestyle intervention involves stopping smoking, making healthier food choices, increasing aerobic physical activity and achieving optimal weight and weight distribution. The ABCDE checklist may be helpful.

A = Aspirin and ACE inhibitor

Aspirin is recommended in all patients following an acute coronary syndrome. If aspirin is contra-indicated, or there are side effects, then clopidogrel 75 mg daily is appropriate. Anticoagulation with warfarin should be considered for selected people at risk of systemic embolisation (large myocardial infarctions, heart failure, left ventricular aneurysm, atrial fibrillation).

An angiotensin-converting enzyme (ACE) inhibitor should always be prescribed for patients with diabetes, heart failure or evidence of asymptomatic left ventricular dysfunction. An angiotensin II receptor blocker (ARB) is an alternative to an ACE inhibitor if there are side effects.

The situation in patients with normal left ventricular function is controversial. While studies comparing ACE inhibitors with placebo-based treatment and usual care showed improved outcomes with ACE inhibitor treatment (HOPE Study Investigators, 2000; PROGRESS Collaborative Group, 2001), recent studies have shown no special benefit of ACE inhibition, beyond that which can be attributable to blood pressure lowering (Williams, 2005). In the HOPE trial, there was no benefit to patients with unstable angina. Short-term treatment in unselected patients with STEMI (started within 36 hours and continued for at least 4 weeks) reduces mortality, mostly in the first few days (ACE Inhibitor Myocardial Infarction Collaborative Group, 1998).

B = Beta-blockers and blood pressure

A beta-blocker is recommended for all people following an acute coronary syndrome, unless there are contraindications. The blood pressure must be maintained below 130/80 mmHg. This target will usually need a combination of antihypertensive drugs, which should include a beta-blocker and ACE inhibitor (or ARB).

C = Cholesterol, clopidogrel and cigarettes

Statins reduce serum cholesterol concentrations and protect patients from further heart attacks, strokes and death. They may additionally reduce vascular inflammation and stabilise vascular endothelium, although these effects do not seem to improve short-term outcomes for patients with acute coronary syndromes (Briel et al, 2006). However, it is usual to prescribe statins earlier rather than later, as it does no harm, and starting treatment in hospital improves future compliance. Hence, a statin should be prescribed as part of the normal treatment of an acute coronary syndrome, regardless of the admission cholesterol concentration. A fasting lipid profile should be estimated at least 8 weeks after the acute event and, if necessary, the dose of statin uptitrated to achieve the total and low-density lipoprotein (LDL) cholesterol targets. High-density lipoprotein (HDL) cholesterol and fasting triglycerides should be measured and considered at the same time. The total cholesterol target is less than 4.0 mmol/L with an LDL cholesterol of under 2.0 mmol/L. Alternatively, there should be a 25% reduction in total cholesterol and/or a 30% reduction in LDL cholesterol, whichever gets the individual to the lowest absolute value.

For people with unstable angina or NSTEMI, clopidogrel with aspirin has been shown to reduce cardiovascular death, myocardial infarction and stroke during the year following hospitalisation (CURE, 2001).

Smoking must stop completely, and suitable advice on nicotine replacement therapy is needed. This is safe in ACS patients. Passive smoking also increases risk, so the family will need to play their part. The risk attributable to smoking falls within 2–3 years to the level of those people with coronary disease who have never smoked.

D = Diet and diabetes

Dietary intervention must aim to maintain a body mass index (BMI) of 20–25 kg/m^2 and avoid central obesity.

The total dietary intake of fat should make up no more than 30% of total energy intake, with specific reduction of saturated fats, being replaced by monounsaturated fats. Dietary cholesterol should be less than 300 mg/day. Fresh fruit and vegetables (at least five portions per day), a regular intake of omega-3 fatty acids and less salt are also advisable. Alcohol should be restricted to under 21 units/week for men and under 14 units/week for women.

The optimal fasting glucose is less than 6.0 mmol/L. If the fasting glucose is abnormal, an oral glucose tolerance test (OGTT) may be needed to exclude dysglycaemia or diabetes (see Chapter 3). For people with impaired glucose regulation, the aim is to prevent progression to diabetes by weight control and encouraging exercise.

Patients will require follow-up annually to reassess glucose tolerance. In known diabetics, rigorous control of glycaemia (and other risk factors) is needed.

E = Education and exercise

Regular aerobic physical activity of at least 30 minutes/day, most days of the week, should be taken (e.g. brisk walking, swimming). An organised programme of cardiovascular prevention and rehabilitation for patients recovering from an acute coronary syndrome, which addresses smoking, diet and physical activity, together with the management of other risk factors, and the use of cardioprotective drug therapies, will reduce mortality. Misconceptions about cardiac illness are common and affect compliance with treatment and rehabilitation. Addressing these reduces stress in both the patients and their family. Patients will require specific advice on driving and return to work.

References

ACE Inhibitor Myocardial Infarction Collaborative Group (1998) Indications for ACE inhibitors in the early treatment of acute myocardial infarction. Systematic overview of individual data from 100 000 patients in randomized trials. ACE inhibitor myocardial infarction collaborative group. *Circulation* 97: 2202–2212.

de Araujo Goncalves P, Ferreira J, Aguiar C et al (2005) TIMI, PURSUIT, and GRACE risk scores: sustained prognostic value and interaction with revascularization in NSTE-ACS. *European Heart Journal* 26: 865–872.

Bahr RD (2000) Chest pain centers: moving toward proactive acute coronary care. *International Journal of Cardiology* 72: 101–110.

Briel M, Schwartz GG, Thompson PL et al (2006) Effects of early treatment with statins on short-term clinical outcomes in acute coronary syndromes. A meta-analysis of randomized controlled trials. *Journal of the American Medical Association* 295: 2046–2056.

Brophy JM, Bogaty P (2004) Primary angioplasty and thrombolysis are both reasonable options in acute myocardial infarction. *Annals of Internal Medicine* 141: 292–297.

Burke AP, Farb A, Malcom GT et al (1999) Plaque rupture and sudden death related to exertion in men with coronary artery disease. *Journal of the American Medical Association* 281: 921–926.

Canto JG, Rogers WJ, Bowlby LJ et al (1997) The pre-hospital electrocardiogram in acute myocardial infarction: is its full potential being realized? National Registry of Myocardial Infarction 2 Investigators. *Journal of the American College of Cardiology* 29: 498–505.

Carbajal EV, Deedwania P (2005) Treating non-ST-segment elevation ACS: pros and cons of current strategies. *Postgraduate Medicine* 118: 23–32.

Collinson J, Flather M, Fox KA et al (2000) Clinical outcomes, risk stratification and practice patterns of unstable angina and myocardial infarction without ST elevation: Prospective Registry of Acute Ischaemic Syndromes in the UK (PRAIS-UK). *European Heart Journal* 21: 1450–1457.

Cucherat M, Bonnefoy E, Tremeau G (2003) Primary angioplasty versus intravenous thrombolysis for acute myocardial infarction. *Cochrane Database of Systematic Reviews* CD001560.

CURE (2001) Effects of clopidogrel in addition to aspirin in patients with acute coronary syndromes without ST elevation. *New England Journal of Medicine* 345: 494–502.

Dauerman HL, Lessard D, Yarzebski J et al (2000) Ten-year trends in the incidence, treatment, and outcome of Q-wave myocardial infarction. *American Journal of Cardiology* 86: 730–735.

Dorsch MF, Lawrance RA, Sapsford RJ et al for the EMMACE Study Group (2004) An evaluation of the relationship between specialist training in cardiology and implementation of evidence-based care of patients following acute myocardial infarction. *International Journal of Cardiology* 96: 335–340.

ESC/ACC (2000) Myocardial infarction re-defined – consensus document of the joint European Society of Cardiology/American College of Cardiology. *European Heart Journal* 21: 1502–1513.

Farkouh ME, Smars PA, Reeder GS et al (1998) A clinical trial of a chest-pain unit for patients with unstable angina. *New England Journal of Medicine* 339: 1882–1888.

Fox KAA, Goodman SG, Klein W et al (2002) Management of acute coronary syndromes. Variations in practice and outcome: findings from the global registry of acute coronary events (GRACE). *European Heart Journal* 23: 1177–1189.

Fox KAA, Birkhead J, Wilcox, R et al (2004) British Cardiac Society Working Group on the definition of myocardial infarction. *Heart* 90: 603–609.

Fromm R, Meyer D, Zimmerman J et al (2001) A double-blind, multicentered study comparing the accuracy of diagnostic markers to predict short- and long-term clinical events and their utility in patients presenting with chest pain. *Clinical Cardiology* 24: 516–520.

Herlitz J, Karlson BW, Sjölin M et al (2001) Ten year mortality in subsets of patients with an acute coronary syndrome. *Heart* 86: 391–396.

Heeschen C, Dimmeler S, Hamm CW et al (2003) Soluble CD-40 ligand in acute coronary syndromes. *New England Journal of Medicine* 348: 1104–1111.

HOPE Study Investigators (2000) Effects of an angiotensin-converting-enzyme inhibitor, ramipril, on cardiovascular events in high-risk people. *New England Journal of Medicine* 342: 145–153.

ISIS-2 (1988) Randomized trial of intravenous streptokinase, oral aspirin, both, or neither among 17,187 cases of suspected acute myocardial infarction. ISIS-2 (Second International Study of Infarct Survival) Collaborative Group. *Journal of the American College of Cardiology* 12(6 suppl A): 3A–13A.

JBS-2 (2005) Joint British Societies' guidelines on prevention of cardiovascular disease in clinical practice. Prepared by: British Cardiac Society, British Hypertension Society, Diabetes UK, HEART UK, Primary Care Cardiovascular Society, The Stroke Association. *Heart* 91: 1–52.

Jowett NI (1997) *Cardiovascular Monitoring.* London: John Wiley.

Keeley E, Boura JA, Grines CL (2003) Primary angioplasty versus intravenous thrombolytic therapy for acute myocardial infarction: a quantitative review of 23 randomised trials. *Lancet* 361: 13–20.

McKenna CJ, Forfar JC (2002) Was it a heart attack? *British Medical Journal* 324: 377–378.

Mehta SR, Cannon CP, Fox KAA et al (2005) Routine vs selective invasive strategies in patients with acute coronary syndromes: a collaborative meta-analysis of randomized trials. *Journal of the American Medical Association* 293: 2908–2917.

Morrison LJ, Verbeek PR, McDonald AC et al (2001) Mortality and pre-hospital thrombolysis for acute myocardial infarction: a meta-analysis. *Journal of the American Medical Association* 283: 2686–2692.

Morrow DA, Cannon CP, Rifai N et al TACTICS-TIMI 18 Investigators (2001) Ability of minor elevations of troponins I and T to predict benefit from an early invasive strategy in patients with unstable angina and non-ST elevation myocardial infarction: results from a randomized trial. *Journal of the American Medical Association* 286: 2405–2412.

Mueller C, Neumann FJ, Perach W et al (2004) Prognostic value of the admission electrocardiogram in patients with unstable angina/non-ST-segment elevation myocardial infarction treated with very early revascularization. *American Journal of Medicine* 117: 145–150.

Ng SM, Krishnaswarmy P, Morissey R et al (2001) Ninety-minute accelerated critical pathway for chest pain evaluation. *American Journal of Cardiology* 88: 611–617.

Novis DA, Jones BA, Dale JC et al (2004) Biochemical markers of myocardial injury test turn-around time: A College of American Pathologists Q-Probes study of 7020 troponin and 4368 creatine kinase-MB determinations in 159 institutions. *Archives of Pathology and Laboratory Medicine* 128: 158–164.

Panteghini M, Cuccia C, Bonetti G et al (2002) Single-point cardiac troponin T at coronary care discharge after myocardial infarction correlates with infarct size and ejection fraction. *Clinical Chemistry* 48: 1432–1436.

PROGRESS Collaborative Group (2001) Randomised trial of a perindopril-based blood-pressure-lowering regimen among 6105 individuals with previous stroke or transient ischaemic attack. *Lancet* 358: 1033–1041.

Turner AM (2003) Troponin levels should be viewed in their clinical context. *Nursing Times* 99: 16.

Watt J, Davie AP, Cruickshank A (2005) Elevation of troponin I in acutely ill medical patients: a pilot study and literature review. *British Journal of Cardiology* 12: AIC9–AIC14.

Williams B (2005) Recent hypertension trials: implications and controversies. *Journal of the American College of Cardiology* 45: 813–827.

de Winter RJ, Windhausen F, Cornel JH et al for the Invasive versus Conservative Treatment in Unstable Coronary Syndromes (ICTUS) Investigators (2005) Early invasive versus selectively invasive management for acute coronary syndromes. *New England Journal of Medicine* 353: 1095–1104.

World Health Organization (1979) Report of the Joint International Society and Federation of Cardiology/World Health Organisation Task Force on Standardisation of Clinical Nomenclature and criteria for diagnosis of ischaemic heart disease. *Circulation* 59: 607–609.

Chapter 7

Management of ST elevation myocardial infarction

Despite improvements in the prevention and treatment of coronary heart disease (CHD), acute myocardial infarction is responsible for between one-third and half of all cardiovascular deaths, and is the major cause of death in most developed countries. In 2004, 231 500 people in the UK suffered a heart attack, and about 105 000 died from the various manifestations of CHD (Allender et al, 2006). Most cardiac deaths occur out of hospital, so our experience of acute myocardial infarction in the coronary care unit (CCU) is based on caring for survivors of a devastating clinical event that has already taken a major toll (Table 7.1). Within hospital, percutaneous intervention, thrombolytic

therapy, aspirin, beta-blockers, statins and angiotensin-converting enzyme (ACE) inhibitors may favourably influence prognosis. Unfortunately, many patients still do not receive these evidence-based interventions, and 10–15% of the patients who reach hospital die before discharge, and another 15–20% will die during the following year (Gandhi, 1997).

Minimising the delay in coming under medical care for those with an evolving myocardial infarction reduces the chance of death from ventricular fibrillation, and maximises the potential benefit from reperfusional strategies to salvage myocardium at risk. The ambulance service has a major role in stabilising the patient and then starting the diagnostic work-up. Performing an ECG prior to hospital admission reduces in-hospital delay, and may enable the administration of prehospital thrombolysis to limit or abort significant myocardial infarction (Task Force of the European Society of Cardiology and the European Resuscitation Council, 1998). Once in hospital, patients are best managed on CCUs rather than on general medical wards, because patients are more likely to receive evidence-based treatment, and the chances of successful resuscitation are two to three times higher. Inpatient mortality fell by about 10% following the introduction of CCUs in the 1960s, mainly thanks to the prompt recognition and treatment of potentially fatal dysrhythmias. Patients admitted to medical wards are not considered soon enough for thrombolytic therapy

Table 7.1 Percentage distribution of 28-day fatalities expressed as median (range) for patients aged 35–64 years in the MONICA Project, 1985–1990. Data from Chambless et al, 1997.

Time	Male (%)	Female (%)
Prehospital	70 (58–80)	64 (42–75)
Hospital < 24 h	22 (15–36)	27 (19–46)
1–28 days	14 (8–21)	16 (11–30)

or for other secondary interventions (Lawson-Matthew et al, 1994). Reductions in hospital mortality following myocardial infarction have mainly been achieved by faster admission procedures, infarct limitation with thrombolysis and primary angioplasty, and enhanced therapies for cardiogenic shock and heart failure (Tunstall-Pedoe et al, 2000). All patients with a suspected acute coronary syndrome should be assessed and cared for by appropriately trained staff on a designated chest pain or coronary care unit.

IMMEDIATE MANAGEMENT IN HOSPITAL

The journey to hospital is usually brief, but delays can occur during admission procedures and in the radiograph and emergency departments. Direct admission to coronary care and/or rapid triage and treatment policies in the emergency department must exist if cardiac mortality and morbidity are to be minimised. Direct admission to the CCU does not lead to congestion, provided there are robust arrangements for rapid stepdown for those not requiring high dependency. Our experience also shows that most direct admissions are appropriate, with 81% of cases having a primary cardiac diagnosis.

Up to one-fifth of patients attending emergency departments have chest pain, yet only 10–15% of these will have a myocardial infarction. There have been several different approaches to organising the management of these patients outside the normal CCU from simple triage to more formal assessment in a chest pain unit. Rapid diagnosis

and early risk stratification are important to identify those in whom early therapy can improve outcome. A 'fast track' admission system can reduce in-hospital delay if patients present to the emergency department or medical admission unit. Targeted clinical examination with a 12-lead ECG on arrival helps to select patients for thrombolytic therapy, and routine evaluation by the admitting medical team is bypassed. The electrocardiogram (ECG) is a powerful tool for triage, and should be reported within 5 minutes of arrival in hospital. Medical rather than computerised interpretation of the ECG is vital.

Patients may be classified as:

- *fast track*: myocardial infarction, ECG showing ST elevation or bundle branch block;
- *slow track*: probable acute coronary syndrome with other ECG changes;
- *no track*: acute coronary syndrome unlikely.

Adopting a fast track system should not require any additional staff or resources, and may halve the in-hospital delay to thrombolysis.

As around half the patients admitted to hospital with chest pains do not have a cardiac illness, slow track or no track patients may be better cared for on an acute chest pain unit, rather than on coronary care. Such units have been shown to be a safe, effective and cost-saving means of ensuring appropriate care of patients at intermediate risk of adverse cardiac events.

ADMISSION TO THE CORONARY CARE UNIT

Patients with ongoing pain, ischaemic ECG changes, haemodynamic instability, left ventricular failure or positive troponin form a high-risk group who should always be admitted to a specialist unit.

There are several interventions that need immediate consideration following admission to the CCU. Many of these will happen simultaneously, and the usual medical sequence of history, examination, investigation and treatment is not usually the most effective way of patient management. If triage has not already been carried out, a rapid clinical appraisal is the first step to assess the likelihood of myocardial infarction and the need for reperfusion.

History and examination of the patient

Taking a history from patients on a CCU is often easy. Somebody somewhere must have thought the history was suggestive of an acute coronary syndrome or other cardiac emergency. The initial enquiry should be brief and serve to answer two questions:

- Is this an acute coronary syndrome needing reperfusion?
- Are there any contraindications for thrombolysis?

Taking a more complete clinical history will still be needed, but this can usually wait until a decision is made for early mechanical or pharmacological reperfusion. Obtaining essential information in the acute phase of the illness when the patient is in pain or nauseated is not ideal, and the complete story often becomes clearer when the patient has been settled with analgesia and antiemetics. While it is essential that there is no delay in instigating treatment, it is important to appreciate the psychological stress placed upon the patient who has been rushed into hospital via an emergency ambulance to be delivered to the high-technology world of the CCU. Autonomic imbalance or impaired left ventricular function may result in nausea, vomiting, sweating, peripheral vasoconstriction and varying degrees of dyspnoea. The typical patient will, therefore, be cool, clammy, in pain and often frightened. Both verbal and tactile communication are important.

The physical appearance and clinical findings in patients suffering from acute myocardial infarction are variable, and alter with time and the presence of any co-existent complications. There are often no physical abnormalities at all. The general appearance of the coronary patient is dependent upon the physical and psychological impact that the illness has upon the particular individual. Hence, although some patients will appear quiet and anxious, others may appear excessively agitated and restless. The situation will be ameliorated or aggravated if the patient has had a previous hospital admission or myocardial infarction,

depending upon his clinical and social course in hospital.

Pulse and blood pressure

Variations in pulse rate and blood pressure usually depend on the amount of pain, the size of the infarct and the degree of left ventricular dysfunction, but may be influenced by overactivity of the autonomic nervous system. Inferior and posterior myocardial infarctions are usually associated with parasympathetic overactivity (bradycardia, hypotension and heart block), whereas anterior and lateral myocardial infarctions are associated with sympathetic stimulation (tachycardia and hypertension). In some patients, profound hypotension may follow the administration of nitrates.

The jugular venous pressure

The jugular venous pressure (JVP) is usually normal unless there has been pre-existing heart failure, pulmonary disease or right ventricular infarction.

The heart sounds

The first heart sound is often diminished and muffled as a result of left ventricular dysfunction, and reversed splitting of the second sound is common, reflecting conduction delay within the ischaemic left ventricle. Fourth heart sounds are usual, so that their absence makes a large myocardial infarction unlikely. Third heart sounds are less common, and will reflect left ventricular failure. As such, a third heart sound implies a poorer prognosis. Detecting these low-pitched sounds is often difficult in patients who are obese or have hyperinflated chests, such as those with emphysema. Auscultation over the carotid or subclavian vessels may then amplify the heart sounds.

Cardiac murmurs

The murmur of mitral incompetence is present in many patients in the early stages of myocardial infarction because of papillary muscle dysfunction or dilatation of the mitral annulus in association with left ventricular failure. Other murmurs may indicate pre-existing valvular disease, which may or may not have predisposed the individual to myocardial infarction. For example, aortic stenosis may cause myocardial infarction in the presence of little or no coronary atherosclerosis.

Intravenous access and blood sampling

Insertion of an intravenous line will allow the administration of an analgesic and an antiemetic by injection. Intramuscular routes are inadequate, as drug absorption from vasoconstricted muscle capillary beds in the 'shutdown' patient is erratic. In addition, this route is contraindicated if thrombolysis is being considered because of the risk of intramuscular haematomas. The use of topical antiseptics such as Betadine does not reduce the risk of cannula-related infection, and cleaning the skin with an alcohol wipe is sufficient (Thompson et al, 1989). This has the added advantage of removing skin oils and allowing the cannula to be fixed more securely to the skin with adhesive tape. The cannula needs to be flushed every 8–12 hours with normal saline and before and after every intravenous drug. The use of a heparin solution does not prolong cannula patency or reduce infection (Jowett et al, 1986).

Baseline blood tests are often taken at the same time as cannula insertion, but care is required if blood samples are withdrawn through the cannula; too small a cannula or too rapid aspiration can cause haemolysis of the blood sample, with misleading results. Near-patient testing with bedside biochemical analysis kits may save time compared with more precise laboratory testing.

Blood should be sent to the laboratory for analysis of the following.

Full blood count

This will detect anaemia or polycythaemia. The white cell count (WBC) and erythrocyte sedimentation rate (ESR) are initially normal but rise in response to muscle necrosis. The WBC peaks at about 15 000 cells/mm^3 after 2–4 days, and higher levels suggest complications, such as infection or pericarditis. The height of the initial WBC count is an independent predictor of hospital death and the development of heart failure (Furman et al, 2004). The ESR often remains elevated for 2–3 weeks.

Renal function tests

Assessment of renal function and the potassium concentration is particularly important in patients taking digoxin or diuretics. Hypokalaemia appears to be associated with high levels of circulating catecholamines, and may reflect the severity of the infarct. Hypokalaemia reduces the threshold for ventricular fibrillation, so maintaining the serum potassium over 4 mmol/L is recommended. An assessment of creatinine clearance may be helpful to detect early signs of renal failure, especially where drugs excreted by the kidneys are being used. Creatinine levels depend on muscle bulk, and a normal serum creatinine is maintained until the glomerular filtration rate (GFR) is less than 50%. Urea concentrations depend upon the state of hydration, protein metabolism and steroid use.

The UK National Service Framework for Renal Services has recommended estimation of kidney function by serum creatinine concentration together with a formula-based estimation of glomerular filtration rate (eGFR), calculated and reported automatically by all biochemistry laboratories. Normal eGFR is approximately 100 mL/minutes/1.73m^2.

Serum cardiac biomarkers

Blood for serum cardiac biomarker determination should be obtained during the initial evaluation, but is not needed for decisions on reperfusion. Modern cardiac biomarkers are more sensitive than previously used 'cardiac enzymes', and are useful for diagnosis, risk stratification and prognosis. An elevated troponin level correlates with an increased risk of death, and the greater the elevation, the greater the risk of an adverse outcome (Antman et al, 1996).

Troponin estimation is insensitive for diagnostic purposes in the first 4–6 hours, unless stuttering pain has been present in the previous few hours. CK-MB and myoglobin may be used in the first 4–6 hours, but are not as sensitive for detecting myocardial infarction.

Random serum lipid levels

Early assessment of random serum lipid concentrations will give an indication of pre-existing dyslipidaemia (Brugada et al, 1996). If not carried out within 24 hours, a formal lipid profile assessment will not be possible for many weeks, as cholesterol concentrations are suppressed and triglyceride concentrations elevated for about 3 months following acute myocardial infarction. The use of statin therapy within the first 24 hours reduces early complications and in-hospital mortality (Fonarow et al, 2005).

Blood glucose level

Diabetic patients comprise up to 25% of patients presenting with myocardial infarction (Bartnik et al, 2004), and around 10% of admissions to coronary care are found to have previously undiagnosed diabetes (Tenerz et al, 2001). Patients with diabetes and hyperglycaemia presenting with acute coronary syndromes have a hospital and long-term mortality nearly twice that of those with normal glucose tolerance (Otter et al, 2004). The admission blood glucose level is a strong, independent predictor of mortality, and the 28-day mortality is higher in those with an admission blood glucose of more than 6.7 mmol/L, compared with patients with lower levels, independently of a previous diagnosis of diabetes (Sala et al, 2002). It is likely that this results from impaired myocardial function caused by metabolic changes that occur in the early stages of acute myocardial infarction. The release of stress hormones (cortisol, catecholamines, growth hormone and glucagon) produces insulin resistance with hyperglycaemia, and endogenous insulin release is suppressed. The combination of low insulin levels with high catecholamine concentrations associates with the release of free fatty acids that increase myocardial oxygen requirements and depress mechanical performance. Controlling the plasma glucose and fatty acid concentrations by insulin infusion could help to preserve myocardial function and reduce morbidity and mortality.

The DIGAMI trials (Malmberg, 1997, Malmberg et al, 2005) assessed the effect of tight control of blood glucose in the peri-infarction period. Whereas the first DIGAMI trial concluded that an insulin–glucose infusion followed by an insulin-based regime reduced mortality, this was not confirmed in DIGAMI-2, which showed that insulin treatment is not any better than any other therapeutic option to control the blood glucose. In addition, high-dose glucose–potassium–insulin (GKI) infusions do not reduce mortality following acute myocardial infarction in patients with or without diabetes (CREATE-ECLA Investigators, 2005). Nevertheless, initiating treatment with an insulin infusion to attain control of the blood glucose and improve the patient's general biochemical status is supported by observations on general intensive care units (Krinsley, 2004). Capillary blood sampling to monitor glucose concentrations is usual, but care is needed in patients who received thrombolytic agents. Excessive bleeding into the finger pulp may be both painful and a source of infection (Jowett, 2006).

Much of the excess mortality in patients with diabetes is due to the high incidence of cardiac failure that is not explained by infarct size or the extent of coronary arterial disease, and has been attributed to a specific diabetic cardiomyopathy (Francis, 2001). All diabetic patients should be treated with an ACE inhibitor, and conventional post-infarction treatment with beta-blockers, aspirin and statins reduces mortality in patients with diabetes but remains underutilised (Rutherford, 2001).

Aspirin

Aspirin should be given at the earliest opportunity, unless there is a clear history of a major bleeding risk or aspirin hypersensitivity. Even in the absence of fibrinolytic treatment, the administration of aspirin has been shown to improve survival, but administration prior to thrombolysis may associate with greater reduction in mortality compared with later treatment (Friemark et al, 1998). The initial dose should be at least 300 mg, either in a soluble form or by being chewed and held in the mouth rather than being swallowed. This enhances absorption and prevents it being regurgitated. Subsequent daily administration of aspirin reduces the 30-day vascular mortality rate by 23% without risk of stroke, and should be continued for life (Anti-platelet Trialists' Collaboration, 1994).

Clopidogrel

Clopidogrel is a useful alternative to aspirin, and using both drugs together further reduces overall mortality and major vascular events, with no increased risk of serious bleeding even in those who do not receive thrombolysis (COMMIT Collaborative Group, 2005a). In patients who are thrombolysed, the addition of clopidogrel to aspirin improves coronary patency in the infarct-related artery and reduces ischaemic complications (Sabatine et al, 2005). The loading dose of clopidogrel is 300 mg, followed by 75 mg daily until hospital discharge.

Nitrates

Coronary arterial spasm is a common associate of acute coronary thrombosis, and nitrates should be of benefit, although ISIS-4 (1995) and GISSI-3 trials (1994) have thrown some doubt on routine use. The high crossover rate to nitrates for post-infarction angina in these trials may have diluted the true value of nitrates, and early administration of sublingual or buccal nitrate is recommended in those with ST segment elevation on the ECG to relieve vasospasm and anginal pain. Intravenous nitrates may be of particular value in patients with large anterior infarcts, hypertension, peri-infarction heart failure or recurrent pain. The intravenous route allows minute-to-minute titration, depending upon heart rate and blood pressure. Caution is required if the patient is hypotensive or already taking nitrate therapy.

Analgesia

The provision of early and adequate pain relief is of major importance. Intravenous diamorphine is the drug of choice, and is well tolerated following myocardial infarction. Diamorphine relieves both pain and anxiety, which may stimulate catecholamine release and cause vasoconstriction and increase cardiac work, making dysrhythmias more likely. An initial intravenous dose of diamorphine,

2.5–5.0 mg, should be given at 1 mg/minute, followed by further 2.5-mg doses until pain is relieved. Intravenous beta-blockers and/or nitrates may be added if pain relief is not complete.

The most common side effects of opiate therapy are nausea and vomiting, which can be reduced by simultaneous administration of an antiemetic such as metoclopramide. Cyclizine causes vasoconstriction, and prochlorperazine can only be given by mouth or intramuscularly, so cannot be recommended. Opiates must be used with care in patients with severe chronic obstructive pulmonary disease, as respiratory depression may occur within minutes and last for many hours. Opiate therapy also reduces gastric and intestinal motility, so oral absorption of important drugs such as diuretics may be impaired.

The rapid and complete relief of pain that accompanies early reperfusion suggests that the pain that accompanies acute myocardial infarction is due to continuing ischaemia in threatened, but still viable, myocardium, rather than from already infarcted cardiac muscle.

Oxygen

Following acute myocardial infarction, it is usual practice to administer continuous low-flow oxygen for 24–48 hours (100% oxygen at 5 L/minutes) for the relief of known or presumed hypoxaemia, although there is little evidence to support its benefits. In one of the few randomised, double-blind, controlled trials of oxygen therapy in patients with uncomplicated myocardial infarction, those treated with oxygen tended to have a higher mortality and more ventricular tachycardia than those randomised to receive air (Rawles & Kenmure, 1976). Too much oxygen causes reflex vasoconstriction in arteriolar smooth muscle, and can reduce cardiac output, increase blood pressure and affect coronary blood flow, particularly to areas of ischaemia (Kenmure et al, 1968), so oxygen must be used with care.

Oxygen is a drug and should be administered in a dose just sufficient to produce the desired effect; additional oxygen is wasteful and potentially dangerous, particularly following acute myocardial infarction. Poor prescribing and monitoring of oxygen therapy is common, and the use

Table 7.2 Efficiency of low-flow oxygen delivery devices [approximate concentration of delivered oxygen (%)].

Oxygen flow rate (L/min)	Nasal prongs	Simple face mask	Partial rebreathing mask	Non-rebreathing mask
1	24			
2	28			
4	32			
5	36	35	50	
6	40	40	60	
7	44	50	70	
8		60	80	80
9				85
10				90

Oxygen concentrations vary widely depending upon the fit of the mask and the respiratory rate.
Flow rates > 4 L/min via nasal prongs irritate the nasopharynx.
Flow rates < 5 L/min with face masks cause rebreathing of carbon dioxide.
Reservoir bags should be kept 30–50% filled on inspiration.

of oxygen prescription charts is desirable (Dodd et al, 2000). Pulse oximetry is the easiest way to assess the need for oxygen, and oxyhaemoglobin saturation (SaO_2) should be documented before and during oxygen therapy to achieve a SaO_2 of above 95%. Continuing oxygen therapy should then be based on achieving target saturations rather than on giving predetermined concentrations or inspired flow rates.

For stable patients with slightly low oxygen saturations, nasal cannulae are preferred to face masks, which spend most of their time oxygenating the forehead. If higher concentrations of oxygen are required, there are two choices of mask:

- Low flow masks deliver oxygen at less than the peak inspiratory flow rate (i.e. less than 15 L/minutes). The concentration of oxygen delivered varies, depending on the patients' breathing pattern. The oxygen should be set to a minimum of 5 L/minutes to prevent rebreathing of carbon dioxide, which can occur if exhaled air is not flushed from the mask. The oxygen flow rate will need to be adjusted to vary the approximate concentration of inspired oxygen (Table 7.2). Low flow masks can sometimes produce unexpectedly high concentrations of inspired oxygen, particularly from masks that incorporate a reservoir bag (partial or non-breathing masks),

so they should not be used in patients with chronic obstructive airway disease unless being monitored by blood gases. Pulse oximetry only gives information on blood oxygen saturation, and not adequacy of ventilation.

- High flow masks (*Venturi masks*) deliver oxygen at a rate above the peak inspiratory flow rate, and can be identified by their noise as oxygen is being forced through a short constriction in the mask to increase gas flow (Venturi effect). By delivering a constant mixture of oxygen and air at above the maximum inspiratory flow rate, changes in breathing do not affect the oxygen concentration delivered. To change the oxygen concentration, the mask and flow rate need to be changed (Table 7.3).

Table 7.3 Guide to the venturi masks.

Colour	Oxygen flow rate (L/min)	Oxygen delivered
Blue	2	24%
White	4	28%
Yellow	6	35%
Red	8	40%
Green	12	60%

Chest radiographs

It is still common practice for a portable antero-posterior (AP) chest film to be taken on admission to the CCU. The clinical value of this is dubious in most cases, as most are performed under subopti-mal conditions and have inherent limitations caused by the AP projection and the inability to position the patient properly. While it may serve to help to exclude other causes of chest pain, such as aortic aneurysm, pneumonia and pneumothorax, the chest radiograph is most often requested to detect heart failure. However, this indication is also limited. There may be a 12-hour lag between haemodynamic dysfunction and the radiographic appearances of cardiac failure. Furthermore, radiological heart failure may take up to 4 days to resolve following haemodynamic stabilisation. A normal chest radiograph usually excludes significant heart failure.

A chest film should be carried out following prolonged resuscitation or after central catheteri-sation to exclude pneumothorax and/or check the catheter position.

Electrocardiographic monitoring

Careful monitoring of cardiac rhythm and the prompt treatment of dysrhythmias has reduced hospital deaths from myocardial infarction, and all patients should be connected to a suitable car-diac monitor as soon as possible (Jowett et al, 1985). If the patient is being transferred from the emergency medicine department, a portable mon-itor/defibrillator must accompany the patient to the CCU.

Standard 12-lead electrocardiography (ECG)

A standard 12-lead ECG should be carried out immediately on arrival in hospital to confirm the diagnosis and assess the suitability for thromboly-sis. The ECG can change within seconds of coro-nary occlusion but, in the early stages of acute myocardial infarction, the ECG may be normal or near normal. Less than half of patients with acute myocardial infarction have clear diagnostic changes on their first ECG trace, and about 10% of patients do not develop ST segment elevation or depression. Serial ECGs or continuous 12-lead ECG monitoring may be very helpful, particularly if there is recurrent pain. There is no single ECG change produced by myocardial ischaemia and infarction, and changes depend upon the duration and location of the ischaemic insult. Proximal coronary arterial occlusions produce the most obvious and widespread electrocardiographic abnormalities.

ECG changes of acute transmural myocardial infarction

There is usually a typical evolving sequence of ST–T wave ECG changes following acute myocar-dial infarction (Fig. 7.1).

T wave changes

The earliest ECG sign of acute myocardial infarc-tion is usually seen in the T waves, which become tall, peaked and symmetrical, particularly in the anterior chest leads. These changes are usually present in the first 30 minutes after the onset of the myocardial infarction, and precede any ST seg-ment changes. These 'hyperacute' T wave changes are often subtle and may be missed, although they are more obvious if compared with previous electrocardiograms.

Early T wave normalisation is associated with myocardial stunning but, if they become inverted, myocardial infarction is likely to have occurred.

ST segment changes

ST segment elevation is usually the first obvious sign of acute myocardial infarction, and is usually evident within hours of the onset of symptoms. The degree of ST segment elevation varies between subtle and gross. Sometimes, a single monophasic giant R wave is seen (a 'tombstone' complex) produced by fusion of the QRS complex, the ST segment and the T wave (Fig. 7.2).

Initially, the ST segment straightens, losing its normal concavity. As the T wave broadens, the ST segment begins to elevate and becomes convex upwards. Without reperfusion, these acute ST–T wave changes may take hours or days to resolve.

Figure 7.1   Evolution of ECG changes following acute transmural myocardial infarction.

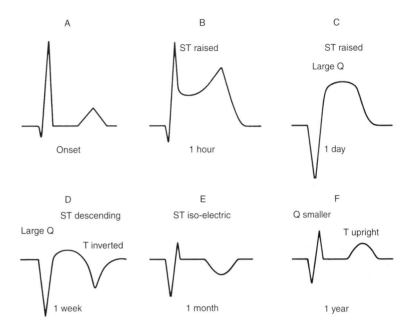

ST segment elevation associated with an inferior myocardial infarction tends to resolve within 2 weeks but, with anterior myocardial infarction, ST elevation may persist for even longer and, if a left ventricular aneurysm develops, may remain elevated indefinitely.

ST segment depression is often seen in leads facing away from the affected area (about 70% of inferior and 30% of anterior infarctions).

These 'reciprocal' changes were thought to be arte-factual, mirroring ST elevation in the other leads, but are more likely to indicate ischaemic myocardial tissue away from the infarction site. As such, extensive reciprocal ST segment depression indi-cates widespread coronary arterial disease, and consequently carries a worse prognosis (Krone et al, 1993). Patients with acute myocardial infarc-tion presenting with ST depression alone do not

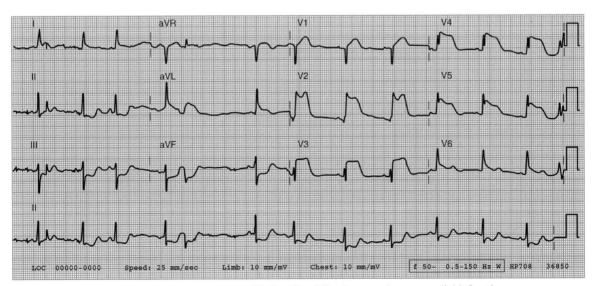

Figure 7.2   ECG: 'tombstone complexes' – gross ST elevation following anterior myocardial infarction.

appear to benefit from thrombolysis and have a bad prognosis.

The Q wave

The electrocardiographic hallmark of transmural myocardial infarction is the Q wave. Transmural necrosis produces an electrical 'window' in the ventricle, so that an overlying skin electrode records an impulse as if the electrode were placed inside the heart. Because the ventricles are depolarised from the inside outwards, an electrode in the heart would record a large negative deflection (a Q wave) as the impulse travels from within the heart to the skin.

Normally, small septal Q waves are seen in the left ventricular leads (V3–6), caused by depolarisation of the septum from left to right. Pathological Q waves are more than 0.04 seconds in duration and are 2 mm or more in depth in the standard leads. A Q wave in standard lead III should only be considered abnormal if it exceeds 0.03 seconds and is accompanied by Q waves in leads II and aVF. The 'normal' Q wave in lead III usually diminishes or disappears on deep inspiration, but a pathological Q wave will remain. In the left ventricular leads, pathological Q waves are more than 4 mm in depth in V4 and V5, and more than 2 mm in V6. Q wave formation does not always imply myocardial infarction, and may be produced by any process that forms a myocardial window, such as myocardial infiltration by cardiac tumours, cardiomyopathies or amyloidosis. Q waves are sometimes seen in patients with left ventricular hypertrophy.

Infarction Q waves usually develop within the first 12–24 hours in those leads facing the area of necrosis, although they may sometimes develop earlier. The presence of pathological Q waves, however, does not necessarily indicate a completed infarct and may simply reflect acute ischaemia. If the history is recent and the ST segments are still elevated, the patient may still benefit from thrombolysis or angioplasty.

When there has been extensive myocardial infarction, Q waves are usually permanent. With less damage, myocardial scar tissue may contract, pulling the electrically inert area away from the overlying ECG skin electrodes. As a result, the Q waves may disappear.

Diagnosing acute myocardial infarction in the presence of bundle branch block

Acute myocardial infarction in the presence of bundle branch block (whether old or new) associates with a poor outcome.

Right bundle branch block usually associates with coronary artery disease, but may be a normal variant. Right bundle branch block usually causes little ST segment displacement on a routine ECG, so will usually interfere with the diagnosis of acute myocardial infarction, unless there is posterior myocardial infarction.

The left branch of the bundle of His usually receives blood from the left anterior descending branch of the left coronary artery and from the right coronary artery. When new left bundle branch block occurs in the context of an acute myocardial infarction, the infarct location is usually anterior, and mortality is extremely high. The electrocardiographic changes of acute myocardial infarction can be difficult to recognise when left bundle branch block is present, but there may be some features suggesting acute ischaemia, such as:

- ST segment elevation of > 1 mm in association with a positive QRS complex (V4–6);
- ST segment depression of > 1 mm in leads V1, V2 or V3 ('inappropriate concordance');
- extreme ST segment elevation (> 5 mm) with negative QRS complex in leads V1 and V2.

Determining the site of infarction

Correlating the ECG findings with knowledge of the coronary circulation may help to determine the site of the coronary occlusion, although normal coronary vasculature varies widely from person to person, so it is only possible to make generalisations (Box 7.1).

The three major coronary vessels are:

- the right coronary artery (RCA);
- the left anterior descending artery (LAD);
- the left circumflex artery (LCx).

Right coronary artery (RCA)

Right atrium
Right ventricle
Inferior left ventricle
Sinus node
Atrio-ventricular node
Posterior interventricular septum

Left anterior descending (LAD) coronary artery

Anterior wall of left ventricle
Anterior interventricular septum
Apex of left ventricle
Bundle of His and bundle branches

Left circumflex (LCx) coronary artery

Left atrium
Lateral and posterior left ventricle
Posterior interventricular septum

The RCA supplies the right atrium, the right ventricle and the inferior left ventricle. Blood is also conveyed to the sinus node, the AV node and the posterior portion of the ventricular septum. Hence, occlusion of the RCA can produce infarction of the inferior and posterior left ventricle and, sometimes, the right atrium and ventricle. Ischaemia or oedema of the sinus and AV nodes may produce bradycardia and heart block (Fig. 7.3).

The main stem of the left coronary artery divides into two main branches, the left anterior descending (LAD) artery and the left circumflex (LCx) artery. The former supplies the anterior left ventricular wall, the apex and the interventricular septum. Septal perforating branches supply the bundle of His and bundle branches. Occlusion of the LAD leads to infarction of the anterior left ventricular wall, the cardiac apex and the interventricular septum. This usually associates with ST elevation in V1–4 or new bundle branch block. The LCx artery supplies the remainder of the left ventricle and, sometimes, the posterior part of the

interventricular septum. In some people, it also supplies the sinus and AV nodes. Occlusion of the LCx leads to lateral infarction, sometimes associated with conduction problems.

Left main stem occlusion effectively leads to infarction of the entire left ventricle and is usually fatal.

Common ECG patterns of infarction

The following ECG patterns of infarction may be seen in the standard 12-lead ECG.

- *Anterior myocardial infarction* (Fig. 7.4) gives rise to changes in leads V1–V4 (antero-septal infarction), standard leads I and aVL and V4–V6 (antero-lateral infarction).
- *Inferior myocardial infarction* produces changes in the inferior leads II, III and aVF (Fig. 7.5).
- *High lateral myocardial infarction* may be seen only in leads I and aVL.
- *Apical infarction* can be seen in leads V5 and V6.
- *Posterior myocardial infarction* involves the postero-basal wall of the left ventricle. The diagnosis is often missed, as there are no ECG leads that cover this part of the heart. Changes may be seen in the anterior leads (V1 to V3) but, as these leads record from the opposite side of the heart, the changes in posterior infarction are reversed, with the R waves increasing in size, becoming broader and dominant and associated with ST depression and upright T waves (Fig. 7.6). Right ventricular hypertrophy and right bundle branch block should be excluded. Leads V7–V9 (precordial leads placed further round the chest) may show ST segment elevation, and may help in identifying the patients who may benefit from thrombolysis.
- *Right ventricular infarction* usually results from occlusion of the right coronary artery proximal to the right ventricular marginal branches, hence its association with inferior infarction. About one-third to one-half of patients with inferior infarction sustain some damage to the right ventricle, and most regain normal right ventricular function over a period of weeks to months even in the absence of reperfusion, suggesting that right ventricular stunning is more common than necrosis. Less commonly, right

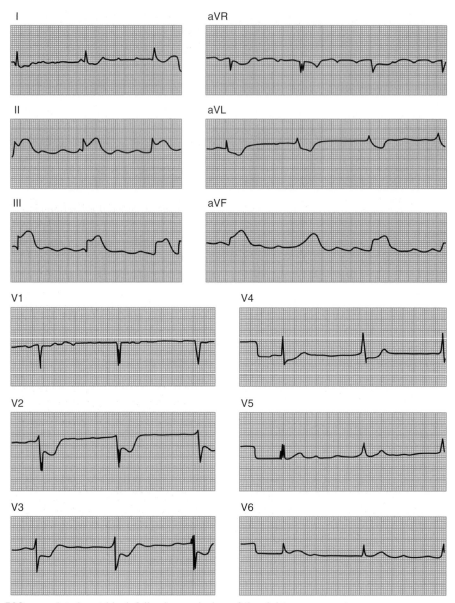

Figure 7.3 ECG: complete heart block following occlusion of the right coronary artery.

ventricular infarction is associated with occlusion of the left circumflex artery and, if this vessel is dominant, there may be an associated infero-lateral wall infarction. Right ventricular infarction is often overlooked, as standard 12-lead ECG is not a particularly sensitive indicator of right ventricular damage, but failure to recognise it may lead to inappropriate management. Right ventricular infarction should be suspected when there are ECG changes of inferior infarction, associated with ST segment elevation in lead V1. Right-sided chest leads are much more sensitive, where > 1 mm ST segment elevation in lead $V4_R$ (right fifth intercostal space in the mid-clavicular line) is the single most important ECG sign of right ventricular ischaemia. Changes may also be seen in $V5_R$ and $V6_R$, with resolution in over half of cases

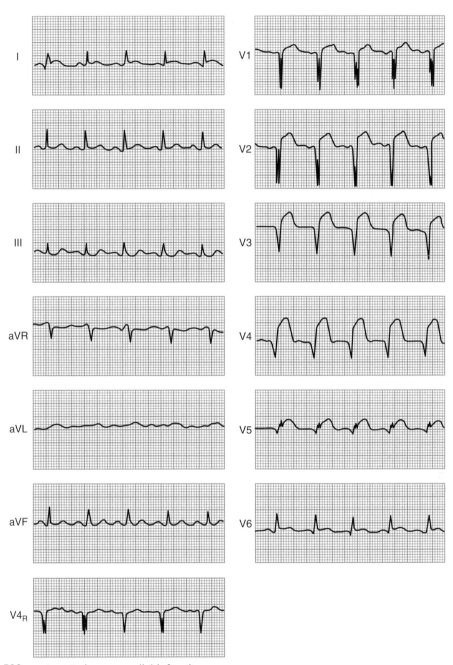

Figure 7.4   ECG: acute anterior myocardial infarction.

within 10 hours of the onset of chest pain. Right ventricular leads should be recorded as soon as possible in all patients with inferior infarction, as changes may be short lived. ST elevation in $V4_R$ is a strong predictor of short-term complications and death (Zehender et al, 1993).

- *Atrial infarction* occurs in about 10% of cases of myocardial infarction, but is often not noticed. It may be recognised by altered P wave morphology on the ECG, with deviation of the PR segment. Atrial dysrhythmias are a common complication, particularly atrial fibrillation.

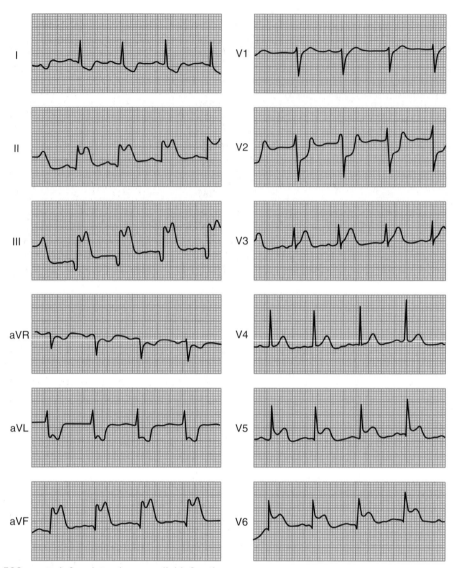

Figure 7.5   ECG: acute infero-lateral myocardial infarction.

ECG changes do not always appear in the 'classical' leads, and additional leads may be required to locate infarcts at unusual sites. For example, V7 and V8 (placed further round the chest) are useful for diagnosing lateral infarcts, and leads in the second and third intercostal spaces may locate high lateral infarcts. With the passage of time following myocardial infarction, the Q waves may regress or even disappear because the scar contracts away from the surface electrode, or because small intraventricular conduction pathways are established in relation to the infarct.

Non-transmural (subendocardial) myocardial infarction

The subendocardium is especially prone to ischaemia, because the high intraventricular pressure limits perfusion. Q wave development usually requires more than 50% of the wall thickness to be involved, so myocardial infarction limited to the inner part of the ventricular wall (subendocardium) will not give rise to Q waves. Subendocardial infarction interferes with repolarisation rather than depolarisation,

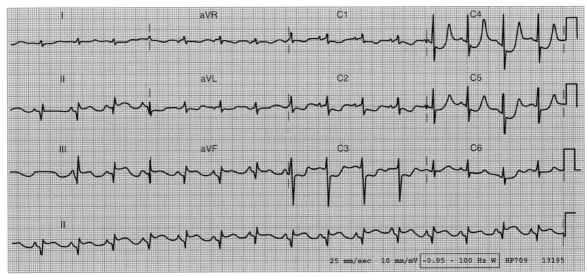

Figure 7.6 ECG: posterior myocardial infarction.

and produces ST depression and deep symmetrical T wave inversion (Fig. 7.7).

ECG changes that mimic myocardial infarction (pseudo–infarction)

There are many circumstances in which ECG appearances may be confused with those of myocardial infarction. ST segment elevation may be a variant of normal or due to non-cardiac disease, so interpretation should always be made in the light of the clinical history and examination findings.

Benign early repolarisation

A degree of ST segment elevation is often present in many healthy individuals (especially young adults and people of African descent). This ST segment elevation is most commonly seen in the precordial leads, especially in lead V4. It is usually subtle, but can sometimes be pronounced and can easily be mistaken for pathological ST segment elevation. Other clues that the cause is benign are:

- elevation of the J point above the isoelectric line (often with a distinct notch);
- concavity of the ST segment;
- large, symmetrical, upright T waves.

Other normal variants are T wave inversion in leads V1 and V2 (and V3 in negroes), and poor R wave progression across the chest leads. QS complexes occasionally occur in V1 and V2 as a normal variant in tall, thin individuals or in those with chest wall deformities (e.g. pectus excavatum).

Pericarditis

Acute pericarditis is commonly mistaken for acute myocardial infarction as both cause chest pain and ST segment elevation on the ECG. In pericarditis, however, ST segment elevation is diffuse rather than localised, and the ST segments are concave upwards, sometimes giving a 'saddle' appearance. Depression of the PR segment may also be seen. Widespread reciprocal changes are unusual, but may occasionally be seen in leads aVR and V1. The ST segment elevation is caused by subepicardial myocarditis, with the injured tissue causing ST elevation in the leads facing the epicardial surface, whereas those facing the ventricular cavity (leads aVR and V1) record ST segment depression.

Metabolic influences

Transient Q wave formation may follow metabolic insults such as hyperkalaemia or hypoglycaemia.

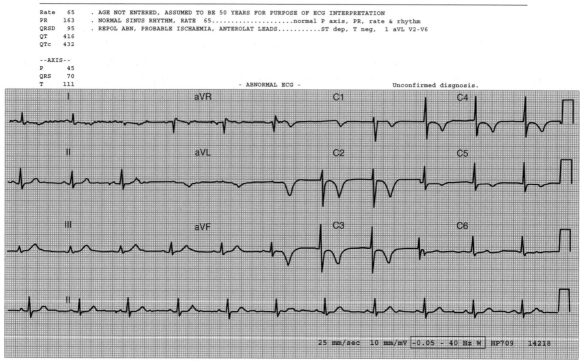

```
Rate   65    . AGE NOT ENTERED, ASSUMED TO BE 50 YEARS FOR PURPOSE OF ECG INTERPRETATION
PR     163   . NORMAL SINUS RHYTHM, RATE 65....................normal P axis, PR, rate & rhythm
QRSD   95    . REPOL ABN, PROBABLE ISCHAEMIA, ANTEROLAT LEADS..........ST dep, T neg,  1 aVL V2-V6
QT     416
QTc    432

--AXIS--
P      45
QRS    70
T      111                          - ABNORMAL ECG -              Unconfirmed disgnosis.
```

25 mm/sec 10 mm/mV -0.05 - 40 Hz W HP709 14218

Figure 7.7   ECG: non-transmural (subendocardial) myocardial infarction.

ST–T wave changes are characteristic of hypo- and hyperkalaemia.

Left ventricular hypertrophy

Left ventricular hypertrophy secondary to hypertension or aortic stenosis may produce poor R wave progression in leads V1–V3. There may also be left axis deviation. The small R wave and deep S waves may be confused with pathological Q waves, particularly if there are co-existent ST–T wave changes of left ventricular strain.

Pulmonary embolism

QR waves in leads V1–V3 are seen in right ventricular hypertrophy or strain. The classic $S_1/Q_3/T_3$ pattern described in acute pulmonary embolism is associated with non-infarction Q waves in standard leads III and aVF. Widespread T wave inversion and a sinus tachycardia are more usual.

Brugada syndrome

This is recognised by a characteristic ECG appearance of right bundle branch block and ST segment elevation in the right precordial leads. The condition is sometimes familial, often in young men and associates with malignant ventricular dysrhythmias and sudden death (Brugada, 2000). It appears to be most prevalent in South-east Asia and Japan, where the disorder is a leading cause of natural death among young men. Finding of Brugada-type ECG in asymptomatic individuals without a family history of sudden death is a growing problem in clinical decision-making.

Coronary arterial spasm

Printzmetal angina is associated with transient ST segment elevation. ST segment abnormalities may be seen in association with cocaine use, and are probably due to a combination of vasospasm and atheroma.

Miscellaneous conditions

Very deep inverted T waves are sometimes found after intracerebral bleeds, probably due to altered autonomic tone, and may be confused with the changes of subendocardial myocardial infarction. Similar T wave changes are often seen after prolonged tachycardias or Stokes–Adams attacks. T wave inversion sometimes occurs in normal hearts as a result of catecholamine stimulation, and can be reversed with beta-blockade. Hyperventilation may also produce transient ST–T wave changes.

TREATMENT OF CORONARY THROMBOSIS BY THROMBOLYSIS

Myocardial infarction is virtually always associated with the presence of fresh thrombus in the affected coronary artery, in a dynamic interaction involving coronary artery spasm, platelet aggregation and a fissured atheromatous plaque. Complete absence of blood flow in the infarct-related artery is usual, although small platelet emboli are shed before the artery becomes occluded, causing multiple, small, distal occlusions in the area supplied by the coronary vessel ('microinfarcts'). Spontaneous thrombolysis may take place to a varying degree in about 30% of patients within the first 12–24 hours (de Wood et al, 1980). Hence, there may be varying consequences of acute coronary thrombosis, ranging from microinfarcts to full transmural infarction.

Thrombolysis was one of the most significant advances in the treatment of acute myocardial infarction in the twentieth century. Ironically, the observation in the 1930s that streptokinase, a breakdown product of some *Streptococcus* strains, could liquefy clotted blood came long before CCUs, bedside monitors and defibrillators existed. It was another 25 years before attempts to reopen coronary arteries with streptokinase were reported in the treatment of acute myocardial infarction (Dewar et al, 1963).

Thrombolytic agents are actually *fibrinolytic* agents that activate plasminogen to form plasmin, which degrades fibrin and breaks down fresh thrombus. Intracoronary administration of streptokinase in acute myocardial infarction was used experimentally in the late 1970s, but it was the GISSI Study Group (1987) which showed that thrombolysis could be effective when given systemically, meaning that administration did not require coronary angiography. The second International Study of Infarct Survival (ISIS-2) confirmed the beneficial effects of thrombolysis, and nearly half a million patients have since been randomised in different thrombolytic trials, making it one of the most extensively researched medical therapies. It is interesting to reflect on the fact that primary angioplasty requires a return to specialist invasive intervention, again limiting availability.

Thrombolytic guidelines

Before therapeutic intervention with thrombolytic agents, there are certain considerations including:

- who should be treated;
- when and how to administer the drug;
- the choice of thrombolytic agent;
- what to do after thrombolysis.

Who should be treated?

It must be remembered that not all patients derive the same benefit from thrombolysis and, in some, the benefits may be marginal or even harmful. Risk/benefits to the individual must be considered. Those patients likely to derive most benefit are those with anterior infarcts, diabetes, the elderly and those in cardiogenic shock. The Fibrinolytic Therapy Trialists' Collaborative Group (1994) analysed all randomised fibrinolytic therapy trials of more than 1000 patients and found that the benefits of fibrinolytic therapy only applied to patients with ST segment elevation or bundle branch block on the presenting ECG (Table 7.4). Benefit was seen at all time intervals within the first 12 hours of symptom onset, with greater benefit the earlier treatment is begun. Within the first 6 hours, 30 deaths are prevented per 1000 patients treated, falling to 20 prevented deaths in the

Table 7.4 Benefits of thrombolysis in different patient groups (Fibrinolytic Therapy Trialists' Collaborative Group, 1994).

Group	Mortality at 35 days without thrombolysis	Lives saved/1000 patients treated[a]
Males	10.1%	19
Females	16.0%	18
Age (years)		
< 55	4.6%	11
55–64	8.9%	18
65–74	16.1%	27
> 75	25.3%	10
Previous myocardial infarction		
Yes	14.1%	16
No	10.9%	20
Diabetes		
Yes	17.3%	37
No	10.2%	15
Presenting ECG		
Bundle branch block[b]	23.6%	49
ST elevation		
Anterior	16.9%	37
Inferior	8.4%	8
Other	13.4%	27
ST depression	13.8%	−14
Other abnormalities	5.8%	6
Normal	2.3%	−7

a A minus sign denotes an increased mortality.
b Unspecified.

7- to 12-hour period. The value of thrombolysis in those presenting more than 12 hours after symptom onset has not been confirmed.

Confusion still exists regarding some ECG criteria for fibrinolysis, particularly that of bundle branch block (BBB). The GISSI and ISIS-2 studies made no distinction between right, left, atypical, old and new BBB, and neither did the Fibrinolytic Therapy Trialists' Collaborative Group's meta-analysis, although most of the trials considered used left bundle branch block (LBBB) as an entry criterion. The ECG diagnosis of acute myocardial infarction in the presence of LBBB is often difficult and sometimes impossible. As a result, the 1999 American College of Cardiology/American Heart Association (ACC/AHA, 1999) guidelines recommend 'BBB (obscuring ST segment analysis) and history suggesting AMI' as an indication for fibrinolytic therapy.

Patients with ST segment depression on the initial ECG have an increased mortality if treated with fibrinolytic therapy but, when marked ST segment depression is confined to leads V1–V4, this usually reflects a posterior current of injury due to circumflex artery occlusion, for which thrombolytic therapy is appropriate. Obtaining posterior ECG leads when one sees anterior ST segment depression and right ventricular leads when one sees lateral ST segment depression is recommended. Alternatively, routinely recording an 18-lead ECG (12-lead ECG + V7–V9 and V4R–V6R) increases the chances of detecting all cases that will benefit from thrombolysis (Zalenski et al, 1997).

Contraindications to the administration of thrombolytic drugs

The main contraindications to the administration of thrombolytic drugs are:

- previous haemorrhagic stroke;
- ischaemic stroke within 6 months;
- active bleeding, but not menstruation;
- suspected aortic dissection;
- intracranial neoplasm or structural vascular lesion;
- closed head trauma within 3 months;
- major trauma or surgery in the previous 3 weeks.

Relative contraindications include:

- chronic severe uncontrolled hypertension;
- blood pressure > 180/110 mmHg on presentation;
- following traumatic resuscitation;
- cerebrovascular surgery;
- anticoagulant therapy [the higher the international normalised ratio (INR), the higher the risk];
- aortic aneurysm;
- advanced liver disease;
- recent internal bleeding (< 28 days);
- active peptic ulceration;
- pregnancy.

Genuine contraindications to thrombolysis exist in between 7% and 10% of patients (French et al, 1996), but many more patients are denied therapy, particularly those with diabetes and the elderly, because of perceived rather than actual problems.

Complications of thrombolysis

The major risks of thrombolysis are intracranial haemorrhage, systemic haemorrhage, immunological complications, dysrhythmias and hypotension.

Intracranial haemorrhage is the most life-threatening complication of fibrinolysis, with reported rates of around 1%. This leads to death in about half of patients, with another third being permanently disabled. Fibrin-specific agents seem to increase this complication, and risk is greater with tissue plasminogen activator (tPA) and reteplase than for streptokinase, especially in elderly patients.

Overall, there are about four additional strokes (mostly cerebral haemorrhage) per 1000 patients treated, mostly in the first 24 hours. Predictors of intracranial haemorrhage are age over 65 years, low body weight (under 70 kg), previous or presenting hypertension and history of cerebrovascular disease.

Major systemic haemorrhage affects about 7 cases per 1000 patients treated, and may require intravenous tranexamic acid or fresh frozen plasma to reverse the effects of thrombolysis. Temporary pacemakers and Swan–Ganz catheters should be inserted via the antecubital fossa or femoral vein to prevent possible occult bleeding following central catheterisation.

Fever and allergic reactions are frequent with streptokinase. Anaphylaxis is a rare complication, and symptoms may be mistaken for cardiogenic shock. Routine pretreatment with hydrocortisone and antihistamines has been advocated in the past, but is no longer used. Hypotension is a frequent accompaniment of thrombolytic therapy with streptokinase, and may require slowing of the infusion, elevating the feet, atropine or intravenous fluids.

Dysrhythmias may accompany reperfusion of the ischaemic myocardium. These 'reperfusion dysrhythmias' are usually without clinical significance. Idio-ventricular rhythm is the most frequent abnormality, although some patients will develop ventricular tachycardia or ventricular fibrillation (Verheugt, 1996).

When and how to administer the drug

For myocardial salvage to be optimised, thrombolysis must be attempted as early as possible. There is a gradual reduction in benefit with delay in administration of thrombolytic therapy, with each hour of delay translating into 1.6 additional lives lost per 1000 patients treated. However, survival benefits are not linear, and are twice as great in those treated in the first 2 hours as in those treated after 2 hours (Boersma et al, 1996). In contrast to early therapy, the benefits of late thrombolysis are less clear. Too few patients presenting more than 12 hours after the onset of symptoms have been studied to allow benefits to be determined (Collins et al, 1997).

The choice of thrombolytic agent

The most commonly chosen thrombolytic agents have been streptokinase (a first-generation thrombolytic agent) and the second-generation alteplase (tPA). Third-generation derivatives of alteplase (reteplase, tenecteplase and lanoteplase) are now established in clinical practice and gaining popularity. Anisoylated plasminogen–streptokinase activator complex (APSAC) was withdrawn because the adverse effects and reperfusion rates were no different from those of streptokinase.

One of the world's largest therapeutic trials compared streptokinase, APSAC and tPA against each other in 41 299 patients with suspected acute myocardial infarction (ISIS-3, 1992). There was no difference in mortality between the treatment groups, but there were fewer cerebral bleeds with streptokinase and, overall, this was found to be the safest drug. As a result, streptokinase has generally been used as the agent of first choice based on the results of the ISIS-3 trial, as well as cost.

The strongest predictor of survival following thrombolysis is the presence of early brisk, antegrade flow in the affected coronary artery – the so-called TIMI (thrombolysis in myocardial infarction) grade 3 flow. Practice changed slightly in favour of tPA following the GUSTO-1 trial (1993), in which TIMI 3 flow was achieved in 54% of patients receiving tPA vs. 32% in those who received streptokinase, using a new tPA regimen referred to as *front-loaded* or *accelerated tPA*. Benefits from this regime were more marked in younger patients treated within 4 hours of the onset of symptoms, especially if the infarct was large and involved the anterior wall. Based on these insights, the new thrombolytic agents (reteplase and tenecteplase) were designed to further improve survival, although no additional improvement in clinical outcome has yet been observed. Reteplase and weight-adjusted tenecteplase (TNK) are equivalent to accelerated tPA in terms of 28-day mortality, but TNK may associate with less bleeding. The major advantage of these third-generation agents is that they may be given by bolus rather than by infusion. This makes administration much easier, and is a particular advantage for prehospital thrombolysis.

Streptokinase Streptokinase is a metabolic product of the group C beta-haemolytic *Streptococcus*, which causes activation of plasminogen, leading to lysis of the fibrin within the fresh thrombus. Unfortunately, it is not clot-specific and causes a systemic thrombolytic state by depleting fibrinogen and alpha-2 antiplasmin concentrations. Streptokinase is also antigenic and may produce allergic side effects, such as fever, rash and even anaphylactic shock. Previous infections with streptococci may induce antibodies to streptokinase, and predispose the patient to allergic reactions and reduced clinical efficacy. Antistreptolysin titres begin to develop from the third day following administration of streptokinase and persist for years (Squire et al, 1999). Many patients presenting with myocardial infarction will have had a previous infarct, are likely to have been exposed to streptokinase and should not receive the drug again. About one-third of patients with acute myocardial infarction have contraindications to streptokinase.

The usual dose of streptokinase is 1.5 million units in 100 mL of 5% dextrose (or saline) infused over 60 minutes. Streptokinase in combination with enoxaparin (intravenous bolus 30 mg followed by 1 mg/kg twice daily) for up to a week is associated with better ST segment resolution and better early angiographic patency, but no increased bleed risk (Simoons et al, 2002).

An accelerated streptokinase regimen (1.5 million units over 20 minutes or as a double infusion of 0.75 million units over 10 minutes, separated by 50 minutes) was used in the ASENOX study (Tatu-Chitoiu et al, 2004), and was shown to be safe, with significantly higher rates of coronary reperfusion and a lower in-hospital mortality compared with the traditional streptokinase therapy.

Tissue plasminogen activator (tPA) Tissue plasminogen activator (tPA) is a naturally occurring protein with greater clot specificity than streptokinase, and fibrinogen and alpha-2 antiplasmin concentrations are less likely to become depleted. Cloning of the tPA gene has provided large quantities of the drug for clinical use but, despite price reductions, it remains relatively expensive (£600 for the standard 100-mg dose). The thrombolytic 'gold standard', *accelerated tPA*, is given as a 15-mg bolus, followed by 50 mg over 30 minutes and the remainder over 60 minutes. The standard infusion is 10 mg by intravenous bolus, followed by 50 mg over 1 hour and the remaining 40 mg over 2 hours. It is indicated up to 6 hours following symptom onset.

Reteplase (recombinant plasminogen activator)

Reteplase (rPA) has a longer plasma half-life than tPA (14–18 minutes vs. 3–4 minutes), allowing it to be administered as a double bolus of 10 units, each 30 minutes apart. It is thus easier to give, and does not need dose adjustment for weight. It is expensive (£666). There are only marginal benefits over streptokinase in terms of outcome, although it may associate with fewer complications such as atrial fibrillation and cardiogenic shock. It may be given up to 12 hours after symptom onset.

Tenecteplase (TNK) Tenecteplase also has a longer plasma half-life than tPA (approximately 17 minutes), which allows for single bolus application, and it does not need refrigeration. This makes it particularly attractive for use prehospital and in the emergency department, and it may be used up to 6 hours after symptom onset. The ASSENT studies confirm similar efficacy to accelerated tPA, but with a wider safety margin (ASSENT-2 Investigators, 1999). The dose must be given according to body weight, and is given as a bolus injection over 10 seconds. It is expensive (£735).

Choice of agent

The choice of fibrinolytic regimen is probably not as important as the speed with which it can be given. Overall, the choice of thrombolytic agent appears to make little difference to overall survival, because the regimens that resolve coronary thrombi more rapidly produce greater risks of cerebral and systemic haemorrhage (Collins et al, 1997). In comparison to accelerated tPA, reteplase and tenecteplase are equal in their efficacy but superior in their ease of administration (Menon et al, 2004). These three agents are preferable if the patient presents within 6 hours of the onset of symptoms, particularly those under the age of 75 years and those with high-risk infarcts:

- anterior myocardial infarction;
- myocardial infarction with BBB;

- inferior myocardial infarction:
  - with anterior ST depression;
  - with right ventricular involvement;
  - with lateral extension.

THROMBOLYSIS IN THE ELDERLY

Although about a third of myocardial infarcts occur in people over the age of 75 years, 70% of these elderly patients will not have ST segment elevation on their presenting ECG. As a result, firm conclusions on the risk and benefits of thrombolysis in the elderly have been difficult because numbers involved in the trials have been small. Long-term data from the ISIS-2 trial show that the absolute survival advantage following thrombolysis is as least as good for older as for younger patients (Baigent et al, 1998). While there is a decreasing relative benefit of fibrinolysis in elderly patients, there is an absolute gain in terms of lives saved (Estess & Topol, 2002).

The major concern over thrombolysis in the elderly is the risk of stroke, which, unlike the benefits of saving myocardium, is not time-dependent. The risk of stroke increases with age, and is more notable with tPA, but less obvious (if at all) with streptokinase. Those at particular risk are females (particularly of low body weight), those with a systolic blood pressure over 160 mmHg and those with a prior history of cerebrovascular disease (Brass et al, 2000). Streptokinase remains the thrombolytic agent of first choice in the elderly, although initial clinical trial data with TNK (tenecteplase) suggest decreased rates of intracranial bleeding for elderly females, when compared with tPA (Barron et al, 1999).

When considering thrombolysis in the elderly, risk can be minimised by restricting its use to those with early presentation (under 6 hours) and clear-cut ST elevation, especially if in the anterior leads or new bundle branch block. Age in itself should not be a considered a contraindication for fibrinolysis; biological age and co-morbid conditions are more important than the chronological age.

Thrombolysis in patients with diabetes

Patients with diabetes derive greater benefit from thrombolysis than those without diabetes, but are often not treated with fibrinolytic agents, perhaps because of fear of inducing intraocular bleeding (Shotliff et al, 1998). However, none of the 300 patients with proliferative retinopathy in the GUSTO-1 trial suffered retinal bleeding (Mahaffey et al, 1997).

Summary guidelines for thrombolysis are shown in Box 7.2.

Box 7.2   Guidelines for thrombolysis in acute myocardial infarction (AMI).

Patients with clinical presentation suggestive of acute myocardial infarction plus:

ST segment elevations > 0.1 mV in two or more contiguous leads (exclude benign early repolarisation, pericarditis or repolarisation abnormality from left ventricular haemorrhage)

Bundle branch block of any type (right, left, paced, new or old)

ST segment depressions of 1 mm or more with upright T waves in two or more contiguous anterior precordial leads suggestive of posterior MI

ST elevations of 1 mm or more in two or more contiguous non-standard leads (V4R–V6R, V7–V9) in patients with clinical presentation suggestive of isolated right ventricular or posterior AMI

Time since onset of symptoms

0–6 h – greatest benefit
6–12 h – possible benefit
> 12 h – little benefit unless continuing or stuttering pain

Age

Biological rather than chronological age is more important (risk increases with more co-morbidities)

Clear-cut benefits are seen in those under 75 years

Very elderly patients have few clear-cut benefits

Streptokinase is a safer agent in the elderly

What to do after thrombolysis

To achieve the best outcome of thrombolysis, the infarct-related artery must be opened fully and quickly, and patency must be maintained. Although the new plasminogen activators have been shown to achieve more rapid or complete infarct vessel patency than tPA, this has not resulted in an improvement in survival, which suggests that the relationship between coronary artery patency and survival is not direct. A possible explanation lies in microvascular obstruction, as patency of the infarct-related epicardial artery does not assure microvascular flow or normal myocardial perfusion. Platelet microemboli from the unstable plaque produce transient microvascular occlusion, or microinfarcts, and are likely to be responsible for the 'no flow' phenomenon often seen at coronary angiography following successful recanalisation. Anterior infarcts are more prone to this than inferior infarcts. Microvascular obstruction carries a fourfold increase in adverse events including death, reinfarction or the development of heart failure in a group of patients after myocardial reperfusion treatment (Wu et al, 1998). It is not clear whether the additive and independent benefits of aspirin relate to the enhancement of thrombolysis or the limiting of the microvascular effects of platelet activation. Underlying the coronary thrombotic event is a fissured atherosclerotic plaque, which initially leads to the formation of a platelet thrombus that is seen angioscopically as 'white' thrombus (Van Belle et al, 1998). Surrounding this area of platelet aggregation is the 'red' thrombus that is fibrin rich. Current thrombolytic agents actually attack not thrombin, but fibrin in the red thrombus. Thrombin, previously enmeshed in the red thrombus, is exposed, and exerts potent platelet proaggregatory effects, promoting microvascular embolisation. So, rather than aiming to achieve complete dissolution of the thrombus alone, approaches to prevent embolisation of part of the thrombus into the microcirculation should be considered.

Heparin does not enhance immediate clot breakdown, but is of value in maintaining vessel patency in the days following fibrinolysis, particularly when fibrin-specific agents have been used. It is usual for an intravenous bolus of sodium heparin (60 units/kg – maximum 4000 units) to be given before thrombolysis, and for heparin cover to continue for varying periods afterwards. Low-molecular-weight heparin (LMWH) offers both practical and pharmacological advantages over infused unfractionated heparin (UFH), not least because of more predictable bioavailability. LMWH given for 4–8 days following thrombolysis reduces reinfarction by about 25% and death by about 10% compared with placebo (Eikelboom et al, 2005), and direct comparisons of UFH and enoxaparin suggest that reinfarction may be reduced by a third using the latter (Antman et al, 2006). The usual regime is enoxaparin 30 mg intravenously then 1 mg/kg twice daily for a minimum of 72 hours.

Utilising a more aggressive antiplatelet approach may also allow a reduced fibrinolytic dose, thereby minimising the prothrombotic state and the risk of intracerebral haemorrhage. This is known as *combination therapy*, and is most often used to describe the combined use of reduced-dose thrombolytics and full-dose glycoprotein (Gp) IIb/IIIa inhibitors, such as abciximab, eptifibatide and tirofiban. Microvascular reperfusion was re-established more often with the combination therapy than with alteplase treatment alone (De Lemos et al, 2000). The combination of full-dose abciximab and half-dose reteplase reduces non-fatal complications of myocardial infarction, but has a similar mortality rate to reteplase alone.

Facilitated percutaneous coronary intervention (PCI) for ST segment elevation myocardial infarction uses various drugs prior to early planned intervention to improve coronary patency. Starting reperfusion while the catheter laboratory is being prepared seems sensible, but giving the thrombolytic agent before PCI removes the advantage of reduction in stroke and haemorrhagic complications (McClellan et al, 2004). Facilitated PCI with thrombolysis has not been shown to offer any benefit over primary PCI alone, and should be avoided (Keeley et al, 2006).

FAILED THROMBOLYSIS

Acute thrombotic coronary artery occlusion rapidly results in severe transmural ischaemia, contractile dysfunction and a wavefront of myocardial injury and necrosis progressing from the endocardium to the epicardium. Coronary artery patency and flow are important and independent prognostic predictors in patients following thrombolysis, and the prognosis in patients who do not reperfuse is worse than that in those who do. Epicardial coronary flow may be classified by the TIMI (thrombolysis in myocardial infarction) flow grade (Table 7.5). This semi-quantitative tool has shown that early failure of thrombolytic treatment is associated with a 30-day mortality of over 15%. At least 30% of patients fail to recanalise by 2 hours following treatment, although only a minority show signs of continuing ischaemia. Why thrombolysis fails in some cases is not clear. Those at risk are generally older, non-smokers, those with a previous infarct and, of course, those where there has been a delay in treatment. Local vascular problems, such as a large thrombus or a large degree of fixed stenosis, may reduce the efficacy of thrombolysis.

Residual atheromatous stenoses may be found by angiography in 80–90% of cases following thrombolysis, and reaccumulation of thrombus

Table 7.5 Classification of coronary artery flow and myocardial perfusion seen at angiography (TIMI and TMP grading system).

Grade	
TIMI flow	
0	No penetration of contrast past the clot in the infarct-related artery
1	Contrast flows past vessel occlusion, but does not fill to the end of the vessel
2	Infarct-related vessel fills to full length, but flow is slower than that down normal adjacent vessels
3	Normal filling of infarct-related artery in comparison to adjacent vessels
TMP perfusion	
0	No or minimal blush
1	Dye does not leave myocardium; blush persists to next injection
2	Dye strongly persists at end of washout, but gone by next injection
3	Normal myocardial blush; mildly persistent at the end of washout

may occur in up to 40% within the first week, although these are not usually totally obstructive, nor accompanied by symptoms. Symptomatic reocclusion of the infarct-related artery occurs in about 5–8% of patients, mostly within the first 3 days. These patients have a more complicated clinical course and a higher mortality.

Vessel patency means there is some flow down the vessel however effective, and the term *recanalisation* is used when a previously occluded vessel has been reopened. Unfortunately, demonstrating an open vessel does not necessarily imply that flow is occurring down to tissue level. Patients with TIMI-2 and TIMI-3 flow have open arteries, but those with TIMI-2 flow have a worse prognosis, probably because of impaired microvascular circulation. It has become clear that it is actually tissue perfusion, and not just an open artery, that is critical to myocardial salvage. The term *reperfusion* refers to re-establishing circulation at capillary level, which cannot be easily determined. Full reperfusion following thrombolysis fails in 60–75% of cases and associates with a mortality of 16–20% (de Belder, 2001). The *no flow phenomenon* arises because of platelet emboli and other atheromatous debris occluding flow in the microvasculature, with ischaemia-induced endothelial swelling and distal vessel vasoconstriction also playing a part (Blows et al, 2005). Microvascular perfusion is considered to be a key factor in the preservation of left ventricular function and prognosis. Perfusion defects following acute myocardial infarction may be visualised by myocardial contrast echocardiography, and relate closely to lack of contractile recovery and irreversible myocyte damage (Reffelmann & Kloner, 2002). Once no flow is established, treatment is often ineffective, and associates with both short- and long-term outcomes. The transmural extent of myocardial and microvascular necrosis is highly variable from patient to patient. The major determinants are the presence and adequacy of collateral circulation, time to treatment and therapeutic efficacy.

Just as TIMI flow grades are important in assessing epicardial artery flow, the TIMI myocardial perfusion (TMP) grading system may be used to define myocardial perfusion (Appleby et al, 2001). Like TIMI flow, perfusion is graded TMP-0 to TMP-3, based on myocardial 'blushing' as angiographic dye passes in and out of the myocardium (Table 7.5). This provides independent risk stratification among patients with normal TIMI-3 epicardial flow.

Diagnosing failed reperfusion

It is not known when to decide that thrombolysis has failed, or even how best to determine that it has failed (Kovlack & Gershlick, 2001). Deciding that thrombolysis has failed too early may lead to unnecessary further interventions, but waiting too long may allow further myocardial damage. Helpful clues may be:

1 *Clinical.* Cessation of chest pain may indicate success in reperfusion, although analgesia may mask this, so it is not of value on its own. Other factors may also raise the pain threshold, such as age and diabetes. Conversely, continuing chest pain does not imply failure to achieve TIMI-3 epicardial flow, possibly because of poor tissue perfusion. Chest pain may also occur during reperfusion, especially in those with large infarcts.

2 *Reperfusion dysrhythmias.* Although frequent, the appearance of so-called reperfusional dysrhythmias does not necessarily indicate success. Idio-ventricular rhythm is perhaps the most common marker of reperfusion, but the relief of chest pain, resolution of ST segments and appearance of dysrhythmias occur in only 15% of patients.

3 *The 12-lead electrocardiogram.* Patients whose ECG returns to normal in the early period following thrombolysis have preserved left ventricular function and a low mortality, whereas non-resolution of ST segment elevation associates with a poor outcome. The best ECG marker of reperfusion is a greater than 50% decrease in ST segment elevation at 60 minutes in the single lead with the maximum ST elevation at presentation (Oldroyd, 2000; Sutton et al, 2000). However, reperfusion by ECG voltage criteria depends on the location of the infarct so, while an anterior infarct should show a > 50% resolution, a > 70% resolution is more appropriate for inferior infarcts. This degree of resolution plus

the resolution of chest pain are more likely to predict patency (De Lemos & Braunwald, 2001). Repeated 12-lead ECGs may be helpful in identifying these patients, although continuous ST monitoring allows this to be done more easily (Klootwijk et al, 1996).

4 *Biochemical markers*. A rapid peak in myoglobin concentrations is a marker of recanalisation, and can be assessed at the bedside with near-patient testing kits. There are no cardiac markers that can differentiate between TIMI-2 and TIMI-3 flow. Detection of reperfusion by most biochemical markers may be too late to allow a change in therapy.

What to do if thrombolysis fails

- *Further thrombolysis* is probably the most often tried intervention, particularly in hospitals without catheter facilities. Unfortunately, there is no good evidence that it works (Gershlick et al, 2005). Potential benefits may be offset by increased bleeding risks, particularly when performed more than 6 hours after initial fibrinolysis.
- *Rescue angioplasty* describes PCI to open the coronary artery that has remained occluded despite thrombolysis. Such intervention is helpful, but not without problems, particularly bleeding from the sheath insertion site (Ellis et al, 2000). Salvage angioplasty rates are about 85% compared with rates of 95% with primary angioplasty, and the patient still has the usual risks of systemic haemorrhage. In-hospital mortality in this group is over 25% (Ross et al, 1998). The REACT trial looked at 427 patients,

who, after a 90-minutes ECG, failed to achieve under 50% resolution of ST changes, and found that rescue PCI is superior to repeat thrombolysis or conservative treatment in terms of event-free survival (Gershlick et al, 2005). The European Society of Cardiology recommends rescue PCI if thrombolysis has failed within 45–60 minutes of fibrinolytic therapy (Silber et al, 2005).

- *Emergency bypass surgery* (CABG) seems unlikely to emerge as a form of treatment for failed thrombolysis. There are no trials in this group of patients, and angioplasty is less risky and easier to deliver.

Inappropriate administration of thrombolytic therapy

While thrombolysis has become standard care for myocardial infarction, apprehension over complications often limits its use. The risk of bleeding and stroke are well appreciated, and reports of a haemorrhagic pericardial effusion in patients with aortic dissection, or unassociated with cardiac rupture, strengthen this concern (Heymann & Culling, 1994). Serious consequences of misdiagnosis were observed in the ASSET trial, where patients with non-coronary chest pain who underwent thrombolysis had a mortality of 9.5%, against a mortality of 1.2% in those treated with placebo (Wilcox et al, 1988). Given the high incidence and multiple aetiologies of chest pain, one needs to guard against inappropriate administration of thrombolytic agents. Using simple guidelines, as in Table 7.6, associates with a low rate of inappropriate thrombolysis.

Table 7.6 Superiority of primary angioplasty compared with thrombolysis. Data from Hartwell et al, 2005.

Cardiac event	Thrombolysis	Primary angioplasty	Relative risk reduction
Mortality (4–6 weeks)	8%	5%	36%
Mortality (4–18 months)	8%	5%	38%
Reinfarction	8%	3%	59%
Recurrent ischaemia	18%	7%	59%
Need for bypass surgery	13%	8%	36%
Stroke	2%	< 1%	64%

Thrombolysis and complete heart block

Complete heart block is a common complication of acute inferior myocardial infarction. Provided there are no contraindications, thrombolysis should be given immediately, as for other cases of myocardial infarction, along with atropine. Atrio-ventricular conduction usually improves, and many cases of complete heart block may be tolerated without the need to insert a temporary pacemaker (Jowett et al, 1989).

TREATMENT OF CORONARY THROMBOSIS BY PRIMARY ANGIOPLASTY

There is little doubt that primary angioplasty is the logical and preferred choice of reperfusion (Table 7.6), but it currently has three major drawbacks:

- lack of availability (catheter labs open 24/7);
- lack of technical expertise (available 24/7);
- a suitable transport infrastructure for getting the right patient to the right place within a short timeframe.

A massive restructuring of cardiac services would be required to give all patients with acute myocardial infarction equal access to primary angioplasty. Modern trials of mechanical reperfusion strategies have not considered these 'real world' logistics, and PCI protocols need to be judged against the outcome achievable by early thrombolysis. For patients presenting within 3 hours of symptoms, thrombolysis results are similar to those achieved by PCI (Widimsky et al, 2000). On the other hand, patient delays are common, as are long journeys to district hospitals in remote areas. Distance transport to a tertiary PCI centre is safe, and immediate intervention decreases mortality in patients presenting over 3 hours after symptom onset. If a reliable prehospital diagnosis can be made, patients with acute myocardial infarction should not necessarily be taken to the most local hospital, but to one that can deliver optimal treatment. Strategies to enable rapid transfer to interventional centres of relatively small numbers of patients should be explored.

OTHER IMPORTANT INTERVENTIONS

Beta–blockade

Intravenous beta-blockade following acute myocardial infarction reduces pain, recurrent ischaemia and mortality in patients with acute myocardial infarction, with a two- to threefold reduction in the risk of cardiac rupture (Freemantle et al, 1999). Despite these benefits, intravenous beta-blockade has not become routine therapy in most countries, and is likely to reduce even further since the publication of the COMMIT Collaborative Group (2005b) trial. In this large study of nearly 46 000 patients, early use of metoprolol (three doses of metoprolol 5 mg intravenously over the course of 15 minutes) did not reduce the risk of in-hospital death, and actually increased the risk of cardiogenic shock, particularly within 24 hours. This cancelled out the benefits of a significant reduction in the risk of dysrhythmic death.

It is now clear that the risk/benefits of acute beta-blockade should be assessed on an individual basis. Low- to medium-risk patients will benefit from intravenous blockers, especially those with persistent sinus tachycardia (unrelated to heart failure), hypertension and those still in pain despite opiates. Early beta-blocker therapy should be avoided in patients with signs of left ventricular dysfunction, bradycardia or hypotension. Low-dose oral beta-blockade can be introduced in these patients when they are stable, and the dose can be titrated upwards if tolerated. Treatment should be continued for at least 2–3 years to achieve maximal benefit, and most would continue the drug indefinitely.

Angiotensin–converting enzyme (ACE) inhibitors

Routine use of ACE inhibitors in unselected patients following acute myocardial infarction reduces mortality and serious cardiovascular events. While the benefits are most marked in those patients with overt cardiac failure or an ejection fraction of less than 40%, there is general agreement that all patients should be started on an ACE inhibitor within the first 36 hours of myocardial infarction.

The ACE inhibitor should be introduced at a low dose with titration over the next few days to maximal doses if tolerated. The ACE inhibitor doses employed in post-infarction trials were captopril (50 mg three times daily), lisinopril (10–40 mg daily), enalapril (20 mg twice daily), ramipril (5 mg twice daily) and trandolapril (4 mg daily). The duration of therapy is unknown, but should continue in the presence of ongoing left ventricular dysfunction.

Magnesium

Magnesium was commonly given to heart attack victims in the 1970s and 1980s, but the ISIS-4 (1995) trial showed there is no mortality benefit in patients receiving fibrinolytic therapy. This was confirmed in the MAGIC trial, in which early administration of magnesium in high-risk patients with STEMI had no effect on 30-day mortality (Antman, 2002). There is thus no indication for the routine administration of intravenous magnesium in patients with STEMI, but measuring and correcting the magnesium level may be advisable if there is hypokalaemia or patients have been on high doses of diuretics, particularly if there are recurrent ventricular dysrhythmias.

Anticoagulants

The routine use of anticoagulants in acute myocardial infarction should be of benefit in:

- preventing deep vein thrombosis and pulmonary emboli;
- preventing left ventricular thrombi and peripheral embolisation;
- possibly limiting infarct size.

Venous thromboembolism and fatal pulmonary emboli are common in all medical patients, and many do not receive prophylaxis. For patients with myocardial infarction, the risk is at least moderate, with a 10–40% risk of a deep vein thrombosis and an approximate 1% risk of fatal pulmonary embolism (THRIFT II Consensus Group, 1998). Subcutaneous low-molecular-weight heparin should be given to all patients from admission until the patient is fully ambulant.

Adding warfarin to aspirin is beneficial in the secondary prevention of myocardial infarction, although the treatment has not been adopted widely. A meta-analysis of 10 trials involving over 11 000 patient–years of observation found that the combination of warfarin and aspirin given after an acute coronary syndrome led to about a halving of risk of myocardial infarction and ischaemic stroke compared with aspirin alone (Rothberg et al, 2005). While the risk of major bleeds more than doubled, this did not affect mortality and, for patients who are at low or intermediate risk for bleeding, the cardiovascular benefits of warfarin outweigh the bleeding risks. The target INR was greater than 2, and most benefits were seen in the first 3 months.

If routine anticoagulant treatment of all post-infarction patients is not practicable, it should be considered in 'high-risk' patients, including those with:

- active thromboembolic phenomena;
- prolonged cardiac failure;
- atrial fibrillation;
- left ventricular aneurysm;
- cardiogenic shock;
- severe obesity;
- an inability to ambulate;
- extensive anterior myocardial infarction.

Antidysrhythmic therapy

Patients are at increased risk of potentially fatal dysrhythmias following acute myocardial infarction. The first 48 hours constitute the highest risk period, although ventricular tachycardia and fibrillation account for almost three-quarters of sudden deaths in the first 12 months following discharge from hospital. Early trials on prophylactic suppression of these dysrhythmias using drugs such as lidocaine and flecainide actually increased mortality, and the routine use of class 1 agents is not recommended. For sustained ventricular tachycardia or repeated short salvos of ventricular tachycardia, lidocaine remains widely used, but intravenous amiodarone is preferable, particularly in those with heart failure and recurrent ventricular ectopic activity (Cairns et al, 1997). Implantation of automatic cardiodefibrillators may offer improved survival over antidysrhythmic drugs in high-risk groups with late ventricular dysrhythmias following acute myocardial infarction (see Chapter 13).

IMPORTANT PHYSICAL FINDINGS IN THE POST-INFARCTION PATIENT

A low-grade fever is often seen in the first 3 days after myocardial infarction, and is more common with large myocardial infarctions. Other causes of fever, such as deep vein thrombosis and infection, should be excluded, especially if the pyrexia exceeds 38°C. Chest and urinary tract infections are common, and bacteraemia may be caused by intravenous cannulae, pacing wires or urinary catheters. Occasionally, drugs may be the cause of late or unusual fevers.

Hypertension

Many patients with myocardial infarction are found to be hypertensive on admission to coronary care. This may represent pre-existing hypertension, or may simply be a response to the stress of myocardial infarction with sympathetic overactivity. Mortality is higher in hypertensive patients, and a systolic blood pressure of more than 160 mmHg persisting for more than 3 hours after admission predisposes to cardiac rupture. If the blood pressure does not settle after relief of pain and anxiety, drug treatment should be commenced, and should be considered as urgent when ischaemic pain continues. Intravenous beta-blockade is recommended first-line treatment unless there is heart failure, in which case intravenous nitrates should be used.

Respiratory system

Pulmonary embolism

Thromboembolic phenomena have become less frequent since the introduction of thrombolysis, prophylactic low-dose heparin therapy and early mobilisation. The diagnosis of pulmonary embolism must be considered in any patient with recurrent chest pain, particularly if associated with dyspnoea, tachycardia and fever. Physical examination is often unhelpful, unless there is pulmonary infarction and a pleural rub.

Respiratory tract infections

Respiratory infections are common, especially in the elderly, the obese and smokers. Pulmonary congestion and left ventricular failure predispose to infection, and opiate therapy is associated with small areas of atelectasis and ventilation/perfusion abnormalities in the lungs. Aspiration pneumonia may follow cardiopulmonary resuscitation.

Pneumothorax

This complication may follow central venous catheterisation, temporary cardiac pacing or cardiopulmonary resuscitation. Aspiration should be carried out if required.

Gastrointestinal tract

Gastric dilatation may sometimes result from nasal administration of oxygen, leading to discomfort, nausea or vomiting. Constipation and occasional paralytic ileus may result from bedrest or opiate therapy. Straining at stool must be avoided to prevent excessive vagal stimulation by the Valsalva manoeuvre.

Gastro-oesophageal reflux is a common co-existent cause of chest pain, and even endoscopic evidence of oesophagitis does not exclude the diagnosis of concomitant myocardial ischaemia. Stress ulceration of the oesophagus, stomach or duodenum may occur, sometimes causing gastrointestinal haemorrhage. This latter complication may be occult, presenting with tachycardia, hypotension and shock in a previously stable patient. This may be misdiagnosed as cardiac failure or cardiogenic shock.

Urinary tract

Urinary problems may result from drug therapy or bladder catheterisation. Atropine and opiates may precipitate urinary retention, especially in the elderly male, which is often exaggerated by a sudden response to diuretics. Catheterisation may be necessary, although it is not without the risk of introducing infection and vagal stimulation. Acute renal failure may result from prolonged hypotension or renal arterial embolisation from left ventricular mural thrombi.

Urinary albumin excretion increases following acute myocardial infarction, and high excretion levels associate with heart failure and increased mortality (Berton et al, 2001).

Nervous system

Alterations in mental state are common on intensive care units, where there may be anxiety or even hostility arising as a response to psychological stress. Decreased cerebral perfusion may give rise to psychiatric symptoms and is predisposed to by pre-existing cerebrovascular disease. Hypoxaemia and deteriorating left ventricular function will exaggerate these effects. Narcotics and anxiolytic drugs may alter perception, and intravenous lidocaine can produce hallucinations and seizures. Mural thrombi may give rise to cerebral embolisation and stroke, and cerebral haemorrhage is a recognised complication of thrombolytic therapy, particularly in the elderly.

The metabolic system

Myocardial infarction, cardiogenic shock or cardiac arrest associate with a metabolic acidosis, because hypoxia associates with accumulation of organic acids, particularly lactic acid (Box 7.3). The clinical picture of lactic acidosis is usually dominated by shock, with hyperventilation and a low arterial pH. Sodium bicarbonate may be used to correct the acidaemia, and is best given in small hypertonic concentrations (e.g. 50–100 mL of 8.4% solution). Great care is needed because of sodium and fluid overload.

Myocardial infarction may precipitate or worsen hyperglycaemia. The blood glucose concentration should be checked routinely and treated if elevated.

POST-INFARCT CARE

Most CCUs have guidelines for a gradual return to physical activity (Box 7.4). The usual period on the unit is about 24–48 hours, although longer admissions will be needed for those patients with extensive myocardial infarction, severe heart failure or

---

Box 7.3 Some causes of lactic acidosis.

Due to impaired tissue oxygenation

Myocardial infarction
Left ventricular failure
Pulmonary embolism
Shock
Sepsis
Pancreatitis

Other causes

Diabetes mellitus
Renal failure
Liver disease
Drugs
    Biguanides
    Alcohol
    Cyanide (sodium nitroprusside)
    Aspirin

Box 7.4 Typical physical activity plan following acute myocardial infarction.

Time	Activity
Day 1	Bed/chair rest
Day 2	Sit out of bed or chair; discharge from coronary care unit
Day 3	Walk around ward and to toilet
Day 4	Try stairs
Days 5–7	Discharge home
Days 7–14	Exercise within home and garden
Days 14–28	Gradual increased walking outside home
	Enrol in rehabilitation programme
Days 28–35	Exercise stress test[a]
Weeks 4–6	Outpatient review
	Return to work
	Recommence driving (in line with DVLA regulations)

a Predischarge exercise stress testing may be preferable if resources allow.

recurrent serious dysrhythmias. About half of the coronary admissions will have an uncomplicated course and probably need little intensive care.

An assessment of prognosis should be made prior to discharge, aided by exercise stress testing, echocardiography and Holter monitoring (Van der Werf et al, 2003). Risk assessment is considered in Chapter 15.

Cardiac rehabilitation is started on an inpatient basis, with discussions that include appropriate physical activity, meal planning, stress management and smoking cessation. Education and support for family members should be enlisted, with the development of a home activity programme, emotional support and a planned return to work.

References

ACC/AHA (1999) Guidelines for the management of patients with acute myocardial infarction: executive summary and recommendations. *Circulation* 100: 1016–1030.

Allender S, Peto V, Scarborough P et al (2006) *Coronary Heart Disease Statistics*. London: British Heart Foundation Statistics database. www.heartstats.org.

Anti-platelet Trialists' Collaboration (1994) Overview I: Prevention of death, myocardial infarction and stroke by prolonged anti-platelet therapy in various categories of patients. *British Medical Journal* 308: 81–106.

Antman EM (2002) Early administration of intravenous magnesium to high-risk patients with acute myocardial infarction in the Magnesium in Coronaries (MAGIC) Trial: a randomised controlled trial. *Lancet* 360: 1189–1196.

Antman EM, Tanasijevic MJ, Thompson B et al (1996) Cardiac-specific troponin I levels to predict the risk of mortality in patients with acute coronary syndromes. *New England Journal of Medicine* 335: 1342–1349.

Antman EM, Morrow DA, McCabe CH for the ExTRACT-TIMI 25 Investigators (2006) Enoxaparin versus unfractionated heparin with fibrinolysis for ST-elevation myocardial infarction. *New England Journal of Medicine* 354: 1477–1488.

Appleby MA, Angeja BG, Dauterman K et al (2001) Angiographic assessment of myocardial perfusion: TIMI myocardial perfusion (TMP) grading system. *Heart* 86: 485–486.

ASSENT-2 Investigators (1999) Single-bolus tenecteplase compared with front-loaded alteplase in acute myocardial infarction: the ASSENT-2 double-blind randomised trial. *Lancet* 354: 716–722.

Baigent C, Collins R, Appleby P on behalf of the ISIS-2 Collaborative Group (1998) ISIS-2: 10 year survival among patients with suspected myocardial infarction in randomised comparison of intravenous streptokinase, oral aspirin, both or neither. *British Medical Journal* 316: 1337–1343.

Barron HV, Fox NL, Berioli S (1999) Comparison of intracranial hemorrhage rates in patients treated with rt-PA and TNK-tPA: impact of gender, age and low body weight. *Circulation* 100(suppl I): I–II.

Bartnik M, Rydén L, Ferrari R et al (2004) The prevalence of abnormal glucose regulation in patients with coronary artery disease across Europe. The Euro Heart Survey on diabetes and the heart. *European Heart Journal* 25: 1880–1890.

de Belder MA (2001) Acute myocardial infarction: failed thrombolysis. *Heart* 85: 104–112.

Berton G, Coriano R, Palmieri R et al (2001) Microalbuminuria during acute myocardial infarction. *European Heart Journal* 22: 1466–1475.

Blows L, Perera D, Redwood S (2005) The 'no-flow' phenomenon. *British Journal of Cardiology (Acute Interventional Cardiology)* 12: AIC92–97.

Boersma E, Maas ACP, Deckers JW et al (1996) Early thrombolytic treatment in acute myocardial infarction: reappraisal of the golden hour. *Lancet* 348: 771–775.

Brass LM, Lichtman JH, Wang Y et al (2000) Intracranial hemorrhage associated with thrombolytic therapy for elderly patients with acute myocardial infarction. Results from the cooperative cardiovascular project. *Stroke* 31: 1802–1811.

Brugada P (2000) Brugada syndrome: an electrocardiographic diagnosis not to be missed. *Heart* 84: 1–2.

Brugada R, Wenger NK, Jacobson TA et al (1996) Changes in plasma cholesterol levels after hospitalization for acute coronary events. *Cardiology* 87: 194–199.

Cairns JA, Connolly SJ, Roberts R et al for the CAMIAT Investigators (1997) Randomised trial of outcome after myocardial infarction in patients with frequent or repetitive ventricular premature depolarisations. *Lancet* 349: 675–682.

Chambless L, Keil U, Dobson A et al (1997) Population versus clinical view of case fatality from acute coronary disease. Results from the WHO MONICA Project 1985–1990. *Circulation* 96: 3849–3859.

Collins R, Peto R, Baigent C et al (1997) Aspirin, heparin and fibrinolytic therapy in suspected acute myocardial infarction. *New England Journal of Medicine* 336: 847–860.

COMMIT (ClOpidogrel and Metoprolol in Myocardial Infarction Trial) Collaborative Group (2005a) Addition of clopidogrel to aspirin in 45,852 patients with acute myocardial infarction: randomised placebo-controlled trial. *Lancet* 366: 1607–1621.

COMMIT (ClOpidogrel and Metoprolol in Myocardial Infarction Trial) Collaborative Group (2005b) Early intravenous then oral metoprolol in 45,852 patients with acute myocardial infarction: randomised placebo-controlled trial. *Lancet* 366: 1622–1632.

CREATE-ECLA Investigators (2005) Effect of glucose–potassium–insulin infusion on mortality with acute ST-segment elevation myocardial infarction. *Journal of the American Medical Association* 293: 437–446.

De Lemos JA, Antman EM, Gibson CM et al (2000) Abciximab improves both epicardial flow and myocardial reperfusion in ST-elevation myocardial infarction. Observations from the TIMI 14 trial. *Circulation* 101: 239–243.

De Lemos JA, Braunwald E (2001) ST segment resolution as a tool for assessing the efficacy of reperfusion therapy. *Journal of the American College of Cardiology* 38: 1283–1294.

Dewar HA, Stephenson P, Horler AR et al (1963) Fibrinolytic therapy of coronary thrombosis. *British Medical Journal* 1: 915–920.

Dodd ME, Kellet F, Davis A et al (2000) Audit of oxygen prescribing before and after the introduction of a pre-scription chart. *British Medical Journal* 321: 864–865.

Eikelboom JW, Quinlan DJ, Mehta SR et al (2005) Unfractionated and low molecular weight heparin as adjuncts to thrombolysis in aspirin treated patients with ST elevation acute myocardial infarction: a meta-analysis of randomised trials. *Circulation* 112: 3855–3867.

Ellis SG, Da Silva ER, Spaulding CM et al (2000) Review of immediate angioplasty after fibrinolytic therapy for acute myocardial infarction: insights from the RESCUE I, RESCUE II, and other contemporary clinical experiences. *American Heart Journal* 139: 1046–1053.

Estess JM, Topol EJ (2002) Fibrinolytic treatment for elderly patients with acute myocardial infarction. *Heart* 87: 308–311.

Fibrinolytic Therapy Trialists' Collaborative Group (1994) Indications for fibrinolytic therapy in suspected acute myocardial infarction: collaborative overview of early and major morbidity results from all randomised trials of more than 1000 patients. *Lancet* 343: 311–322.

Fonarow GC, Wright RS, Spencer FA et al and the National Registry of Myocardial Infarction 4 Investigators (2005) Effect of statin use within the first 24 hours of admission for acute myocardial infarction on early morbidity and mortality. *American Journal of Cardiology* 96: 611–616.

Francis GS (2001) Diabetic cardiomyopathy: fact or fiction? *Heart* 85: 247–248.

Freemantle N, Cleland J, Young P et al (1999) Beta-blockade after myocardial infarction: systematic review and meta-regression analysis. *British Medical Journal* 318: 1730–1737.

French JK, Williams BF, Hart HH et al (1996) Prospective evaluation of eligibility for thrombolytic therapy in acute myocardial infarction. *British Medical Journal* 312: 1637–1641.

Friemark D, Behar S, Matetsky S et al (1998) Time dependent effect of treatment with ASA during thrombolytic therapy in acute myocardial infarction. *Journal of the American College of Cardiology* 31: 231A.

Furman MI, Gore JM, Anderson FA et al GRACE Investigators (2004) Elevated leukocyte count and adverse hospital events in patients with acute coronary syndromes: findings from the Global Registry of Acute Coronary Events (GRACE). *American Heart Journal* 147: 42–48.

Gandhi MM (1997) Clinical epidemiology of coronary heart disease in the UK. *British Journal of Hospital Medicine* 58: 23–27.

Gershlick AH, Stephens-Lloyd A, Hughes S et al (2005) REACT: Rescue angioplasty after failed thrombolytic therapy for acute myocardial infarction. *New England Journal of Medicine* 353: 2758–2768.

GISSI Study Group (1987) Long-term effects of intravenous thrombolysis in acute myocardial infarction: final report of the GISSI study. *Lancet* ii: 871–874.

GISSI-3 (1994) Effects of lisinopril and transdermal glyceryl trinitrate singly and together on 6-week mortality and ventricular function after acute myocardial infarction. Gruppo Italiano per lo Studio della Sopravvivenza nell'infarto Miocardico. *Lancet* 343: 1115–1122.

GUSTO (1993) An international randomised trial comparing 4 strategies for acute myocardial infarction. *New England Journal of Medicine* 329: 673–682.

Hartwell D, Colquitt J, Loveman E et al (2005) Clinical effectiveness and cost-effectiveness of immediate angioplasty for acute myocardial infarction: systematic review and economic evaluation. *Health Technology Assessment* 9: 1–99.

Heymann TD, Culling W (1994) Cardiac tamponade after thrombolysis. *Postgraduate Medical Journal* 10: 455–456.

ISIS-3 (Third International Study of Infarct Survival) Collaborative Group (1992) A randomised comparison of streptokinase vs tissue plasminogen activator vs anistreplase and of aspirin plus heparin vs aspirin alone among 41,299 cases of suspected myocardial infarction. *Lancet* 339: 753–770.

ISIS-4 Collaborative Group (1995) A randomised trial assessing early oral captopril, oral mononitrate and intravenous magnesium sulphate in 58,050 patients with suspected acute myocardial infarction. *Lancet* 345: 669–685.

Jowett NI (2006) Thrombolysis and capillary glucose sampling. *Practical Diabetes International* 23: 94.

Jowett NI, Thompson DR, Bailey SW (1985) Electrocardiographic monitoring. I. Static monitoring. *Intensive Care Nursing* 2: 71–76.

Jowett NI, Stephens JM, Thompson DR et al (1986) Do indwelling cannulae on coronary care need a heparin flush? *Intensive Care Nursing* 2: 16–19.

Jowett NI, Thompson DR, Pohl JEF (1989) Temporary transvenous cardiac pacing: 6 years experience in one coronary care unit. *Postgraduate Medical Journal* 65: 211–215.

Keeley EC, Boura JA, Grines CL (2006) Comparison of primary and facilitated percutaneous coronary interventions for ST-elevation myocardial infarction: quantitative review of randomised trials. *Lancet* 367(9510): 579–588.

Kenmure AC, Murdoch WR, Beattie AD et al (1968) Circulatory and metabolic effects of oxygen in myocardial infarction. *British Medical Journal* 4: 360–364.

Klootwijk P, Langer A, Meij S et al (1996) Non-invasive prediction of reperfusion and coronary artery patency by continuous ST monitoring in the GUSTO-1 trial. *European Heart Journal* 17: 689–698.

Kovlack JD, Gershlick AH (2001) How should we detect and manage failed thrombolysis? *European Heart Journal* 22: 450–457.

Krinsley JS (2004) Effect of an intensive glucose management protocol on the mortality of critically ill adult patients. *Mayo Clinic Proceedings* 79: 992–1000.

Krone RJ, Greenberg H, Dwyer EM (1993) Long-term prognostic significance of ST segment depression during acute myocardial infarction. *Journal of the American College of Cardiology* 22: 361–367.

Lawson-Matthew PJ, Wilson AT, Woodmansey PA et al (1994) Unsatisfactory management of patients with acute myocardial infarction admitted to general medical wards. *Journal of the Royal College of Physicians of London* 28: 49–51.

McLellan CS, Le May MR, Labinaz M (2004) Current reperfusion strategies for ST elevation myocardial infarction: a Canadian perspective. *Canadian Journal of Cardiology* 20: 525–533.

Mahaffey KW, Granger CB, Toth CA et al (1997) Diabetic retinopathy should not be a contraindication to thrombolytic therapy in acute myocardial infarction: review of ocular hemorrhage incidence and location in the GUSTO-1 trial. *Journal of the American College of Cardiology* 30: 1606–1610.

Malmberg K for the DIGAMI Study Group (1997) Prospective randomised study of intensive insulin treatment on long-term survival after acute myocardial infarction in patients with diabetes mellitus. *British Medical Journal* 314: 1512–1515.

Malmberg K, Ryden L, Wedel H et al (2005) Intense metabolic control by means of insulin in patients with diabetes mellitus and acute myocardial infarction (DIGAMI 2): effects on mortality and morbidity. *European Heart Journal* 26: 650–661.

Menon V, Harrington RA, Hochman JS (2004) Thrombolysis and adjunctive therapy in acute myocardial infarction. *Chest* 126: 549s–575s.

Oldroyd KG (2000) Identifying failure to achieve complete (TIMI 3) reperfusion following thrombolytic treatment: how to do it, when to do it, and why it's worth doing. *Heart* 84(2): 113–115.

Otter W, Kleybrink S, Doerig W et al (2004) Hospital outcome of acute myocardial infarction in patients with and without diabetes mellitus. *Diabetic Medicine* 21: 183–187.

Rawles JM, Kenmure AC (1976) Controlled trial of oxygen in uncomplicated myocardial infarction. *British Medical Journal* 1: 1121–1123.

Reffelmann T, Kloner RA (2002) The 'no-flow' phenomenon: basic science and clinical correlates. *Heart* 87: 162–168.

Ross AM, Lundergan CF, Rohrbeck SC et al (1998) Rescue angioplasty after failed thrombolysis: technical and clinical outcomes in a large thrombolysis trial (GUSTO-1). *Journal of the American College of Cardiology* 31: 1511–1517.

Rothberg MB, Celestin C, Fiore LD et al (2005) Warfarin plus aspirin after myocardial infarction or the acute coronary syndrome: Meta-analysis with estimates of risk and benefit. *Annals of Internal Medicine* 143: 241–250.

Rutherford JD (2001) Diabetes and coronary artery disease – therapy and outcomes. *Coronary Artery Disease* 12: 149–152.

Sabatine MS, Cannon CP, Gibson CM et al CLARITY-TIMI 28 Investigators (2005) Addition of clopidogrel to aspirin and fibrinolytic therapy for myocardial infarction with ST-segment elevation. *New England Journal of Medicine* 352: 1179–1189.

Sala J, Masiá R, González de Molina F-J for the REGICOR Investigators (2002) Short-term mortality of myocardial infarction patients with diabetes or hyperglycaemia during admission. *Journal of Epidemiology and Community Health* 56: 707–712

Shotliff K, Kaushal R, Dove D et al (1998) Withholding thrombolysis in patients with diabetes mellitus and acute myocardial infarction. *Diabetic Medicine* 15: 1028–1030.

Silber S, Albertsson P, Avilès FF et al (2005) Guidelines for percutaneous coronary interventions. The Task Force for Percutaneous Coronary Interventions of the European Society of Cardiology. *European Heart Journal* 26: 804–847.

Simoons M, Krzeminska-Pakula M, Alonso A et al (2002) Improved reperfusion and clinical outcome with enoxaparin as an adjunct to streptokinase thrombolysis in acute myocardial infarction: the AMI-SK study. *European Heart Journal* 23: 1282–1290.

Squire IB, Lawley W, Fletcher S et al (1999) Humoral and immune responses up to 7.5 years after administration of streptokinase for acute myocardial infarction. *European Heart Journal* 20: 1245–1252.

Sutton AG, Campbell PG, Price DJ et al (2000) Failure of thrombolysis by streptokinase: detection with a simple electrocardiographic method. *Heart* 84: 113–115.

Task Force of the European Society of Cardiology and the European Resuscitation Council (1998) The pre-hospital management of acute heart attacks. *European Heart Journal* 19: 1140–1164.

Tatu-Chitoiu G, Teodorescu C, Capraru P et al (2004) Accelerated streptokinase and enoxaparin in ST-segment elevation acute myocardial infarction (the ASENOX study). *Kardiologia Polska* 60(5): 441–446.

Tenerz A, Lonneberg I, Berne C et al (2001) Myocardial infarction and prevalence of diabetes mellitus: is increased casual blood glucose at admission a reliable criterion for the diagnosis of pre-existing diabetes? *European Heart Journal* 22: 1102–1110.

Thompson DR, Jowett NI, Folwell AM et al (1989) A trial of povidone-iodine antiseptic solution for the prevention of cannula-related thrombo-phlebitis. *Journal of Intravenous Nursing* 12: 99–102.

THRIFT II (Thrombo-embolic Risk Factors) Consensus Group (1998) Risk of and prophylaxis for venous thrombo-embolism in hospital patients. *Phlebology* 13: 87–97.

Tunstall-Pedoe H, Vanuzzo D, Hobbs M et al (2000) Estimation of contribution of changes in coronary care to improving survival, event rates, and coronary heart disease mortality across the WHO MONICA Project populations. *Lancet* 355: 688–700.

Van Belle E, Lablanche JM, Bauters C et al (1998) Coronary angioscopic findings in the infarct-related vessel within 1 month of acute myocardial infarction: natural history and the effect of thrombolysis. *Circulation* 97: 26–33.

Van der Werf F, Ardissino D, Betriu A (2003) Management of acute myocardial infarction in patients presenting with ST segment elevation. The task force on the management of acute myocardial infarction of the European Society of Cardiology. *European Heart Journal* 24: 28–66.

Verheugt FW (1996) Thrombolysis-associated ventricular fibrillation: is it reperfusion, the drug or what? *European Heart Journal* 17: 172–173.

Widimsky P, Groch L, Zelízko M et al (2000) Multicentre randomized trial comparing transport to primary angioplasty vs immediate thrombolysis vs combined strategy for patients with acute myocardial infarction presenting to a community hospital without a catheterisation laboratory. The PRAGUE study. *European Heart Journal* 21: 823–831.

Wilcox RG, Olsson CG, Skene AM et al (1988) Trial of tPA for mortality reduction in acute myocardial infarction (ASSET). *Lancet* ii: 525–530.

de Wood MA, Spores J, Notske R et al (1980) Prevalence of total coronary occlusion during the early hours of transmural myocardial infarction. *New England Journal of Medicine* 303: 897–902.

Wu KC, Zerhouni EA, Judd RM et al (1998) Prognostic significance of micro-vascular obstruction by magnetic resonance imaging in patients with acute myocardial infarction. *Circulation* 97: 765–772.

Zalenski RJ, Rydman RJ, Sloan EP et al (1997) Value of posterior and right ventricular leads in comparison to the standard 12-lead electrocardiogram in evaluation of ST-segment elevation in suspected acute myocardial infarction. *American Journal of Cardiology* 79: 1579–1585.

Zehender M, Kasper W, Kauder E et al (1993) Right ventricular infarction as an independent predictor of prognosis after acute inferior myocardial infarction. *New England Journal of Medicine* 328: 981–988.

Chapter 8

Unstable coronary syndromes: management of unstable angina and non-ST elevation myocardial infarction

The majority of patients presenting with an acute coronary syndrome will have either unstable angina (UA) or non-ST elevation myocardial infarction (NSTEMI), conditions that currently account for more than 130 000 admissions to UK hospitals every year. These two conditions may be considered together as their pathogenesis and presentation are similar, but they differ in the severity of the ischaemic insult. In those with NSTEMI, this has been sufficient to produce detectable myocardial injury. Although the degree of myocardial damage is usually smaller following NSTEMI than in cases of acute transmural infarction, the long-term mortality is higher (Herlitz et al, 2001). This probably relates to persistence of the underlying unstable plaque, which, unless modified, may be involved in another

acute coronary syndrome. Around 5–10% of these cases progress to transmural myocardial infarction or death within 30 days (Collinson et al, 2000). Prognosis is particularly bad for those who present with ST depression on the electrocardiogram (ECG), as these patients often have multivessel coronary disease or pre-existing myocardial damage.

Because the unstable coronary syndromes are high-risk conditions, patients require urgent admission to coronary care for stabilisation. Even with optimal medical treatment, up to half the patients will experience recurrent ischaemia and require revascularisation. An overview of management is shown in Figure 8.1.

DIAGNOSIS

Unstable coronary syndromes are a heterogeneous group of disorders that may present in many different ways. About half the patients have warning symptoms, the commonest of which is worsening angina. The severity of anginal symptoms has been graded by the Canadian Cardiovascular Society (CCS) (Box 8.1). Most present following an episode of prolonged anginal pain at rest (over 20 minutes). In other cases, there has been recent destabilisation of angina to at least CCS III or a change in the character of the anginal symptoms.

The condition may be missed in patients with no previous history of cardiac disease, as the diagnosis may not be considered. Atypical presenting

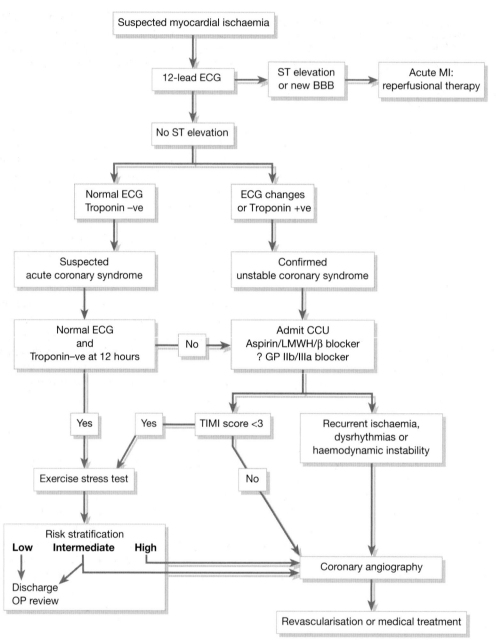

Figure 8.1   Management of patients with suspected acute coronary syndrome without ST segment elevation on the presenting ECG. BBB, bundle branch block; GP IIb/IIIa blocker, glycoprotein IIb/IIa inhibitor; LMWH, low-molecular-weight heparin; OP, outpatient; TIMI, Trials in Myocardial Infarction risk score (see Box 8.2).

Box 8.1 Canadian Cardiovascular Society (CCS) grading of angina. Adapted from Campeau, 1976.

Class I	Angina occurring with strenuous, but not with ordinary, activities
Class II	Slight limitation of ordinary activities, e.g. angina after two flights of stairs
Class III	Marked limitation of ordinary activities, e.g. angina after one flight of stairs
Class IV	Angina precipitated by any activity or at rest

symptoms are more common in women, younger men and those with diabetes, such as stabbing or pleuritic chest pain, indigestion, epigastric pain or increasing dyspnoea (Lee et al, 1985). Elderly patients are a particularly difficult diagnostic group and may present with unexplained dyspnoea, fatigue, nausea, vomiting or sweating. Sometimes, these 'angina equivalents' may have no relation to exertion.

Physical examination is often normal, but it may help to exclude non-cardiac causes of the chest pain such as aortic dissection, pneumonia or pneumothorax. Anxiety, sweating and a tachycardia are usual. Signs of haemodynamic instability or left ventricular failure indicate poor left ventricular function and indicate high risk. Cardiogenic shock may develop in up to 5% of patients with NSTEMI, and carries a mortality of over 60%.

ECG CHANGES

An early 12-lead ECG is vital to make the diagnosis and provide prognostic information. During pain, the ECG may show ST elevation indicating transmural ischaemia but, more usually, there is planar or downsloping ST depression. T waves may be flattened, peaked or inverted. These ECG changes may be transitory, and serial ECGs may show both ST elevation and depression. A normal ECG in pain does not exclude an unstable coronary syndrome. Between episodes of ischaemic

pain, the ECG may be normal, although non-specific changes are often present. If the patient has a previously abnormal ECG, further recordings should be made during pain or other symptoms and then compared with tracings taken when symptom-free.

The appearance of Q waves usually implies infarction, although they may simply be a transitory manifestation of ischaemia (Goldberger, 1979). The changes in the ECG during pain do not always predict subsequent angiographic findings, but widespread ST depression and anterior T wave inversion usually associate with severe coronary disease and a poorer outcome. Deep symmetrical T waves in the anterior leads often relate to a proximal stenosis in the left anterior descending coronary artery (Wellen's sign).

Each ECG provides a brief view of a dynamic process, and continuous 12-lead ECG monitoring may identify abnormalities not captured on the standard ECG. Many ischaemic episodes in unstable angina are brief and painless and thus unlikely to be recorded unless there is continuous multi-lead electrocardiographic monitoring.

TROPONIN

Troponin positivity associates with increased risk of infarction or death, and the higher the value, the greater the risk (Ohman et al, 1996). This is independent of other risk factors. In addition, troponin positivity identifies those who will benefit from treatment with low-molecular-weight heparin and glycoprotein inhibitors. Troponin testing therefore provides diagnostic, therapeutic and prognostic information at the same time. An initial rise in troponin may be detectable in the blood as early as 3–4 hours after the onset of chest pain and persists for up to 2 weeks.

RISK ASSESSMENT

Patients who present with an acute coronary syndrome (ACS) are a heterogeneous group of individuals with varying degrees of severity and extent of coronary atheroma, and differing degrees of acute 'thrombotic' risk. It is important to determine those who are most at risk of myocardial infarction or death, as these patients generally need, and may benefit from, an early intervention strategy. Such evaluation needs to be made early and repeated in the light of clinical, ECG and biochemical evaluation. Patients are already at risk if there is a prior history of coronary heart disease, heart failure or hypertension, or if they are already taking aspirin. Elderly patients, particularly men, are more likely to have established and extensive coronary disease.

The two most important high-risk features are ST segment depression on the presenting ECG and troponin positivity. Additional risk factors include advanced age, pain at rest, haemodynamic instability and serious dysrhythmias. Patients at intermediate risk include those with post-myocardial infarction angina (i.e. within 2 months), patients with recurrent pain after admission, those with diabetes and patients with established coronary disease, especially if they have had previous bypass surgery. Patients are at intermediate levels of risk if they have one but not all of the high-risk features.

Low-risk patients are usually younger and have no rest pain, a normal presentation ECG and a negative troponin. They may declare themselves at higher risk if they become unstable during observation or have a positive exercise stress test.

Several risk scores, based on clinical, ECG and laboratory variables, have been developed and appear to be useful for evaluating the risk of subsequent adverse outcomes (de Araujo Goncalves et al, 2005). In general, these risk scores assess short-term outcomes (in hospital and up to 6 weeks) after an ACS event, although the thrombolysis in myocardial infarction (TIMI) score (Box 8.2) may also indicate risk of death, recurrent ischaemia and myocardial infarction at 1 year (Scirica et al, 2002).

TREATMENT

Treatment of the unstable coronary syndromes requires deactivation of the platelets and dissolution of the thrombus, with measures to 'calm' the plaque. Additional therapy is needed to relieve the symptoms and effects of myocardial ischaemia. Oxygen therapy is usual, although not all patients will need it. Patients with obvious cyanosis or dyspnoea should be treated with oxygen during

---

> **Box 8.2**   TIMI risk score for UA/NSTEMI.
>
> ### Score one point for each of the following:
>
> Age over 65 years
> Three or more coronary risk factors
>   (hypertension, hypercholesterolaemia,
>   diabetes, family history, smoking)
> Aspirin use within the last 7 days
> Known coronary disease (> 50% stenosis at
>   angiography)
> More than two anginal events in previous 24 h
> Raised troponin (or other cardiac biomarker)
> ST deviation (depression or transient elevation)
>
> ### Risk of major coronary event in 14 days
>
> 0–2 points = low risk (5–8%)
> 3–4 points = medium risk (13–20%)
> 5–7 points = high risk (26–41%)

---

initial assessment and others if arterial saturation falls below 90%.

ANALGESIA

Intravenous diamorphine should be used for those whose pain does not respond to initial sublingual nitrates. Diamorphine has potent analgesic and anxiolytic effects, as well as haemodynamic effects that may be valuable in unstable coronary syndromes. It produces venodilation, reduces the blood pressure and slows the heart rate by increasing vagal tone. The fall in blood pressure reduces myocardial oxygen demand, although care is required as blood pressure reduction may be profound if there is volume depletion or in the presence of other vasodilators. Doses of 2.5–5 mg may be given every 5–30 minutes until pain is relieved and to maintain comfort. Significant respiratory depression is unusual, but may be reversed with naloxone 0.4–2.0 mg intravenously. Diamorphine is not a substitute for anti-ischaemic agents.

ANTI-ISCHAEMIC AGENTS

These are used to reduce myocardial oxygen consumption by decreasing heart rate, depressing contractility or lowering blood pressure. Most of this effect is due to dilatation of venules, but some agents may vasodilate the coronary arteries to promote oxygen delivery.

Beta-blockers

Beta-blockers are the mainstay of therapy for unstable angina, and will control pain in about three-quarters of patients and produce a 13% reduction in the risk of myocardial infarction (Yusuf et al, 1988). Beta-blockers act predominantly at beta-1 receptors and reduce the heart rate, blood pressure, myocardial contractility and, hence, myocardial oxygen consumption. In the absence of bradycardia, hypotension and heart failure, beta-blockers should be given as early as possible.

Nitrates

Nitrates work predominantly by venodilation, with arteriolar dilatation at higher doses. They thus relieve cardiac preload and afterload, and thereby reduce myocardial oxygen consumption. Subendocardial blood flow is also improved by dilatation of normal, collateral and atherosclerotic coronary arteries. Some of these effects may be offset by an increase in heart rate, so that nitrates should be co-prescribed with a beta-blocker or diltiazem. The intravenous route may be used initially to allow rapid titration. The starting dose of intravenous nitrate should be low, and may be increased every 3–5 minutes until symptoms are relieved or until the blood pressure is affected. Once a partial blood pressure response is observed, the rate of increase should be slowed. The systolic blood pressure should not be allowed to fall below 100 mmHg or by more than 25% of the initial blood pressure, or coronary perfusion pressures will fall, which may worsen myocardial ischaemia. If hypotension develops at low doses of nitrate therapy, hypovolaemia should be suspected. A fluid challenge may be used to ensure that the patient has an adequate left ventricular filling pressure. Abrupt cessation of intravenous nitrates may produce rebound ischaemia, and the dose should be weaned rather than stopped abruptly. Tolerance of the effects of nitrates is duration-dependent, and patients who require more than 24 hours of intravenous therapy may require periodic increases in the infusion rate to maintain efficacy. Oral nitrates may be commenced before stopping the infusion.

Nicorandil is a potassium channel activator with nitrate-like action, and may be used as an alternative to isosorbide. Tolerance does not occur and, when given with beta-blockers or calcium channel blockers, it reduces the frequency of angina, ischaemia and dysrhythmias in patients with unstable angina (Patel et al, 1999).

Calcium channel blockers

The calcium channel blockers work by producing vasodilatation, and some will affect heart rate and atrio-ventricular conduction. They are used for symptom relief in patients already on beta-blockers and nitrates. They may also be of benefit in those who cannot tolerate beta-blockade, and both verapamil and diltiazem have been shown to be useful agents in reducing ischaemic episodes in patients with unstable angina. Calcium channel blockers have not been shown to reduce mortality, but diltiazem may reduce reinfarction and the need for revascularisation in patients with non-ST elevation myocardial infarction (Boden et al, 2000). The main groups of calcium blockers are the dihydropyridines (e.g. nifedipine), the phenyl-alkylamines (e.g. verapamil) and the benzothiazepines (e.g. diltiazem). Short-acting dihydropyridines, such as nifedipine and nicardipine, should not be used unless the patient is already on a beta-blocker, because they induce a tachycardia. Amlodipine and felodipine appear to be well tolerated if there is left ventricular dysfunction, but verapamil is not.

ANTITHROMBIN THERAPY

Intracoronary thrombus consists of fibrin and platelets, and formation and dissolution may be promoted by inhibition of thrombin, fibrinolytic drugs and antiplatelet agents.

Heparin

Intravenous unfractionated heparin (UFH) and subcutaneous low-molecular-weight heparin

(LMWH) are both effective in reducing risk when given in combination with aspirin. Subcutaneous LMWH is easier to administer, has a more constant antithrombin effect, does not need routine anticoagulant monitoring and improves outcomes (Califf et al, 2005). The OASIS 5 trial has shown that the synthetic Xa inhibitor fondaparinux is superior to enoxaparin, reducing mortality and bleeding complications (Yusuf et al, 2006).

LMWH is of greatest benefit in those with positive troponin concentrations, and should be given for at least 2 days and longer in cases of recurrent ischaemia. In high-risk patients, LMWH should be continued until angiography is undertaken and, if revascularisation is judged not to be feasible, LMWH should be continued for a period of at least 2 weeks (Wallentin et al, 2000).

Aspirin

Unstable angina is associated with enhanced platelet reactivity and increased production of the powerful vasoconstrictor, thromboxane A_2. Aspirin is an irreversible inhibitor of platelet cyclo-oxygenase-1 which prevents the formation of thromboxane A_2 and thus reduces platelet aggregation.

Aspirin reduces death and progression to myocardial infarction in patients with unstable angina by 36% (Anti-platelet Trialists' Collaboration, 1994). This effect is maintained for up to 2 years. Low-dose treatment (75 mg) is probably sufficient, provided a loading dose of at least 300 mg has been given. Aspirin should be given as soon as the diagnosis of an acute coronary syndrome is considered, either dissolved in water or chewed to enhance absorption.

Clopidogrel

Clopidogrel is a platelet adenosine diphosphate (ADP) inhibitor that helps to prevent platelet aggregation, and is often used as an alternative to aspirin. Co-prescribing clopidogrel with aspirin in unstable angina significantly reduced the risk of myocardial infarction and recurrent ischaemia. The benefits start early, so all patients presenting with an unstable coronary syndrome should be given aspirin 300 mg and clopidogrel 300 mg

immediately. Both drugs should be continued at 75 mg/day for at least 12 months (Walsh et al, 2005).

Glycoprotein IIb/IIIa receptor blockers

The glycoprotein IIb/IIIa receptor provides the final common pathway to platelet aggregation, and is found in abundance on platelet membrane surfaces. When activated, the receptor attracts fibrinogen, which sticks platelets together. Blocking these sites with glycoprotein IIb/IIIa inhibitors will inhibit platelet aggregation by antagonising the formation of the fibrinogen bridges between activated platelets. Three agents are available for use: abciximab, eptifibatide and tirofiban.

Abciximab is a monoclonal antibody used at the time of percutaneous coronary intervention (PCI). *Tirofiban* and *eptifibatide* are small molecules suitable for repeated intravenous administration, but their value in those who are already destined to receive abciximab is unclear. Both tirofiban and eptifibatide may be given intravenously, in addition to heparin, clopidogrel and aspirin, to reduce complications (Knight, 2001). Oral IIb/IIIa inhibitors have not been found to be beneficial. Abciximab is not used outside the catheter laboratory. Very early use of glycoprotein inhibitors will reduce ischaemic events in all high-risk patients until a decision is made regarding angiography (Boersma et al, 2002). In patients managed without PCI, the benefits of GPIIb/IIIa infusions are less clear (Carbajal & Deedwania, 2005).

Direct thrombin inhibitors

Bivalirudin and lepirudin are direct thrombin inhibitors that specifically and reversibly bind to both circulating and clot-bound thrombin. Direct thrombin inhibitors produce a more predictable anticoagulant response to heparin. The ACUITY trial (Stone et al, 2006) showed that bivalirudin was superior to the combination of heparin and glycoprotein inhibitors in high-risk patients with acute coronary syndromes, with fewer bleeding complications. The drug may therefore simplify anticoagulation in these patients.

Thrombolysis

Fibrinolytic therapy is not recommended for acute coronary syndromes without ST segment elevation. The Fibrinolytic Therapy Trialists' overview (1994) showed that mortality following thrombolysis in patients with suspected myocardial infarction and ST depression was 15.2%. Mortality in those not treated with thrombolysis was 13.8%.

Oxygen

Supplementary oxygen may be helpful. Oxygen should be given at 2–4 L/minutes via nasal prongs until stability, particularly if there is hypotension or heart failure, and should aim to ensure that the SaO_2 is over 90%.

LIPID-LOWERING THERAPY

Reduction in plasma lipids has profound effects on plaque morphology. Apart from reducing the size of the lipid pool, macrophage numbers are reduced, and smooth muscle cell numbers and collagen content rise. These plaque-stabilising effects can take up to 18 months, and may explain why the secondary prevention trials do not show survival benefits until 1–2 years after starting statin therapy. However, observational studies have suggested improvements in outcome in statin-treated patients compared with untreated patients in the course of an acute coronary syndrome (Waters & Hsue, 2001). Improved outcome would be too quick to relate to atherosclerosis regression, but may be due to reversal of endothelial dysfunction and inflammation or a decrease in prothrombotic factors. Intensive cholesterol lowering administered immediately after hospitalisation for unstable angina or NSTEMI has been shown to reduce the incidence of recurrent ischaemic events over the next 4 months (Schwartz et al, 2001).

Stabilisation

While the majority of patients settle with conservative management in the first 24 hours, this does not mean the plaque has stabilised. The period of plaque healing is not known, and there is potential for rapid progression of the culprit lesion despite medical intervention. Most recurrent cardiac events occur soon after the initial presentation (Theroux & Fuster, 1998), so at-risk patients need identifying before discharge from hospital.

Risk assessment

Risk assessment is a continuous process. After initial assessment and treatment, increased risk is indicated by:

- a raised cardiac troponin concentration;
- recurrent ischaemic symptoms;
- recurrent ischaemic ST segment changes (with or without symptoms);
- a positive exercise stress test;
- poor left ventricular function.

Patients with the worst prognosis are those with continuing or recurrent symptoms and ischaemic ST segment changes despite anti-ischaemic medical treatment (refractory acute coronary syndrome). This is particularly so if the symptoms occur soon after a myocardial infarction, or where there is evidence of pre-existing coronary heart disease. Most high-risk patients can be identified in the acute phase, but there are some who respond readily to treatment, but remain at high risk. It is important to identify this group before discharge from hospital.

A symptom-limited exercise stress test (using the modified Bruce protocol) is often the simplest way to define residual ischaemia, although inducible ischaemia alone has a low predictive value for death and myocardial infarction in the first year (Shaw et al, 1996). Risk stratification by treadmill testing is enhanced when combined with the troponin T concentration (Table 8.1). Myocardial perfusion scintigraphy or stress echocardiography may be helpful in those unable to use the treadmill (Lin et al, 1998). The other main determinant of long-term risk is left ventricular function, and echocardiography should be carried out in all patients. Those with evidence of left ventricular dysfunction should be treated with an angiotensin-converting enzyme (ACE) inhibitor, and those with an ejection fraction of less than 40% should be considered for early coronary angiography.

Table 8.1 Risk of cardiac death or myocardial infarction at 5 months after an episode of unstable angina (adapted from Lindahl et al, 1997).

ETT risk category	Troponin T < 0.06 µg/L	Troponin T = 0.06–0.2 µg/L	Troponin T > 0.2 µg/L
High	22%	19%	34%
Medium	7%	9%	16%
Low	1%	7%	5%
Unable to exercise	3%	16%	27%

ETT, exercise stress test.

Management according to risk

Guidelines for the management of UA/NSTEMI have been published in the UK, Europe and America (British Cardiac Society, 2001; ACC/AHA, 2002; Bertrand et al, 2002), and present an 'ideal' framework for management, based upon evidence from clinical trials. However, many of these trials focused on selected populations, and subgroups such as the elderly and women are not well represented. Nevertheless, the recommendations are very similar, and should be applied to all patients until there is evidence to the contrary. A contemporary overview of management of the acute coronary syndromes according to risk is shown in Figure 8.2, and may be summarised as follows.

Low risk

If there are no further symptoms after 12 hours, the cardiac troponin result is negative, and the echocardiogram and stress test result indicate a low-risk category, the patient can be discharged from hospital. The diagnosis may remain uncertain, and other non-cardiological investigations may be appropriate. Patients are at low risk of a cardiac event whatever the diagnosis, and subsequent outpatient review is appropriate for further investigations and adjustment or cessation of drug treatment.

Intermediate risk

This includes patients without high-risk features, but a stress test that indicates intermediate risk or

those with a mildly elevated cardiac troponin (troponin T < 1.0 ng/mL), but with a stress test and echocardiogram result indicating a low risk. Early coronary angiography cannot be considered mandatory, as there is currently no evidence that routine investigation improves outcome (Choudhry et al, 2005). A 'wait-and-see' policy might be adopted, with a low threshold for angiography.

High risk

Early angiography and revascularisation is appropriate, although defining 'high risk' remains controversial (Braunwald et al, 2000). Patients require intensive therapy with beta-blockers, aspirin, clopidogrel, LMWH and glycoprotein IIb/IIIa inhibitors. Early coronary angiography (within 48 hours) is needed in those classified at high risk. Delaying intervention does not improve outcome.

Coronary angiography and revascularisation

If major coronary stenoses are demonstrated at angiography, the choice of revascularisation procedure is not very different from patients without unstable angina (Fig. 8.3). Routine stenting of the culprit lesion is usual, and direct stenting associates with a more rapid return of ST segments to normal. An identifiable culprit lesion cannot be identified in more than one-third of patients, and multiple culprit lesions may be seen in 14% of patients (Kerensky et al, 2002).

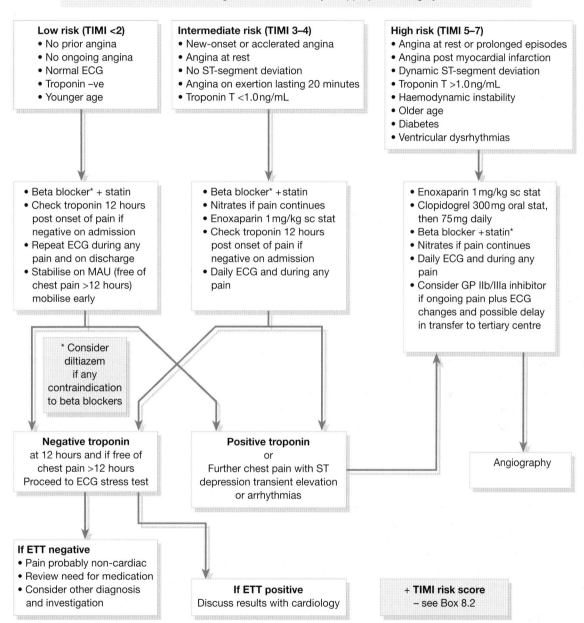

Figure 8.2 Management of patients according to risk.

Between 20% and 25% of patients will be shown to have left main stem disease, severe proximal left anterior descending coronary disease, triple coronary artery disease or ventricular aneurysms, and are usually considered for early bypass surgery (Eagle et al, 2004). If possible, bypass surgery should be delayed until medical stabilisation, as instability associates with a greater risk of perioperative complications. Those previously referred for and awaiting coronary

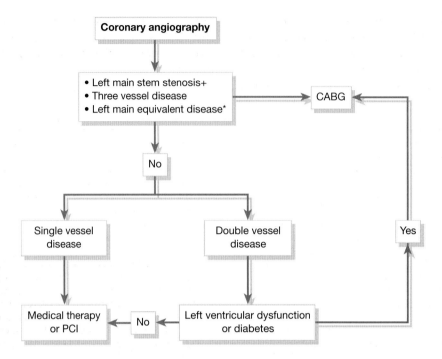

Coronary angiography

- Left main stem stenosis+
- Three vessel disease
- Left main equivalent disease*

→ CABG

No

Single vessel disease

Double vessel disease

Yes

Medical therapy or PCI ← No ← Left ventricular dysfunction or diabetes

+ A significant stenosis is defined as >70% reduction in vessel diameter (>50% in the left main stem)
* Left main equivalent disease = over 70% stenoses in the proximal LAD and proximal left circumflex arteries

Figure 8.3 Revascularisation guide following angiography. CABG, coronary artery bypass surgery; LAD, left anterior descensing coronary artery; PCI, percutaneous intervention.

artery bypass graft (CABG) surgery should be given waiting list priority.

About a quarter of all patients presenting with unstable angina have diabetes and, at angiography, they will be shown to have more severe coronary disease, with more ulcerated plaques and intracoronary thrombus. As a group, patients with diabetes obtain a better outcome with bypass surgery than with PCI.

Up to one-fifth of patients who present with an unstable coronary syndrome will have angiographically normal coronary arteries, or only minor irregularities within the major epicardial vessels. Although the absence of major stenoses does not exclude an acute coronary syndrome, the diagnosis needs to be reviewed. In selected patients, an ergonovine provocation test may detect or exclude important coronary spasm.

LONG-TERM MANAGEMENT

The acute phase of the unstable coronary syndromes is usually about 2 months, during which time there is an increased risk of progression to myocardial infarction or death. After this time, risks decline to those of patients with stable angina. Aggressive risk factor intervention is appropriate for all.

A recurrent acute coronary syndrome is defined as a return of symptoms or ischaemic changes on the ECG despite drug therapy within 2 months of a confirmed acute coronary syndrome. Patients who were initially managed medically should undergo coronary angiography.

A cardiac rehabilitation course should be available to all those recovering from an acute coronary syndrome, and may enhance patient education and compliance with medication. The healthcare team should work with the patient and their family to instruct on specific targets for cholesterol, blood pressure, body weight and exercise levels. Discharge instructions should include a written instruction sheet; both the patient and the family should know what to do if symptoms return. Formal or informal telephone follow-up may provide reassurance.

References

ACC/AHA (2002) Guideline update for the management of patients with unstable angina and non-ST elevation myocardial infarction. *Journal of the American College of Cardiology* 40: 1366–1374.

Anti-platelet Trialists' Collaboration (1994) Overview I: Prevention of death, myocardial infarction and stroke by prolonged anti-platelet therapy in various categories of patients. *British Medical Journal* 308: 81–106.

Bertrand ME, Simoons ML, Fox KAA et al (2002) Management of acute coronary syndromes *without* persistent ST-segment elevation. The task force on the management of acute coronary syndromes of the European Society of Cardiology. *European Heart Journal* 23: 1809–1840.

Boden WE, Van Gilst WH, Scheldewaert RG et al (2000) Diltiazem in acute infarction treated with thrombolytic drugs: a randomised placebo-controlled trial. INTERCEPT. *Lancet* 355: 1751–1756.

Boersma E, Harrington RA, Moliterno DJ et al (2002) Platelet glycoprotein IIb/IIIa inhibitors in acute coronary syndromes: a meta-analysis of all major randomised clinical trials. *Lancet* 359: 189–198.

Braunwald E for the ACC/AHA committee on management of patients with unstable angina (2000) ACC/AHA guidelines for unstable angina and non-ST elevation myocardial infarction. *Journal of the American College of Cardiology* 36: 970–1062.

British Cardiac Society (2001) Guidelines for the management of patients with acute coronary syndromes without ECG ST segment elevation. *Heart* 85: 133–142.

Califf RM, Petersen JL, Hasselblad V et al (2005) A perspective on trials comparing enoxaparin and unfractionated heparin in the treatment of non-ST-elevation acute coronary syndromes. *American Heart Journal* 149: s91–99.

Campeau L (1976) Grading of angina. *Circulation* 54: 522–523.

Carbajal EV, Deedwania P (2005) Treating non-ST-segment elevation ACS: pros and cons of current strategies. *Postgraduate Medicine* 118: 23–32.

Choudhry NK, Singh JM, Barolet A et al (2005) How should patients with unstable angina and non-ST-segment elevation myocardial infarction be managed? A meta-analysis of randomized trials. *American Journal of Medicine* 118: 465–474.

Collinson J, Flather M, Fox KA et al (2000) Clinical outcomes, risk stratification and practice patterns of unstable angina and myocardial infarction without ST elevation: Prospective Registry of Acute Ischaemic Syndromes in the UK (PRAIS-UK) *European Heart Journal* 21: 1450–1457.

de Araujo Goncalves P, Ferreira J, Aguiar C et al (2005) TIMI, PURSUIT, and GRACE risk scores: sustained prognostic value and interaction with revascularization in NSTE-ACS. *European Heart Journal* 26: 865–872.

Eagle KA, Guyton RA, Davidoff R et al (2004) ACC/AHA 2004 guideline update for coronary artery bypass graft surgery: a report of the American College of Cardiology/American Heart Association Task Force on Practice Guidelines. *Circulation* 110: e340–437.

Fibrinolytic Therapy Trialists' (FTT) Collaborative Group (1994) Indications for fibrinolytic therapy in suspected acute myocardial infarction: collaborative overview of early mortality and major morbidity results from all randomised trials of over 1000 patients. *Lancet* 343: 311–322.

Goldberger AL (1979) *Myocardial Infarction: Electrocardiographic Differential Diagnosis*. St Louis: CV Mosby.

Herlitz K, Karlson BW, Sjolin M et al (2001) Ten year mortality in sub-sets of patients with an acute coronary syndrome. *Heart* 86: 391–396.

Kerensky RA, Wade M, Deedwania P et al and the Veterans Affairs Non-Q-Wave Infarction Strategies in-Hospital (VANQWISH) Trial Investigators (2002) Revisiting the culprit lesion in non-Q-wave myocardial infarction. Results from the VANQWISH trial angiographic core laboratory. *Journal of the American College of Cardiology* 39: 1456–1463.

Knight CJ (2001) National Institute for Clinical Excellence guidance: too NICE to glycoprotein IIb/IIIa inhibitors? *Heart* 85: 481–483.

Lee T, Cook F, Erb R (1985) Acute chest pain in the emergency room. *Archives of Internal Medicine* 145: 65–69.

Lin SS, Lauer MS, Marwick TH (1998) Risk stratification of patients with medically treated unstable angina using exercise echocardiography. *American Journal of Cardiology* 82: 720–724.

Lindahl B, Andren B, Ohlsson J and the FRISC study group (1997) Risk stratification in unstable coronary artery disease. Additive value of troponin T determinations and pre-discharge exercise tests. *European Heart Journal* 18: 762–770.

Ohman EM, Armstrong PW, Christenson RH et al (1996) Cardiac troponin T levels and risk stratification in acute myocardial ischemia. *New England Journal of Medicine* 335: 1333–1341.

Patel DJ, Purcell HJ, Fox KM (1999) Cardio-protection by opening of the kATP channel in unstable angina. Is this a clinical manifestation of myocardial preconditioning? Results of a randomised study with nicorandil. *European Heart Journal* 20: 51–57.

Schwartz GG, Olsson AG, Ezekowitz MD et al for the Myocardial Ischemia Reduction with Aggressive Cholesterol Lowering (MIRACL) Study Investigators (2001) Effects of atorvastatin on early recurrent ischemic events in acute coronary syndromes: the MIRACL study: a randomised controlled trial. *Journal of the American Medical Association* 285: 1711–1718.

Scirica BM, Cannon CP, Antman EM et al (2002) Validation of the thrombolysis in myocardial infarction (TIMI) risk score for unstable angina pectoris and non-ST-elevation myocardial infarction in the TIMI III registry. *American Journal of Cardiology* 90: 303–305.

Shaw LJ, Peterson ED, Kesler K et al (1996) A meta-analysis of pre-discharge risk stratification after acute myocardial infarction with stress electrocardiography, myocardial perfusion and ventricular function imaging. *American Journal of Cardiology* 78: 1327–1337.

Stone GW, McLaurin BT, Cox DA et al. Acuity Investigators (2006) Bivalirudin for patients with acute coronary syndromes. *New England Journal of Medicine* 355: 2203–2216.

Theroux P, Fuster V (1998) Acute coronary syndromes: unstable angina and non-ST elevation myocardial infarction. *Circulation* 97: 1195–1206.

Wallentin L, Lagerqvist B, Husted S et al (2000) Outcome at one year after an invasive compared with a non-invasive strategy in unstable coronary artery disease: the FRISC II invasive randomized trial. *Lancet* 356: 9–16.

Walsh SJ, Spence MS, Crossman D et al (2005) Clopidogrel in non-ST segment elevation acute coronary syndromes: an overview submission by the British cardiac Society and the Royal College of Physicians to the National Institute for Clinical Excellence, and beyond. *Heart* 91: 1135–1140.

Waters DD, Hsue PY (2001) What is the role of intensive cholesterol lowering in the treatment of acute coronary syndromes? *American Journal of Cardiology* 88 (suppl): 7J–16J.

Yusuf S, Wittes J, Friedman L (1988) Overview of results of randomised clinical trials in heart disease, II: unstable angina and heart failure. Primary prevention with aspirin and risk factor modification. *Journal of the American Medical Association* 260: 2259–2263.

Yusuf S, Mehta SR, Chrolavicus S for the OASIS 5 investigators (2006) Comparison of fondaparinux and enoxaparin in acute coronary syndromes. *New England Journal of Medicine* 354: 1464–1476.

Chapter 9

Nursing patients with acute coronary syndromes

Nursing management is designed to help the patient overcome various physical and psychological reactions to the myocardial infarction. Therapeutic goals are broadly designed to promote healing of the damaged myocardium, prevent complications and facilitate the patient's rapid return to normal health and lifestyle (Webster & Thompson, 1992). Meeting the basic needs of the patient, such as comfort, rest, sleep and elimination, forms an essential component of nursing intervention. Some will require immediate attention, whereas others will be dealt with in later days. The nurse should be aware of what will be required and anticipate problems, rather than waiting for them to occur.

Patients are usually under a great deal of stress and anxiety, both during their hospital stay and after discharge. There will be uncertainty about their surroundings, fear of what has happened to them and worry about lack of control over what may occur in the following days. The situation may be exacerbated by lack of information, pain, discomfort or inability to obtain adequate rest. Patients' perceptions of the cardiac care unit have been linked to recovery (Proctor et al, 1996). Nurses need to demonstrate a calm, confident approach and, while needing the knowledge and skills to interpret and act on a wide variety of variables, they should also be sensitive to the patient's body language, facial expressions and tone of voice (Klein, 2005).

The acute illness brings changes for the patient and family in terms of usual patterns of living, which, although hopefully only short term, may persist after discharge from hospital. Acute myocardial infarction, in particular, poses major threats to the patient, usually because of the suddenness of the illness, and because of the connotations that heart disease carries. Fear of sudden death is the immediate worry, usually followed by a realisation that the patient will have to cope with a chronic disease. Apart from these changes in self-image, there are also feelings of loss in terms of status within the family unit, working environment and social circle. The secure knowledge of a regular financial income, the ability to care for the family and continuing full physical fitness are no longer present.

The responses that individual patients make to these threats include emotional crisis, defence mechanisms and coping behaviours. The patient's personal beliefs, attitudes, responsibilities, values and experiences will all influence how he or she perceives and responds to the acute illness. In the unfamiliar and frightening environment of the coronary care unit (CCU), the nurse needs to establish a close rapport with the patient and family in order to be effective in reducing anxiety and fear, promoting the resolution of losses, encouraging adjustment to change and planning together for complete recovery and successful rehabilitation. This will include detailed explanations about the significance of the illness, the nature of coronary heart disease and the goals of treatment, including the part that the CCU plays. The personnel involved in the provision of care will need to be introduced, and the roles of these people and the surrounding equipment should be fully explained. The encouragement of independence and the fostering of a realistic but optimistic outlook are of great importance. Such interventions should involve the nurse in providing care in an individualised and flexible fashion, rather than the traditional rigid task-orientated system. The CCU is an ideal setting for the nurse, patient and family to meet and discuss progress and future management. Care plans should be based upon an assessment completed within the initial hours of admission, so that priorities of care can then be established early and modified as the patient improves.

Nursing intervention involves many challenges in the management of acute myocardial infarction. A considerate and sensitive approach to the patient and family will allow full evaluation of present and potential problems, and the establishment of an overall plan of care, which may overcome them.

Care planning for patients on the cardiac care unit should consider the following:

1 The reduction or control of stressful physical (e.g. temperature and pain) and sensory (e.g. noise and lighting) stimuli is desirable. Specific sources should be identified in the assessment plan.

2 The preservation, where possible, of patients' routines. In CCUs, patients' eating, toileting and resting habits will be very different, sometimes resulting in disorientation or physical complications.

3 The adherence to lifestyle changes and drug regimens. The nurse needs to ensure that the patient listens to, understands and retains information and adheres to advice.

4 Encouragement of the patient and family to participate in care planning with the aim of taking responsibility for their own health.

There are many types of format for recording data, defining problems and outlining goals and intervention strategies. Although different units or wards may have their own care plans, it is desirable to have some degree of standardisation to facilitate the transfer of patients between wards, units and hospitals, if required. The care plan is the major tool for communicating instructions and providing a permanent and legal record. Entries should be written concisely, legibly and systematically, avoiding jargon and abbreviations to minimise ambiguity about care. The care plan should be kept up to date and made flexible to meet patients' changing needs.

COMMUNICATION

If nursing intervention is to be effective, then communication between the nurse, the patient, the family and other personnel involved in care has to be effective. Communication can take many forms – structured or informal, verbal or non-verbal – and tends to be a continuous process in situations in which individuals are working within the same environment. Thus, much of nursing management will be directly or indirectly concerned with communication at some level.

There are various reasons why nurse–patient communication is often inadequate in coronary care. These include the short duration of the patient's stay on the unit, the severity of the patient's condition and, often, the nurse's preoccupation with handling technical rather than personal requirements. Staff need to judge the timing and content of their communication with patients (Svedlund et al, 1999). The patient needs to perceive the nurse as friendly, helpful, competent and reliable, and the nurse should recognise the patient's individuality, perceived needs and actual needs.

Coronary care patients are often brought suddenly into the unfamiliar environment of hospital. They change from a position of being in control of their lives to one of having to accept the submissive role of a patient. Effective communication can really only be achieved if patients are allowed to retain their individuality. The nurse should work with the patient to effect positive adaptation and coping mechanisms by education and counselling. Liaison with the patient and family is required to ensure that they are aware of the objective of the cardiac unit and understand the various procedures and treatments. A realistic outlook for the future, based on knowledge and understanding, may then be achieved. It is important for communication to be clear and comprehensible, using language familiar to the patient (at whatever level) and avoiding the use of jargon. Simple explanations need to be reiterated, as retention of verbal information is seldom for long. Reassuring patients that survival and recovery are fully anticipated should encourage an atmosphere of optimism.

Cardiac nurses themselves need to be able to demonstrate credibility in their role as communicators. Communication is a two-way process, and there is a need to interact with the patient, adapting the approach to meet changing needs.

Some patients may not possess the necessary skills to be able to communicate successfully. They may be too ill or anxious, they may be physically disabled or have learning difficulties, or they may lack the knowledge and understanding to be able to make realistic decisions regarding their future. This may equally apply to the relatives, who can find the hospital environment imposing. Nurses have an important role to play as advocates of the patient and relatives, basing advice on experience, knowledge of the illness and the individual patient. As well as structured planned communication to convey specific points, there is also day-to-day conversation, interaction and non-verbal communication. Human contact is important in a technical environment such as coronary care. Patients are likely to appreciate knowing that a nurse is near at hand, especially if they are bedridden, when communication is perhaps the only way in which some patients can influence their environment and routine.

In the highly technical and invasive atmosphere of coronary care, there is sometimes a need to stand back and think carefully about what is the best treatment or strategy for the patient. Allowing a critically ill patient to die with peace and dignity is not a failure and may be a better course of action than prolonging life with multiple therapies, which mislead the relatives into thinking there is hope (Thompson, 1995). Discussing such subjects openly in a constructive fashion with medical colleagues, in a detached and unemotional manner, involves a sensitive and professional approach, which is necessary but seldom easy.

Smooth and effective communication between nurses and other personnel is likely to result in better nurse–patient communication. There is a need in cardiac care units to ensure that the medico-technical aspects do not detract from the physical and emotional requirements of patients.

INFORMATION

In most studies of the self-perceived needs and concerns of post-infarct patients and their families, information needs rank as the highest priority (Moser et al, 1993). Many patients understand little of what has happened to them or how to manage their lives in the aftermath of an acute myocardial infarction (Calkins et al, 1997). Many require information at different times and for different purposes (Turton, 1998). Some items might be readily understood, whereas others might need to be reiterated, especially when a patient's receptivity is limited by physical debility and emotional distress.

Determining the most important information for patients to know and communicating it effectively are crucial elements in improving the quality of healthcare. Healthcare staff should communicate accurate, relevant and timely information to patients at their own level of understanding. Now that patient turnover is becoming more rapid and hospital stay shorter, nurses have less time for verbal information giving. Supplementing advice with written information is helpful, but such materials should be of the highest quality, taking into account issues such as format and presentation as well as content (Walsh & Shaw, 2000).

An important issue in information giving is that of beliefs and misconceptions that patients and relatives may have. Indeed, nurses often have as many, or even more, misconceptions as their patients (Newens et al, 1997). Early, in-hospital counselling, commencing in the cardiac care unit and aimed at correcting misconceptions, dispelling myths and allaying fears, has been shown to be effective in improving knowledge and satisfaction and reducing psychological distress in patients and partners (Thompson, 1990). Delivering routine health information by audiotape is a useful adjunct to personally tailored advice. This would allow the information to be delivered early, in a standardised fashion, and repeated whenever necessary at the patient's convenience. Such an approach is appreciated by patients and reduces the number of misconceptions they may have (Lewin et al, 2002).

ASSESSMENT OF PAIN

Pain is a complex and personal experience, and it is usually the nurse who is near at hand when the patient experiences pain and who is responsible for its evaluation and for providing relief. Yet, pain assessment and management by nurses is often suboptimal (Meurier et al, 1998), but may lend itself to numerical or graphic measurement. Three pain rating scales are in common use, the Visual Analogue Scale, the Verbal Rating Scale and the Numerical Rating Scale, but interpretation of the scales is not always straightforward (Williamson & Hoggart, 2005). All three pain rating scales are valid, reliable and appropriate for use in clinical practice and, although patients usually prefer the Verbal Rating Scale because of simplicity, it lacks sensitivity.

The assessment of pain should include the patient's own description of it and observation of his or her reaction to it. It is not always possible to make this evaluation on admission to coronary care if the patient is critically ill but, later on, it will be important to determine whether the pain the patient is still suffering is ischaemic or pericarditic pain or is just due to anxiety. Each of these will have different specific antidotes, such as

aspirin for pericarditis or diazepam for anxiety, although the disinterested may simply choose to obliterate all possibilities with a large dose of diamorphine.

In addition to the traditional provision of analgesia with drug therapy, there is a wide range of pain-relieving strategies that can be instituted by the nurse:

- ensuring peace and comfort;
- careful positioning of the patient;
- reassurance;
- protection from stressful situations;
- limitation of unnecessary activity;
- promotion of sleep.

If the patient fully understands the pain and its cause, it may then become less distressing.

COMFORT

The promotion of relaxation and comfort is an essential and fundamental component of nursing. Unfortunately, such skills tend to be overlooked on CCUs. Careful positioning of the patient, reassurance and the presence of a caring nurse assume a high priority to ensure complete comfort. Careful bedmaking, regulation of light, temperature and noise, and the provision of hot milky drinks in the evening may seem mundane and obvious, but are often delegated to the most junior nurse as a low priority in the 'high-tech' environment of coronary care. Other comforting strategies such as massage have been shown to be effective in promoting sleep and recovery in critically ill patients (Richards, 1998). The effects of massage and associated therapeutic touch have been shown to reduce anxiety and promote comfort and rest in intensive care units (Cox & Hayes, 1998).

Attached monitoring equipment or frequent disturbances that occur when routine observations are made may compound patient discomfort. Invasive monitoring devices and intravenous lines often result in the general enforced immobilisation of the patient, which carries with it the attendant risk of pressure sores. Thus, frequent changing of the patient's position in bed and the use of pressure-relieving devices are important in reducing discomfort. Consideration should be given to the siting of intravenous cannulae and the use of nasal cannulae rather than oxygen masks.

Rest has to be both physical and mental and can be achieved by a variety of factors including:

- adequate pain relief;
- promotion of relaxation, comfort and sleep;
- ensuring that noise is kept at a low level;
- control of temperature, light and humidity;
- planned rest periods during the day.

A warm, stimulating environment should be encouraged, where patients feel they can relax and chat with fellow patients, staff and relatives. Nursing interventions such as music and relaxation can be comforting and reduce anxiety in patients with myocardial infarction (White, 1999; Biley, 2000).

BEDREST AND ACTIVITY

Bedrest is usual, but recent trends are towards early mobilisation, with slower schedules being reserved for those with complications. Hospitalisation and enforced bedrest can produce their own problems, such as constipation, bone resorption, thromboembolism, pulmonary atelectasis, pressure sores and urinary retention. It is, therefore, important that patients mobilise as soon as possible, particularly the elderly, who fare worse from complications due to enforced rest than they would otherwise do as a result of myocardial infarction alone. Active and passive leg movements should be encouraged, and early chest physiotherapy is advisable, especially in smokers.

Although the CCU should theoretically be the ideal environment for resting, in practice, it rarely is because of the non-stop activity in and around the patients. Among its many other benefits, the purpose of rest following myocardial infarction is to decrease the myocardial demand for oxygen and limit myocardial work. Inactivity is a major problem, in that it serves as a source of frustration and boredom. It is, therefore, important to stress to patients the need for temporary limitation but to reassure them that bedrest is only short term and is in their own best interest. Enforced bedrest will only have adverse effects on people who are normally active, by making them perceive themselves as more seriously ill. Relaxation, deep

breathing and active and passive leg exercises are useful in reducing boredom and mood changes, as well as the risk of the physical complications of bedrest. Such activities will boost patients' morale by making them feel that they are playing an active part in the recovery process.

It is preferable that the patient sits upright in bed rather than lying flat, because the latter requires more myocardial work to pump blood through the excess pool of tissue fluid in the lungs. Thus, patients with uncomplicated infarcts should sit out as early as possible. Some patients may feel reluctant or hesitant to resume activity, whereas others are overzealous.

There is no reason why most patients cannot wash, eat and shave. In fact, it is likely that there is a danger of more stress resulting from not being allowed to do such activities than the actual performance of them. Patients may require some assistance from the nurse if they are severely restricted by equipment, such as short monitor cables, intravenous infusions, pacemaker units, etc., or if they are feeling weak or are generally too ill. The nurse should offer to assist, as some patients may feel unable to ask. If the patient is bed bound, the nurse needs to ensure that he or she has everything needed within easy reach.

EARLY AMBULATION

Only 40 years ago, patients with acute myocardial infarction were kept on strict bedrest for 2 months to allow the heart to heal. All activities were performed by attending nursing staff, with limited mobilisation over the following year to prevent heart failure, rupture of the heart or the formation of a left ventricular aneurysm. However, it soon became apparent that this form of therapy led to an increased incidence of thromboembolic disorders, chest infections and musculoskeletal disorders. Alteration in vasomotor reflexes and hypovolaemia also occur with prolonged bedrest, leading to tachycardia, hypotension and unsteadiness on standing. The highly controversial approach to early mobilisation in the early 1960s was regarded as reckless and dangerous when uncomplicated infarct patients were allowed out of bed after only 15 days (Cain et al, 1961).

The emphasis today is on early mobilisation and discharge, especially for those who have an uncomplicated hospital course. This type of approach minimises physical and psychological disability, and reduces the risk of thromboembolism. The point at which the risk to the individual becomes acceptably low is a matter of judgement, but the risk of a major adverse event declines rapidly after a heart attack, and particularly for patients without heart failure.

Peri-infarction mortality is higher in patients who have had complications such as prolonged or recurrent chest pain, left ventricular failure, significant dysrhythmia (e.g. ventricular tachycardia or fibrillation) or those with complicating disease, particularly diabetes. Early mobilisation should be delayed in these patients, even when the underlying complication has been corrected. However, most of these potential high-risk cases may be identified in the first 24 hours following admission, and provisional selection for early discharge may be made within 48 hours.

Nursing should reflect the current pattern of care for coronary patients, which has been characterised by an increase in physical activity soon after infarction and has led to a decrease in imposed invalidism and an earlier discharge from hospital. Patients with an uncomplicated infarct are kept in bed for a maximum of 24–48 hours only. Indeed, in some units, patients are encouraged to sit out on the day of admission, providing they are free from pain and significant dysrhythmia (Herkner et al, 2003). Gradual but early mobilisation should, certainly, encourage patients to walk around the ward by the end of a few days, and it is important that an individualised approach takes preference over a strict regimen.

When the patient resumes activity, it is helpful if the nurse knows the normal activity levels and habits of the patient. This should have been ascertained during the nursing assessment. A plan can then be developed by the nurse and patient to provide a framework as to what level of activity he can realistically be expected to achieve by a specific time.

Observing heart rate and rhythm, respiratory rate and blood pressure can assess the stress that various activities have on the body. However, these should be monitored in an informal manner to avoid unduly worrying the patient. The development of symptoms such as chest pain, shortness of breath, palpitations or faintness is an indication to cease activity. The patient should be made aware of this and encouraged to inform the nurse if such symptoms occur.

In uncomplicated cases, patients should be encouraged to climb one or two flights of stairs before they are discharged home. They will need to be advised about what they will be able to do at home, including information on eating, drinking and driving. A realistic appraisal of the prospect of a full recovery and early return to work is essential.

SLEEP

The function of sleep is unknown, and there is debate about whether it is concerned with bodily and brain restitution, energy conservation or as an occupier of time. Sleep may be roughly divided into two broad stages:

- *non-REM* (rapid eye movement) or orthodox sleep;
- *REM* or paradoxical sleep.

Non-REM sleep is characterised by lowering of the blood pressure, heart and respiratory rates, whereas REM sleep is characterised by the opposite and is strongly correlated with dreaming. Many people experience onset or worsening of an illness during the night. Cardiovascular events often occur with a high frequency during sleep, especially REM sleep. Patients with nocturnal angina are more likely to suffer their attacks during periods of REM sleep, and there is also an increase in the frequency of ventricular ectopic activity. The onset of symptoms of acute myocardial infarction is more frequent in bed, especially just after falling asleep and on waking (Thompson et al, 1991).

Patients in specialised units experience marked sleep disturbances in hospital, and much of this sleep is desynchronised, being affected by noise, temperature, comfort, pain and anxiety (Webster & Thompson, 1986). The promotion of comfort and relaxation is important, with control of environmental factors (e.g. reduced noise, regulated room temperature and dimmed lights) needed.

Pain relief is, of course, essential. Unnecessary nursing or medical observations or interventions disrupt the continuity and efficiency of patients' sleep, and essential procedures should be organised in a fashion that ensures that patients are only minimally disturbed. With current advanced technology, multichannel monitoring facilities make many routine observations easy to perform without waking the patient.

Nursing assessment should incorporate information about the patient's usual sleeping habits and patterns, such as quality and quantity of normal sleep and the identification of any routines that the patient feels will enhance his or her ability to sleep. Hot milky drinks often form part of the night-time ritual and have been shown significantly to improve sleep. The use of a sleep questionnaire, such as the St Mary's Hospital Sleep Questionnaire (Ellis et al, 1981), is a useful adjunct in the assessment of sleeping habits. Snoring is associated with a significant increased risk of acute myocardial infarction and stroke and should be taken into consideration when treating patients with cardiac disease.

DIET

Although diet is not usually considered in the early stages following myocardial infarction, there are many reasons why adjustments may need to be made. In the early hours following admission, nausea and vomiting are common, and there is a higher risk of cardiorespiratory arrest, which may lead to bronchial aspiration of gastric contents. A liquid diet is, therefore, probably best given initially until a normal diet can be instituted. Caffeine should be avoided because of its possible dysrhythmic effect, and salt intake should be limited in all cardiac patients, but especially in those with hypertension and heart failure. The co-ingestion of grapefruit/grapefruit juice can increase the blood levels of numerous orally administered drugs that undergo cytochrome P-450 oxidative metabolism. The compounds (bioflavanoids and furanocoumarins) that are contained in grapefruit/grapefruit juice inhibit this enzyme system, resulting in higher blood levels of various drugs (Table 9.1). The inhibitory effects can last up to 24 hours. As the degree of interaction can vary from drug to drug, and the type and amount of grapefruit/grapefruit juice consumed, it should not be kept on hospital menus.

Other considerations in relation to diet include:

1 Patients on CCUs feel nauseated or not hungry. Nourishing drinks and small snacks at times other than established meal times may be more appreciated.
2 Patients from ethnic minorities will require special consideration, and relatives need to be consulted, as they can offer valuable advice and assistance by bringing in meals.
3 Fluid restriction may be warranted if the patient is in heart failure. Such patients will require attention to mouth care, including mouthwashes and sips of cold or iced water.

Table 9.1   Grapefruit juice and cardiac medications.

Drug group	Medications substantially boosted by grapefruit juice	Medications that have little or no interaction with grapefruit juice
Calcium channel blockers	Felodipine Nifedipine	Verapamil Diltiazem Amlodipine
Statins	Atorvastatin Simvastatin	Fluvastatin Pravastatin Rosuvastatin
Angiotensin blockers Antidysrhythmic agents	Losartan Amiodarone Aminophylline	

Confiscating the water jug is not sufficient; the patient should be informed of what is being done and why.

4 Nurses play a major role in nutrition education as part of secondary prevention and rehabilitation, yet all too often they seem to ignore their responsibility in this area, prematurely enlisting the help of a dietician. While professional assessment should be provided for the obese (BMI > 30 kg/m^2) or those with impaired glucose regulation or diabetes, the dietary principles needed by most patients are not complex. It is now universally recognised that a diet that is high in fat, salt and free sugars, and low in complex carbohydrates, fruit and vegetables increases the risk of chronic diseases – particularly cardiovascular disease.

Many patients will have preconceived ideas obtained from their relatives and the media about good dietary habits. The major difficulty is not in giving the advice to patients and their relatives, but in achieving the appropriate behavioural responses that should be in their own interests.

ELIMINATION

Prolonged bedrest and general physical inactivity should be avoided, as this inhibits gastrointestinal motility and leads to constipation. The faeces may, additionally, become hardened because of increased water resorption and the use of diuretics. The constipated patient will strain at stool, with excessive isometric work, which leads to vagal stimulation. This is likely to produce bradycardia or heart block, and may severely compromise venous return, with dramatic falls in cardiac output and vasovagal collapse. Similar vasovagal effects may result from the use of bedpans that are uncomfortable and stressful. Using a bedside commode is easier and more comfortable and places the patient in a more familiar position for defecation. Laxatives may be warranted to prevent excessive straining at stool, which may be helped by careful attention to the fluid and fibre content of the diet. The patient needs to be reassured that many patients have altered bowel habits following admission to hospital. This may simply be due to different dietary habits or enforced bedrest, but certain drugs can alter normal elimination habits. For instance, opiates cause constipation, and broad-spectrum antibiotics may cause diarrhoea. Additionally, many patients feel extremely embarrassed about using a commode or urinal in the vicinity of others. This in itself may give rise to constipation or retention. They are more likely to feel at ease in a private room or cubicle than in the middle of an open-plan area, even if they do have the benefit of partially closed curtains through which different faces keep appearing. More patients should be permitted to use a toilet at an earlier stage.

Careful recording of fluid balance is essential for patients on diuretic therapy. Daily weighing of the patient may be more accurate than a fluid balance chart for assessment in congestive cardiac failure. The patient should be warned of the resulting increase in the quantity and frequency of urine. Consideration should be given to the timing of diuretic administration so that the patient is minimally disturbed during the night.

HYGIENE

Bathing and hygiene

Many patients admitted to coronary care have been unprepared for admission because of the sudden onset of symptoms, and may feel acutely embarrassed and uncomfortable, particularly if they are sweating, have vomited or are partly naked. Patients are likely to be feeling too unwell in the immediate stages to look after themselves and, although the nurse will need to assist acutely, he or she should avoid encouraging dependency. The psychological aspects of bathing and hygiene are important. For example, patients feel better after a shower or bath, and appreciate simple things such as being offered hand washing facilities after using the commode, without having to ask.

Oral hygiene

Mouth toilet should be offered to all patients, especially those who wear dentures, are on fluid restriction or have been vomiting. Patients with dentures are often very embarrassed about cleaning them in the presence of others and should be afforded the necessary privacy and facilities.

Use of the bath and shower

It appears that coronary patients move more slowly and deliberately than normal when bathing in order to conserve energy (Winslow et al, 1985). Patients may prefer to shower if this has been their normal domestic routine, particularly during the later stages of their stay in hospital. However, oxygen consumption is higher in patients who shower than in those who use a bath, and this should be taken into consideration. The isometric activity required by some patients to get out of a bath may result in a steep rise in arterial blood pressure, which increases myocardial work. Hence, before a patient is first bathed, the nurse needs to evaluate any potential difficulties. If the patient is weak, obese or generally likely to have difficulties, bathing is probably contraindicated.

EMOTIONAL DISTURBANCES

Emotional disturbances after myocardial infarction may adversely influence subsequent recovery and health outcome. They are extremely common in patients admitted to coronary care. Anxiety is, not surprisingly, very common, especially in women (Kim et al, 2000), and many patients are depressed, agitated or even openly hostile. Many complain of difficulty in concentrating, and nearly half of patients will have difficulty with sleep. If anxiety is unrelieved, depression usually supervenes, and both may persist for long periods of time in many patients (Lane et al, 2002).

The nurse needs to be able to recognise verbal and non-verbal cues to emotional distress and understand the basic mechanisms that the patient is using to cope. Three of the most common acute responses following acute myocardial infarction are fear, dependency and disorientation. These may later be replaced by anxiety and depression.

Fear

The patient's immediate reaction is usually fear, not only of death, but also of the threat the illness poses to his or her lifestyle (Thompson, 1995). This fear can be reduced by an explanation of the purpose of coronary care, the monitoring equipment and the high nurse–patient ratio. Patients need to be warned of and informed about routine observations, investigations and drug administration. Knowing the names of staff and the ease of summoning them increases their security. In general, the unit environment should become more reassuring than frightening to the patient, and later the family too.

Dependency

Encouraging resumption of usual activities as soon as possible will minimise the sense of damage and helplessness. Involving the patient in planning his or her own care helps to increase feelings of self-worth and independence. Involving the partner or other family members is a useful adjunct.

Disorientation

Disorientation, together with social isolation, can be reduced by the provision of a suitable environment, which includes calendars, clocks, radios, televisions, newspapers and windows with a view of the outside world. The additional comforts and provision of items such as personal photographs indicate extra thoughtfulness.

Anxiety

Anxiety is a normal but complex human phenomenon, which is difficult to define exactly. Mild anxiety is part of normal everyday life but, in excess, it impairs physical and mental performance. Empirically, anxiety is used to describe an unpleasant emotional state, although it is also used to describe differences in anxiety proneness as a personal characteristic.

Anxiety is certainly the most common initial response to acute myocardial infarction. Its main source is the prospect of sudden death, and the signs of anxiety are more likely to be noticed during the initial phase of the illness, when recurrent symptoms such as chest pain or shortness of breath develop, or when special procedures such as the insertion of a temporary pacemaker or cardioversion are required. A less obvious symptom that evokes anxiety is the feeling of weakness and complete exhaustion. Patients who have normally been fit and strong, but are now feeling weak as a consequence of an infarct, may experience extreme anxiety and frustration. Anxiety about transfer to the ward and discharge home is likely to be particularly high if the patient is discharged abruptly with little or no warning.

Anxiety can be identified subjectively and objectively. Subjectively, patients will appear tense, apprehensive and restless. They may have a sustained tachycardia, sweat freely and constantly seek reassurance. Care must be taken not to mistake these symptoms for heart failure. Objectively, anxiety can be measured in a variety of ways, including physiological and biochemical indices, such as blood pressure, heart rate and plasma or urinary catecholamine levels. However, in cardiac patients, such methods are more likely to reflect the physical than the psychological state. Questionnaires such as the Hospital Anxiety and Depression (HAD) Scale (Zigmond & Snaith, 1983) or visual analogue scales may prove more practical and quicker to use. The Cardiac Depression Visual Analogue Scale (CD-VAS) is a valid and reliable measure for brief and rapid repeated assessments of depressive symptoms in a cardiac population (Di Benedetto et al, 2005).

Once anxiety has been assessed, intervention can be tailored more specifically to the patient's needs. The patient with a mild level of anxiety is usually alert and able to absorb information and solve problems, even though he may be restless and irritable. In contrast, the patient with a very high level of anxiety is often terrified and much too distressed to perceive and communicate normally.

Considerate, attentive and competent nursing will reduce anxiety, and can provide a major source of reassurance. Close and consistent nurse–patient contact increases the patient's feelings of security (Thompson, 1990). Relaxation techniques involving progressive muscle relaxation may be effective in minimising undue stress.

Depression

Depression is common in coronary patients, particularly in women, and will often follow anxiety, especially if the latter is untreated. It is a reactive rather than endogenous depression and seldom assumes psychotic status. Depression may be triggered by the severity of the myocardial infarction, whereas ongoing and recurrent depression is more related to personality. It is an understandable response to myocardial infarction because of the implied loss of health, loss of earning capacity, impairment of physical activity and diminution of general status within the family and society. It is important that depression is recognised and dealt with promptly, because it may interfere with the recovery process. Patients who are depressed make the poorest long-term recovery, as measured by their ability to return to work and resume sexual activity. They may experience sadness, disinterest, sleep disturbances and loss of appetite. In the acute phase, depression usually appears on the third to fifth day, when the patient is at an emotional low ebb. Denial is the most common coping mechanism and can often be recognised by statements the patient makes. There may be refusal to acknowledge that he has suffered a heart attack and is becoming depressed as a consequence. Denial is usually a temporary phenomenon and may serve to protect the patient from further psychological deterioration. Gradual acceptance of the illness and active participation in recovery usually follow. However, denial is dangerous to the patient when its presence allows him or her to engage in some form of behaviour that threatens his or her welfare, for example trying to take too much exercise too soon. The nurse needs to examine to what extent denial is interfering with the treatment and endangering the patient.

Some patients may be irritable, oversensitive or prone to bouts of tearfulness. Others may experience feelings of hopelessness and helplessness, which results in them forming a generally pessimistic outlook. A full assessment of the patient's situation is required to ascertain whether the depression is part of the normal process of adapting to illness or whether it is related to other events. It may be helpful for the nurse to sit quietly with the patient and attempt to determine the major worries. Many of the fears may be quite realistic and are likely to prove difficult to resolve or alleviate. Some concerns may be unfounded and, once these are identified, the nurse can help to correct any misconceptions that the patient may hold. Having someone to talk with, or to hold or cry with, may enable the patient to organise his or her thinking and help him or her positively to reassess the future. An optimistic but realistic outlook, which conveys hope and gives the patient energy and enthusiasm, is usually what is required. Probably the best antidote is early mobilisation, to counter the physical and psychological problems associated with immobility. The sooner the patient is back on his or her feet, the sooner will feelings of self-worth and self-esteem return. The nurse will need to avoid overprotection or the encouragement of dependency.

Anger and hostility

The experience of a cardiac event is a significant source of stress for both patients and their family members. The acute phase after myocardial infarction reflects a crisis for patients and family members as they attempt to reconcile the effect of the event and adapt to the uncertainties associated with hospitalisation and the initial recovery process.

Once patients are aware of the fact that they have had a heart attack (and what this may imply), it is possible that their reaction may be one of anger, hostility or both. There is much emphasis and media coverage today on healthy living, and patients who consider that they have taken special care of their health may feel cheated that this has happened to them. Anger occurs in response to frustration, threat or injury. It may be expressed actively or passively, or may be self-directed. Active expressions of anger include sarcasm, criticism, irritability and argument. Passively, it may be expressed through non-compliance, boredom, withdrawal or forgetfulness. Self-directed anger is manifested as depression, self-deprecation, accident proneness and somatic symptoms such as headaches and dizziness.

It is often difficult to remain objective, especially when the patient is critical of the care he or she is receiving or of the personnel who provide it. The attending medical staff and others may feel powerless or may experience anger themselves. They need to try to help the patient to clarify his or her ideas and feelings, and explain constructive ways of dealing with such feelings. A consistent approach should be adopted towards the patient, and staff should not allow themselves to be played off against each other.

THE REACTION OF THE FAMILY

Hospital is a frightening place for the majority of the general public, especially cardiac intensive care and high-dependency units, their very titles suggesting danger and bodily assault. The family will have more time to sit and think about the implications of these titles and may actually fear the CCU more than the patient, who is usually too busy being ill. Relatives often feel that their loved one has been taken away and isolated from them. They frequently feel helpless, frightened and unnecessarily excluded from close involvement with their loved one. All members of the family (especially the partner) may fear that the patient may die, and there may be many recriminations and feelings of guilt if there have been recent family arguments or upsets. The course of the illness involves multiple adjustments by patients and family members as they attempt to reconcile the effect of the event and adapt to the uncertainties associated with the acute phase of illness (Fleury & Moore, 1999).

Professional support from nurses and doctors is sadly lacking where the family is concerned, and the support they do get is often inadequate or inappropriate (Thompson et al, 1995). Nursing intervention is aimed at assessing and supporting the family's coping mechanisms by providing information and reassurance and involving other appropriate professional help and opinion. Family members may view the patient's illness as a loss; they may feel they have lost the security of having certain needs, especially economic and emotional security, consistently and reliably met. They are, therefore, likely to need information, reassurance and support, but often feel reluctant to seek out staff and indicate their concerns. Many feel that, by doing so, they may be in the way, stopping important work, or that they may cause friction with the staff, resulting in a deterioration in their relative's care. It is, therefore, important for the coronary care staff to take the initiative in making and maintaining contact with the family, especially the partner, who is most likely to benefit from involvement in the care of the patient. The partner can also provide a unique service by giving insight into the patient's preferences, dislikes and frame of mind, and by generally supporting recovery. Unnecessary distress may be prevented by including the partner in discharge planning and preparing the family for the patient's homecoming. Anticipation of any difficulties will facilitate a smooth and continuous transition from hospital to home.

The reaction of the partner to the illness is likely to be influenced by a number of factors, not least of which will be the general stage of the marriage. Partners will need to be warned that they are likely to experience emotional and physical responses to their loved one's illness, such as fatigue, anxiety, depression, difficulty in sleeping, weight loss and sexual difficulties. These are expected stress reactions to the patient's return home. Partners will often feel that, if they show concern, they may be accused of being overprotective and, if they do not, they may be regarded as callous and unsympathetic.

Once the patient returns home, family members are often afraid to express their true feelings to the patient in case they induce another heart attack. Such cautious suppression of feelings inhibits frank and easy communication within the family and often results in a general atmosphere of tension. Both partners and their families should be invited to follow-up visits to continue education and to provide an opportunity to discuss their problems and receive advice about possible resolution. Groups for the partners of post-infarction patients may be beneficial in offering support, providing information and encouraging changes in lifestyle.

TRANSFER FROM THE CORONARY CARE UNIT

Although transfer to the ward may be interpreted by the patient as evidence of improvement, it may sometimes be viewed as an indication of lack of care or rejection. There is a perception among some patients and family members that units such as coronary care are secure, safe and familiar (Coyle, 2001). Anxiety and even fear about transfer are not uncommon, and these are likely to be compounded if the patient is transferred abruptly or during the night. Careful preparation and explanation at the time of transfer can alleviate such negative reactions.

It is important to warn the patient and family that, after transfer, there is usually a marked change in daily routine, with fewer nurses and doctors on hand and possible changes in medication, diet and activity. Most patients assume that they must have virtually recovered, as they no longer have monitoring equipment, cannulae or high nurse–patient ratios. Ward staff may assume likewise, and there is a real danger that the patients will be left alone to 'self-care', in the belief that they require minimal nursing contact. It is vital that, during handover from the unit to the ward, a full explanation of what has happened to the patient, and what is required in terms of care and treatment, is given. A fully documented up-to-date care plan, with a suggested plan of further management and expected outcome, is highly desirable. Patients may forget the verbal information given to them at the time of transfer and often have limited memory of the CCU. Providing written information as part of a structured discharge plan provides patients and relatives with a resource that they can refer to at any time and that enhances verbal communication (Paul et al, 2004).

Preparing patients for transfer from coronary care forms an important part of nursing management and requires more attention than it is frequently afforded. This is particularly so when patients are being discharged home directly from the CCU (Senaratne et al, 1999).

References

Biley FC (2000) The effects on patient well-being of music listening as a nursing intervention: a review of the literature. *Journal of Clinical Nursing* 9: 668–677.

Cain HD, Frasher WG, Stivelman R (1961) Graded activity program for safe return to self-care after myocardial infarction. *Journal of the American Medical Association* 171: 111.

Calkins DR, Davis RB, Reiley P et al (1997) Patient–physician communication at hospital discharge and patients' understanding of the post discharge treatment plan. *Archives of Internal Medicine* 157: 1026–1030.

Cox C, Hayes J (1998) Experiences of administering and receiving therapeutic touch in intensive care. *Complementary Therapies in Nursing and Midwifery* 4: 128–133.

Coyle MA (2001) Transfer anxiety: preparing to leave intensive care. *Intensive and Critical Care Nursing* 17: 138–143.

Di Benedetto M, Lindner H, Hare DL et al (2005) A Cardiac Depression Visual Analogue Scale for the brief and rapid assessment of depression following acute coronary syndromes. *Journal of Psychosomatic Research* 59: 223–229.

Ellis BW, Johns MW, Lancaster R et al (1981) The St Mary's Hospital Sleep Questionnaire: a study of reliability. *Sleep* 4: 93–97.

Fleury J, Moore SM (1999) Family-centred care after acute myocardial infarction. *Journal of Cardiovascular Nursing* 13: 73–82.

Herkner H, Thoennissen J, Nikfardjam M et al (2003) Short versus prolonged bed rest after uncomplicated acute myocardial infarction: a systematic review and meta-analysis. *Journal of Clinical Epidemiology* 56: 775–781.

Kim KA, Moser DK, Garvin BJ et al (2000) Differences between men and women in anxiety early after acute myocardial infarction. *American Journal of Critical Care* 9: 245–253.

Klein ER (2005) Effective communication with patients. *Pennsylvania Nurse* 60: 14–15.

Lane D, Carroll D, Ring C et al (2002) The prevalence and persistence of depression and anxiety following myocardial infarction. *British Journal of Health Psychology* 7: 11–21.

Lewin RJP, Thompson DR, Elton RA (2002) Trial of the effects of an advice and relaxation tape given within the first 24 hours of admission to hospital with acute myocardial infarction. *International Journal of Cardiology* 82: 107–114.

Meurier CE, Vincent CA, Parmar DG (1998) Perceptions of causes of omissions in the assessment of patients with chest pain. *Journal of Advanced Nursing* 28: 1012–1019.

Moser DK, Dracup KA, Marsden C (1993) Needs of recovering cardiac patients and their spouses: compared views. *International Journal of Nursing Studies* 30: 105–114.

Newens AJ, McColl E, Lewin R et al (1997) Cardiac misconceptions and knowledge in nurses caring for myocardial infarction patients. *Coronary Health Care* 1: 83–89.

Paul F, Hendry C, Cabrelli L (2004) Meeting patient and relatives' information needs upon transfer from an intensive care unit: the development and evaluation of an information booklet. *Journal of Clinical Nursing* 13: 396–405.

Proctor T, Yarcheski A, Oriscello RG (1996) The relationship of hospital process variables to patient outcome post-myocardial infarction. *International Journal of Nursing Studies* 33: 121–130.

Richards K (1998) Effect of a back massage and relaxation intervention on sleep in critically ill patients. *American Journal of Critical Care* 7: 288–299.

Senaratne MP, Irwin ME, Shaben S et al (1999) Feasibility of direct discharge from the coronary/intermediate care unit after acute myocardial infarction. *Journal of the American College of Cardiology* 33: 1040–1046.

Svedlund M, Danileson E, Norberg A (1999) Nurses' narrations about caring for inpatients with acute myocardial infarction. *Intensive and Critical Care Nursing* 15: 34–43.

Thompson DR (1990) *Counselling the Coronary Patient and Partner.* London: Scutari Press.

Thompson DR (1995) Fear of death. In: O'Connor S (ed.) *The Cardiac Patient: Nursing Interventions.* London: Mosby, pp. 117–126.

Thompson DR, Sutton TW, Jowett NI et al (1991) Circadian variation in the frequency of onset of chest pain in acute myocardial infarction. *British Heart Journal* 65: 177–178.

Thompson DR, Ersser SJ, Webster RA (1995) The experiences of patients and their partners 1 month after a heart attack. *Journal of Advanced Nursing* 22: 707–714.

Turton J (1998) Importance of information following myocardial infarction: a study of the self-perceived needs of patients and their spouse/partner compared with the perception of nursing staff. *Journal of Advanced Nursing* 27: 770–778.

Walsh D, Shaw DG (2000) The design of written information for cardiac patients: a review of the literature. *Journal of Clinical Nursing* 9: 658–667.

Webster RA, Thompson DR (1986) Sleep in hospital. *Journal of Advanced Nursing* 11: 447–459.

Webster RA, Thompson DR (1992) *Caring for the Coronary Patient.* Oxford: Butterworth Heinemann.

White JM (1999) Effects of relaxing music on cardiac autonomic balance and anxiety after acute myocardial infarction. *American Journal of Critical Care* 8: 220–230.

Williamson A, Hoggart B (2005) Pain: a review of three commonly used pain rating scales. *Journal of Clinical Nursing* 14: 798–804.

Winslow EH, Lane LD, Gaffney FA (1985) Oxygen uptake and cardiovascular responses in control adults and acute myocardial infarction patients during bathing. *Nursing Research* 34: 164–169.

Zigmond AS, Snaith RP (1983) The Hospital Anxiety Depression Scale. *Acta Psychiatrica Scandinavica* 67: 361–370.

Chapter 10

Complications of acute myocardial infarction and their management

There are numerous complications that may arise as a consequence of acute myocardial infarction. The risk of complications is mostly dependent upon:

- the size of the myocardial infarction;
- the cumulative loss of functional myocardium following previous ischaemic damage;
- the extent and severity of coronary arterial disease.

Abnormal electrical activity within ischaemic or necrotic cardiac tissue can precipitate disturbances in cardiac rate, rhythm and conduction (the 'dysrhythmias'), while the loss of left ventricular myocardium associates with pump malfunction ('heart failure').

Dysrhythmias are the most common complication of myocardial infarction. A classification is shown in Box 10.1. These will need to be treated if there is deterioration in circulatory function with hypotension, heart failure or syncope, or if the rate is increasing myocardial work such that ischaemia is worsened. Many dysrhythmias can be prevented or abolished by relief of pain and anxiety, correction of hypoxaemia and treatment of heart failure.

Heart failure complicates about one-quarter to one-half of cases of acute myocardial infarction, and is caused by loss of contractility of damaged myocardium. The fall in arterial blood pressure reduces perfusion of the vital organs, and this, with arterial hypoxaemia and acidosis, leads to a further reduction in myocardial performance. *Cardiogenic shock* may follow. While the development of heart failure is primarily determined by the extent of myocardial necrosis, poor perfusion of the adjacent surviving myocardium may compromise its contractility (myocardial hibernation) or even extend the area of necrosis in the border zone.

DISTURBANCE OF CARDIAC RHYTHM

Dysrhythmias are particularly common in the first 24 hours after myocardial infarction. Detection and

Box 10.1 A classification of cardiac dysrhythmias.

Abnormal impulse formation and ectopic beats

At the sinus node

Sinus arrhythmia
Sinus bradycardia
Sinus tachycardia
Sinus arrest

In the atria

Atrial ectopic beats
Atrial tachycardia
Atrial flutter
Atrial fibrillation
Wandering atrial pacemaker

In the AV node

Nodal ectopic beats
Junctional rhythm
Junctional tachycardia

In the ventricles

Ventricular ectopic beats
Idio-ventricular rhythm
Ventricular tachycardia
Ventricular fibrillation

Conduction disturbances

In the sinus node

SA block

In the AV node

First-, second- and third-degree AV block

In the bundle of His

Left bundle branch block
Right bundle branch block
Left anterior and posterior hemi-blocks

Others

Intra-atrial block
Ventricular pre-excitation
AV dissociation

AV, atrio-ventricular; SA, sino-atrial.

prompt treatment of these was the primary reason for the creation of coronary care units (CCUs). Most patients will have frequent ectopic beats, 15–20% will have transient atrial fibrillation, and up to a fifth will have potentially life-threatening dysrhythmias. Bradycardia affects about a third of patients, particularly those with inferior myocardial infarction, and about 5–10% will have an episode of heart block. Uncontrolled dysrhythmias are an important cause of heart failure.

Cardiac arrest complicates about 3% of cases that reach hospital, and may be recurrent. Circulatory standstill is usually associated with ventricular fibrillation, ventricular tachycardia, asystole or pulseless electrical activity (PEA), although many other dysrhythmias can have serious haemodynamic consequences during the acute phase of myocardial infarction.

Both the size and the location of the infarction play a part in early phase dysrhythmias. Important contributory factors include electrolyte imbalance, hypoxia, acidosis and free radicals released following reperfusion of ischaemic myocardium. Sympathetic overactivity may be evident through tachycardia and transient hypertension in nearly half of all patients, particularly those with anterior infarction, and this lowers the threshold for ventricular fibrillation.

Clinical consequences of cardiac dysrhythmias are extremely variable, but are always more pronounced in patients with chronic heart disease. While the healthy heart can withstand many abnormal rhythms, the diseased heart cannot, and sustained dysrhythmias may lead to ischaemic pain, heart failure or circulatory collapse. Tachycardias are particularly serious, as increases in heart rate lead to a reduction in diastolic timing. Coronary arterial blood flow takes place during diastole, and a shortened perfusion time reduces oxygen supply to the myocardium at a time when demand is high. Any circulatory embarrassment is serious following acute myocardial infarction, as it may compromise perfusion in areas of marginally ischaemic myocardium. If these then become infarcted, the cycle may be repeated.

Management of acute rhythm disturbances

The treatment of acute rhythm disturbances usually aims to restore normal sinus rhythm and prevent recurrence. Establishment of sinus rhythm is sometimes not possible (e.g. in atrial fibrillation), and treatment is then designed to slow the ventricular rate and improve cardiac output. Treatment is either electrical or pharmacological. If drugs are used, they are usually given intravenously, as absorption by other routes may be slowed because of a low cardiac output, which impairs tissue perfusion in the muscle and gut. Wherever possible, attention should be directed towards the precipitating cause. Pain, fear, hypoxia, acidosis and electrolyte imbalance should be considered. Restoring and maintaining normal cardiac rhythm will be difficult if these factors remain uncorrected.

Sinus tachycardia

Sinus tachycardia is arbitrarily defined as a sinus rhythm > 100 beats/minute and commonly ranges between 100 and 150 beats/minute. The P waves are normal and have a 1:1 relationship with the QRS complexes. The PR and QT intervals decrease as the heart rate increases, so that the P wave tends to merge with the preceding T wave. It may then be difficult to ascertain whether the rhythm is arising from the sinus node or elsewhere, but there may be clues. During sinus tachycardia, the heart rate is usually < 130 beats/minute at rest and varies with respiration (sinus arrhythmia). The tachycardia does not start or finish abruptly. In the absence of an obvious precipitating cause, a persistent sinus tachycardia should suggest an alternative rhythm disturbance. For example, 'sinus' rates of 150 beats/minute are, on closer inspection, usually due to atrial flutter with 2:1 block.

A sinus tachycardia is found in one-third of patients with acute myocardial infarction and represents an attempt to maintain cardiac output in the face of reduced stroke volume. The tachycardia may be worsened by fear, anxiety or pain. The mortality of patients with sinus tachycardia is higher than that of those with sinus bradycardia, and death is usually due to left ventricular failure. Incipient heart failure is suggested by a sinus tachycardia in the presence of tachypnoea, a wide pulse pressure and a loud first heart sound.

Adequate analgesia will often settle a sinus tachycardia following myocardial infarction, and also helps with associated anxiety. The use of beta-blockade has been shown to improve prognosis in patients with acute myocardial infarction by limiting heart rate, myocardial work and infarct size (Freemantle et al, 2001), but should only be given when the patient is haemodynamically stable. The ultra short-acting beta-blocker esmolol is safe and effective if there is any doubt about cardiac decompensation.

Atrial ectopic beats (Fig. 10.1)

Atrial extrasystoles occur when an atrial focus discharges before the sinus pacemaker, and are seen on the electrocardiogram (ECG) as premature, often abnormally shaped P waves, usually followed by normal QRS complexes. The further the ectopic focus is from the sinus node, the greater the abnormality in the shape of the P wave and the shorter the PR interval. An incomplete compensatory pause follows the ectopic beat, because the premature impulse depolarises the SA node, which must recover before it is able to initiate another sinus beat. The PP interval between three consecutive P waves (i.e. two complete PQRST complexes) is therefore only slightly longer than the interval between two normal PQRST complexes. Complete compensatory pauses are a characteristic feature of ventricular ectopic beat, which fails to conduct back to the atria, hence leaving the

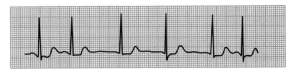

Figure 10.1 ECG: atrial ectopic beats. Note that the ectopic P waves are slightly different from those of SA origin.

sinus node undisturbed. The sum of the coupling interval and the compensatory pause is equal to twice the sinus cycle length, unlike an incomplete compensatory pause that arises if the sinus node is discharged early by the ectopic depolarisation.

Conduction of atrial impulses to the ventricles depends upon the recovery status of the atrio-ventricular (AV) node. If the atrial ectopic beat arises near the AV node (seen as an abnormal P wave and short PR interval), the AV node may be refractory. The impulse is therefore blocked, and no QRS follows. If the AV node is partially refractory, a prolonged PR interval is seen, because conduction of the ectopic beat is delayed. Other parts of the conducting system below the AV node may also be refractory, even when the AV node is able to convey the supraventricular impulse, and an aberrantly conducted impulse is then seen on the ECG.

Aberrant conduction is the term applied when a widened and abnormal QRS complex follows a supraventricular impulse. It is caused by the unequal recovery periods of the right and left bundle branches. If a supraventricular stimulus presents to the bundles before both have recovered, functional bundle branch block will occur. This is usually of the right bundle branch block pattern, as the right bundle has a longer refractory period than the left bundle. In the V1 chest lead, the primary R wave is smaller than the secondary R wave (i.e. the right 'rabbit's ear' is longer). In contrast, ventricular ectopics usually show monophasic or biphasic QRS patterns in V1, and the left 'rabbit's ear' is larger. P waves are not seen, and the ectopic beat is followed by a full, rather than an incomplete, compensatory pause.

Atrial ectopics are very common following acute myocardial infarction, often indicating sympathetic overactivity, hypoxia or anxiety. They are usually asymptomatic and cause no haemodynamic upset. With relief of pain, sedation and beta-blockade, they usually disappear but, where they reflect progressive atrial dilatation, treatment of heart failure is necessary.

Narrow-complex tachycardias

The main narrow-complex tachycardias are junctional tachycardias, atrial flutter and atrial fibrillation. Other atrial causes of fast or irregular pulses include sinus tachycardia and multiple ectopic beats. With the exception of atrial fibrillation, narrow-complex tachycardias are regular, and the P wave may or may not be visible. If seen, it is usually different from the sinus rhythm P wave. AV block may occur during the tachycardia. Sometimes it is not possible to determine the exact atrial rhythm during tachycardias unless specialised ECG leads are used.

The term narrow-complex tachycardia is useful to describe the ECG appearance, but it should be remembered that junctional tachycardias and atrial fibrillation might sometimes appear as a broad-complex tachycardia.

Junctional tachycardias   A junctional tachycardia is characterised by the sudden onset of a tachycardia > 150 beats/minute (Fig. 10.2). In some patients, there may be no symptoms but, in the context of acute myocardial infarction, there is often ischaemic pain, dyspnoea, sweating or presyncope.

Most junctional tachycardias are due to an AV nodal re-entry circuit. The term supraventricular tachycardia (SVT) is often used, but is anatomically incorrect as most narrow-complex tachycardias incorporate parts of the ventricular myocardium within the re-entry circuit (see Chapter 12). The ECG shows rapid normal QRS complexes at a rate of 150–220 beats/minute, with the P wave buried in the QRS complex. The onset is usually associated with a premature atrial beat, which, if recorded, is seen to conduct to the ventricles with a prolonged PR interval.

Atrial tachycardias are much less common and are caused by the rapid discharge of an atrial pacemaker arising from one or more foci in the atria (usually the interatrial septum) at a rate of 150–250/minute (Fig. 10.3). It is thus a true supraventricular tachycardia. An intra-atrial re-entry circuit is usually present, although a few cases of atrial tachycardia may be caused by enhanced automaticity of an

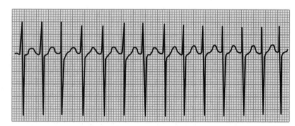

Figure 10.2   ECG: junctional tachycardia.

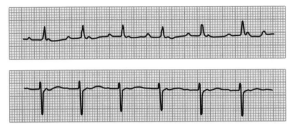

Figure 10.3 ECG: atrial tachycardia with 2:1 block (leads aVF and V1). Atrial rate is 175/min.

atrial focus that speeds up. Second- or third-degree atrio-ventricular block is often present, so the ventricular response is usually not rapid and causes little systemic upset. While 'paroxysmal atrial tachycardia (PAT) with block' is described classically in relation to digitalis toxicity, this is the underlying cause in only about 10% of patients.

The urgency of treatment depends upon symptoms and haemodynamic stability. Ischaemic pain may be produced and, in the peri-infarction period, ventricular work must be limited to prevent infarct extension. Electrical cardioversion is then the treatment of choice, regardless of prior digitalisation.

Carotid sinus massage may terminate re-entry tachycardias or increase AV block to allow differentiation from atrial flutter (Fig. 10.4). Other methods of vagal stimulation are the Valsalva manoeuvre, splashing cold water on the face and stimulation of the soft palate, which causes the gag reflex.

Drug treatment is usually very effective, and long-term treatment should be considered for repeated and poorly tolerated attacks. The drug of choice for terminating acute narrow-complex tachycardias is adenosine, particularly if there is left ventricular dysfunction or hypotension. Adenosine is sometimes used in broad-complex tachycardias too, if they are thought to be due to an aberrantly conducted supraventricular tachycardia. Intravenous adenosine may induce atrial fibrillation or even asystole, but this is usually short lived. Flushing or transient chest pain may occur.

A bolus injection of verapamil (5–10 mg) may be preferable in patients with asthma, as adenosine can cause bronchospasm.

Beta-blockers are often successful, but should be avoided if there is uncontrolled cardiac failure or in patients who have been pretreated with verapamil. Refractory tachycardias usually respond to amiodarone. Overdrive cardiac pacing may be effective in selected cases.

Idio–nodal tachycardia (Fig. 10.5) The normal discharge rate from the AV node is about 50–60 beats/minute. If there is suppression of sinus or atrial pacemaker function, the AV node may take over as the pacemaker. Because of enhanced automaticity, the rate may increase gradually to 70–100 beats/minute. The sinus node often continues to discharge at a slower rate, and there is a propensity to atrio-ventricular dissociation. Idio-nodal rhythm arises as a consequence of sinus node depression following myocardial infarction, or secondary to drugs that may need to be stopped.

Atrial flutter (Fig. 10.6) During atrial flutter, there is a macro re-entry circuit in the right atrium that spreads to the left atrium and causes atrial contraction at a rate of 220–350 beats/minute. The ECG shows flutter (F) waves, which have a sawtooth appearance in the inferior leads. Leads V1 and V2 often appear to show large, discrete biphasic P waves. The QRST complex may obscure flutter waves if the rate is very fast and, because atrial activity is concealed, sinus tachycardia of 150 beats/minute may be diagnosed. In such cases, flutter waves may be revealed by carotid sinus massage, which will transiently increase AV blockade and slow the ventricular response. If this is not effective, alternate F waves should be sought, which are often found hidden in the preceding T wave. This may be confirmed by measuring the interval between the P wave and the following T wave peak. It should be precisely

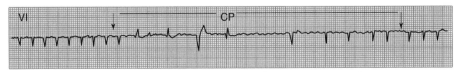

Figure 10.4 ECG: SVT slowed by pressure on the carotid sinus (cp, carotid pressure). This has increased block at the AV node, showing that the underlying rhythm is atrial flutter.

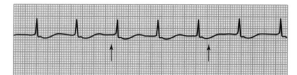

Figure 10.5   ECG: idio-nodal tachycardia. There are P waves seen after the QRS complexes due to retrograde activation of the atria. An occasional sinus beat can be seen (arrows).

the same as the interval between the T wave peak and the following P wave.

Although the AV node can respond to atrial rates of about 300 beats/minute, there is some degree of AV blockade. In the healthy AV node unaffected by drugs, this results in a ventricular rate of about 150 beats/minute (i.e. there is 2:1 block). Higher degrees of AV blockade usually occur in the presence of drugs or when there is damage to the conducting system, although 3:1 conduction is unusual. While the pulse is usually regular, AV conduction ratios may vary, giving rise to varying RR intervals on the ECG and an irregular pulse. Exercise decreases AV blockade and may lead to a doubling of the pulse rate. As a result, the apparently normal patient with a pulse rate of 75 beats/minute may feel faint on exercise when switching from 4:1 block to 2:1 conduction. During 2:1 conduction, ventricular conduction may become aberrant, and the widened QRS complexes may give the appearance of ventricular tachycardia.

Atrial flutter is unstable and should always be converted to sinus rhythm. Carotid sinus massage will not restore sinus rhythm but may reveal the true nature of the atrial dysrhythmia by increasing AV block, allowing flutter waves to be seen more easily. Verapamil can also be used to increase AV block temporarily, and it produces sinus rhythm in 20% of cases. Otherwise, the treatment of atrial flutter is the same as for atrial fibrillation. Low-energy, direct current (DC) cardioversion is especially useful. Rapid atrial pacing is also effective.

Atrial fibrillation (Fig. 10.7)   Atrial fibrillation (AF) associated with acute myocardial infarction is a common occurrence, usually within the first 24 hours. The incidence of AF complicating acute myocardial infarction approaches 20%, but the higher estimates in some reports probably include those with pre-existing AF. It is typically transient, lasting minutes to hours, but may recur. The dysrhythmia occurs for many different reasons, including left ventricular dysfunction, atrial infarction or hypoxia. Patients are more likely to have three-vessel coronary disease. It thus occurs more often in patients with larger infarcts, those whose infarcts are anterior in location and in patients whose hospital course is complicated by heart failure, complex ventricular dysrhythmias, advanced AV block, atrial infarction or pericarditis. Atrial fibrillation may also occur in patients with inferior myocardial infarction due to involvement of the sino-atrial nodal artery, which usually provides the major blood supply to the atria. The incidence of AF after acute myocardial infarction has decreased since routine thrombolysis became available, but is still an indicator of cardiac failure and a poor prognosis (Pizzetti et al, 2001). This negative influence persists for at least 4 years.

During atrial fibrillation, a disorganised and continuous series of irregular fibrillation waves (350–600/minute), caused by multiple and changing micro re-entry circuits, replaces normal atrial contraction. Myocardial contraction is ineffective for atrial emptying, which functionally remains in diastole. Because the ventricles are incompletely filled by loss of atrial systole prior to ventricular contraction, the presence of AF reduces cardiac output by about 10–20%. Although AF makes the heart less efficient, the most important consequence is that of thromboembolism, especially stroke. The incidence of peripheral embolisation is particularly high in patients with paroxysmal AF, atrial infarction or previous rheumatic heart valve disease.

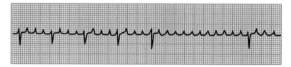

Figure 10.6   ECG: atrial flutter, with varying degrees of AV block.

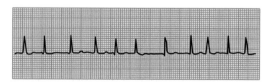

Figure 10.7   ECG: atrial fibrillation.

Stroke is three times more frequent than in those who remain in sinus rhythm following acute myocardial infarction.

The ECG in atrial fibrillation shows the replacement of P waves by small irregular undulations of the baseline (f waves), which represent the only evidence of atrial activity. These are not usually visible in all leads and, at fast heart rates, the ventricular response becomes more regular, and f waves are not visible. Differentiation from a nodal tachycardia may then be difficult and, often, it is only a slight irregularity in the ventricular rate that allows the correct diagnosis to be made. Sometimes, the f waves are very coarse and may be mistaken for normal P waves or flutter waves ('flutter fibrillation'). If the atrial f waves have a rate of more than 350/minute, AF is more likely, particularly if the ventricular response is totally irregular. The ventricular response in the untreated patient is usually at a rate of about 100–180 beats/ minutes, and the QRS is normal, except when the rate is so fast that aberrant conduction occurs. If the ventricular rate is not too fast, no treatment is needed and, in other cases, it may be enough to control the ventricular rate with a small dose of beta-blocker, as episodes are frequently short lived. Digoxin should be avoided in the context of acute ischaemia. It is poor at controlling the ventricular rate following myocardial infarction, does not encourage a return to sinus rhythm and may worsen ischaemia on account of its positive inotropic action. This in turn may lead to ventricular dysrhythmias. Intravenous amiodarone rapidly slows the ventricular rate, and will convert 75% of patients back to sinus rhythm within 4 hours. In patients with AF of more than 1–2 days' duration, the risks of thromboembolisation following cardioversion (either electrically or pharmacologically) are 3–5% unless the patient has been anticoagulated.

If AF is producing haemodynamic deterioration, intravenous amiodarone or DC cardioversion should be considered. The energy required to cardiovert AF is very variable, but in the range of 100–200 J (biphasic).

VENTRICULAR DYSRHYTHMIAS

Ventricular dysrhythmias include ventricular ectopics (VEs), ventricular tachycardia (VT), ventricular flutter and ventricular fibrillation (VF). The detection and prompt treatment of serious ventricular dysrhythmias were the primary reasons for the creation of CCUs.

Common factors predisposing to ventricular dysrhythmias

Myocardial ischaemia

Myocardial ischaemia may result from occlusive or non-occlusive changes in the coronary vasculature that impair the blood supply to the myocardium. Ischaemia predisposes to cardiac dysrhythmias, regardless of whether or not myocardial necrosis takes place. Normal electrical conduction pathways may alter with ischaemia, providing a focus for dysrhythmias. Myocardial irritability following acute myocardial infarction is, of course, the major cause of ventricular dysrhythmia. Necrotic myocardial tissue provides a focus for this ectopic activity, and myocardial hypoxia associated with exaggerated catecholamine release compounds the situation.

Electrolyte and acid/base imbalance

Hypokalaemia (serum potassium less than 3.5 mmol/L) is probably the most common electrolyte disturbance seen on the CCU. It increases the risk of dysrhythmias, particularly in patients with pre-existing heart disease and in those treated with digoxin. It often associates with prior diuretic therapy, although acute myocardial infarction itself may produce a transient fall in the serum potassium. Hypokalaemia is a marker for the severity of the infarct, reflecting a catecholamine-induced shift of potassium into cells.

ECG features of hypokalaemia include ST segment changes, with T wave flattening and prominent U waves. Severe hypokalaemia (< 2.5 mmol/L) associates with complex ventricular ectopic beats, ventricular tachycardia and ventricular fibrillation. The risk of ventricular fibrillation is approximately 10-fold in patients with a serum potassium of < 3 mmol/L following acute myocardial infarction, compared with those whose potassium level is > 4 mmol/L (Campbell et al, 1987).

Potassium replacement depends upon the initial serum level and the urgency of the situation.

Gradual replacement of potassium is preferable but, in more urgent situations, intravenous potassium is required. Bananas are a rich source of oral potassium (500 mg/banana), and more palatable than potassium chloride. The maximum recommended intravenous infusion rate of potassium is 20 mmol/hour, but more rapid infusion (20 mmol over 10 minutes, followed by 10 mmol over the next 10 minutes) may be used when cardiac arrest is considered imminent. Continuous ECG monitoring is essential. Many patients who are potassium deficient are also deficient in magnesium. Correcting the magnesium stores will help in a more rapid correction of hypokalaemia.

Hyperkalaemia (> 5.5 mmol/L) predisposes to cardiac arrest, and may be found in those on angiotensin-converting enzyme (ACE) inhibitors, in renal failure or because of acidaemia following cardiac arrest. The effect of hyperkalaemia on the ECG depends on the serum potassium as well as the rate of increase. When there is severe hyperkalaemia (> 6.5 mmol/L), most patients will show some ECG abnormality, such as first-degree heart block, flattened or absent P waves or tall, peaked (tented) T waves. The QRS widens, indicating an intraventricular conduction block. If untreated, the QRS duration continues to increase, and ventricular fibrillation ensues.

Treatment of hyperkalaemia depends on the serum potassium concentration (Mahoney et al, 2005). If there are toxic ECG changes, the first step is to protect the heart from arrest. Intravenous calcium gluconate (10 mL of a 10% solution given over 3 minutes) will antagonise the toxic effects of hyperkalaemia on the myocardial cell membrane. Strategies to shift potassium into cells and remove potassium from the body are then needed. A dextrose–insulin infusion containing 10 units of a short-acting insulin and 50 g of glucose is usual over 15–30 minutes, and will work within 15 minutes. Nebulised salbutamol (5 mg) repeated may also be used, but may provoke a tachycardia. Sodium bicarbonate, 50 mmol intravenously over 5 minutes is less effective than dextrose–insulin or nebulised salbutamol, but should be used with these measures if a metabolic acidosis is present. It is obviously important to monitor for rebound hyperkalaemia and take any necessary steps to prevent recurrence.

The effect of drugs

Many drugs, both cardiovascular and non-cardiovascular, may predispose the patient to cardiac dysrhythmias. Furthermore, many drugs prescribed as antidysrhythmic agents may sometimes produce serious dysrhythmias (proarrhythmic effect). Drugs that affect the QT interval, such as disopyramide and flecainide, may precipitate torsades-de-pointes. It is likely that severe left ventricular dysfunction predisposes to this dysrhythmia, which is often self-terminating, but may progress to ventricular fibrillation. Treatment with 2 g of 50% magnesium sulphate (4 mL = 8 mmol) intravenously over 1–2 minutes is helpful if hypomagnesaemia is present or likely.

Ventricular ectopics (Fig. 10.8)

Ventricular extrasystoles are universal in the first 24 hours. They occur when an ectopic ventricular focus discharges prematurely anywhere within the His–Purkinje system or the ventricles at any time in diastole. The QRS complex is premature, widened to over 0.12 seconds. slurred and usually notched. There is no preceding P wave, and the following T wave usually points in the opposite direction.

Although infrequent ventricular ectopics do not adversely affect cardiac output, attention has previously been focused on them as 'warning dysrhythmias' (Lown et al, 1967). Ventricular ectopic beats that are frequent, multifocal, occurring in salvoes or showing the R-on-T phenomenon (ventricular ectopics occurring on the apex of the preceding T wave) are termed 'complex', and have been considered to be precursors of cardiac arrest. However, these warning dysrhythmias occur in only about half of patients who develop ventricular fibrillation, but are an indicator of risk of subsequent mortality (total mortality and sudden death).

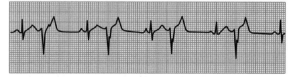

Figure 10.8 ECG: ventricular ectopic beats (ventricular bigeminy).

While no antidysrhythmic drug has yet been shown to decrease mortality when used to suppress ventricular ectopics (apart from beta-blockers), drug therapy should be considered for ventricular ectopics producing haemodynamic disturbances, repetitive short episodes of ventricular tachycardia and, perhaps, R-on-T ectopics. If beta-blockers cannot be used, lidocaine is probably the most frequently, and most controversially, used agent. Prophylaxis with lidocaine reduces the incidence of VF, but may increase mortality. Amiodarone is probably a better choice.

Parasystole (Fig. 10.9)

Parasystole is an uncommon dysrhythmia, but is often seen following myocardial infarction, particularly in patients taking digoxin. It is a dual rhythm, in which two pacemakers concurrently and independently govern the rhythm of the heart. An ectopic ventricular focus discharges regularly and competes with another focus, which may be in either the atria or the ventricles. The competition is usually with normal sinus rhythm, the ventricular rhythm mostly being at a slightly faster rate. The interval between successive ventricular ectopic beats is the same or a multiple of that interval and, as this parasystolic focus is independent of the regular heart rhythm, there is no fixed relationship between the two rhythms, and the coupling interval (i.e. the interval between the ectopic beat and the sinus beat) varies.

It might be expected that the dominant pacemaker would take over cardiac rhythm and suppress the ectopic focus. However, during parasystole, the ectopic focus is protected by 'entrance block', a unidirectional block in the vicinity of the ectopic focus. Outward conduction from the ectopic focus is normal and forms the secondary pacemaker. Two pacemakers therefore exist, each discharging at its own independent rate and depolarising the myocardium if it is in a responsive state. If the two pacemakers discharge simultaneously, each activates the adjacent myocardium, and a 'fusion beat' will arise as the two discharge waterfronts collide. A QRS complex intermediate in appearance between a normal sinus beat and a ventricular ectopic results. No treatment is required, and parasystole normally resolves spontaneously.

Ventricular tachycardia (VT)

Following myocardial infarction, the heart is particularly vulnerable to ventricular dysrhythmias. Risk factors include older age, hypertension, diabetes and cases in which reperfusion has not been attempted. Ventricular dysrhythmias are the commonest cause of death at the time of infarction and the main reason why patients die before reaching medical help. The majority of post-infarction VT occurs within the first 48 hours following the infarct, and seldom recurs. Short bursts of up to five beats of non-sustained VT are particularly common within the first 24 hours, but do not require specific therapy. It does not reflect infarct size or prognosis, and long-term prophylaxis is not indicated. In contrast, late sustained or monomorphic VT at rates < 170 beats/minute deserves careful evaluation, including consideration of electrophysiological studies. Recurrence is likely in the post-infarction period, days, weeks or even months later. Late VT is usually related to re-entry associated with scar tissue at the interface between infarcted and normal myocardium, and associates with larger infarcts. The risk of late VT is difficult to predict, but the likelihood increases with worsening left ventricular function. For patients with significantly reduced left ventricular function (ejection fraction < 35%) and episodes of sustained VT,

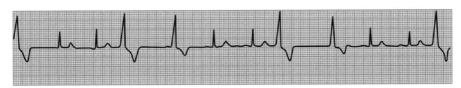

Figure 10.9   ECG: parasystole.

insertion of an implantable defibrillator (AICD) improves survival over and above any protection offered by antidysrhythmic drugs.

Ventricular tachycardia is a re-entry dysrhythmia, and is usually defined as a succession of three or more beats arising from one or more foci in the ventricles at a rate of over 120 beats/minute. The tachycardia may be non-sustained VT (lasting < 30 seconds) or sustained VT (lasting > 30 seconds and/or causes earlier haemodynamic compromise requiring immediate intervention). The term 'accelerated idio- ventricular tachycardia' refers to ventricular rhythms with rates of 100–120 beats/minute. Ventricular tachycardia is described as 'monomorphic' when the QRS complexes have the same general appearance, and 'polymorphic' if there is wide beat-to-beat variation in QRS morphology. Monomorphic ventricular tachycardia is the commonest form of sustained ventricular tachycardia.

During ventricular tachycardia, the ECG will show widened QRS complexes (> 0.16 seconds), which are regular at a rate of 100–250 beats/minute. The atria continue to beat independently from the ventricles, and dissociated P waves may be seen (AV dissociation). The atrial rate is usually slower than the ventricular rate, as it originates at the sinus node. However, there may be co-existent atrial tachycardia, junctional rhythm or atrial fibrillation. Occasionally, ventricular beats may pass back through the AV node to stimulate the atria, and inverted P waves then appear after the QRS complex or concealed in the terminal part of the QRS complex.

Fusion and capture beats may be present, which helps in distinguishing ventricular tachycardia from other broad-complex tachycardias.

- *Fusion beats* occur when a normal supraventricular stimulus meets a ventricular stimulus being conducted back from the ventricles. The resulting

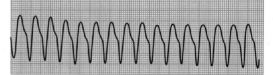

Figure 10.10 ECG: monomorphic ventricular tachycardia.

QRS complex looks partly like a normal QRS complex and partly like a ventricular ectopic beat.
- *Capture beats* occur when an atrial stimulus arrives at a non-refractory AV node and is conducted normally to the ventricles. This results in a normal P wave followed by a normal (narrow) QRS complex in the middle of a run of wide complexes.

There are four types of ventricular tachycardia:

- monomorphic ventricular tachycardia;
- polymorphic ventricular tachycardia;
- accelerated idio-ventricular tachycardia;
- ventricular flutter.

Monomorphic ventricular tachycardia (Fig. 10.10)

This is the most common form of ventricular tachycardia. The ventricular complexes are of uniform appearance (monomorphic), and each episode of ventricular tachycardia continues for a variable time, usually terminating in a long pause before sinus rhythm returns. Each paroxysm of tachycardia starts with a ventricular ectopic beat, which occurs at the same fixed interval from the previous QRS complex.

Polymorphic ventricular tachycardias (Fig. 10.11)

Whereas monomorphic VT consists of QRS complexes of the same configuration, the QRS complexes in a polymorphic VT undulate around the

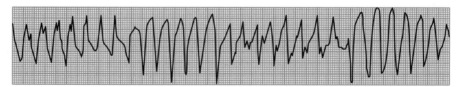

Figure 10.11 ECG: torsades-de-pointes.

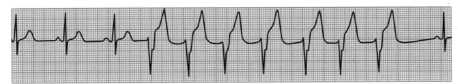

Figure 10.12   ECG: accelerated idio-ventricular tachycardia.

isoelectric line, with a marked change of amplitude occurring every 5–30 beats, changing from one direction to another and back again.

Torsades-de-pointes ('turning of the points') is a dangerous form of polymorphic ventricular tachycardia characterised by paroxysms of ventricular tachycardia when the QT interval is prolonged during sinus rhythm and prominent U waves may be seen. Prolongation of the QT interval implies prolongation of repolarisation. While this may affect the whole myocardium, polymorphic VT is more likely to occur when different regions of the myocardium repolarise at different rates. Transient prolongation of the QT interval may occur in the acute phase of myocardial infarction but, more commonly, this is due to the administration of drugs that prolong the QT interval, such as class 1 antidysrhythmic agents, or electrolyte imbalance.

Episodes of torsades-de-pointes usually terminate spontaneously but may precede ventricular fibrillation. Antidysrhythmic drugs should be stopped, and it may be necessary to increase the heart rate to over 100 beats/minute by pacing to prevent recurrence until the precipitating drugs are metabolised or electrolyte imbalance has been corrected.

Polymorphic ventricular tachycardias unassociated with QT prolongation are uncommon, but have the electrocardiographic characteristics of torsades-de-pointes. If the QT interval in sinus is normal, management is that of monomorphic ventricular tachycardia.

Accelerated idio-ventricular tachycardia
(Fig. 10.12)

When escape rhythms arise in the ventricles or His–Purkinje system, they are called idio-ventricular rhythms. Idio-ventricular rhythm often occurs in association with successful thrombolysis, is benign and requires no treatment. The rate is usually slow, at about 60 beats/minute, sometimes referred to as 'slow VT'. After about 30 beats, sinus rhythm usually takes over. Occasionally, the rhythm accelerates, although the rate does not usually exceed 120 beats/minute. Rarely, sustained ventricular tachycardia or ventricular fibrillation may replace accelerated idio-ventricular tachycardia.

Ventricular flutter (Fig. 10.13)

This is characterised by a rapid ventricular rate of 180–250 beats/minute, in which it is not possible to differentiate the QRS complexes from the ST segments or T waves. The pattern of oscillating waves of large amplitude has been likened to rows of hairpins. It often precedes ventricular fibrillation and, for practical purposes, does not differ from ventricular fibrillation.

The diagnosis of broad–complex tachycardias

Differentiating ventricular tachycardia from other broad-complex tachycardias is important, both in the management of the acute dysrhythmia and for long-term therapy to prevent recurrence. It is often difficult.

Regular broad-complex tachycardias may be due to:

- ventricular tachycardia;
- supraventricular tachycardia (SVT) with pre-existent bundle branch block;
- SVT with rate-related bundle branch block.

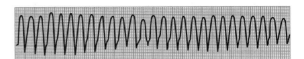

Figure 10.13   ECG: ventricular flutter.

Irregular broad-complex tachycardias may be due to:

- atrial fibrillation with pre-existing bundle branch block;
- atrial fibrillation with rate-related bundle branch block;
- torsades-de-pointes.

Ventricular tachycardia is often misdiagnosed as having a supraventricular origin, which is of major concern as treatment and prognosis are markedly different. Generally speaking, if the patient is known to have a normal heart, the tachycardia is likely to be supraventricular in origin. However, a history of coronary heart disease or congestive cardiac failure is 90% predictive of ventricular tachycardia. A broad-complex tachycardia in patients aged over 35 years is more likely to be ventricular in origin.

Differentiation by ECG relies heavily on the demonstration of independent atrial and ventricular activity (AV dissociation), although VA conduction (from ventricles to atria) may sometimes occur in VT. A full 12-lead ECG should always be recorded, providing the patient is well enough during the tachycardia. If the QRS in sinus rhythm is of normal duration, QRS duration > 160 ms usually indicates a ventricular origin of the tachycardia. VT arising close to the interventricular conducting tissue may have a QRS duration under 140 ms.

Determining the frontal plane QRS axis may be helpful. With the onset of ventricular tachycardia, the mean frontal plane axis changes by more than 40° to the left or right from the usual −30° and +90° sector, and is often extreme. A positive QRS complex in aVR indicates a grossly abnormal axis to either the left or the right ('up in R, axis bizarre'), and will occur if the tachycardia originates close to the apex of the ventricle, with the wave of depolarisation moving upwards towards the base of the heart. Predominantly negative QRS complexes in leads I, II and III suggest VT.

Ventricular concordance (uniformly positive or negative QRS complexes) in the chest leads usually indicates ventricular tachycardia. Positive concordance indicates that the origin of the tachycardia lies on the posterior ventricular wall. The wave of depolarisation moves towards all the chest leads and thus produces positive complexes. A similar pattern may be seen in the Wolff–Parkinson–White syndrome with an antidromic atrio-ventricular tachycardia using a left-sided accessory pathway.

Negative concordance correlates with a tachycardia originating in the anterior ventricular wall and, hence, depolarisation moves away from all chest leads. The absence of an RS complex in any of the chest leads strongly suggests VT.

The RR interval is regular unless there are capture beats and, in contrast to supraventricular tachycardias that are affected by respiration, does not vary by more than 0.04 seconds.

It is important to realise that the clinical condition of the patient is not helpful. Some patients tolerate ventricular tachycardia extremely well, whereas others may be severely haemodynamically compromised by a rapid supraventricular tachycardia. If in doubt, broad-complex tachycardias should be treated as ventricular tachycardia. Summary guidelines for diagnosis are shown in Box 10.2.

Treatment of ventricular tachycardia

Treatment of ventricular tachycardia depends on the haemodynamic status of the patient. Short salvoes of non-sustained VT do not usually require treatment, but most sustained ventricular dysrhythmias are accompanied by moderate to severe haemodynamic decompensation and require immediate termination. The treatment of choice in such circumstances is cardioversion. An initial shock of no less than 120 J (biphasic) should be used as lesser charges may induce ventricular fibrillation. Where a defibrillator is not immediately available, a precordial blow is sometimes effective, as is lying flat with the legs raised. Coughing (cough cardiopulmonary resuscitation) may maintain a cardiac output until cardioversion.

Stable ventricular tachycardia in the presence of good cardiac output and blood pressure can be treated either electrically or with amiodarone 300 mg intravenously over 20–60 minutes followed by an infusion of 900 mg over 24 hours. An approach to the management of regular, acute, broad-complex tachycardias is shown in Figure 10.14.

Box 10.2   Features of ventricular tachycardia.

Clinically

The venous pulse rate is slower than the arterial pulse rate

There are irregular cannon waves seen in the venous pulse

There is varying intensity of the first heart sound

There is a varying systolic blood pressure

In the 12-lead ECG

There is usually left axis deviation (QRS axis less than $-30°$)

The QRS duration is usually > 0.16 s (160 ms)

There are multiple QRS morphologies

There is concordance of the QRS vector in the chest leads (i.e. they are all in the same direction)

Dissociated P waves may be seen (AV dissociation)

Blocked, fusion and capture beats may be present

QRS morphologies in V1 and V6

In an RBBB pattern, a broad monophasic R wave or a qR in V1 and an S wave greater than the R wave in V6 suggest VT.

In the LBBB pattern, a broad R wave (usually > 30 ms) and/or a slow descent to the S wave in V1 and a Q in V6 suggest VT.

ECG, electrocardiogram; AV, atrio-ventricular; RBBB, right bundle branch block; LBBB, left bundle branch block; VT, ventricular tachycardia.

Ventricular fibrillation (Fig. 10.15)

Electrically and mechanically, the heart is completely disorganised when in ventricular fibrillation (VF), and cardiac arrest results. The ECG shows fine or coarse waves of irregular size, shape and rhythm. VF may occur within minutes or hours after the onset of chest pain, so its precise timing in relation to the onset of ischaemia is variable. About 90% of deaths following acute myocardial infarction are due to ventricular fibrillation, most occurring immediately (primary VF).

Primary VF (phase 1 VF) is the term used if the heart was functioning normally when in sinus rhythm, and it normally occurs during the first 30 minutes of ischaemia when most myocardial injury is still reversible. It is usually associated with a good prognosis, as the heart is often in good condition, and those who survive to hospital discharge have the same long-term prognosis as patients who did not experience primary VF.

Reperfusional VF may occur following thrombolysis, but this probably reflects a good prognosis as it implies that the infarct-related artery has been opened.

Secondary or late VF (phase 2 VF) describes fibrillation in hearts whose function has been severely compromised by the infarct. These patients have usually been hypotensive and in heart failure. The prognosis is poor.

The frequency of VF has declined over the last 30 years from 5–10% in the 1970s to under 2% by the 1980s, probably because of greater use of beta-blockers and other cardioprotective therapy (particularly control of blood glucose, electrolytes and oxygenation). The management of cardiac arrest from ventricular fibrillation is discussed in Chapter 11.

Prophylaxis against ventricular fibrillation following acute myocardial infarction

Trials of VF prophylaxis with lidocaine showed a reduction in the incidence of primary VF, but this was offset by a trend towards increased mortality from fatal episodes of bradycardia and asystole. With the high doses required to obtain this result, side effects due to toxicity are frequent. Routine administration of lidocaine to all patients with known or suspected myocardial infarction has been abandoned in most contemporary CCU protocols because of this unfavourable risk–benefit ratio and because it has not been shown to improve survival. Routine administration of beta-blockers in the acute phase of myocardial infarction seems to reduce the incidence of serious dysrhythmias, attributable, in part, to their inherent antidysrhythmic properties, as well as limiting infarct size. Overall, beta-blockers reduce total mortality and the incidence of reinfarction by 25%.

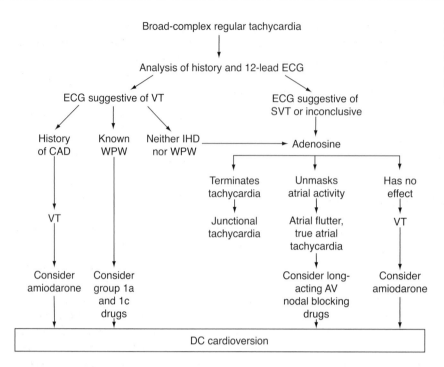

Figure 10.14 An approach to the management of acute broad-complex regular tachycardia. WPW, Wolff–Parkinson–White syndrome.

Following an episode of VF, there is no conclusive data to support the use of lidocaine or any particular strategy for preventing VF recurrence. Amiodarone may be beneficial where recurrent ventricular ectopics, tachycardia or fibrillation have complicated myocardial infarction (Cairns et al, 1997). Many other drugs have been tried as prophylaxis against ventricular dysrhythmias following myocardial infarction, but short-term mortality does not seem to differ with or without treatment (Pratt et al, 1998). Although no trial has specifically looked at the role of implantable defibrillators in the early post-infarction period, it may become the therapy of choice in high-risk patients.

THE BRADYCARDIAS

Slow heart rates (bradycardias) occur as a result of sino-atrial dysfunction, when the generation of the impulse at the sinus node is inhibited or when conduction through the heart is slowed or blocked (heart block). Bradycardia predisposes to cardiac standstill.

Sinus bradycardia

Sinus bradycardia is defined arbitrarily as a sinus rhythm slower than 60 beats/minute. Bradycardia occurs in about 30–40% of patients following acute myocardial infarction and normally indicates parasympathetic overactivity, with release of acetylcholine from autonomic fibres in the atria and atrio-ventricular node. Because afferent vagal fibres are more common on the inferior surface of the heart, vagal overactivity and consequent bradycardia often accompany inferior myocardial infarction, particularly in the first hour. While slowing of the heart is useful in protecting the

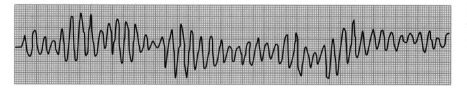

Figure 10.15 ECG: ventricular fibrillation.

injured heart, by limiting myocardial work, it may result in hypotension secondary to a reduced cardiac output. Escape rhythms are also more likely to occur, which can predispose to ventricular tachycardia and fibrillation. Sinus bradycardia may sometimes occur following reperfusion of the right coronary artery. This is due to the Bezold–Jarish reflex, involving a marked increase in vagal (parasympathetic) efferent discharge to the heart, elicited by stimulation of chemoreceptors, primarily in the left ventricle.

Sinus bradycardia is usually asymptomatic, but sudden onset of any bradycardia may result in hypotension or syncope. No treatment is required unless there are signs of low cardiac output, when a small dose of atropine (0.5 mg) is usually sufficient to raise the pulse and restore the blood pressure to normal. Further doses may be given at 2- to 3-minute intervals, to a total dose of 3 mg. Adrenaline (epinephrine) may be used to maintain heart rate, but it increases myocardial work and may precipitate ventricular dysrhythmias. Cardiac pacing should be considered if the sinus rate is poorly tolerated, or there is evidence of ectopic (escape) ventricular activity. This will often control the ectopic rhythm without resort to antidysrhythmic agents. If sinus bradycardia complicates anterior myocardial infarction, external pacing pads should be applied, as sudden complete heart block may follow. Endocardial pacing should be considered (Jowett et al, 1989).

Sino-atrial block

If the sinus node fails to initiate one or more stimuli, or if there is block of transmission of the impulse into the atria, sino-atrial (SA) block is said to occur (Fig. 10.16). The atria and ventricles will not be depolarised, and long pauses in the pulse may result.

Block at the sinus node is classified in the same way as block at the AV node, although first-degree SA block cannot be recognised electrically.

Second-degree SA block may occur in one of two forms:

- The PP interval becomes progressively shorter until a long pause occurs between two beats (sino-atrial Wenckebach). This is very similar in appearance to sinus arrest.
- Long pauses occur regularly following multiple normal PP cycles. While this most frequently happens every three or four beats and has little effect on the pulse rate, the pulse rate will be halved if it occurs with alternate beats.

Third-degree SA block (sinus arrest) is characterised by cardiac standstill for varying periods of time. Escape beats from the atria, AV node or ventricles then take over pacemaker function. As the right coronary artery usually supplies the sinus node, SA block is particularly common following inferior myocardial infarction. Drugs may sometimes be implicated.

No treatment is required if the pauses are short and asymptomatic. If drugs are responsible, they should be stopped or the dose reduced. Atropine, adrenaline and pacing may be required, as for sinus bradycardia.

Junctional bradycardia (Fig. 10.17)

The atrio-ventricular (AV) node is the second major site of impulse formation. If the sinus node fails to initiate an impulse, and no other focus arises in the atria, the AV junction takes over pacemaker function. This most commonly arises following acute myocardial infarction, particularly

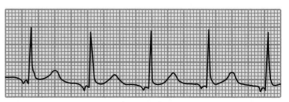

Figure 10.17 ECG: junctional bradycardia, lead aVF. The junctional focus has also activated the atria, as shown by the fact that each ventricular complex is preceded by an inverted P wave.

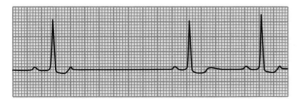

Figure 10.16 ECG: SA block.

if the patient is acidotic or hypoxic. AV junctional rhythms are relatively slow (40–60 beats/minute), but may speed up by enhanced automaticity.

If junctional rhythm is present, the nodal pacemaker may stimulate the atria and ventricles at the same time. The stimulus passes normally into the ventricles, producing a normal QRS complex, but there is also retrograde activation of the atria by the same impulse, such that a P wave may appear slightly before, after or buried in the QRS complex, depending upon the velocity of forward (antegrade) and backward (retrograde) conduction. The retrograde spread of the atrial impulse may also be recognised by the shape of the P wave, which is abnormal and usually inverted.

Because the atria and ventricles beat simultaneously, atrial contraction takes place against closed mitral and tricuspid valves. Blood is then pumped backwards into the superior vena cava, resulting in giant venous 'v' waves in the venous pulse. Junctional rhythm is usually short lived, and no treatment is required apart from stopping any medication that may be depressing the sinus node. Atropine may restore sinus rhythm, if necessary.

HEART BLOCK

Heart block exists when conduction from the atria to the ventricles is either slowed down or completely blocked. The conduction disturbance may arise within or just below the AV node (high block) or below the divisions of the bundle of His and involving the bundle branches (low block). Inferior infarction is usually associated with high block, and anterior infarction is associated with low block. Inter-His and multisite block may occur. Heart block usually results in bradycardia, with or without hypotension and reduced cardiac output. Alternatively, ventricular standstill and sudden death may follow.

Heart block develops in approximately 10% of patients with acute myocardial infarction and associates with an increased risk of in-hospital death, which relates more to the extent of myocardial damage rather than to the conduction problem. This probably explains why temporary cardiac pacing has not been shown to reduce mortality.

Atrio–ventricular (AV) block

Atrio-ventricular heart block may be transient, intermittent or permanent, and the dysfunction has been classified as first-, second- or third-degree AV block.

First-degree heart block (Fig. 10.18)

During first-degree heart block, the impulse passing from the atria to the ventricles is delayed at the AV node (or rarely in the atria or bundle of His), resulting in prolongation of the PR interval on the ECG. The PR interval increases with age, but does not usually exceed 0.2 seconds. First-degree heart block is asymptomatic, because it produces no change in heart rate, and the abnormality may only be appreciated electrocardiographically. It is more common with inferior myocardial infarction, and approximately 40% will progress to higher degrees of AV block.

Any cause of increased vagal tone can delay AV conduction and prolong the PR interval. Drugs, such as digoxin, diltiazem and beta-blockers, which affect the AV node, may also produce first-degree heart block.

Second-degree heart block

This is a partial AV block, which results in some atrial impulses failing to reach the ventricles. It is usually asymptomatic, unless it is associated with a slow ventricular rate. There are two electrocardiographically recognised types of second-degree heart block.

Mobitz type I (Wenckebach) AV block (Fig. 10.19)   About 90% of cases of second-degree heart block are Mobitz type I, in which each successive stimulus from the atria finds it more difficult to pass through the AV junction, reflected as a

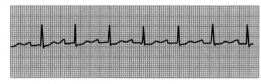

Figure 10.18   ECG: first-degree AV block.

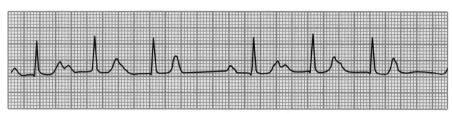

Figure 10.19   ECG: second-degree AV block (Mobitz type I).

progressive prolongation of the PR interval on the ECG. Eventually, the stimulus is completely blocked, and a QRS complex does not follow the atrial P wave. When the next atrial impulse reaches the AV junction, it is able to pass through normally, as conductivity is restored, and the cycle then repeats. The frequency of dropped beats varies, and may be numerous or very few.

This dysrhythmia often complicates inferior myocardial infarction, and may precede complete heart block. It is usually responsive to atropine but, if complicating anterior myocardial infarction, temporary pacing pads should be applied, with consideration of prophylactic endocardial pacing. Other causes of Mobitz I block include electrolyte imbalance or drugs that suppress AV conduction, such as digoxin and diltiazem. It may also be benign, particularly if observed during sleep, when it associates with increased vagal tone.

Mobitz type II AV block (Fig. 10.20)   Here, the AV junction does not respond to every atrial stimulus because of infranodal blockade in the bundle of His or bundle branches, rather than in the AV node. The observed rhythm may be called 2:1 or 4:1 heart block to denote the ratio of atrial to ventricular beats. The pulse is regular but slow. The QRS complex is often widened, denoting blockade

is at the level of the bundle branches. This is why this form of block is more serious, as bundle branch disease associates with slow ventricular rates, Stokes–Adams attacks and sudden death. Temporary pacemaker prophylaxis is advisable.

Third-degree (complete) heart block (Fig. 10.21)

In complete heart block, atrial impulses are totally blocked, either at or below the AV junction (nodal or infranodal block). An escape rhythm takes over from within the distal AV node, the His–Purkinje system or the ventricles. P waves occur regularly but have no relationship to the slower ventricular QRS complexes. Complete heart block can also occur with atrial fibrillation, in which case there are no P waves, and it can then be recognised only by appreciation of the ectopic ventricular pacemaker, which will be slow and with abnormal QRS morphology. The heart rate and QRS morphology vary in complete heart block, depending upon the origin of the secondary pacemaker. If the block is within the AV node, the QRS complex is usually normal, unless there is co-existent bundle branch block. However, if the block is infranodal, the ectopic pacemaker usually arises in either the left or the right bundle, producing widened QRS complexes at a slower rate. In general, the lower down the conducting system that the secondary pacemaker arises, the slower the rate, the wider the complex and the higher the associated mortality. Lower pacemakers are often irregular, with a propensity to interposed ventricular ectopic beats and ventricular standstill.

Complete AV block complicates about 8% of patients following acute inferior infarction, and these cases have higher in-hospital mortality. Heart block usually develops slowly following

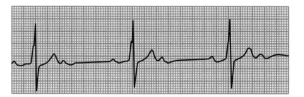

Figure 10.20   ECG: second-degree AV block (Mobitz type II), with 2:1 AV conduction.

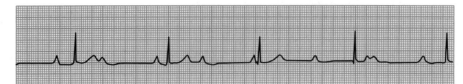

Figure 10.21   ECG: third-degree AV block.

first- and second-degree heart block. The pacemaker is usually high nodal rate producing a regular and haemodynamically stable rhythm at 40–60 beats/minute. Recovery of the AV node function usually occurs within a few hours or days, although it may take up to 3 weeks.

Complete heart block following acute anterior myocardial infarction is far more serious, and usually results from massive septal necrosis and infarction of the bundle branches. The onset often occurs without warning with escape rhythms originating low down in the ventricles. As such, they are slow (less than 45 beats/minute), irregular and often precede ventricular standstill. Most patients who develop complete heart block following anterior myocardial infarction die within 3 weeks as a result of associated extensive myocardial damage. The hospital mortality in this group is about 63% compared with 19% mortality in anterior infarction without heart block. Urgent insertion of a temporary pacemaker is usual, but does not seem to alter prognosis. If sinus rhythm does return, bifascicular block often persists, and complete heart block may recur weeks or months later.

Complete heart block may be asymptomatic if there is an efficient ventricular escape rhythm, and most cases of AV block complicating acute myocardial infarction do not require temporary pacing (Jowett et al, 1989). Drugs affecting AV conduction, such as digoxin, diltiazem and beta-adrenergic blocking agents, should be stopped.

TRIFASCICULAR DISEASE

Patients with conduction problems in all three fascicles of the conducting tissues are said to have *trifascicular disease*. At any one time, one of the three fascicles is capable of intermittent conduction, and this is recognised on the ECG as sinus rhythm with bifascicular block. As a result, trifascicular disease is usually suggested by:

- left bundle branch block with a prolonged PR interval;
- new right bundle branch block and left posterior hemi-block;
- new right bundle branch block with left anterior hemi-block and a prolonged PR interval;
- alternating right and left bundle branch block.

Following acute myocardial infarction, patients with evidence of trifascicular disease should be paced temporarily, because progress to complete heart block is very common. Prognosis depends upon the extent of coronary disease and left ventricular function.

Indications for temporary and permanent cardiac pacing are discussed in detail in Chapter 13.

MANAGEMENT OF PUMP FAILURE – HEART FAILURE AND CARDIOGENIC SHOCK

Acute coronary occlusion affects left ventricular function within seconds, even before there has been any myocardial damage. Subsequent myocardial infarction causes loss of myocardial tissue, and the effects on cardiac output may be compounded by dysrhythmias or by drugs that either depress myocardial contractility or produce salt and water retention. Patients with heart failure or asymptomatic left ventricular systolic dysfunction after acute myocardial infarction have a poor short- and long-term prognosis, and there is a close relationship between the degree of left ventricular dysfunction and subsequent mortality (Wu et al, 2002). The Killip classification is widely used (Killip & Kimball 1967) (Table 10.1).

Although this classification was only based on observations in 250 patients, and before modern

Table 10.1   The Killip classification.

Killip class	Clinical status	Mortality
Class 1	No failure	6%
Class 2	Mild/moderate heart failure	17%
Class 3	Severe heart failure	38%
Class 4	Cardiogenic shock	81%

interventions with thrombolysis, beta-blockade and ACE inhibition, Killip class still predicts mortality (Madias, 2000).

Acute left ventricular failure may present suddenly, with marked breathlessness, anxiety and tachycardia. When accompanied by hypotension, peripheral hypoperfusion and oliguria, the syndrome constitutes cardiogenic shock. Left ventricular failure may lead to frank pulmonary oedema as a result of transudation of fluid into the pulmonary alveoli. There is decreased airflow to and from the alveoli, because oedema of the pulmonary membranes causes airway narrowing. The lung compliance ('stiffness') increases, making breathing more difficult, and alveolar flooding reduces gaseous exchange within the alveoli. This leads to dyspnoea with arterial hypoxaemia. Increased mucus production may precipitate cough and wheeze (cardiac asthma), and the sputum may be tinged with blood from small haemorrhages in the congested bronchial mucosa.

Mild heart failure should not be based upon a few crackles at the lung bases alone, as this may simply reflect prior lung disease. A prominent third heart sound, especially with a tachycardia (gallop rhythm), is usually diagnostic, particularly when it occurs with crackles at the lung bases that do not clear with coughing. The chest radiograph appearances may be supportive, but an echocardiogram is definitive.

Treating acute heart failure

The aims of treatment are to relieve symptoms by:

- reducing intracardiac pressures and volume overload;
- increasing salt and water excretion.

Although assisting impaired left ventricular contraction with positive inotropes would seem logical, myocardial stimulation increases oxygen consumption in the areas of borderline perfusion, and also increases the potential for dysrhythmias. Treatment is therefore aimed at reducing volume overload with diuretics and increasing capacitance with vasodilators.

The patient should be sat upright and given high concentrations of oxygen to breathe. This is particularly important following acute myocardial infarction, as hypoxaemia will worsen already impaired left ventricular function by increasing areas of critical myocardial ischaemia. Ventilatory function will already be compromised by the combined action of reduced pulmonary compliance, pulmonary vascular congestion and respiratory depression from injected opiates. Oxygen saturation should be maintained at > 95% to maximise tissue oxygenation.

Loop diuretics work by decreasing cardiac preload, mostly by venodilatation and partly by volume depletion. Intravenous bumetanide and furosemide reduce pulmonary venous pressure within 15 minutes. Relief of symptoms occurs before the onset of diuresis, probably due to a direct vasodilator effect on the capillary beds.

Diamorphine may be an important adjunct in certain cases by relieving anxiety and pain and reducing myocardial oxygen demand. Opiates produce transient venodilation, which may be helpful, but may aggravate bradycardia and suppress ventilation, and should be used sparingly.

Nitrates are venodilators that reduce cardiac filling pressures. As most episodes of cardiac failure are due to fluid redistribution rather than fluid overload, high-dose nitrates, preferably given as repeated intravenous boluses, may be very beneficial in early treatment (Northridge, 1996; Sharon et al, 2000). They improve the haemodynamic status and help to prevent remodelling. Provided they do not provoke tachycardia, nitrates may also help to limit infarction size by increasing collateral blood flow. Continued treatment with high-dose nitrates and furosemide is better than high-dose furosemide alone.

Sodium nitroprusside is a potent dilator of arteries and veins that acts by direct action on vascular smooth muscle, with a rapid onset and rapid cessation of action when infusions are turned on and off. The major side effect is cyanide toxicity, and limiting infusions to less than 48 hours can reduce cyanide levels. Hydroxocobalamin (vitamin B12) infusions reduce cyanide concentrations and may be given concurrently. Administration requires close supervision.

Nesiritide is a recombinant brain peptide that has potent vasodilator properties (arterial, venous and coronary), and has benefits similar to intravenous nitrates, but with fewer side effects.

ACE inhibitors reduce mortality in all patients following myocardial infarction and are particularly beneficial in those with heart failure, anterior infarction and asymptomatic left ventricular dysfunction (ACE Inhibitor Myocardial Infarction Collaborative Group, 1998). Early administration is advised (< 36 hours) to prevent ventricular remodelling, which starts very early in the course of myocardial infarction.

Angiotensin receptor blockers (ARBs) have not been shown to be superior to ACE inhibitors, but the VALIANT trial did show that valsartan was as effective as captopril, providing an alternative for patients unable to tolerate an ACE inhibitor (Pfeffer et al, 2003).

Aldosterone blockade is of proven value in both acute and chronic heart failure. Aldosterone plays an important role in the pathophysiology of myocardial and vascular hypertrophy, fibrosis and remodelling. The precise mechanisms for this are unknown. Clinical benefits of aldosterone inhibition have been seen with both eplerinone and spironolactone. *Eplerinone* 25 mg/day started in hospital significantly reduces all-cause mortality as well as readmissions for cardiovascular reasons when prescribed in addition to conventional therapy in patients with a left ventricular ejection fraction of under 40%, those with signs of heart failure or in patients with diabetes (Pitt et al, 2005). The optimum duration of treatment in post-infarct patients is not known. Long-term aldosterone blockade is certainly important in those with persistent left ventricular dysfunction, but a switch to less expensive *spironolactone* for chronic therapy is probably not harmful. For those who improve (perhaps to an ejection fraction > 40%), it may be possible to discontinue this treatment. The risk of serious hyperkalaemia is the primary safety concern with the aldosterone antagonists, and they should only be used in patients with heart failure if serum potassium is regularly monitored.

Beta-blockade was the first evidence-based treatment for myocardial infarction over 25 years ago, but there is still reluctance to prescribe beta-blockers in patients with heart failure. Bisoprolol, metoprolol, nebivolol and carvedilol may be used with good effect in those with impaired left ventricular dysfunction after acute myocardial infarction. It is essential that the patient is haemodynamically stable before beta-blockade is started.

Assisted ventilation

Assisted ventilation should be considered in severe cardiogenic pulmonary oedema. Formal intubation and ventilation may have detrimental cardiovascular effects due to sedation, hypotension and reduced cardiac output secondary to high intrathoracic pressures. Non-invasive positive pressure ventilation can be very helpful in the management of ventilatory failure complicating acute pulmonary oedema. It improves pulmonary compliance, decreases diaphragmatic activity and reduces both cardiac preload and afterload. The decreased alveolar pressure reduces the work of breathing. Oxygenation is improved, with correction of any acidosis, and left ventricular function improves (Cooper & Jacob, 2002).

Further management

Bedrest is valuable until signs and symptoms of cardiac failure improve. Recumbency reduces metabolic demand and increases renal perfusion, and thus decreases myocardial work and improves diuresis. Passive leg exercises and low-molecular-weight heparin are recommended to prevent deep vein thrombosis. Anticoagulation with warfarin should be considered for patients with enlarged hearts, atrial fibrillation and anterior myocardial infarction or generally poor left ventricular function. This last group is prone to deep vein thrombosis, pulmonary emboli, left ventricular thrombus and peripheral embolisation. Strategies for the management of patients with heart failure including specialised follow-up by a multidisciplinary team will reduce readmission and also reduce mortality (McAlister et al, 2004).

CARDIOGENIC SHOCK

Shock is a complex syndrome associated with inadequate perfusion of vital organs, most significantly the brain, the kidneys and the heart. Cardiogenic shock is the commonest cause of in-hospital death after acute myocardial infarction, and is essentially a disease of inadequate pump function associated with massive cardiac damage (more than 40% of the left ventricular myocardium). Cardiogenic shock can also occur with major pulmonary emboli, cardiac tamponade or following cardiac surgery. The presence of diabetes, established cardiovascular disease, increasing age and the female sex all place the patient at risk. It occurs in 7% of patients with ST segment elevation myocardial infarction and 3% with non-ST segment elevation myocardial infarction. Some patients are admitted to coronary care already in shock, and most cases develop the syndrome within 24 hours. About 15% may develop shock more than 7 days later. In the GUSTO-I study (1993), 7% developed cardiogenic shock, 11% on admission and 89% in the subsequent 2 weeks. Almost all of those who developed cardiogenic shock did so by 48 hours after the onset of symptoms, and their overall 30-day mortality was 57%, compared with an overall study group mortality of just 7%.

Preshock is a cardiological emergency that requires aggressive management aimed at preventing deterioration into established cardiogenic shock, which is difficult to reverse (Box 10.3). Despite advances in the treatment of acute myocardial infarction with thrombolysis and other reperfusion therapies, there has been no significant change in the incidence of cardiogenic shock, which has remained at between 7% and 10% for the last 20 years. Hospital mortality was over 90% in the 1970s and is still in the region of 45–80% (Goldberg et al, 1999). It is thus a major contributor to overall cardiovascular morbidity and mortality.

There are typically four types of conditions that predispose to cardiogenic shock.

Box 10.3   Key management of cardiogenic shock.

Rapid admission to a coronary care unit
Reperfusion (primary angioplasty or thrombolysis)
Control dysrhythmias
Echocardiography
Invasive haemodynamic assessment
Haemodynamic stabilisation (fluids/inotropic support/vasodilators)
Intra-aortic balloon pumping
Cardiac catheterisation, to define coronary anatomy and mechanical defects
Cardiac surgery or PCI

PCI, percutaneous coronary intervention.

---

1   Recent massive myocardial infarction. The affected vessel is usually the main stem of the left coronary artery, which will generally result in 40–50% of the left ventricular myocardium being damaged.

2   Acute-on-chronic infarction. This occurs when a smaller myocardial infarction takes the cumulative damage to more than 40% of the ventricular myocardium. These patients are more likely to have pre-existing hypertension and multicoronary artery disease.

3   Myocardial infarction with mechanical complication. Here, acute myocardial infarction is complicated by a mechanical defect, such as a ruptured mitral valve, ruptured septum or acute left ventricular aneurysm.

4   Myocardial infarction with recurrent dysrhythmias. Dysrhythmias, especially ventricular dysrhythmias, reduce cardiac output and increase myocardial work and oxygen consumption, so they may extend the size of the originally infarcted area. Extension of the infarction is common in patients who die from cardiogenic shock.

The syndrome of cardiogenic shock presents with:

- systemic hypotension (systolic blood pressure < 90 mmHg);
- oliguria (< 20 mL urine per hour);
- arterial vasoconstriction, leading to hypoperfusion of the vital organs and peripheries.

The patient is cold, sweaty and cyanosed, with rapid shallow respiration, hypotension and tachycardia. Mental changes reflecting poor cerebral perfusion are usually present, including irritability, restlessness and, later, coma. Shunting of blood occurs, particularly in the lungs, and the resulting decreased tissue flow causes hypoxia, anaerobic metabolism and a propensity to lactic acidosis, which further embarrasses left ventricular function. In an attempt to maintain cardiac output, the remaining non-ischaemic myocardium becomes hypercontractile, and its oxygen consumption increases. The falling blood pressure increases catecholamine levels, leading to systemic arterial and venous constriction, which in turn compromises coronary flow and worsens the ischaemia to the rest of the myocardium, thus worsening function. A vicious cycle is set up, whereby arterial hypotension leads to coronary hypoperfusion and poor myocardial perfusion, which produces left ventricular dysfunction. This in turn results in worsening heart failure, hypoxia, acidosis and hypotension, and so on. Additional factors, such as the severity of disease in the other coronary arteries, dysrhythmias and infarct expansion, all come into play. The frequent finding of infarct extension in these patients is relevant. Salvage of the border zone of infarction by revascularisation, even late after coronary occlusion, may prevent infarct expansion and aneurysm formation, and may salvage enough myocardium to provide an adequate contractile mass.

Management

Unfortunately, patients are seldom seen early enough and, once cardiogenic shock is established, the prognosis is dire, even with aggressive intervention. Early reperfusion of the ischaemic or infarcting myocardium to arrest the inevitable progress to loss of left ventricular myocardium is needed (Ryan et al, 1999). Thrombolysis has been proven to reduce development of cardiogenic shock, but is unlikely to benefit those who present with cardiogenic shock (Fibrinolytic Therapy Trialists' Collaborative Group, 1994). Successful fibrinolysis depends on drug delivery to the clot but, as blood pressure falls, optimal reperfusion becomes less likely. Special attention is needed in

the relief of ischaemia, control and prevention of dysrhythmias and optimisation of haemodynamic variables by inotropic support. The use of glucose–potassium–insulin (GKI) infusions to support viable myocardial function has not been shown to be of value (CREATE-ECLA Investigators, 2005).

High-concentration oxygen should be given, and some patients will benefit from non-invasive ventilation. Immediate echocardiography is vital to assess the major haemodynamics, which may later be confirmed by insertion of a Swan–Ganz catheter (Stokes & Jowett, 1985). The abrupt loss of myocardial contractility usually results in a significant rise in intracardiac pressures and a critical fall in arterial blood pressure and cardiac output. However, left ventricular filling pressures and the cardiac index can vary widely, and it is not wise to assume that cardiac output is low or the filling pressures high. Hypovolaemia and low filling pressures may be found in patients with unsuspected right ventricular infarction and patients taking diuretics or antihypertensive agents. The left ventricular filling volume should be optimised and, in the absence of pulmonary congestion, a saline fluid challenge of at least 250 mL should be administered over 10 minutes. Echocardiography will also exclude pericardial tamponade and provides information about left ventricular function and size. Mechanical defects may also be defined. A chest radiograph can give information about heart size, lung fields and aortic root size. An increase in the last may suggest aortic dissection as a cause of the shock.

All drugs commonly prescribed during acute myocardial infarction need reviewing. Opiates, ACE inhibitors, beta-blockers, nitrates and calcium antagonists need to be used very cautiously in these patients because they can worsen hypotension and cardiogenic shock (Williams et al, 2000).

Inotropic support with drugs such as dopamine and dobutamine may provide temporary stabilisation until other measures can be instituted, although they are unlikely to affect outcome alone. If the blood pressure on maximal inotropic stimulation fails to exceed 100/70 mmHg and the patient is still clinically hypoperfused (i.e. oliguric, peripherally shut down), the patient is unlikely to survive on medical treatment alone. The greatest mortality benefit is seen after intra-aortic balloon pumping, urgent coronary angiography and revascularisation (Hochman et al, 1999).

Intra-aortic balloon pumping

Since its introduction in the 1960s, intra-aortic balloon counterpulsation has been recognised as an effective treatment for patients with unstable ischaemic syndromes and cardiogenic shock (Kantrowitz et al, 1968). Modern intra-aortic balloons are inserted percutaneously without arterial cut-down. Fluoroscopy is generally used, but blind insertion is possible. The narrow balloon catheter is inserted via the femoral artery and advanced to lie in the descending aorta, just below the aortic arch (Fig. 10.22). The two phases of counterpulsation are inflation during diastole and deflation during systole. During systole, sudden deflation allows blood to be ejected from the left ventricle around the deflated balloon. Before deflation, the balloon protects the aortic outflow, so afterload is low, which promotes left ventricular emptying. At the onset of diastole, an ECG-activated trigger causes the balloon to inflate with helium, just after the dicrotic notch of aortic valve closure, thus occluding the aorta. Approximately 50 mL of blood is pushed up towards the closed aortic valve, and actively propels blood into the coronary arteries to promote myocardial perfusion and, additionally, improve cerebral blood supply. When the balloon deflates again, the intra-aortic

pressure is low, and blood is ejected with minimal extra cardiac work and oxygen consumption. Pulmonary congestion is relieved, and global myocardial perfusion, often including collateral circulation to the infarcted area, is improved. Cardiac output may increase by up to 50%, allowing improved blood flow to the vital organs. The mean arterial blood pressure increases as myocardial function improves by about 15 mmHg, and shock quickly stabilises.

Counterpulsation was first used as a stand-alone modality to treat patients with post-infarct cardiogenic shock, but it is used today as a stabilising device or bridge to facilitate diagnostic angiography and revascularisation or repair (Kumar & Roberts, 2001). Recommendations for intra-aortic balloon counterpulsation include:

- cardiogenic shock not quickly reversed with pharmacological therapy as a stabilising measure before angiography and revascularisation;
- acute mitral regurgitation or septal rupture complicating myocardial infarction, as a stabilising therapy for angiography and repair/revascularisation;
- recurrent intractable ventricular arrhythmias with haemodynamic instability;
- refractory post-infarct angina as a bridge to angiography and revascularisation.

Unfortunately, although balloon pumping may improve the initial mortality for patients in

Figure 10.22 Intra-aortic balloon counterpulsation in (A) diastole and (B) systole

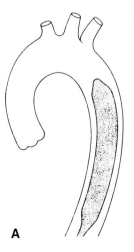 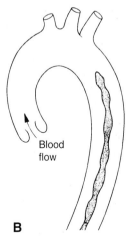

Blood flow

A   B

cardiogenic shock, 'balloon dependence' is common, so that, when this support is withdrawn, shock returns. Insertion should only be considered where myocardial stunning is thought to play a major part, or where surgical intervention is possible. Left ventricular assist devices (LVADs) have also been used as holding measures until surgery can be performed (see Chapter 16). Balloon pumping alone does not reduce mortality.

Balloon pumping is currently underutilised outside tertiary centres. District hospitals need to develop a suitable programme so that treatment may be initiated before transfer whenever possible.

RIGHT VENTRICULAR INFARCTION

Although myocardial infarction usually results in left ventricular dysfunction, the right ventricle may also be involved, either alone or with the left ventricle. Clinical consequences vary from none to cardiogenic shock. Isolated right ventricle infarction is uncommon, but involvement with acute inferior myocardial infarction is very common (Goldstein, 1998). Some degree of right ventricular ischaemia may be demonstrated in half of all inferior infarcts, but only 10–15% will develop clinically important abnormalities. In most cases, the right ventricle becomes stunned, with normal function returning over a period of weeks to months. However, where there is right ventricular necrosis in association with inferior infarction, there is increased mortality.

The right coronary artery usually supplies most of the right ventricular myocardium, and right coronary occlusion proximal to the right ventricular (marginal) branches will lead to right ventricular ischaemia. However, there is usually little haemodynamic consequence, as the right ventricle is relatively protected against the effects of acute ischaemia through extensive collateral flow from left to right, with coronary perfusion that occurs in both systole and diastole. Oxygen demand is also not as high as for the left ventricle because the right ventricle has a much smaller muscle mass, with a lower vascular resistance pulmonary circuit. These factors explain why right ventricular ischaemia usually passes unnoticed in most patients with proximal right coronary artery occlusion.

The clinical triad of hypotension, clear lung fields and elevated jugular venous pressure in the setting of an inferior myocardial infarction is characteristic of right ventricular infarction, but not very sensitive. Distended neck veins alone or the presence of Kussmaul's sign (distended neck veins that fail to empty on inspiration) are both sensitive and specific clinical clues for right ventricular involvement in these patients.

Electrocardiography is usually unhelpful unless right-sided chest leads are used. Demonstration of 1-mm ST segment elevation in the right precordial lead $V4_R$ is the single most predictive electrocardiographic finding in patients with right ventricular infarction, but it may be transient (Andersen et al, 1989). This ECG lead should be recorded in all cases of shock following myocardial infarction if not included in routine electrocardiography.

Echocardiography is necessary to exclude cardiac tamponade, and may show right ventricular dilatation and hypokinesia, with abnormal interventricular and interatrial septal motion. There is often marked tricuspid regurgitation secondary to dilatation of the tricuspid annulus. The acutely ischaemic right ventricle dilates, but it is restrained by the pericardium. The increased intrapericardial pressure reduces the right ventricular systolic pressure and output, which in turn decreases left ventricular preload and stroke volume. There is paradoxical movement of the interventricular septum into the right ventricle during systole, providing a piston-like movement that helps right ventricular emptying. This compensatory mechanism will be lost if there is concomitant septal infarction that may result in a major diminution of right ventricular output. The intra-atrial septum also bows towards the left atrium because of raised intra-atrial pressure.

Treatment of right ventricular infarction aims to maintain the right ventricular filling pressure, while reducing the right ventricular afterload. Drugs used routinely in the management of myocardial infarction, such as nitrates and diuretics, which reduce preload, may diminish cardiac output and produce severe hypotension. Volume loading with normal saline alone often resolves accompanying hypotension and improves cardiac output. However, in some patients, volume loading further elevates the right-sided filling pressure and right dilatation, resulting in decreased left ventricular output. So, while volume loading (0.5–1 L of normal saline) is a critical first step in the management of hypotension, inotropic support with dobutamine should be initiated promptly if cardiac output fails to improve after fluids have been given. Sodium nitroprusside or an intra-aortic balloon pump is often necessary to unload the heart, and measurement of intracardiac pressures with a Swan–Ganz catheter is of major value in balancing therapy to optimise cardiac output. Early percutaneous coronary intervention (PCI) may result in rapid haemodynamic improvement, and seems to produce better outcomes than thrombolysis.

Atrial fibrillation occurs in up to one-third of patients with right ventricular infarction and may have profound haemodynamic effects. Prompt cardioversion should be considered. Similar haemodynamic deterioration may develop if there is complete heart block, which is a common complication of right coronary occlusion. Sequential atrio-ventricular pacing is preferable to ventricular pacing to maintain cardiac output.

Clinical and haemodynamic right ventricular dysfunction may persist for weeks or months following acute myocardial infarction. Recovery is helped by a gradual stretching of the pericardium, which relieves its restraining effect on the heart. Any improvements in left ventricular dysfunction help to reduce right ventricular afterload.

CARDIAC RUPTURE

After dysrhythmias and cardiogenic shock, the most common cause of death following acute myocardial infarction is cardiac rupture. It used to occur in the healing stages following infarction (3–5 days) but, following thrombolysis, the maximum risk is in the first 24–48 hours (ISIS-2 Collaborative Group, 1988). Noticeably, early institution of thrombolysis (under 6 hours) reduces the risk of cardiac rupture, whereas a delay (> 12 hours) increases the risk. The risk of cardiac rupture may be decreased by early treatment with beta-blockers. Rupture is predisposed to by extensive infarction, prior hypertension or smoking, diffuse coronary heart disease, diabetes and anticoagulant therapy. It is four times more common in women, especially older women.

Free wall rupture

The most common site for rupture is through the free left ventricular wall, producing chest pain, hypotension, dyspnoea and distended neck veins. Death is rapid and caused by an acute haemopericardium, leading to cardiac tamponade. Recurrent chest pain without ECG changes may warn of imminent rupture, and cardiac collapse in the presence of normal complexes on the electrocardiogram is typical (PEA). Free wall rupture is probably responsible for 10–20% of in-hospital deaths following acute myocardial infarction.

A high index of suspicion is required to identify patients with subacute rupture. Small quantities of blood leak into the pericardial cavity, and signs of tamponade develop slowly. These patients often remain hypotensive with recurrent pain suggestive of reinfarction. There is nausea or repetitive vomiting, and the patient is restless. There are no specific ECG clues, but ST elevation in leads not previously involved in the prior infarction may herald rupture (Birnbaum et al, 2003). Echocardiography may demonstrate pericardial fluid (haemopericardium), but this is not specific, as small pericardial effusions are fairly common following myocardial infarction. However, if a thrombotic mass is seen, urgent surgery is indicated.

Ventricular septal rupture

Rupture of the interventricular septum complicates about 1–2% of cases of acute myocardial infarction. It produces an intracardiac shunt with blood being forced from the powerful left ventricle into the lower pressure right ventricle, resulting in a marked fall in cardiac output, with pulmonary circuit overload and severe pulmonary oedema. A loud pan-systolic murmur is audible at the left sternal edge, with a systolic thrill. If left ventricular function is poor, the murmur may be very soft or even absent. The site of perforation depends on the site of myocardial infarction, and can affect the surgical repair. Inferior myocardial infarction involves the posterior or basal septum and is often more complex. Anterior infarcts usually produce a single apical defect. Both may easily be identified by echocardiography.

Acute mitral regurgitation

Minor mitral regurgitation is a fairly common finding at echocardiography in patients following acute myocardial infarction (40%), although it is not so frequent at angiography (19%). It is a marker of poorer outcome. Early reperfusion reduces the frequency of mitral regurgitation, and improvements may be dramatic following emergency PCI. There are three causes of acute mitral regurgitation:

- dilatation of the mitral annulus;
- papillary muscle dysfunction;
- papillary muscle rupture.

Dilatation of the mitral annulus occurs secondary to left ventricular dilatation and often improves with reperfusion and ACE inhibitors.

The papillary muscles may become ischaemic and infarcted, like any other part of the ventricular myocardium. This usually associates with inferior and posterior rather than anterior myocardial infarction. Occlusion of the right or circumflex coronary artery typically causes ischaemia of the postero-medial papillary muscle. *Papillary muscle dysfunction* usually occurs in the healing stages.

Acute severe mitral regurgitation results from complete *rupture of the papillary muscle*, with a dramatic fall in cardiac output, acute pulmonary oedema and, often, cardiogenic shock. An apical pan-systolic murmur develops, which radiates to the axilla or sometimes to the left sternal edge (the regurgitant jet is often eccentric). Milder degrees of mitral dysfunction will occur with partial rupture, and transoesophageal echocardiography may be necessary to make the diagnosis. The prognosis is better than for septal rupture and depends upon the degree of left ventricular dysfunction. Treatment with arterial vasodilators may support the circulation until surgery can be performed.

Management of cardiac rupture

The management of mechanical defects following acute myocardial infarction is surgical (see Chapter 16); without operation, most patients with cardiac rupture will die.

LEFT VENTRICULAR ANEURYSM

Left ventricular aneurysms develop more commonly following acute myocardial infarction in the presence of diffuse coronary heart disease, in hypertensive patients or where there has been extensive myocardial damage. The site is usually antero-lateral (60%), while 20% occur in the inferior wall. The apex and septum may also be affected. Patients are often identified because of refractory left ventricular failure or persistent ST elevation on the ECG that persists weeks after the infarct (a non-specific sign). While there may be no related symptoms, the aneurysm may act as a focus for recurrent ventricular tachycardia, and also as a site for thrombus formation. Systemic embolisation complicates about 5% of cases of left ventricular aneurysm, mostly in the first few weeks following myocardial infarction. Diagnosis may be confirmed by echocardiography or ventriculography. Where possible, surgical excision is usually combined with revascularisation procedures, and is particularly advised where heart failure is difficult to control or embolic episodes are continuing despite anticoagulation (Chapter 16).

A *pseudoaneurysm* is a rare complication, where a partial rupture is sealed off by adherent pericardium. It will have a narrow neck that distinguishes it from a true aneurysm. Many patients have no related symptoms; otherwise, there may be chest pain or breathlessness. A systolic murmur may be heard. Urgent surgery is required.

LEFT VENTRICULAR THROMBUS

Left ventricular mural thrombus may develop over areas of acutely inflamed endocardium in the first 3 weeks following myocardial infarction, particularly in association with large anterior infarcts and left ventricular aneurysms. Echocardiographic screening is not always helpful, and a quarter of emboli occur in patients without echodetectable ventricular thrombus. Prophylactic anticoagulation helps to prevent mural thrombus and, if a thrombus develops, helps to prevent embolisation. Without intervention, up to 15% of patients with mural thrombus will have embolic episodes, mostly resulting in stroke. Overall, cerebral embolism affects 1–3% of patients with myocardial infarction, and usually occurs within the first 10 days, although the risk may continue for many weeks, depending on left ventricular function. Large mesenteric emboli are generally fatal. Limb emboli may need to be removed surgically. Coronary emboli causing reinfarction are fortunately uncommon. Mortality in patients with mural thrombus reflects the large myocardial infarct rather than any embolic complication (Keeley & Hillis, 1996).

Anticoagulation for at least 6 months is recommended if left ventricular thrombus is detected. Short-term anticoagulation should also be considered in those with extensive anterior infarcts and poor cardiac function. The risk of stroke following myocardial infarction is in the region of 2.3% in the first month, falling dramatically thereafter, but remaining at two to three times the expected rate for 2–3 years.

DEEP VEIN THROMBOSIS AND PULMONARY EMBOLISM

There are many reasons why deep vein thrombosis (DVT) is more likely following myocardial infarction, including immobility, increasing age, obesity and heart failure. DVT is thought to complicate as many as one-third of cases of myocardial infarction, most of which are asymptomatic. Post-mortem examinations have found pulmonary emboli in 8% of deaths associated with acute myocardial infarction (Griffin, 1996). Prophylaxis is therefore of major importance.

DVT prophylaxis

Patients on the CCU are at least at moderate risk of venous thromboembolism. Prophylaxis with subcutaneous low-molecular-weight heparin should be used routinely in all patients, and full anticoagulation should be considered for those with prolonged immobilisation and heart failure. Graded pressure (TED) stockings may also be useful. Early mobilisation is desirable for all patients, especially the elderly, provided there are no contraindications.

Diagnosis of established DVTs

Clinical signs of DVT are not always reliable, but may include swelling, tenderness and redness of the affected limb. These signs are not specific, and clinical diagnosis is less than 50% accurate. The role of D-dimer measurement following recent coronary thrombosis is limited, but a negative result may rule out active thrombosis, especially if clinical suspicion is low. *Compression ultrasound* of the legs is sensitive for detecting proximal DVT when carried out by an experienced practitioner. *Venography* may be used to demonstrate thrombosis in the deep veins up to the inferior vena cava. The investigation is invasive and has the risk of producing thrombophlebitis in some patients.

Management

For initial treatment of DVT, low-molecular-weight heparin is effective and easier to administer than unfractionated heparin. Heparin should be continued for 4–5 days, and oral anticoagulants given at the same time. The international normalised ratio (INR) should be 2–3 for at least 2 days before heparin is discontinued. The optimum duration of anticoagulation is not clear, and depends upon the clinical status of the patient and reversible risk factors. Typically, warfarin is continued for 6 weeks to 6 months (Jowett, 1999).

Physical measures are very important, but often forgotten. Bedrest is unnecessary, and indeed may be harmful in promoting venous stasis. Adequate analgesia is required, and walking should be encouraged in class II graduated compression stockings. In patients with severe oedema, high elevation of the affected leg will help to reduce the swelling until a stocking can be worn. When not walking, the patient should return to bed with the leg elevated at a level higher than the heart. Sitting for long periods should be avoided as it encourages venous stasis and increases calf compartment pressures, predisposing to limb ischaemia.

Thrombolysis is an attractive alternative to anticoagulation for DVT, as it will clear veins more quickly and preserve valve function (Jowett et al, 1998), but there have been concerns about precipitating pulmonary embolism when the clot breaks up (Armon & Hopkinson, 1996).

POST-INFARCT ANGINA

If flow in the infarct-related artery is not fully restored, there is a risk of reocclusion. Cases of reinfarction are more likely to develop cardiogenic shock and have a poor prognosis and a 2.5 times greater risk of death or further myocardial infarction within 1 year. Symptomatic coronary reocclusion usually occurs within 24 hours, although asymptomatic reocclusion may occur later (Ohman et al, 1990).

Post-infarction chest pain may be due to many causes, such as pericarditis, pulmonary embolism or dyspepsia, so a definite diagnosis of angina is needed. Transient ECG changes and response to glyceryl trinitrate (GTN) are the main confirmatory features. About 20% of patients develop angina while still in hospital. These often have multivessel coronary disease, are 10 times more likely to suffer further infarction while in hospital and have a poor long-term prognosis. Early coronary angiography is important in this high-risk group, followed by PCI or bypass surgery to improve prognosis. Surgery is usually delayed following transmural infarction to reduce perioperative risk.

PERICARDITIS AND DRESSLER SYNDROME

Post-infarction pericarditis affects about 25% patients in the first week following acute transmural myocardial infarction, and is more common in those with larger infarcts and left ventricular failure. As such, it associates with a poorer long-term prognosis. Thrombolytic therapy has reduced the incidence of this complication, probably by limiting the size of infarction. Around 9% of those with non-ST elevation myocardial infarction (NSTEMI) may also develop pericarditis. A friction rub may be heard in about 50% of patients. The erythrocyte sedimentation rate (ESR) and white cell count may be elevated, and a small pericardial effusion can be seen on echocardiography.

Sometimes, pericarditis and pleurisy recur 2–12 weeks after myocardial infarction, a condition called *Dressler syndrome* (Dressler, 1956). Pericardial pain is accompanied by systemic symptoms such as fever and malaise. Large pleural and pericardial effusions may develop. The mechanism is thought to be autoimmune, triggered by blood in the pericardial cavity or from antibodies to necrotic myocardium. There has been a marked reduction in this complication in recent years.

Treatment of pericarditis is with a single high dose of a non-steroidal anti-inflammatory agent and bedrest. Long-term analgesia is seldom required. Echocardiography should be repeated to check for increasing pericardial effusion, particularly if the ECG shows progressive low-voltage reduction. The condition is self-limiting but may recur. It is best to discontinue anticoagulants, because of the risk of a haemorrhagic pericardial effusion. More resistant cases may need corticosteroid therapy.

PERICARDIAL EFFUSION AND TAMPONADE

A small pericardial effusion may be found in up to 25% of patients following acute transmural myocardial infarction, often in those with heart failure. Tamponade is very rare. Larger effusions indicate a poorer prognosis.

SHOULDER–HAND SYNDROME

The shoulder–hand syndrome presents with stiffness and pain in the shoulder (usually the left side) 2–8 weeks after acute myocardial infarction, sometimes accompanied by pain and swelling of the hand. Physiotherapy and analgesia are all that is required. With early mobilisation of the post-coronary patient, this has become a rare complication.

PSYCHOSOCIAL COMPLICATIONS

Between 20% and 50% of post-infarct patients have high levels of stress, anxiety and hostility. Depression is particularly common, and may result from denial or being too frightened to admit to problems. Depression associates with adverse outcomes following acute myocardial infarction, perhaps due to poor compliance with treatment.

Early mobilisation, with prompt involvement of the rehabilitation team, can prevent depression. While trials of psychosocial interventions have shown inconsistent results, functional status and quality of life may be improved.

SUDDEN DEATH

Sudden cardiac death (SCD) can occur at any stage following the onset of an acute coronary syndrome. Most of these deaths associate with malignant ventricular dysrhythmias, although they may be due to pulmonary embolism or acute cardiac rupture. Primary ventricular fibrillation often occurs before admission to hospital, typically within the first 2 hours following the onset of symptoms. Reperfusional therapy has a clear role in reducing in-hospital mortality by reduction in cardiogenic shock and dysrhythmic death. Furthermore, early perfusion limits infarct size and ventricular enlargement and preserves left ventricular function, all of which help to reduce late ventricular dysrhythmias.

Late ventricular dysrhythmias occur 10 days or more after myocardial infarction, at a time when most patients have been discharged from hospital. The patient has often made normal post-infarction progress, and then suddenly collapses at home. Trying to identify this group of patients is difficult. Some of these patients are predisposed to ventricular dysrhythmias because of electrolyte imbalance, particularly hypokalaemia, which must be avoided in the peri-infarction period. Early exercise testing or Holter monitoring before discharge in selected high-risk cases (large infarcts, heart failure, diabetes) may help to identify those prone to SCD.

Owing to the complex mechanisms leading to SCD, a variety of therapeutic targets may be considered. The terms primary and secondary prophylaxis are used in the context of ventricular dysrhythmias. 'Primary' intervention is applied to patients at high risk who have not yet had a ventricular dysrhythmia. Secondary prophylaxis is applied to those who have already had a VF arrest or ventricular tachycardia associated with hypotension and presyncope.

Primary prophylaxis

ACE inhibition following acute myocardial infarction decreases progression to overt or worsening heart failure, and may reduce mortality from SCD by as much 30–54% (Kober et al, 1995). Antidysrhythmic drugs have a limited role in prophylaxis against SCD post infarction. The suppression of spontaneous non-sustained ventricular tachycardia does not affect outcome, and certain agents may be harmful (e.g. class I agents). Treatment with beta-blockers reduces all-cause mortality, some of which is related to reductions in SCDs. The greatest benefits of beta-blockade have been shown in those with poor left ventricular function and heart failure, a subgroup who have traditionally been denied this therapy. Amiodarone may be safely administered for symptomatic non-sustained VT where beta-blockers are contraindicated.

Primary intervention trials of automatic implantable cardiodefibrillators (AICDs) show a reduction in all-cause mortality when compared with medical therapy, and implantation is suggested in:

- patients with a history of previous myocardial infarction (> 4 weeks) with:
  - left ventricular dysfunction (ejection fraction < 35%); *and*
  - non-sustained ventricular tachycardia on Holter monitoring; *and*
  - inducible ventricular tachycardia on electrophysiological testing;
- patients with a history of previous myocardial infarction (> 4 weeks) with:
  - left ventricular dysfunction (ejection fraction < 30%); *and*
  - QRS duration > 120 ms.

The second group of patients may benefit from a combined AICD/biventricular pacing unit.

Secondary prophylaxis

Patients who have a cardiac arrest or demonstrate sustained VT following acute myocardial infarction are most usefully treated by amiodarone or sotalol, but the recent trials with AICDs may suggest that this approach is not necessarily the best. A meta-analysis of the major trials of secondary prevention showed a clear benefit of AICDs over amiodarone over a 6-year follow-up (Connolly et al, 2000). An AICD should be considered when there is:

- spontaneous ventricular tachycardia producing syncope or significant haemodynamic compromise;
- sustained ventricular tachycardia with left ventricular dysfunction (ejection fraction < 35%);
- patients with secondary (late) cardiac arrest.

The role of AICDs is discussed in Chapter 13.

References

ACE Inhibitor Myocardial Infarction Collaborative Group (1998) Indications for ACE inhibitors in the early treatment of acute myocardial infarction: systematic overview of individual data from 100,000 patients in randomized trials. *Circulation* 97: 2202–2212.

Andersen HR, Falk E, Nielsen D (1989) Right ventricular infarction: diagnostic accuracy of electrocardiographic right chest leads $V3_R$ to $V7_R$ investigated prospectively in 43 consecutive fatal cases from a coronary care unit. *British Heart Journal* 61: 514–520.

Armon MP, Hopkinson BR (1996) Thrombolysis for acute deep vein thrombosis. *British Journal of Surgery* 83: 580–581.

Birnbaum Y, Chamoun AJ, Anzuini A et al (2003) Ventricular free wall rupture following acute myocardial infarction. *Coronary Artery Disease* 14: 463–470.

Cairns JA, Connolly SJ, Roberts R et al (1997) Randomised trial of outcome of myocardial infarction in patients with frequent or repetitive ventricular depolarizations: Canadian Amiodarone Myocardial Infarction Arrhythmia Trial (CAMIAT). *Lancet* 349: 675–682.

Campbell RWF, Higham D, Adams P et al (1987) Potassium – its relevance for arrhythmias complicating acute myocardial infarction. *Journal of Cardiovascular Physiology* 10: S25–S27.

Connolly SJ, Hallstrom AP, Cappato R et al (2000) Meta-analysis of the implantable cardioverter defibrillator secondary prevention trials. *European Heart Journal* 21: 2071–2078.

Cooper N, Jacob B (2002) Biphasic positive pressure ventilation in acute cardiogenic pulmonary oedema. *British Journal of Cardiology* 9: 38–41.

CREATE-ECLA Investigators (2005) Effect of glucose-potassium-insulin infusion on mortality with acute ST-segment elevation myocardial infarction. *Journal of the American Medical Association* 293: 437–446.

Dressler W (1956) A post-myocardial infarction syndrome: preliminary report of a complication resembling idiopathic, recurrent, benign pericarditis. *Journal of the American Medical Association* 160: 1379–1383.

Fibrinolytic Therapy Trialists' Collaborative Group (1994) Indications for fibrinolytic therapy in suspected acute myocardial infarction: collaborative overview of early and major mortality from all randomised trials of more than 1000 patients. *Lancet* 343: 311–322.

Freemantle N, Cleland JG, Young P et al (2001) Beta-blockade after myocardial infarction: systematic review and meta-regression analysis. *British Medical Journal* 318: 1349–1355.

Goldberg RJ, Samad NA, Yarzebski J et al (1999) Temporal trends in cardiogenic shock complicating acute myocardial infarction. *New England Journal of Medicine* 340: 1162–1168.

Goldstein JA (1998) Right heart ischemia: patho-physiology, natural history, and clinical management. *Progress in Cardiovascular Diseases* 40: 325–341.

Griffin J (1996) *Deep Vein Thrombosis and Pulmonary Embolism*. London: Office of Health Economics.

GUSTO-I (1993) The effects of tissue plasminogen activator, streptokinase, or both on coronary-artery patency, ventricular function, and survival after acute myocardial infarction. The GUSTO Angiographic Investigators. *New England Journal of Medicine* 329: 1615–1622.

Hochman JS, Sleeper LA, Webb JG et al (1999) Early revascularization in acute myocardial infarction complicated by cardiogenic shock. SHOCK Investigators. *New England Journal of Medicine* 341: 625–634.

ISIS-2 Collaborative Group (1988) Randomised trial of intravenous streptokinase, oral aspirin, both or neither amongst 17,187 cases of suspected acute myocardial infarction. *Lancet* ii: 349–360.

Jowett NI (1999) Use of anti-coagulants in the treatment of deep vein thrombosis. *Prescriber* 6: 57–74.

Jowett NI, Thompson DR, Pohl JEF (1989) Temporary transvenous endocardial pacing: six years experience in one coronary care unit. *Postgraduate Medical Journal* 65: 211–215.

Jowett NI, Robinson CGF, Clow WM (1998) Invasive management of deep vein thrombosis. *Postgraduate Medical Journal* 74: 311–312.

Kantrowitz A, Tjonneland S, Freed PS et al (1968) Initial clinical experience with intra-aortic balloon pumping in cardiogenic shock. *Journal of the American Medical Association* 203: 113–118.

Keeley EC, Hillis LD (1996) Left ventricular mural thrombus after acute myocardial infarction. *Clinical Cardiology* 19: 83–86.

Killip T, Kimball JT (1967) Treatment of myocardial infarction in a coronary care unit: two years experience with 250 patients. *American Journal of Cardiology* 20: 457–464.

Kober L, Torp-Pedersen C, Carlsen JE et al (1995) A clinical trial of the angiotensin-converting-enzyme inhibitor trandolapril in patients with left ventricular dysfunction after myocardial infarction with clinical evidence of heart failure. Trandolapril Cardiac Evaluation (TRACE) study. *New England Journal of Medicine* 333: 1670–1676.

Kumar S, Roberts DH (2001) Intra-aortic balloon pulsation: an overview. *British Journal of Cardiology* 8: 658–663.

Lown B, Fakhro AM, Hood WB et al (1967) The coronary care unit: new perspectives and developments. *Journal of the American Medical Association* 199: 188–198.

McAlister FA, Stewart S, Ferrua S et al (2004) Multidisciplinary strategies for the management of heart failure patients at high risk for admission: a systematic review of randomized trials. *Journal of the American College of Cardiology* 44: 810–819.

Madias JE (2000) Killip and Forrester classifications. Should they be abandoned, kept, re-evaluated, or modified? *Chest* 117: 1223–1226.

Mahoney B, Smith W, Lo D et al (2005) Emergency interventions for hyperkalaemia. *Cochrane Database Systematic Reviews* CD003235.

Northridge D (1996) Furosemide or nitrates for acute heart failure? *Lancet* 347: 667–668.

Ohman EM, Califf RM, Topol EJ et al (1990) Consequences of re-occlusion after successful reperfusion therapy in acute myocardial infarction. *Circulation* 82: 781–791.

Pfeffer MA, McMurray JJ, Velazquez EJ for the Valsartan in Acute Myocardial Infarction Trial Investigators (2003) Valsartan, captopril, or both in myocardial infarction complicated by heart failure, left ventricular dysfunction, or both. *New England Journal of Medicine* 349: 1893–1906.

Pitt B, White H, Nicolau J et al (2005) Eplerinone reduces mortality 30 days after randomisation following acute myocardial infarction in patients with left ventricular systolic dysfunction and heart failure. *Journal of the American College of Cardiology* 46: 425–431.

Pizzetti F, Tarazza FM, Franzosi MG et al on behalf of the GISSI-3 Investigators (2001) Incidence and prognostic significance of atrial fibrillation in acute myocardial infarction: the GISSI-3 data. *Heart* 86: 527–532.

Pratt CM, Waldo AL, Camm AJ (1998) Can anti-arrhythmic drugs survive survival trials? *American Journal of Cardiology* 81: 24D–34D.

Ryan TJ, Anderson JL, Antman EM (1999) ACC/AHA guidelines for the management of patients with acute myocardial infarction. A report of the American College of Cardiology/American Heart Association task force on practice guidelines (Committee on management of acute myocardial infarction). *Circulation* 100: 1016–1030.

Sharon A, Shipirer I, Kaluski E et al (2000) High dose intravenous isosorbide dinitrate is safer and better than Bi-PAP ventilation combined with conventional treatment for severe pulmonary oedema. *Journal of the American College of Cardiology* 36: 832–837.

Stokes PH, Jowett NI (1985) Haemodynamic monitoring with the Swan–Ganz catheter. *Intensive Care Nursing* 1: 9–17.

Williams G, Wright DJ, Tan LB (2000) Management of cardiogenic shock complicating acute myocardial infarction: towards evidence based medical practice. *Heart* 83: 621–626.

Wu AH, Parsons L, Every NR et al (2002), Second National Registry of Myocardial Infarction. Hospital outcomes in patients presenting with congestive heart failure complicating acute myocardial infarction: a report from the second national registry of myocardial infarction (NRMI-2). *Journal of the American College of Cardiology* 40: 1389–1394.

Chapter **11**

Cardiopulmonary resuscitation

CARDIAC ARREST

Cardiorespiratory arrest occurs when there is sudden cessation of spontaneous respiration and circulation. In clinical practice, this implies either ventricular standstill (asystole) or ventricular fibrillation (VF), although there may be virtual circulatory arrest with profound bradycardias or ventricular tachycardia (VT). Pulseless electrical activity (PEA) describes a state in which normal electrical complexes continue to show on the electrocardiogram, but there is no effective pulse or blood pressure. This may occur in many conditions, including cardiac rupture or tamponade, severe haemorrhage, pulmonary embolism and electrolyte imbalance. During cardiac arrest, there is no effective cardiac contraction with a consequent lethal fall in cardiac output.

The majority of cardiac arrests occur outside hospital, and sudden death is usually due to a ventricular dysrhythmia, which may result from problems arising within the heart (e.g. acute coronary occlusion) or elsewhere in the body (e.g. hypovolaemia, hypoxia, stroke). Although most sudden and unexpected deaths in middle-aged and elderly individuals are attributed to cardiac disease, post-mortem examinations suggest that only about two-thirds of such deaths are cardiac in origin, with coronary artery disease and its complications accounting for the majority of deaths (Zheng et al, 2001). Common precipitating causes are acute myocardial ischaemia, valvular heart disease (especially aortic stenosis), cardiomyopathy, chronic obstructive airways disease and drugs.

In hospital, the three most common reasons for cardiac arrest in adults are cardiac dysrhythmias, acute respiratory failure and shock. An important and growing theme in resuscitation is that of *preventing* cardiac arrest rather than responding to this common medical emergency. A pattern of deterioration is often seen in the hours, or even days, before cardiopulmonary arrest, but is often unrecognised. Early warning scores, or 'calling criteria', have been adopted by many hospitals to assist in the early detection of prearrest deterioration (McArthur-Rouse, 2001), with personnel skilled in the care of the seriously ill actively seeking out, assessing and managing patients whose clinical state threatens cardiac arrest (Hodgetts et al, 2002). Once identified, these patients should be moved to areas where the level of care provided is matched to the level of sickness. Trying to manage severely ill patients on general wards increases morbidity and mortality (McQuillan et al, 1998). Outreach teams of critical care nurses can be effective in reducing ward deaths, postoperative events and the need for intensive care (Department of Health, 2003). In some hospitals, the traditional cardiac arrest team has been replaced by a medical emergency team (MET) of intensive care staff and acute physicians that responds, not only to patients in cardiac arrest, but also to those who become acutely unwell (Lee et al, 1995). Such teams may reduce the number of inappropriate cardiac arrest calls by improving the education of ward staff and identifying those cases in which resuscitation attempts would be futile (Smith & Nolan, 2002).

Coronary care units (CCUs) were developed primarily to treat ventricular fibrillation and other serious dysrhythmias in the first few hours following myocardial infarction. Unfortunately, most of these episodes occur before admission to hospital, and around three-quarters of all deaths from myocardial infarction occur after cardiac arrest in the community. This proportion is even higher in people under 55 years of age, in whom 91% of sudden cardiac deaths occur outside hospital. Many victims can survive if bystanders act immediately while ventricular fibrillation is still present, because successful resuscitation is unlikely once the rhythm has deteriorated to asystole. For every minute without cardiopulmonary resuscitation (CPR), survival decreases by 7–10%. When bystander CPR is provided, the decline in survival is more gradual and averages 3–4% per minute, and doubles or triples survival from witnessed cardiac arrest (Waalewijn et al, 2001).

Patients who suffer cardiac arrest outside hospital are relatively healthy, and are more likely to survive, whereas those in hospital usually have a serious underlying illness. On the other hand, many more cardiac arrests in hospital are monitored, and the speed to defibrillation is obviously faster. This is particularly so on coronary care, as well as on high-dependency and intensive treatment units (ITUs). Cardiac arrests occurring on the hospital wards do not have such a good outcome.

Simulated cardiac arrests may help in identifying any deficiencies or difficulties in resuscitation where patients are not being monitored (Sullivan & Guyatt, 1986). Although the chances of resuscitation should be optimal within hospital, there are often deficiencies in the knowledge of basic resuscitation skills in both nursing and medical staff (David & Prior-Willeard, 1993). One of the functions of the CCU and its specialist staff must be to help train personnel in the basic resuscitation procedures (Jowett & Thompson, 1988a). All hospital staff, whatever their work, need to learn the rudiments of CPR as it is one of the main life-saving procedures that can be carried out by everybody. In addition, junior medical staff and those in specialist areas (e.g. CCU, ITU or the emergency department) need to be checked on their proficiency at these basic skills, the use of simple equipment (oxygen, suction and airways) and defibrillation procedures (Royal College of Physicians, 1987). As staff become more senior and more experienced at attending arrests, increased confidence is not necessarily matched by an increase in skills, so that periods of retraining and retesting are required (Brown et al, 2006). The appointment of a resuscitation training officer (RTO) to address these problems helps to improve survival to discharge following cardiac arrest (McGowan et al, 1999).

In 2004, the Royal College of Anaesthetists, the Royal College of Physicians of London, the Intensive Care Society and the Resuscitation Council (UK) published 'Cardiopulmonary resuscitation standards for clinical practice and training in the UK', which provides hospitals with guidance on delivering an effective resuscitation service (Gabbott et al, 2005).

THE ETHICS OF RESUSCITATION

In 2001, the British Medical Association, the Resuscitation Council (UK) and the Royal College of Nursing updated their statement 'Decisions Relating to Cardiopulmonary Resuscitation' as a framework on which health trusts may build their own more detailed guidelines (see British Medical Association et al, 2001). The guidance avoids the term 'DNR' (do not resuscitate) in favour of 'DNAR' (do not attempt resuscitation) to highlight the fact that CPR is frequently unsuccessful and should not even be attempted in many, if not most, cases. Resuscitation should not be an automatic response to all cases of cardiorespiratory failure; it should be considered where it represents an appropriate part of a patient's management, but should not limit any other medical or nursing care (Shepardson et al, 1999).

Public education is essential to prevent misunderstanding over what resuscitation can achieve. Despite the best medical efforts, most resuscitation attempts fail and, while emergency cardiovascular care aims to preserve life and restore health, it must also relieve suffering and limit disability. CPR decisions made in haste may conflict with a patient's desires or best interests. Written information about resuscitation policies should be included in the general literature that is provided to patients at the time of, or prior to, admission, allowing them to express views on their care.

When is resuscitation inappropriate?

All life ends with cardiopulmonary arrest, and CPR is not a treatment for those who are dying. Resuscitation should never be attempted if a patient is found dead or if they are known to have a distressing or inevitably fatal illness. The age of the patient is immaterial. CPR is at best traumatic and invasive, and failed attempts do little to enhance the dignity of death and may subject the patient and relatives to added pain and misery (Candy, 1991). Those who have come to the end of their natural lives should be allowed to die as peacefully as possible. There are three common situations in which resuscitation is obviously inappropriate:

- when CPR is very unlikely to be effective;
- when it is known that the patient does not wish to receive CPR;
- where successful CPR would not result in a length or quality of life that would be in the patient's best interest.

Chances of success

The likelihood of survival following cardiac arrest is dependent on many variables, the most important of which are:

- where cardiac arrest takes place;
- the patient's overall physical fitness;

- the underlying pathology;
- the patient's condition after return of spontaneous circulation (ROSC).

CPR may succeed in as many as half of the patients in a CCU, but fails in 85–90% of patients in general medical wards, sometimes causing substantial damage to the victim. Survival in 2121 cases of adult cardiac arrest in one UK hospital was initially 38%, falling to 25% at 24 hours, 16% at discharge and 11% at 1 year (Cooper et al, 2006). The USA National Registry of Cardiopulmonary Resuscitation recorded an initial return of spontaneous circulation in 44% of 14 720 adult victims, with 17% surviving to hospital discharge (Peberdy et al, 2003). Of those who survive the initial cardiac arrest, half the long-term survivors of aborted sudden cardiac death are cognitively intact 6 months after resuscitation, but 25% have moderate to severe impairment in memory that often compromises independent life (Berek & Aichner, 1999). Memory loss and depression are common in resuscitated victims, with continuing anxiety over another cardiac arrest and an undignified death. Most surveys show that the general public have an unrealistic view of what can be achieved by modern CPR and the generally poor outcome even in those who survive (Jones et al, 2000).

Advance directives and living wills

Patient wishes with regard to treatment and resuscitation should always be respected, assuming that the individual can understand what it involves and can give valid consent or refusal. Advance directives can be used as an expression of a person's preferences, usually in the form of a written 'living will', rather than by recollections of conversations. Any advanced directive should constitute clear evidence of the individual's wishes, so that both carers and relatives may respect it and it permits legal enforcement if necessary.

DNAR orders

Current NHS guidelines suggest that staff should involve patients and their families in resuscitation decisions in accordance with local policies

(Department of Health, 2000). However, the practicalities of discussing resuscitation may be difficult, inappropriate or a source of anxiety to those nominated to do so. While discussion may help to improve communication and transparency, it is often not appropriate to burden the patent or family with such decisions when the clinical team is certain that resuscitation cannot help the patient (Regnard & Randall, 2005). Patients are often designated for resuscitation by default to avoid lengthy discussions or accusations of discrimination (Diggory et al, 2003).

All NHS establishments are required to have a policy on resuscitation and are expected to provide CPR unless a written decision has been made to the contrary. DNAR policies are usually poorly adhered to because they often do not make clinical sense and are operationally impossible (Aarons & Beeching, 1991). Patients do not have a right to futile interventions, nor do doctors have a duty to provide them on demand if there is no reasonable prospect of success (Saunders, 2001). Many European countries have no formal policy for recording DNAR decisions, and discussion with patients and their families is uncommon. Laws governing the use of DNAR forms and advance directives vary by jurisdiction, so providers should be aware of local regulations. The attending doctor must make the initial decision in the best interests of the patient, and should not refrain from making a DNAR order because full discussions have not taken place. While the views of the patient and their relatives may need to be considered, they cannot insist on provision of care that will not increase length or quality of life (Ebrahim, 2000). It is good practice to record DNAR orders in both medical and nursing notes, with the rationale for the order and details of any patient consultation. Such orders should be reviewed frequently and changed if there is any relevant change in the patient's condition or circumstances.

STANDARDS FOR CARDIOPULMONARY RESUSCITATION

The American Heart Association first published 'Standards for Cardiopulmonary Resuscitation and Emergency Cardiac Care' in 1973 and, despite little evidence base for the recommendations, they were generally followed around the world. In 1986, a group representing five Nordic countries joined the UK Resuscitation Council in producing guidelines more suited to European practice. The European Resuscitation Council (ERC) was officially established in 1989 as a multidisciplinary group representing many European countries, and it produced four sets of guidelines between 1992 and 1998. The International Liaison Committee On Resuscitation (ILCOR) was founded in 1992 with representatives from around the world, to provide international consensus, with resuscitation guidelines first published in August 2000 (AHA/ILCOR, 2000). The interpretation of these guidelines varies in different countries on the basis of local custom and availability of resources, but essentially uniform CPR guidelines now exist throughout the world. The latest consensus statement (ILCOR, 2005) and the guidelines drawn from it have been adopted by the Resuscitation Council (UK) without modification.

The major changes in this most recent guideline are:

- emphasis on delivery of effective chest compressions;
- a compression-to-ventilation ratio of 30:2;
- rescue breaths being given over 1 second and sufficient to produce visible chest movement;
- a single 200-J biphasic shock, rather than three stacked monophasic shocks for VF/VT arrest, followed by immediate CPR rather than a pulse or rhythm check.

The guidelines have become more comprehensive, dealing with cardiac arrest in a wide range of special circumstances, and emphasising prevention with recognition of the common prodromata of cardiac arrest. Ethical and legal aspects and the support of relatives are also covered.

PRINCIPLES OF RESUSCITATION

The basic resuscitation components of airway management, rescue breathing and external chest compression have been in practice for only 50 years. While early manual methods of ventilation (e.g. Holger–Neilson) were soon surpassed by 'mouth-to-mouth' resuscitation (Safar et al, 1958), support of the arrested circulation has changed little since early descriptions of closed chest cardiac massage (Kouwenhoven et al, 1960). Initially, it was believed that the heart was 'emptied' by being squeezed between the sternum and the thoracic spine, but we now know that it is actually compression of the whole chest that makes the heart and great vessels behave like a giant pump, propelling blood forward by the production of an intermittent pressure gradient between the inside of the chest and the rest of the body. The mitral and aortic valves remain open, but partial closure of the pulmonary valve, with collapse of the great veins, helps to prevent retrograde blood flow. The heart fills passively on chest recoil.

There are no reliable clinical criteria that can be used to assess the efficacy of chest compression. At best, chest compressions produce a coronary and cerebral perfusion that is only 30% of normal. Feeling for arterial pulses is common during resuscitation attempts but, because there are no valves in the inferior vena cava, retrograde blood flow into the venous system may produce pulsations that do not indicate arterial flow. Measuring end-tidal carbon dioxide in the intubated patient may be used as an indicator of cardiac output produced by chest compressions. During cardiac arrest, carbon dioxide continues to be generated throughout the body. When the circulation slows during CPR, not so much carbon dioxide is delivered to the lungs for excretion, and the end-tidal carbon dioxide concentration is low. If chest compressions are producing effective circulation and providing ventilation is reasonably constant, an increase in the end-tidal carbon dioxide concentration may reflect an improved cardiac output.

The quality of manual chest compression (both speed and depth) is limited by fatigue, so mechanical aids have been developed that rhythmically depress the sternum or circumferentially compress the chest to offer relief to rescuers during prolonged resuscitation attempts.

*Load-distributing band*s squeeze the chest by a pneumatically or electrically activated constricting band. The *Lund University cardiac arrest system* (LUCAS) depresses the sternum by means of a compressed gas-powered plunger mounted on a backboard. Active decompression is achieved by a suction cup that pulls the anterior chest upwards.

This increases venous return to the heart and, hence, increases cardiac output and subsequent coronary and cerebral perfusion pressures during the following compression phase.

Such devices may improve haemodynamics or short-term survival when used by well-trained providers, although no mechanical aid has consistently been shown to be superior to conventional CPR.

Defibrillation

Defibrillation works by depolarisation of a sufficiently large myocardial mass ahead of the intrinsic ventricular fibrillation (VF) depolarisation wave, making it refractory to conduction. With the application of a big enough electric shock, the whole myocardium is suddenly depolarised and waits for intrinsic pacemaker function to return, hopefully from the sino-atrial node. The use of an electric current to terminate VF in man was first reported in 1947 by Beck and colleagues, who applied a 120-volt shock directly to the ventricles. Later, an alternating current (AC) defibrillator was developed for terminating VF by passing a 720-volt shock across the chest (Zoll et al, 1956). By the 1960s, it was apparent that an alternating current physically harmed the heart, and Lown developed the first modern direct current (DC) defibrillator in 1962. This was smaller, rechargeable and (because lower currents were being employed) less likely to cause myocardial damage or precipitate dysrhythmias. These *monophasic* defibrillators have been the mainstay of external defibrillation for over four decades.

The necessity to reduce the size of defibrillators for implantation has now led to the development of *biphasic* defibrillators. This technology has not only allowed smaller units, but has also demonstrated that they are equally effective at reduced energies (Amato-Vealey, 2005). Unlike previous defibrillators that sent a high-energy electrical charge in a single direction, biphasic defibrillators use a self-reversing waveform. The current first flows in one direction for a specified duration and then reverses. On average, 65% less current is required for the equivalent effect, and biphasic shocks of 200 J are as safe and effective as monophasic shocks of 360 J (Tang et al, 2001).

The devices are smaller, lighter, less expensive and less demanding of batteries, with fewer maintenance requirements. Biphasic defibrillators are thus more efficient than monophasic defibrillators and, because fewer shocks are needed, skin burns are much less common (Page et al, 2002). Modern defibrillation does not damage the heart (Rao et al, 1999). Monophasic defibrillators are no longer being manufactured, although many remain in use.

Resistance to the electrical current (otherwise known as transthoracic impedance) is now widely accepted as an important predictor of successful defibrillation, and recent defibrillator development has therefore focused on overcoming this resistance, and enhancing the delivery of energy to the myocardium. Transthoracic impedance (TTI) varies considerably between patients as a result of many factors, including the energy selected, electrode size, paddle–skin coupling material and the distance between the skin electrodes (size of the chest). Modern biphasic defibrillators can alter the waveform delivered to the patient based on the patient's TTI using an impedance-compensated biphasic waveform. The defibrillator titrates the 'dose' by adjusting the amount and duration of current delivered, based on impedance measurements performed twice during every shock. This eliminates the need for increasing the energy for persistent VF recommended for monophasic defibrillators, although the optimal energy for the first shock has not yet been agreed. Current resuscitation guidelines suggest that initial energies of 150–200 J should be used, and the same or higher energies can be chosen for second and subsequent shocks. This wording is likely to cause much confusion. We would suggest that:

- All monophasic defibrillators should be taken out of service.
- All biphasic shocks for VF should start at 200 J.
- Higher energies are not mandatory.

Defibrillator design

The basic appearance of the defibrillator has not changed over many years, comprising a large capacitor for storing electrical energy and two conductive paddles for delivering a shock to the heart.

The energy delivered is measured in joules (volts × amps × time), and output is displayed on a meter. The two handheld paddles usually have buttons built into the handles for selection and delivery of the defibrillating shock. These paddles can act simultaneously as electrodes for electrocardiogram (ECG) monitoring ('quick-look paddles'). To help reduce TTI, improve contact and reduce skin burns, conductive gel pads are used. The paddles need to be placed firmly against the gel pads with at least 8 kg of pressure to prevent loss of current. It may be necessary to shave the chest prior to elective cardioversion. Hairy chests produce a higher TTI, because air is trapped between the electrode and skin.

Handheld defibrillator paddles are usually applied in the antero-anterior (AA) position, with one paddle applied close to the sternum over the right second–third intercostal space and the other just below the apex of the heart in the mid-axillary line (V6 electrode position). TTI is minimised when the apical electrode is under rather than over the female breast. Paddle position is important and, in particular, adequate separation of the paddles is needed to maximise the energy delivered through the heart, rather than across the skin (Fig. 11.1). Observational studies suggest that paddles are not positioned optimally in many cases, with a tendency to place the apical paddle anteriorly rather than laterally (Heames et al, 2001). With the introduction of defibrillator pads, electrode position can be varied, and other configurations may be used.

Defibrillator pads

Self-adhesive monitor/defibrillator electrode pads are an alternative to paddles, and can be used for monitoring and for rapid administration of a defibrillatory shock when necessary (Perkins et al, 2002). These allow 'hands-free' defibrillation of the patient from a safe distance rather than by leaning over them, with the additional advantage of conforming well to the chest contour to improve conduction. Although most pads are labelled left and right, or carry a diagram for their correct placement, it does not matter if they are reversed.

The electrode pads are usually positioned in the conventional AA position, with the right

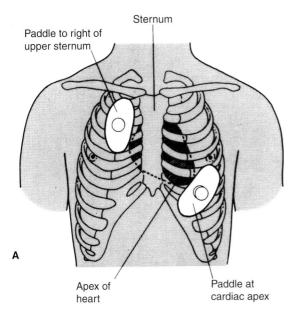

A

Sternum

Paddle to right of upper sternum

Apex of heart

Paddle at cardiac apex

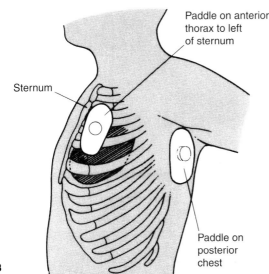

B

Paddle on anterior thorax to left of sternum

Sternum

Paddle on posterior chest

Figure 11.1 Positioning of defibrillation paddles for (A) a normal weight patient and (B) an obese patient (from Jowett and Thompson, 1988b; reproduced by kind permission of Churchill Livingstone).

(sternal) chest pad on the right infraclavicular region and the left pad placed lateral to the left breast. The left pad should be placed with its long axis vertical to improve efficiency (Deakin et al, 2003). An alternative configuration is the apico-posterior (AP) position placing one pad at the cardiac apex and the other to the right of the spine below the scapula. AP electrode placement may be more effective than the AA position in elective cardioversion of atrial fibrillation and in obese patients, but electrode position is probably much less important when using biphasic defibrillators (Kirchhof et al, 2002). Other variations have been described, such as right anterior to left posterior chest, and with the pads on the right and left lateral chest wall (bi-axillary), but there are no data showing the superiority of one configuration over the other.

Defibrillation in pacemaker patients

Modern pacemakers and implanted defibrillators have circuitry to protect against external defibrillation, although reports of pacemaker damage have been reported. Defibrillation pads should be placed away from the pulse generator (over 10 cm), or use the antero-posterior paddle positions if the generator is in the right infraclavicular area. Pacemaker function should be checked prior to discharge from hospital.

Automated external defibrillators (AEDs)

Automated external defibrillators are computerised devices that use auditory and visual prompts to guide rescuers to safe and appropriate defibrillation. Advances in technology, particularly with respect to battery capacity, and software dysrhythmia analysis have enabled the mass production of these reliable and easily operated portable defibrillators. The AED can be semi-automated (when the machine advises the responder to deliver a shock) or fully automated (where the device delivers the shock automatically). An algorithm for use of an AED during cardiac arrest is shown in Figure 11.2.

Healthcare providers should consider the use of an AED to be an integral part of basic life support. Public access defibrillation and first responder AED programmes may increase the number of victims who receive bystander CPR and early defibrillation, thus improving survival from out-of-hospital cardiac arrest (Public Access Defibrillation Trial Investigators, 2004).

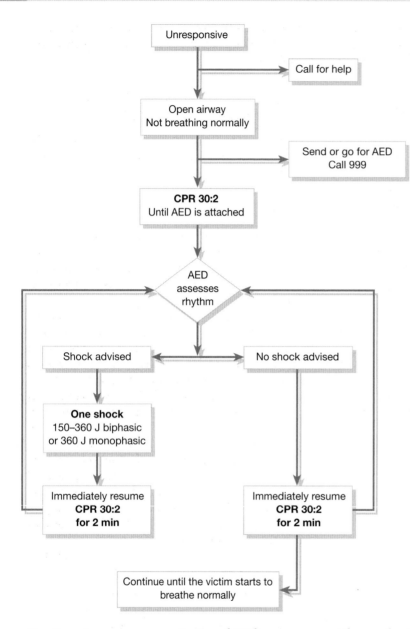

Figure 11.2 Management of cardiac arrest using an automated external defibrillator. Courtesy of the Resuscitation Council (UK).

Cardiopulmonary resuscitation (CPR)

There are four vital steps needed for successful resuscitation, sometimes referred to as the 'chain of survival'. The links in this chain are:

1 early recognition of cardiac arrest (or pre-arrest) and calling for help;
2 early basic life support;
3 early defibrillation;
4 early advanced life support and post-resuscitation care.

The emphasis in all phases is on 'early'. Prompt CPR and defibrillation instituted within 3–5 minutes of cardiac arrest can produce survival rates as high as 75%, but with each minute of delay in defibrillation, the probability of survival to discharge is reduced by 10–15% (Peberdy et al, 2003).

BASIC LIFE SUPPORT

Basic life support (BLS) refers to maintaining airway patency and supporting breathing and the circulation without the use of supportive equipment. It may include the use of protective devices, although the safety and effectiveness of barrier devices during basic life support is unknown. If simple airways or facemasks are used, the term 'BLS with airway adjunct' is sometimes used (Jowett & Thompson, 1988b).

Most patients who suffer a sudden cardiac arrest are found to be in ventricular fibrillation (VF), although many will have been in ventricular tachycardia (VT) at the time of collapse. With delay, the rhythm usually deteriorates into asystole. Many victims can survive if bystanders act immediately while VF is still present, but successful resuscitation is unlikely once the rhythm has deteriorated to asystole. The main objective of BLS is to provide oxygen to the vital organs (brain, heart and kidneys) until return of spontaneous circulation (ROSC) or until advanced life support can be initiated. While, at best, BLS in adults only provides 30% of normal cardiac output, this may be sufficient to protect the brain and extend the time window for effective defibrillation. The lungs can withstand long periods of anoxia, and the heart and kidneys can survive for 30 minutes before irreversible ischaemic changes result, but the cerebral cortex can only withstand anoxia for about 5 minutes. The critical factor in BLS, therefore, is speed.

The basic life support sequence in adults

If more than one person is present at the scene of a cardiac arrest, several actions can take place simultaneously. One or more rescuer can begin CPR while another telephones the arrest team and retrieves a defibrillator. The cardiac arrest team is usually summoned using a standard telephone number, although this has often varied in different hospitals. The UK Resuscitation Council and the National Patient Safety Agency (NPSA) have advised that a standard number for use in all NHS acute trusts should be 2222.

Basic life support has traditionally been taught by the 'ABC' sequence of airway, breathing and circulation but, as most patients who arrest have been breathing normally until collapse, arterial and tissue oxygenation will be near normal, and

initial resuscitation attempts should concentrate on establishing circulation. The ABC sequence now applies to:

1   opening the AIRWAY;
2   checking for spontaneous BREATHING;
3   starting chest COMPRESSIONS.

Within our hospital, we use another ABC reminder first to emphasise that safety and getting help are vital.

A = Ascertain arrest

An assessment phase must start with ensuring the safety of rescuer and patient. The next stage is the recognition and confirmation of cardiopulmonary arrest. The alternative term 'assess responsiveness' is sometimes used.

During cardiac arrest, there is ineffective mechanical activity of the heart, a reduced cardiac output and cerebral hypoperfusion. Confirmation of cardiac arrest may be difficult and often wastes time. Loss of consciousness, apnoea and loss of pulses occur within seconds, but other signs, such as cyanosis and dilatation of the pupils, take much longer and cannot be awaited. Heavy, noisy or gasping breathing (agonal gasps) occur in 40% of patients following cardiac arrest and may be mistaken for normal breathing. Checking arterial pulses is an inaccurate method of confirming the presence or absence of circulation. Following prolonged palpation in one study, 45% of carotid pulses were pronounced absent in normal volunteers (Priori et al, 2001). Hence, cardiac arrest must be assumed to have occurred with:

- any sudden loss of consciousness;
- seizure in a non-epileptic patient;
- acute onset of respiratory distress.

Other causes of sudden collapse may be responsible (e.g. syncope, cerebrovascular accidents, haemorrhage or epilepsy), but immediate CPR should still be instituted and is unlikely to be harmful.

B = Bang on chest

The *precordial thump* is not included in recommendations for BLS, but can be remarkably effective for witnessed or monitored cardiac arrests as might occur on the coronary care unit. It is often used by more experienced rescuers while the defibrillator is charging.

A sharp blow is delivered to the lower half of the sternum with the ulnar border of the fist from a height of about 20 cm (followed by immediate retraction), which creates an impulse wave and will convert about 40% of patients with ventricular tachycardia and 2% of patients with ventricular fibrillation into sinus rhythm.

Conscious patients with ventricular tachycardia may be returned to sinus rhythm by quickly raising the legs or placing the patient in the Trendelenberg position. A similar mechanical stimulus may be given by forceful coughing every 1–3 seconds for up to 90 seconds (cough CPR). Even if cardioversion does not occur, pressure changes in the chest can produce arterial pressures of 100 mmHg (Criley et al, 1976).

C = Call for help ('call first, call fast')

If a cardiac arrest is suspected, help will be required for basic and advanced resuscitation. The person first on the scene should immediately shout for help and make sure that an 'arrest call' is put out. If no one responds, it is better to leave the victim to get help, because it is the defibrillator that will save life. BLS is just a holding measure until help arrives.

The second ABC of basic life support

The second ABC refers to the basic resuscitation skills of opening the airway, checking for spontaneous breathing and initiating chest compressions.

A = Opening the airway

Effective CPR requires the patient to be supine and on a flat, firm surface (i.e. an arrest board or the floor) during chest compressions to optimise the effectiveness of compressions. The head must not be raised above the level of the thorax or the brain will not be perfused. If in bed, pillows and the backrest need to be removed, cot sides lowered and bed-brakes engaged.

The most important initial action is to open the airway (Fig. 11.3). The upper airway will be

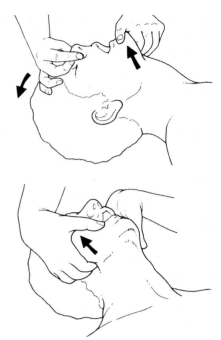

Figure 11.3 Opening the airway: the head-tilt/chin-lift and head-tilt/jaw-thrust methods.

obstructed in 90% of unconscious patients, usually by the tongue, which falls back into the pharynx when muscle tone is lost. As the tongue is attached to the lower jaw, moving the jaw forward will lift the tongue away from the back of the throat and open the airway. There are two main ways of doing this:

Head–tilt/chin–lift manoeuvre The head is tilted back by firm backward pressure on the patient's forehead with the palm of the hand. The fingers of the other hand are used to lift the chin forward so that the teeth almost close together. This supports the jaw and helps to hold the head back.

Head–tilt/jaw–thrust Grasping the angle of the jaw on both sides and tilting the head back will pull the mandible forward. This may be made easier if the rescuer's elbows are allowed to rest on the floor close to the patient's head.

The simplest method is the head-tilt/chin-lift method, although medically trained staff may find the head-tilt/jaw-thrust method more efficient. It is technically more difficult and tiring, but is highly effective and especially useful if neck injury is suspected, as it may be used without hyperextending the neck.

B = Check for spontaneous Breathing ('look–listen–feel').

The absence of respiration is deduced by the lack of chest movement and by listening and feeling for expired air from the patient's mouth and nose. It should take only a few seconds to:

- *look* for chest movement;
- *listen* at the victim's mouth for breath sounds;
- *feel* for air on your cheek.

If these are absent, resuscitation should start with chest compressions.

During the first few minutes after cardiac arrest, blood oxygen saturations remain high, and the immediate problem is delivery of blood to the vital organs, rather than problems with oxygenation. If there is no spontaneous breathing, artificial ventilation can wait, as it is less important than chest compressions in the early phase of cardiac arrest.

C = Chest compressions

Chest compression is considered to be the key to survival when defibrillation cannot be given within 4 or 5 minutes. After such a delay, defibrillation is not so effective because the myocardium becomes hypoxic and acidotic, with ventricular dilatation that hinders effective contraction. Chest compressions generate a small, but vital amount of blood flow to the myocardium and increase the likelihood that defibrillation will be successful. Hence, when resuscitation has been delayed by more than a few minutes, it is probably better to give compressions for up to 3 minutes before attempting defibrillation.

The key elements for chest compressions are:

- push hard, push fast;
- allow full chest recoil after each compression;
- do not allow (or minimise) any interruptions to continuous chest compressions.

Optimal chest compressions can produce systolic arterial pressure peaks of around 70 mmHg, although diastolic pressure remains low, and mean arterial pressure in the carotid artery seldom exceeds 40 mmHg. On stopping chest compressions, the coronary flow decreases substantially, and several compressions are necessary before the coronary flow recovers to its previous level (Kern et al, 2002). Chest compressions must be given without pauses.

The heel of the dominant hand is placed over the centre of the chest, and the non-dominant hand placed over the top, with the fingers either extended or interlocked (but not in contact with the chest). Pressure of the fingers on the ribs or lateral pressure increases the possibility of rib fractures or costochondral separation. The arms should be kept straight, with the elbows locked, so that pumping action is delivered in a straight line from the shoulders by pivoting at the hips to depress the sternum 4–5 cm in adults. The same amount of time should be allowed for compression and relaxation, and the chest should be allowed to recoil completely after each compression to allow the heart to refill. If pressure is not taken off the sternum, blood flow during the next compression will be reduced because the heart will not have filled adequately. Compressions should be smooth, regular and uninterrupted, at a rate of about 100/minute. All steps must be taken to minimise interruptions in chest compression. When more than one rescuer is present, rescuers should change 'compressor' roles about every 2 minutes or five cycles of CPR (one cycle of CPR = 30 compressions and two rescue breaths) to minimise fatigue, which may compromise high-quality CPR. Inadequate chest compression (rate or depth) and inadequate chest recoil may develop in as little as 1–2 minutes, although the rescuer may not appreciate this. Rescuers should try to complete the change over in less than 5 seconds. There is a need for training to avoid unnecessary interruptions to chest compressions such as pauses for ventilations, rhythm analysis and any additional time required by automated defibrillators to analyse rhythms.

If a co-ordinated heart rhythm is not achieved by immediate defibrillation, compressions should continue for a further 2 minutes to assist the recovery of effective cardiac contractions, rather than pausing to check cardiac rhythm. Subsequent shocks should only be given after additional cycles of chest compressions. The ratio of compressions to ventilations of 30:2 is recommended to give more time for chest compressions. Using a one-shock strategy may improve outcome by reducing interruption of chest compressions and maintaining a cardiac output.

Initial rescue breaths

After 30 chest compressions, mouth-to-mouth ventilation should commence, and many rescuers find this the most difficult intervention. Not only does the sight of vomit and blood usually deter the most hardened resuscitator, the theoretical transmission of infectious diseases such as serum hepatitis and AIDS (the acquired immune deficiency syndrome) have to be contended with, although there is actually very little evidence of disease transmission during mouth-to-mouth ventilation. Where there is reluctance to perform mouth-to-mouth ventilation, *chest compression-only CPR* may be as effective as combined ventilation and compression in the first few minutes (because of maintained oxygen saturations), and chest compression without ventilation is significantly better than doing nothing at all (Kern et al, 2002).

While maintaining the airway using the head-tilt/chin-lift technique, the victim's nose is pinched, and two slow breaths are delivered in succession (1 second each), with the lips sealed over the patient's mouth. Because blood flow to the lungs is substantially reduced, adequate ventilation perfusion ratios can be maintained with lower tidal volumes, and around 500–600 mL in an adult should be adequate, which is enough just to raise the chest visibly. Attempts at faster inflation simply force air down the oesophagus, leading to gastric dilatation, which promotes vomiting and limits full expansion of the lungs. It is therefore unnecessary to deliver a full, forced expiration, but rather a slow exhalation over 1–2 seconds to make the chest rise. Expiration of air should be heard when the chest falls. If chest movement does not occur despite adequate airway control, an obstruction, such as vomit or foreign bodies (e.g. dentures), may be present. Blind finger sweeping is unhelpful, but solid material in the airway should be removed if it can be seen.

While the use of equipment may be useful, basic resuscitation should never be neglected because of the absence of medical aids. The design of BLS does not require the use of equipment, although the highest priority must be given to early defibrillation. Once instituted, therapy should be continued until admission to a specialist unit or until a decision is made for life support to be terminated. An algorithm for basic life support is shown in Figure 11.4.

In hospital, there is often no clear division between BLS and advanced life support, and the exact sequence of actions after in-hospital cardiac arrest depends upon where the arrest takes place (clinical or non-clinical areas; monitored or unmonitored), the number and skill levels of the responders and what equipment is immediately

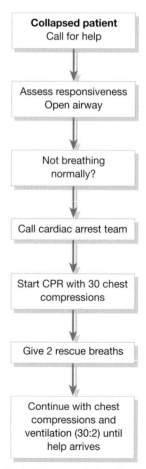

Figure 11.4   Basic life support algorithm.

available. Simple basic measures remain important until help arrives (Fig. 11.5). The presence of other members of staff nearby means it is usually possible to undertake several actions simultaneously depending upon their training and experience. The arrival of help should lead to advanced resuscitative measures, including:

- securing an airway (preferably with an endotracheal tube);
- augmentation of oxygenation with portable oxygen;
- recognition of cardiac rhythms with an ECG;
- treatment of dysrhythmias with drugs and electrical defibrillation;

- cardiovascular stabilisation to allow transport of the patient to a high-dependency unit.

ADVANCED LIFE SUPPORT

Advanced life support (ALS) combines BLS with the use of specialist techniques and equipment for maintaining circulation and respiration. The key components are:

- early defibrillation;
- ensuring an adequate airway;
- establishing intravenous access;
- electrocardiographic monitoring;
- pharmacological therapy.

On coronary care and other high-dependency units, the arrest is likely to be witnessed or monitored, and the usual response here is therefore:

- Confirm cardiac arrest and shout for help.
- Give a precordial thump (if the rhythm is VF/VT) while the defibrillator is being charged.
- Defibrillate immediately (200 J biphasic).

Immediate defibrillation has always been a key to successful resuscitation but, outside specialised units, this is usually not possible. When the delay to defibrillation exceeds 5 minutes, a period of chest compressions before defibrillation may improve survival (Eftestol et al, 2004).

Airway management

The airway can be cleared in most patients by correct positioning of the head and neck and suction. A wide-bore rigid sucker (Yankauer) may be used to remove blood, saliva and gastric contents from the upper airway, although this may provoke vomiting if the patient has an intact gag reflex. Oropharyngeal and nasopharyngeal airways may be used to overcome backward displacement of the soft palate and tongue in an unconscious patient, but head-tilt and jaw-thrust may also be required. Oropharyngeal airways should be used only in unconscious patients, as they may otherwise induce vomiting. In patients who are not deeply unconscious, a nasopharyngeal airway is tolerated better than an oropharyngeal airway.

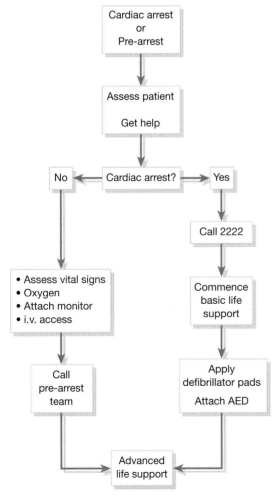

Figure 11.5   Management of in-hospital cardiac arrest.

Care and practice is required for correct insertion, or the tongue may be displaced backwards into the pharynx and obstruct the airway.

As expired air has fractional inspired oxygen (FiO_2) of only about 18%, enrichment with portable oxygen is required. A standard oxygen mask with a high flow of oxygen will deliver a concentration of about 50–60%, but a mask with a reservoir bag is preferable, giving concentrations of 80–90% with oxygen flows of around 10 L/minute. Bag-mask ventilation is particularly helpful during the first few minutes of resuscitation, but requires adequate training and frequent practice. Other than anaesthetists, many rescuers find that successful application of bag-mask ventilation needs two people to be effective. One rescuer maintains the jaw-thrust position and ensures a tight seal between the mask and the patient's face, while the other inflates the lungs by squeezing the bag with a tidal volume sufficient to make the chest rise when delivered over 1 second (400–600 mL). During the first phase of CPR, two inflations are given during a brief (about 3–4 seconds) pause after every 30 chest compressions. The main disadvantage of mask ventilation is gastric distension, leading to diaphragmatic splinting and oesophageal regurgitation.

Advanced airways

There are risks and benefits of insertion of an advanced airway during resuscitation. Because insertion of an advanced airway may require interruption of chest compressions for many seconds, the rescuer should weigh the need for continued compressions against the need for insertion of an advanced airway. It is better to perform about five cycles of CPR after shock delivery before attempts to insert an advanced airway.

The optimal method of managing the airway during cardiac arrest is by endotracheal intubation, but this requires training and repeated practice to maintain speed and success. Alternative airways are available that can be inserted without direct visualisation of the upper airway, and these may therefore be appropriate when the endotracheal route has failed or the expertise or equipment for its use is not to hand.

The laryngeal mask airway (LMA) consists of a plain flexible tube with a distal inflatable silicone ring attached (Fig. 11.6A). The ring is designed to obliterate the hypopharynx and oesophagus, achieving a low-pressure seal between the tube and trachea and reducing the risk of gastric regurgitation and aspiration. The LMA is relatively easy to insert, and is valuable for those unskilled in endotracheal intubation, and may even be chosen as an alternative in cases of difficult intubation because of anatomical problems (Baskett, 2001). The ProSeal LMA is a modification to the standard LMA. It is slightly more difficult to insert, but an improved seal to the larynx enables ventilation at higher airway pressures.

The Combitube is a double-lumen tube, with two balloons, one helping to stabilise the tube in the trachea for ventilation and the other larger proximal balloon occluding the hypopharynx (Fig. 11.6B). The Combitube is inserted blindly along the tongue, rather than along the palate as with the LMA, and gives similar airway protection (Urtubia et al, 2000).

Endotracheal intubation

An endotracheal tube is the best means of securing and maintaining an airway, ensuring delivery of high concentrations of oxygen and providing an alternative route for drug administration. The main problem with endotracheal intubation is that it requires skill, and unsuccessful attempts may delay or interrupt chest compressions. Misplaced tubes may also pass unrecognised. The risks and benefits of intubation need to be weighed against the interruption to effective chest compressions.

Endotracheal tubes are labelled with the internal diameter in millimetres. Female patients will require the 7.0- to 8.0-mm size, and male patients the 8.0- to 9.0-mm. Passage of the tube may sometimes be aided by external pressure on the cricoid cartilage (the Sellick manoeuvre), which occludes the upper part of the oesophagus and prevents the aspiration of gastric contents (Sellick, 1961). Cricoid pressure should only be applied by trained personnel, as excessive force can make intubation more difficult. The position of the tube should be verified by watching for equal expansion of both sides of the chest and listening over the lungs with a stethoscope.

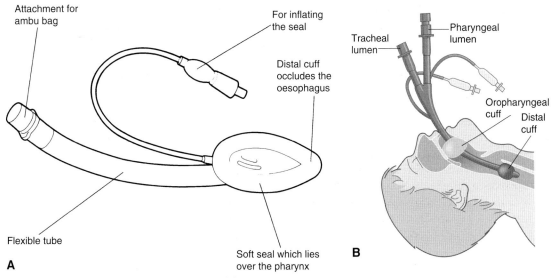

Figure 11.6   (A) The laryngeal mask airway. (B) The Combitube.

When an advanced airway is in place, rescuers should deliver 8–10 breaths/minute during CPR. Each breath is delivered over about 1 second, while chest compressions are delivered at a rate of 100/minute without pauses. It is not necessary to attempt to synchronise the compressions with the ventilations. If a perfusing heart rhythm is achieved, the respiratory rate can be increased to 10–12/minute (one breath every 6–7 seconds). Key aspects of performing CPR after insertion of the advanced airway are shown in Box 11.1.

Intravenous access

Intravenous access is needed for the administration of fluids and drugs. Peripheral lines are the simplest, as peripheral veins are easily seen, despite their tendency to collapse following cardiac arrest. The site of choice is the antecubital fossa, as cannulation of the subclavian and neck veins needs practice and may require a temporary halt to CPR. Peripheral administration of drugs may take between 1 and 2 minutes to reach the heart, even with optimal chest compressions. The process may be made faster by flushing with at least 20 mL of 0.9% saline, followed by elevation of the extremity for 10–20 seconds to facilitate delivery into the central circulation.

A central line provides the optimal route for delivering drugs into the central circulation, but placement may be difficult and could cause complications. *Intraosseous (IO) cannulation* provides access to a non-collapsible venous plexus, enabling drug delivery similar to that achieved by central venous access. Commercially available kits can facilitate IO access in adults if intravenous access is unavailable (Macnab et al, 2000). It provides effective vascular access for fluid resuscitation, drug delivery and blood sampling in all age groups.

Regardless of the aetiology of the arrest, increased vascular permeability allows plasma proteins and water to pass into the extravascular spaces, leading to intravascular hypovolaemia. However, in the absence of hypovolaemia, infusion of an excessive volume of fluid is likely to be harmful by causing an increase in right atrial pressure relative to aortic pressures, which reduces coronary arterial perfusion pressures. Expansion of circulating blood volume is, of course, critical in patients with severe acute blood loss, and cardiac arrest in these patients is often marked by pulseless electrical activity (see below). There are no clear advantages in using colloids over crystalloids. Dextrose should be avoided as it rapidly redistributes away from the intravascular space

---

Box 11.1 Key aspects of resuscitation after insertion of an advanced airway.

- Ensure the advanced airway is in the right position:

Helpful	**Unhelpful**
Equal chest expansion	Chest movement
Equal breath sounds in both axillae	Breath sounds close to sternum
No breath sounds in epigastrium	Condensation in tube

- Continuous chest compression at a rate of 100/minute without pauses for ventilation (8–10/minute)
- Excessive ventilation (rate or volume) may compromise venous return and cardiac output
- Those providing chest compression should change approximately every 2 min to prevent fatigue and deterioration in the quality and rate of chest compressions

---

and may contribute to hyperglycaemia, which can worsen neurological outcome after cardiac arrest.

Drug therapy

The value of drug therapy for the treatment of cardiac arrest is minimal, and the importance of BLS with early defibrillation cannot be stressed enough. Few drugs are needed during the immediate management of a cardiac arrest. Given that there is now international agreement, the contents of cardiac arrest boxes can be rationalised and standardised with regard to content and appearance (Jowett et al, 2001).

Pharmacological intervention may be used to:

- correct hypoxia and acidosis;
- accelerate or reduce the heart rate;
- suppress ectopic activity;
- stimulate the strength of myocardial contraction.

Because of the haemodynamic changes during CPR, the administration of drugs into the central circulation is preferable, although gaining access is often difficult and should not be allowed to hinder BLS or defibrillation.

Adrenaline (epinephrine)

Adrenaline has strong alpha- and beta-adrenergic agonist activity. Alpha-agonist action causes peripheral vasoconstriction, which helps to divert blood to the brain and coronary vessels. The beta-agonist

properties (positive chronotropic and inotropic effects) help myocardial function following attainment of sinus rhythm. Regardless of the arrest rhythm, adrenaline 1 mg (10 mL of a 1:10 000 solution) is given every 3–5 minutes.

Vasopressin

Vasopressin was first suggested as an alternative vasopressor agent 10 years ago, but evidence has not yet shown any advantage over adrenaline (Aung & Htay, 2005). Where conventional adrenergic vasopressor drugs are ineffective (e.g. noradrenaline, dopamine), a continuous infusion of vasopressin may be beneficial.

Sodium bicarbonate

With effective BLS, deterioration in blood gases and pH is slow in previously well patients. With prolonged resuscitation, particularly in those who may have been unwell prior to cardiac arrest, an effort to combat the metabolic acidosis that accompanies poor tissue perfusion is needed. Acidosis results from the build up of lactic acid and, with increased levels of carbon dioxide, depresses myocardial contractility, produces vasodilatation and capillary leakage and inhibits catecholamine activity, increasing the likelihood of dysrhythmias.

Intravenous sodium bicarbonate has been widely used in the past for correcting the metabolic acidosis during cardiac arrest, but there is little evidence that this therapy improves outcome. Hence, routine administration of sodium bicarbonate is no longer recommended because of the frequent occurrence of deleterious side effects, including increasing carbon dioxide levels, hypernatraemia, inactivation of concurrently administered catecholamines and tissue necrosis if accidentally given extravascularly.

Critically ill patients in hospital may warrant early therapy with sodium bicarbonate if there is developing hyperkalaemia or acidosis that might precede a cardiac arrest, for example:

- severe acidosis (pH < 7.1);
- cardiac arrest associated with hyperkalaemia;
- cardiac arrest associated with tricyclic antidepressant overdose;
- blind administration after prolonged resuscitation (10–20 minutes).

The principal method of correcting acidosis is by establishing adequate ventilation. Hyperventilation corrects respiratory acidosis by removing carbon dioxide, which diffuses freely across cellular membranes. Optimal oxygenation, ventilation and airway control are therefore vital.

Antidysrhythmic agents

When considering these drugs, there are certain basic principles:

- Electrical cardioversion is preferable in most cases, and especially if the patient is unstable.
- All drugs used for treating dysrhythmias are potentially pro-arrhythmic.
- Most drugs impair myocardial function.
- Cocktails of different agents are dangerous.

Amiodarone

Amiodarone (300 mg bolus) is used in refractory ventricular fibrillation (i.e. after three shocks). A further dose of 150 mg may be given for recurrent or refractory VF/VT. Prefilled syringes are available. These initial doses may be followed by an infusion of 1 mg/minute for 6 hours and then 0.5 mg/minute to a maximum of 1.2 g in 24 hours. Intravenous amiodarone may worsen hypotension, related to both the rate of delivery and its solvent (Polysorbate 80), which causes histamine release. Aqueous amiodarone is relatively free from these side effects, but is not widely available.

Magnesium

Magnesium should be given for refractory VF or VT if there is any suspicion of hypomagnesaemia. This may be assumed if patients have been taking potassium-losing diuretics. Magnesium also has a role in digoxin toxicity and torsades-de-pointes. The intravenous dose is 2 g (4 mL of 50% magnesium sulphate) peripherally over 1–2 minutes, repeated if required after 10–15 minutes.

Lidocaine

Lidocaine has been used for many years for the control of ventricular dysrhythmias complicating cardiac arrest and myocardial infarction. Its major action during cardiac arrest is to inhibit the initiation of re-entry dysrhythmias in the ischaemic myocardium, but its use makes defibrillation more difficult. Until 2000, lidocaine was the antidysrhythmic drug of choice for VT/VF, but it is now recommended only when amiodarone is unavailable. Lidocaine should not be given in addition to amiodarone.

When used, bolus therapy at a dose of 0.5 mg/kg every 10 minutes is usual. Reduced hepatic circulation may make lidocaine toxicity more likely, and no more than 3 mg/kg should be administered.

Atropine

Atropine is indicated in:

- asystole;
- pulseless electrical activity (PEA) with a rate under 60 beats/minute;
- bradycardia causing haemodynamic problems.

Atropine lowers vagal tone, although its value after the first few minutes following cardiac arrest is unclear, as significant vagotonia is unlikely to be present. However, a single dose of 3 mg is still recommended in asystolic and bradycardic arrest to ensure that vagal tone is fully blocked. Repeat doses should be avoided, as they may reduce the electrical stability of the heart, making ventricular fibrillation more likely (Cooper & Abinader, 1979). For symptomatic bradycardia, aliquots of 500 µg may be given to a total dose of 3 mg.

Aminophylline

Aminophylline causes release of adrenaline from the adrenal medulla, and it has chronotropic and inotropic actions. Its value in cardiac arrest is debatable, but 250 mg given by slow intravenous injection may be tried in asystolic cardiac arrest or periarrest bradycardia refractory to atropine (Abu-Laban et al, 2006).

Calcium

Although calcium ions play a critical role in myocardial contractility and impulse formation, no benefit has been shown from the administration of calcium during CPR. An initial dose of 10 mL of 10% calcium chloride is suggested in PEA associated with:

- hyperkalaemia;
- hypocalcaemia;
- overdose of calcium channel-blocking drugs.

Transbronchial administration of drugs

If intravenous access cannot be established, some drugs can be given by the tracheal route, although unpredictable plasma concentrations are achieved, and the optimal tracheal dose of most drugs is unknown. Drug absorption is impaired by pulmonary oedema, atelectasis and, perhaps, the drugs themselves; for example, adrenaline causes local vasoconstriction. After instillation of transbronchial drugs, five inflations should be given to aid distribution and absorption.

Adrenaline can be given down the endotracheal tube using three times the intravenous dose (3 mg), diluted with 5–10 mL of water. Lidocaine can also be given in this way. Its onset of action is as rapid as an intravenous bolus, and its effect is twice as long. Other agents that can be given transbronchially are atropine and naloxone. Bicarbonate, calcium carbonate, amiodarone and noradrenaline must not be given via the endotracheal tube, as they are very irritant to the tissues.

Putting it all together – the resuscitation algorithm

The current adult advanced life support resuscitation algorithm is shown in Figure 11.7. Each step assumes that the preceding step has been unsuccessful. Attention must be focused on high-quality, uninterrupted basic life support, which should be instituted if the defibrillator arrival is delayed (Jowett & Thompson, 1988a). As soon as the defibrillator arrives, the arrest rhythm may be confirmed by applying paddles or self-adhesive pads to the chest.

The treatment pathways essentially follow one of two directions: 'shockable rhythms (VF/VT)' or 'non-shockable rhythms (PEA/asystole).

Shockable rhythms

Defibrillation is the cornerstone of advanced resuscitation (Zoll et al, 1956), and the earlier this is performed, the more likely sinus rhythm is to result. Any delay allows further myocardial ischaemia, anoxia and acidaemia, which will inhibit the restoration of normal rhythm. A period of chest compressions before defibrillation is desirable if there has been a delay in getting the machine to the patient. All initial shocks are given at 200 J biphasic, followed by 2 minutes of chest compressions before additional shocks are delivered. If VT/VF persists, further shocks are given at 200 J or more. There is no evidence to support either a fixed or an escalating energy protocol.

Irrespective of the outcome of defibrillation, chest compressions and ventilations should be resumed immediately to maintain circulation. Time should not be wasted in waiting to see the results on the monitor or feeling for pulses. If the patient is still in VF/VT, any delay in compressions will further compromise the myocardium. On the other hand, if cardioversion has been successful, additional compressions will not do any harm, and will support circulation until co-ordinated contraction is established. CPR (30:2 compressions to breaths) is continued for a further 2 minutes before the rhythm is rechecked.

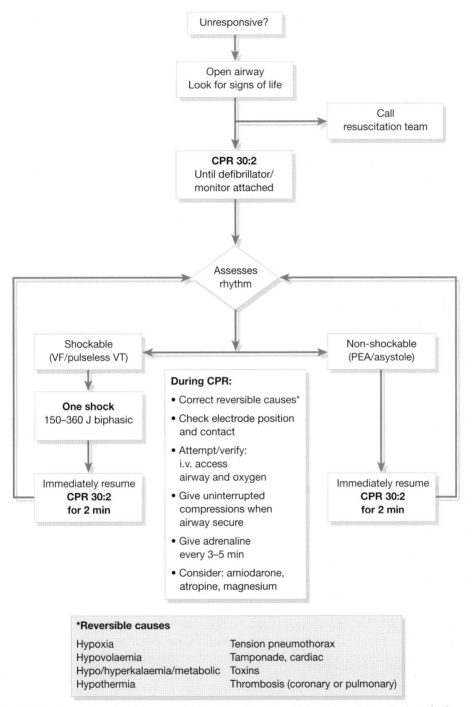

Figure 11.7 Adult advanced cardiac life support algorithm. Courtesy of the Resuscitation Council (UK).

If an advanced airway (e.g. endotracheal tube) has been inserted, ventilations should be given at 8–10 ventilations/minute with continuous compressions at 100/minute. If the patient is still in VF/VT after 2 minutes, a second shock is given, and CPR is started again without delay. If the dysrhythmia persists after a further 2 minutes of CPR, 1 mg of adrenaline is given followed by further chest compressions to circulate the adrenaline, followed by the third shock.

If normal rhythm has not returned after the initial three shocks, the chances of recovery are less than 20%. If it is thought appropriate to continue resuscitation, priorities must change to preserving cerebral and myocardial perfusion. This is best done by administration of adrenaline, combined with CPR. The ventricular fibrillation algorithm, therefore, enters a loop, which includes administration of 1 mg of adrenaline every 3 minutes, further ventilation and further shocks. It is important that potential causes or aggravating factors such as toxins or electrolyte imbalance are considered (Box 11.2).

Life beyond the third cycle?   Regardless of the arrest rhythm, adrenaline 1 mg should be given every 3–5 minutes; this will be once every two loops of the algorithm.

- If VT/VF persists after three shocks, an intravenous bolus of amiodarone 300 mg should be given, followed by a brief rhythm analysis before delivery of the next shock.
- If a rhythm check reveals an organised rhythm (complexes appear regular or narrow), a palpable output should be sought, although chest

compressions should not be stopped (unless the patient shows signs of recovery).

- If the patient's rhythm changes to asystole or PEA, the non-shockable recommendations should be followed.

Non-shockable rhythms

Asystole is characterised by ventricular standstill due to suppression of the cardiac pacemakers by myocardial disease, anoxia, electrolyte imbalance or drugs. Strong cholinergic activity may depress the sinus and AV nodes following myocardial infarction or episodes of myocardial ischaemia. Asystole may occur without warning, or may be preceded by various degrees of heart block, and is found in about 25% of hospital cardiac arrest (10% outside hospital). It often represents massive cardiac damage and sometimes appears as the last dying rhythm of the heart following prolonged ventricular fibrillation. Survival is less than 4%. The ECG shows a flat trace, which must be differentiated from faulty connection of the leads and problems with the gel pads. Modern defibrillators often show loose leads by a 'broken line' trace but, after one or more defibrillatory shocks, an electrical peculiarity may occur within the gel, so that the monitor may show a continuous or broken straight line, even when ventricular fibrillation is still present.

While previous recommendations have emphasised differentiation of asystole from fine VF, this is no longer considered important. If the VF is difficult to distinguish from asystole, it will not be coarse enough to cardiovert into a perfusing rhythm. Continuing good-quality CPR may improve the amplitude and frequency of the VF and improve the chance of successful defibrillation. Delivering repeated shocks in an attempt to defibrillate what is thought to be fine VF will increase myocardial injury, both directly from the electricity and indirectly from the interruptions in coronary blood flow.

Whenever a diagnosis of asystole is made, the ECG should be checked carefully for the presence of P waves, indicating ventricular standstill rather than asystole. External cardiac percussion ('thump' pacing) involves soft blows over the cardiac apex (not the sternum) at 100/minute that may

---

Box 11.2   The '4 H's' and '4 T's' – common precipitants of cardiac arrest.

Hypoxia
Hypovolaemia (e.g. severe haemorrhage)
Hyperkalaemia, hypocalcaemia, acidaemia
Hypothermia (e.g. drowning)

Tension pneumothorax
Tamponade
Toxins
Thromboembolism

generate QRS complexes with cardiac output if cardiac contractility is not severely compromised (Dowdle, 1996). This may be utilised until pacing can be instituted. There is no benefit in attempting to pace true asystole.

Pulseless electrical activity (PEA) is characterised by regular complexes on the ECG in the absence of any palpable pulse. It was previously known as electromechanical dissociation (EMD). The occurrence of PEA following myocardial infarction usually signifies a terminal event, such as rupture of the heart or cardiac tamponade. PEA is rare outside hospital practice, but occurs in about 5% of hospital cardiac arrests. The prognosis is very poor. The patient's best chances of survival depend upon identification and treatment of the underlying problem.

Treatment of non-shockable rhythms If the rhythm is unshockable (asystole, fine VF or PEA), CPR is commenced as usual with a compression/ventilation ratio of 30:2, and adrenaline 1 mg is given as soon as intravascular access is achieved. This should be followed by a single dose of atropine 3 mg at the end of the first CPR cycle. After 2 minutes of CPR, the rhythm may be checked.

- If there is no change in the ECG appearance, CPR should continue, with adrenaline being give every 3–5 minutes. One dose of vasopressin (40 U intravenously) may be substituted for either the first or the second dose of adrenaline.
- If the rhythm changes to VF, the 'shockable rhythm' protocol should be followed (the left side of the algorithm).
- If an organised rhythm is present, an effective pulse should be sought. If no pulse is present (or if there is any doubt about the presence of a pulse), CPR is continued. If a pulse is present, begin post-resuscitation care.

WHEN TO STOP

The decision to terminate resuscitation is a medical one, and should be made by the most senior physician present, in consultation with other members of the resuscitation team. This decision should follow an assessment of the patient's cerebral and cardiovascular status, as well as prognosis. Witnessed collapse or monitored cardiac arrest with a short time to arrival of professional CPR improves the chances of a successful resuscitation.

A poor outcome is usual in:

- unwitnessed arrests;
- delay to BSL of over 6 minutes;
- delay to first shock of more than 8 minutes;
- no response after 20 minutes of ALS;
- asystole/PEA.

Patients with non-VF arrests seldom recover after 15–20 minutes unless the arrest was associated with drugs or hypothermia. For those with persistent VF, the situation is potentially reversible, but outcome remains poor. Prolonged resuscitation is seldom justified; the mortality following an arrest of over 15 minutes is 90%.

Patients with hypothermia are a special group, and may still recover after prolonged resuscitation, and attempts should continue until the core temperature is over 36°C and the arterial pH and serum potassium are normal. Some drug overdose patients may also warrant prolonged resuscitation attempts.

Family members are usually excluded during attempted resuscitation despite suggestions that many wish to be present (Boyd, 2000). Those who have been at an unsuccessful resuscitation attempt may gain solace from being present at the moment of death, easing their own grieving. Resuscitation team members should be sensitive to the presence of family members during resuscitative efforts, and should assign a team member to answer questions and provide emotional support.

Periarrest dysrhythmias

Cardiac dysrhythmias are a common complication of acute myocardial infarction. They may precede VF or follow successful defibrillation. Dysrhythmias in the periarrest period may need treatment to prevent recurrent cardiac arrest or to obtain haemodynamic stability after resuscitation. The choice of treatment depends on the nature of the dysrhythmia and the overall status of the patient. The presence or absence of adverse signs or symptoms will dictate the appropriate treatment for most rhythm disturbances. Treatment is usually advised if there is excess tachycardia or bradycardia, and particularly if there is evidence of low cardiac output or heart failure. Oxygen is always needed in the periarrest period, and close attention should be paid to the correction of electrolyte abnormalities.

If the patient is stable, a 12-lead ECG should be obtained and evaluated. It is sometimes better to await expert consultation, because pharmacological treatment often has the potential for harm. Management of peri-infarction rhythm disturbances is covered in Chapter 10, and dysrhythmias unassociated with recent myocardial infarction in Chapter 12.

POST-ARREST MANAGEMENT

Full recovery from cardiac arrest is rarely immediate, and can only be said to have occurred when the patient is fully conscious, with full cardiac, cerebral and renal function. These will be more likely if prompt CPR and defibrillation are carried out and if the underlying dysrhythmia was ventricular fibrillation. Following successful resuscitation, the patient's condition may be broadly classified into four groups:

- Immediate recovery with no sequelae.
- Unconscious for a few hours. These patients will often suffer anxiety, confusion, delusions and difficulty in concentrating for several months.
- Unconscious for more than 24 hours. These patients often exhibit signs of spasticity, stroke or inco-ordination. The prognosis is variable.
- Decerebrate. Death is usual within a few days.

After stabilisation, all standard care should be given (preferably in a high-dependency environment), although the amount of care patients require following a cardiac arrest varies enormously (Box 11.3). Interventions in the post-resuscitation period can influence the prognosis significantly (Langhelle et al, 2003). Following the return of a spontaneous circulation, it is neurological function that usually influences survival. Two-thirds of those who arrest outside hospital and a quarter of those who arrest in hospital die from neurological injury. Most post-resuscitation deaths occur during the first 24 hours.

Box 11.3 First steps after resuscitation.

1 Check ventilation is adequate:
   - Endotracheal tube is correctly placed
   - 100% oxygen
2 Obtain blood gases and potassium
3 Insert urinary catheter
   - Measure hourly output
4 Insert nasogastric tube
   - Aspirate gas and fluid
5 Obtain ECG and chest radiograph
6 Consider the need for low-dose dopamine infusion

The post-resuscitation period is associated with a marked increase in blood cytokine concentrations, resulting in multiple organ dysfunction. The patient should be examined to assess haemodynamic status and to look for complications of the resuscitation procedure, such as bleeding (especially in thrombolysed patients) or aspiration of gastric contents or pneumothorax (secondary to rib fracture or central venous catheterisation). An underlying cause for the arrest, such as hypoxia, electrolyte imbalance or drug toxicity, should be considered. Elective ventilation and prophylactic drug therapy may be required. The post-resuscitation period is often marked by haemodynamic instability as well as biochemical and haematological abnormalities. Sepsis is a potentially fatal complication. Renal failure and pancreatitis are common and transient, but require recognition and appropriate treatment.

Special attention should be given to the following.

Cardiovascular system

The ischaemia and reperfusion following cardiac arrest and the effects of electrical defibrillation can cause global myocardial stunning and dysfunction that usually lasts 24–48 hours, but can last for several days or weeks. Haemodynamic instability is common, with hypotension and recurrent dysrhythmias, and early death due to multiorgan failure is more likely where there is a persistently low cardiac output in the first 24 hours after resuscitation. An adequate blood pressure and cardiac output must be obtained to allow renal, coronary and cerebral perfusion. Cerebral autoregulation will be impaired, and both cerebral hypoperfusion and oedema need to be avoided. Invasive monitoring may be necessary to measure blood pressure accurately and to determine the most appropriate combination of medications to optimise blood flow and distribution (Stokes & Jowett, 1985).

Respiratory system

Ventilation/perfusion (VQ) defects are common in both lungs following resuscitation, and oxygen therapy is usual. Hypoxia and hypercapnoea both increase the likelihood of a further cardiac arrest and may contribute to secondary brain injury. Pulse oximetry is helpful, but arterial blood gases and pH should be measured immediately, and periodically afterwards. Some patients will remain dependent on mechanical ventilation. There is no evidence that hyperventilation protects the brain or other vital organs from further ischaemic damage after cardiac arrest. A chest radiograph is needed to exclude pneumothorax, aspiration or bleeding into the pleural cavity.

Renal system

Adequate renal perfusion must be obtained as a priority and should produce 40–50 mL of urine per hour. Catheterisation of the bladder will usually be required, with urine output measured at hourly intervals to detect early signs of renal failure. Careful titration of intravenous fluids, vasoactive (e.g. noradrenaline), inotropic (e.g. dobutamine) and inodilator (e.g. enoximone) drugs are needed to support blood pressure, cardiac index and systemic perfusion. Low-dose dopamine, furosemide infusions and mannitol have all been used to prevent renal shutdown and/or cerebral oedema. Renal failure should be treated along conventional lines. Careful consideration must be given to the use of drugs excreted by the kidneys and those with potential nephrotoxic side effects.

Central nervous system

Primary cerebral damage may be caused by hypoxia during the arrest. Secondary damage may also occur after circulation is restored if the injured brain becomes oedematous. A flat trace on the electroencephalogram (EEG) is seen within 10 seconds of loss of cerebral circulation, and cerebral glucose is depleted within 1 minute. Microthrombi may form in the small cerebral vessels when blood flow ceases, which compromises cerebral perfusion when circulation is restored. Microemboli may also be ejected from the heart and great vessels during cardiac massage. Cerebral blood flow is reduced even if perfusion pressures are normal as a result of microvascular dysfunction.

Adequate arterial oxygenation is of great importance, if necessary using mechanical ventilation, and cerebral perfusion pressure should be maintained by ensuring a normal or slightly elevated mean arterial pressure. Cerebral oedema may be relieved by limitation of intravenous fluids and elevation of the head to 30° to increase venous drainage. Intravenous mannitol (200 mL of a 20% solution) and dexamethasone (10 mg intravenously, followed by 4 mg orally every 6 hours) may be needed. Convulsions and pyrexia increase cerebral metabolic requirements, contributing to brain damage, and should be controlled by hypothermia and anticonvulsants. There is a strong association between high blood glucose after resuscitation from cardiac arrest and poor neurological outcome (Langhelle et al, 2003), but there have been no trials on strict glycaemic control and outcome.

Acid–base status

The acid–base balance must be assessed urgently, and plasma potassium measured immediately and frequently after the arrest. Both should be corrected as required. Immediately after a cardiac arrest, there is often a period of hyperkalaemia, followed by hypokalaemia as endogenous catecholamine release promotes intracellular transportation of potassium. The serum potassium should be maintained above 4 mmol/L to prevent ventricular dysrhythmias. Hyperkalaemia over 6.5 mmol/L should be treated with a glucose–insulin infusion. Giving 10 mL of 10% calcium chloride intravenously over 5 minutes will offer some cardioprotection. Any significant metabolic acidosis should be treated by hyperventilation. Care is required in the administration of sodium bicarbonate, as it can lead to a rapid fall in plasma potassium levels and a rise in $p\text{CO}_2$, thereby worsening cerebral oedema.

Therapeutic hypothermia

Mild therapeutic hypothermia is thought to suppress many of the chemical reactions associated with reperfusion injury, and may improve outcome for patients remaining unconscious following return of spontaneous circulation (Nolan et al, 2003). External and/or internal cooling techniques can be used. Intravascular cooling (using cold saline at 4°C) enables more precise control of core temperature than external methods (e.g. cooling blankets and ice bags). Cooling to between 32 and 34°C should be started as soon as possible, and continued for at least 12–24 hours.

Blood glucose and magnesium levels

Hyperglycaemia and electrolyte abnormalities are common, including hypomagnesaemia. Blood glucose should be monitored frequently and hyperglycaemia treated with an insulin infusion. The optimal blood glucose target in critically ill patients has not been determined, and hypoglycaemia must be avoided. There is no evidence for giving magnesium routinely during cardiopulmonary arrest, but magnesium treatment is indicated if there is documented hypomagnesaemia or with torsades-de-pointes, regardless of the blood magnesium level (2 g of 50% magnesium sulphate intravenously over 5–10 minutes).

Prognosis

Four clinical signs strongly predict death or poor neurological outcome within 24 hours of the cardiac arrest:

- absent corneal reflex;
- absent pupillary response;
- absent withdrawal response to pain;
- no motor response.

An EEG performed at 24–48 hours after resuscitation can help to define prognosis (Ajisaka, 2004), and raised serum concentrations of neuron-specific enolase (NSE) may provide an additional indication of a poor outcome.

The period after resuscitation is often stressful for family members (and carers), as questions arise about prognosis. Unfortunately, we have no reliably predictors of outcome, yet some survivors of prolonged cardiac arrest have the potential to lead normal lives (Booth et al, 2004).

References

Aarons EJ, Beeching NJ (1991) Survey of 'do not resuscitate' orders in a district general hospital. *British Medical Journal* 303: 1504–1506.

Abu-Laban C, McIntyre J, Christenson C et al (2006) Aminophylline in brady-asystolic cardiac arrest: a randomised placebo-controlled trial. *Lancet* 367: 1577–1584.

AHA/ILCOR (2000) Guidelines 2000 for cardiopulmonary resuscitation and emergency cardiovascular care – an international consensus on science. *Resuscitation* 46: 1–448.

Ajisaka H (2004) Early electroencephalographic findings in patients with anoxic encephalopathy after cardiopulmonary arrest and successful resuscitation. *Journal of Clinical Neuroscience* 11: 616–618.

Amato-Vealey E (2005) Demystifying biphasic defibrillation. *Nursing* 35: 6–11.

Aung K, Htay T (2005) Vasopressin for cardiac arrest: a systematic review and meta-analysis. *Archives of Internal Medicine* 165: 17–24.

Baskett PJF (2001) The respiratory system during resuscitation: a review of the history, risk of infection during assisted ventilation, respiratory mechanics, and ventilation strategies for patients with an unprotected airway. *Resuscitation* 49: 123–134.

Beck CS, Prilchard WH, Feil HS (1947) Ventricular fibrillation of long duration abolished by electric shock. *Journal of the American Medical Association* 135: 985–986.

Berek K, Aichner F (1999) Prognosis of cerebral hypoxia after cardiac arrest. *Current Opinion in Critical Care* 5: 211–215.

Booth CM, Boone RH, Tomlinson G et al (2004) Is this patient dead, vegetative, or severely neurologically impaired? Assessing outcome for comatose survivors of cardiac arrest. *Journal of the American Medical Association* 291: 870–879.

Boyd R (2000) Witnessed resuscitation by relatives. *Resuscitation* 43: 171–176.

British Medical Association, the Resuscitation Council (UK) and the Royal College of Nursing (2001) *Decisions relating to Cardiopulmonary Resuscitation*. A joint statement from the British Medical Association, the Resuscitation Council (UK) and the Royal College of Nursing, London.

Brown TB, Dias JA, Saini D et al (2006) Relationship between knowledge of cardiopulmonary resuscitation guidelines and performance. *Resuscitation* 69: 253–261.

Candy CE (1991) 'Not for resuscitation': a student nurse's viewpoint. *Journal of Advanced Nursing* 16: 138–146.

Cooper MJ, Abinader EG (1979) Atropine-induced ventricular fibrillation: case report and review of the literature. *American Heart Journal* 99: 225–228.

Cooper S, Janghorbani M, Cooper G (2006) A decade of in-hospital resuscitation: outcomes and predictors of survival. *Resuscitation* 68: 231–237.

Criley JM, Blaufuss AH, Kissel GL (1976) Cough-induced cardiac compression. *Journal of the American Medical Association* 236: 1246–1250.

David J, Prior-Willeard PF (1993) Resuscitation skills of MRCP candidates. *British Medical Journal* 306: 1578–1579.

Deakin CD, Sado DM, Petley GW et al (2003) Is the orientation of the apical defibrillation paddle of importance during manual external defibrillation? *Resuscitation* 56: 15–18.

Department of Health (2000) *HSC 2000/028: Resuscitation Policy*. Health Service Circular. London: Department of Health.

Department of Health (2003) *National Outreach Report*. London: Department of Health and National Health Service Modernisation Agency.

Diggory P, Cauchi L, Griffith D et al (2003) The influence of new guidelines on cardiopulmonary resuscitation (CPR) decisions. Five cycles of audit of a clerk proforma which included a resuscitation decision. *Resuscitation* 56: 159–165.

Dowdle JR (1996) Ventricular standstill and cardiac percussion. *Resuscitation* 32: 31–32.

Ebrahim S (2000) Do not resuscitate decisions: flogging dead horses or a dignified death? *British Medical Journal* 320: 1155–1156.

Eftestol T, Wik L, Sunde K et al (2004) Effects of cardiopulmonary resuscitation on predictors of ventricular fibrillation defibrillation success during out-of-hospital cardiac arrest. *Circulation* 110: 10–15.

Gabbott D, Smith G, Mitchell S et al (2005) Cardiopulmonary resuscitation standards for clinical practice and training in the UK. *Resuscitation* 64: 13–19.

Heames RM, Sado D, Deakin CD (2001) Do doctors position defibrillation paddles correctly? Observational study. *British Medical Journal* 322: 1393–1394.

Hodgetts TJ, Kenward G, Vlackonikolis I et al (2002) The identification of risk factors for cardiac arrest and formulation of activation criteria to alert a medical emergency team. *Resuscitation* 54: 125–131.

ILCOR (2005) International consensus on cardiopulmonary resuscitation and emergency cardiovascular care science with treatment recommendations. *Resuscitation* 67: 181–341.

Jones GK, Brewer KL, Garrison HG (2000) Public expectations of survival following cardiopulmonary resuscitation. *Academic Emergency Medicine* 7: 48–53.

Jowett NI, Thompson DR (1988a) Basic life support. The forgotten skills? *Intensive Care Nursing* 4: 9–17.

Jowett NI, Thompson DR (1988b) Advanced cardiac life support: current perspectives. *Intensive Care Nursing* 4: 71–81.

Jowett NI, Turner AM, Hawkins D et al (2001) Emergency drug availability for the cardiac arrest team: a national audit. *Resuscitation* 49: 179–181.

Kern KB, Hilwig RW, Berg RA et al (2002) Importance of continuous chest compressions during cardiopulmonary resuscitation: improved outcome during a simulated single lay-rescuer scenario. *Circulation* 105: 645–649.

Kirchhof P, Eckardt L, Loh P et al (2002) Anterior-posterior versus anterior-lateral electrode positions for external cardioversion of atrial fibrillation: a randomized controlled trial. *Lancet* 360: 1275–1279.

Kouwenhoven WB, Jude JR, Knickerbocker GG (1960) Closed chest cardiac massage. *Journal of the American Medical Association* 173: 1064–1067.

Langhelle A, Tyvold SS, Lexow K et al (2003) In-hospital factors associated with improved outcome after out-of-hospital cardiac arrest. A comparison between four regions in Norway. *Resuscitation* 56: 247–263.

Lee A, Bishop G, Hillman K et al (1995) The medical emergency team. *Anaesthesia and Intensive Care* 23: 183–186.

McArthur-Rouse F (2001) Critical care outreach services and early warning scoring systems: a review of the literature. *Journal of Advanced Nursing* 36: 696–704.

McGowan J, Graham CA, Gordon MW (1999) Appointment of a resuscitation training officer is associated with improved survival from in-hospital ventricular fibrillation/ventricular tachycardia cardiac arrest. *Resuscitation* 41: 169–173.

MacNab A, Christenson J, Findlay J et al (2000) A new system for sternal intra-osseous infusion in adults. *Pre-hospital Emergency Care* 4: 173–177.

McQuillan P, Pilkington S, Allan A et al (1998) Confidential inquiry into quality of care before admission to intensive care. *British Medical Journal* 316: 1853–1858.

Nolan JP, Morley PT, Vanden Hoek TL et al (2003) Therapeutic hypothermia after cardiac arrest. An advisory statement by the Advancement Life Support Task Force of the International Liaison Committee on Resuscitation. *Resuscitation* 57: 231–235.

Page RL, Kerber RE, Russell JK for the BiCard Investigators (2002) Biphasic versus monophasic shock waveform for conversion of atrial fibrillation. *Journal of the American College of Cardiology* 39: 1956–1963.

Peberdy MA, Kaye W, Ornato JP et al (2003) Cardiopulmonary resuscitation of adults in the hospital: a report of 14 720 cardiac arrests from the National Registry of Cardiopulmonary Resuscitation. *Resuscitation* 58: 297–308.

Perkins GD, Roberts C, Gao F (2002) Delays in defibrillation: influence of different monitoring techniques. *British Journal of Anaesthesia* 89: 405–408.

Priori SG, Aliot E, Blomstrom-Lundqvist C et al (2001) Task force on sudden cardiac death of the European Society of Cardiology. *European Heart Journal* 22: 1374–1450.

Public Access Defibrillation Trial Investigators (2004) Public-access defibrillation and survival after out-of-hospital cardiac arrest. *New England Journal of Medicine* 51: 637–646.

Rao ACR, Naeem N, John C (1999) Direct current cardioversion does not cause cardiac damage: evidence from cardiac troponin T estimation. *Heart* 81: 576–579.

Regnard C, Randall FA (2005) A framework for making advanced decisions on resuscitation. *Clinical Medicine* 5: 354–360.

Royal College of Physicians (1987) Resuscitation from cardiopulmonary arrest. Training and organisation. *Journal of the Royal College of Physicians* 21: 175–182.

Safar P, Escarra L, Elam J (1958) A comparison of the mouth to mouth and mouth to airway methods of artificial respiration with the chest pressure arm-lift method. *New England Journal of Medicine* 258: 671–677.

Saunders J (2001) Perspectives on CPR: resuscitation or resurrection? *Clinical Medicine* 1: 457–460.

Sellick BA (1961) Cricoid pressure to control regurgitation of stomach contents during induction of anaesthesia. *Lancet* ii: 404–406.

Shepardson LB, Youngner SJ, Speroff T et al (1999) Increased risk of death in patients with do-not-resuscitate orders. *Medical Care* 37: 722–726.

Smith GB, Nolan J (2002) Medical emergency teams and cardiac arrests in hospital. *British Medical Journal* 324: 1215.

Stokes PH, Jowett NI (1985) Haemodynamic monitoring using the Swan–Ganz catheter. *Intensive Care Nursing* 1: 9–17.

Sullivan MJ, Guyatt GH (1986) Simulated cardiac arrests for monitoring quality of in-hospital resuscitation. *Lancet* ii: 618–620.

Tang W, Weil MH, Sun S et al (2001) A comparison of biphasic and monophasic waveform defibrillation after prolonged ventricular fibrillation. *Chest* 120: 948–954.

Urtubia RM, Aguila CM, Cumsille MA (2000) Combitube: a study for proper use. *Anesthesia and Analgesia* 90: 958–962.

Waalewijn RA, De Vos R, Tijssen JGP et al (2001) Survival models for out-of-hospital cardiopulmonary resuscitation from the perspectives of the bystander, the first responder, and the paramedic. *Resuscitation* 51: 113–122.

Zheng ZJ, Croft JB, Giles WH et al (2001) Sudden cardiac death in the United States, 1989 to 1998. *Circulation* 104: 2158–2163.

Zoll P M, Linenthal A J, Gibson W et al (1956) Termination of ventricular fibrillation in man by externally applied counter shock. *New England Journal of Medicine* 254: 727–732.

Chapter 12

Management of other conditions presenting to the coronary care unit

Patients are usually admitted to the coronary care unit because of chest pain, breathlessness, a rhythm disturbance or sometimes all three.

HEART FAILURE

Heart failure is a complex syndrome that results from any structural or functional disorder that impairs the ability of the heart to operate as a pump. As a result, the heart is unable to provide an adequate cardiac output for the body's metabolic needs and patients will have:

- symptoms of heart failure (at rest or during exercise); *and*
- objective evidence of cardiac dysfunction (usually by echocardiography); *and*
- a response to heart failure therapy.

Many patients with chronic heart failure (CHF) have breathlessness, fatigue and poor exercise tolerance, but little evidence of fluid retention, so the older term, congestive cardiac failure (CCF), is usually inappropriate.

CHF is a major and rapidly increasing problem in industrialised countries, where 1–2% of the population is affected. The prevalence of heart failure increases steeply with age, so that while around 1% of men and women aged under 65 years have heart failure, this increases to about 7% of those aged 75–84 years and 15% of those aged 85 years and above (Allender et al, 2006).

With increased survival of heart attack victims, the number of patients with heart failure is rising. In addition, the elderly population is increasing, and this group has the highest incidence of cardio-vascular diseases, including the commonest precursors of heart failure, coronary artery disease and hypertension. The risk of heart failure is higher in men than in women, and the median age at first diagnosis is now 76 years.

Apart from known cases of heart failure, there are probably an equal number of people with asymptomatic left ventricular dysfunction who are at risk of sudden death or developing overt heart failure (Wang et al, 2003). At-risk groups include patients with hypertension, diabetes mellitus, coronary artery disease and those with a family history of cardiomyopathy.

Chronic heart failure punctuated by acute exacerbations is the most common form of heart failure seen in hospital, and patients are often admitted

> **Box 12.1** Some causes of worsening heart failure in patients with CHF.
>
> **Cardiac**
>
> Dysrhythmias
> - New onset atrial fibrillation
> - Paroxysmal tachycardias
> - Bradycardia
>
> Acute coronary syndromes
> Valvular disease
>
> **Non-cardiac**
>
> Infection
> Non-compliance
> Alcohol
> Introduction of new drugs (especially NSAIDs)
> Thromboembolism
> Anaemia
> Thyroid disease (especially with amiodarone)

directly to the coronary care unit (CCU). Common reasons for deterioration are shown in Box 12.1. An average district general hospital can be expected to manage over 1000 deaths and discharges related to heart failure every year, with an average length of stay of nearly 2 weeks (Cleland et al, 2000).

The prognosis of CHF is very poor. Many patients die within 3 months of diagnosis, and approximately 60% will die within 5 years (McMurray & Stewart, 2000). The Seattle Heart Failure Model provides an accurate estimate of survival from individual clinical, pharmacological and laboratory characteristics (Levy et al, 2006).

Aetiology

Heart failure is a syndrome, not a diagnosis, and it is important to define the underlying cardiac abnormality. The majority of cases of CHF are secondary to myocardial ischaemia or myocardial infarction. This results in *systolic heart failure*, where the left ventricular pump is weakened and cannot eject enough blood during ventricular systole. Other causes of CHF include:

- hypertension;
- cardiomyopathy;
- valve disease;
- cardiac dysrhythmias (e.g. heart block and atrial fibrillation);
- pericardial disease (e.g. pericardial effusion, constrictive pericarditis);
- infection [e.g. rheumatic fever, viral myocarditis, human immunodeficiency virus (HIV)];
- alcohol and drugs (e.g. cancer chemotherapy).

In the UK, over 80% of cases of heart failure are secondary to coronary artery disease. Ischaemic injury to the left ventricular myocardium initiates a progressive process of worsening cardiac function, even in the absence of further identifiable insults. Progression is marked by left ventricular remodelling, causing the left ventricle to dilate and/or hypertrophy. This increases the stresses on the ventricular wall and depresses mechanical performance. Mitral regurgitation is frequent, and often prompts further remodelling. Other conditions, such as diabetes mellitus, hypertension or the onset of atrial fibrillation, may also contribute to the progression of CHF.

Diastolic heart failure is often diagnosed when there are signs and symptoms of heart failure, but the resting left ventricular systolic function is normal (Wu & Yu, 2005). This situation is seen predominantly in the elderly, particularly those with hypertension or other fibrotic heart diseases that increase the stiffness of the ventricular wall. Inadequate myocardial relaxation in diastole compromises ventricular filling. *Diastolic dysfunction* therefore refers to a disturbance in ventricular distensibility, regardless of whether the ejection fraction (EF) is normal or depressed and whether the patient is asymptomatic or symptomatic.

High-output heart failure is uncommon, but may occur in sepsis, anaemia, thyrotoxicosis and Paget's disease. There is a high cardiac output, but signs of heart failure because the high metabolic needs are not being fulfilled. The underlying cause needs treatment.

The response to heart failure

The symptoms of heart failure are not usually due to the low left ventricular ejection fraction itself but, rather, to the compensatory mechanisms that the body employs to maintain an adequate cardiac output. The fall in blood pressure caused by a diminished cardiac output stimulates the baroreceptors, which leads to increased catecholamine secretion, with tachycardia, increased myocardial contractility and a rise in systemic vascular resistance. Selective arterial vasoconstriction redistributes the cardiac output, so that flow to the gut and liver is reduced, with preferential perfusion of the brain and heart. The heart dilates, increasing myofibril stretch, which increases the force of myocardial contraction (Starling's law) and augmenting cardiac output. A further adaptation is seen in the arterioles, particularly those supplying skeletal muscle and kidneys, where the vessel walls become oedematous and less responsive to circulating vasodilators. Reduced renal blood flow stimulates the renin–angiotensin– aldosterone system (RAAS) with the release of high levels of angiotensin II and aldosterone, causing widespread vasoconstriction with sodium and water retention. Activation of other endogenous neurohormonal systems also plays an important role in cardiac remodelling and thus the progression of CHF, with elevated circulating or tissue levels of noradrenaline, angiotensin II, aldosterone, vasopressin and inflammatory cytokines.

Adverse circulatory effects are antagonised by *natriuretic peptides*, which produce many effects including diuresis, vasodilatation and increased sodium excretion. The natriuretic peptide family comprises atrial natriuretic peptide (ANP), brain natriuretic peptide (BNP), C-type natriuretic peptide (CNP) and D-type natriuretic peptide (DNP). ANP and BNP are synthesised in the heart, CNP is produced mainly in vessels, and DNP has been isolated in the atrial myocardium.

The plasma concentrations of BNP and the co-secreted, but inactive, N-terminal (NT) pro-BNP are raised in patients with heart failure. In general, the more severe the underlying cardiac abnormality, the higher the concentration, so measurement of plasma BNP or NT pro-BNP concentrations may aid decision-making in the diagnosis of heart failure or in predicting outcome in those with established heart failure (Latini et al, 2001; Januzzi et al, 2006). Serial BNP levels can provide prognostic information in compensated and decompensated heart failure patients, and may allow

titration of treatment to reduce BNP levels and optimise CHF therapy.

Investigations

There is no single diagnostic test for heart failure, and many other conditions may mimic the condition (Box 12.2). The resting 12-lead electrocardiogram (ECG) is usually abnormal (> 90%), so normality suggests an alternative diagnosis. A chest radiograph will detect cardiac enlargement and pulmonary congestion, but is of most value in ruling out other causes of breathlessness. A normal chest radiograph does not exclude heart failure.

Echocardiography is mandatory to give objective evidence of cardiac dysfunction, and exclude valvular disease and intracardiac shunts. Nuclear scanning can also be used to assess cardiac function and myocardial perfusion. Thyroid function tests and a blood count will exclude thyroid disease and anaemia as precipitants of worsening heart failure. Baseline renal function tests should be taken before long-term treatment with diuretics and angiotensin-converting enzyme (ACE) inhibitors. Liver function tests may be abnormal, reflecting hepatic congestion, and a raised serum urate associates with a poor prognosis.

As the symptoms and signs of heart failure are not very specific, BNP testing can assist in the

---

Box 12.2   Other conditions confused with heart failure.

Obesity
Chest disease
Ankle oedema due to:
    Venous insufficiency
    Drugs (e.g. calcium channel blockers, NSAIDs)
Anaemia
Thyroid disease
Hypoalbuminaemia (renal or hepatic disease)
Pulmonary emboli

Notes: (1) most people with ankle oedema do not have heart failure; (2) elderly patients are more likely to have heart failure, but may have combinations of the above diagnoses; (3) a normal ECG makes these diagnoses more likely.

diagnosis of heart failure in the ambulatory as well as in the emergency setting. Assays are now straightforward, with turnaround times of < 20 minutes. A normal BNP concentration virtually excludes heart failure, although high concentrations do not necessarily confirm it. Raised levels of BNP are found in the elderly, females and those with other conditions such as pulmonary disease, hypertension and renal failure (Cowie, 2004). The use of BNP testing is therefore most valuable as a test for ruling out heart failure (NICE, 2003). Those with a positive test do not necessarily have heart failure, but will require further evaluation. BNP levels can be used to assess prognosis in patients with confirmed heart failure.

Coronary angiography has only limited value, as revascularisation in the absence of angina does not affect prognosis. In patients with refractory idiopathic heart failure or valvular disease, cardiac catheterisation may be helpful.

Clinical features of heart failure

The most common symptoms of CHF are breathlessness, fatigue, exercise intolerance and fluid retention, although the severity of symptoms may fluctuate even in the absence of changes in medication. Other non-specific symptoms of heart failure include nocturia, anorexia, abdominal discomfort, constipation and cerebral symptoms such as confusion, dizziness and memory impairment. There is a poor relationship between symptoms and the severity of heart dysfunction, although marked symptoms usually indicate a poor prognosis, particularly if they persist after therapy.

Dyspnoea is probably caused by increased pulmonary vascular engorgement, with decreased compliance of the lungs. In contrast to patients with acute heart failure, those with chronic heart failure do not have increased lung water content (O'Dochartaigh et al, 2005). Pulmonary oedema is therefore unlikely to contribute to the exertional dyspnoea characteristic of the condition. Blood gases remain normal or near normal during exercise, but ventilatory reflexes are exaggerated. *Paroxysmal nocturnal dyspnoea* is common when nocturnal absorption of oedema fluid increases the intravascular volume, waking the patient with breathlessness, cough and wheeze. Fatigue and lethargy are marked, caused by low blood flow to exercising muscles. A specific skeletal myopathy, with structural and metabolic changes in the muscles, may cause weakness and wasting, and indicates a poor prognosis (cardiac cachexia). Swelling of the ankles is common, but does not always result from heart failure.

Right ventricular failure usually occurs secondary to left heart failure, but can occur in isolation following right ventricular infarction or pulmonary embolism, and may complicate pulmonary valve disease or chronic lung disease (cor pulmonale). Symptoms are due to high systemic venous pressure. Oedema, with elevation of the jugular venous pressure, is usual. The liver becomes engorged and enlarged and may be tender. Functional tricuspid incompetence occurs, and the dilated right ventricle often produces a right parasternal heave. Pleural effusions and ascites are common.

A variety of approaches have been used to quantify the degree of functional limitation imposed by CHF. The most widely used scale is the New York Heart Association (NYHA) classification, although this is subject to considerable interobserver variability.

- *NYHA I (asymptomatic).* No limitation to physical activity (asymptomatic left ventricular dysfunction is included in this category).
- *NYHA II (mild symptoms).* People have slight limitation of physical activity. They are comfortable at rest and during most ordinary exertion, but more strenuous activity (e.g. hills, stairs) may cause shortness of breath. Most can live life normally, including working.
- *NYHA III (moderate symptoms).* People have marked limitation to physical activity. They are comfortable at rest, but less than ordinary physical activity causes symptoms that interfere with their lives. Walking on the flat makes them breathless. Many are unable to work. *Class IIIa* heart failure means there is no dyspnoea at rest but, with *Class IIIb* failure, there has been recent dyspnoea at rest.
- *NYHA IV (severe symptoms).* People are unable to carry out any physical activity without discomfort. Symptoms are present at rest. Most patients are housebound.

Treating heart failure

The aims of treatment are to improve life expectancy and the quality of life (NICE, 2003). Symptom relief alone may be more appropriate in many elderly patients. The general aims of treatment are:

- increasing salt and water excretion;
- reducing intracardiac pressures and volume overload;
- increasing myocardial contractility.

Bedrest reduces metabolic demand, increases renal perfusion and is valuable until symptoms improve. Thereafter, regular aerobic exercise (such as brisk walking) and even resistive exercise (such as weight training) will improve symptoms, exercise performance and quality of life without deleterious effects on left ventricular performance. It also improves skeletal muscle function and exercise tolerance, and may be more effective when part of a rehabilitation programme. Inactivity should be avoided, as it leads to physical deconditioning and muscle weakness, with worsening of symptoms and exercise performance.

For hospital inpatients, passive leg exercises are recommended to prevent deep vein thrombosis, and subcutaneous low-molecular-weight heparin should be given as CHF patients are at high risk of thromboembolism. Formal anticoagulation with warfarin is recommended for patients with atrial fibrillation and/or very poor left ventricular function.

Diuretics

Diuretics provide the mainstay of treatment for heart failure, giving symptomatic relief and improving exercise capacity. They do not improve prognosis. Diuretics inhibit sodium resorption by the kidney, reduce intravascular volume and, hence, reduce cardiac preload. Loss of sodium from arteriolar walls causes vasodilatation and a reduction in afterload. Potassium intake needs to be increased to prevent hypokalaemia and its consequences. Loop diuretics are the first choice, and thiazides can be added if the glomerular filtration rate is less than 30 mL/minute. Combination therapy is superior to simply increasing the dose of

the loop diuretic in terms of efficacy and side effects, but there may be worsening of renal function and/or hyponatraemia.

In severe heart failure, the gut wall becomes oedematous, limiting the absorption of orally administered drugs. Intravenous diuretics can get round this problem, switching to oral therapy once the diuresis has started. Overdiuresis should be avoided, as depleting the plasma volume will reactivate the RAAS and stimulate fluid retention and vasoconstriction. The dose of diuretic must be reduced to just sufficient to prevent salt and water retention, and should be titrated (up and down) according to need.

Aldosterone blocking agents have both diuretic and antihypertensive effects, but exhibit other valuable non-renal effects, including prevention of myocardial fibrosis, improvement of endothelial function and helping to reduce vascular inflammation (Pitt, 2003). Spironolactone 25 mg should be used in patients with moderate to severe chronic heart failure (Pitt et al, 1999). Its value in NYHA classes I and II cardiac failure is unknown.

Hyperkalaemia is more frequent when spironolactone is combined with ACE inhibitors, and the serum electrolytes need to be checked at least weekly until they are stable, and then 3- to 6-monthly thereafter. An increase in the serum potassium up to 6 mmol/L is usually acceptable.

Vasodilators

Many episodes of pulmonary oedema that punctuate CHF are not caused by fluid overload, but rather fluid redistribution that is directed to the lungs. Episodes of acute-on-chronic heart failure are characterised by a sudden reduction in stroke volume that triggers increased sympathetic activity, resulting in tachycardia and an abrupt increase in systemic vascular resistance (Kramer et al, 2000). The combination of tachycardia and increased peripheral resistance shifts fluid from the peripheries into the central circulation. Because of impaired left ventricular function, the heart cannot cope with this sudden fluid overload, and pulmonary oedema results, even though there is no excess fluid retention (Northridge, 1996). This is why treatment with vasodilators rather than escalating doses of diuretics is so effective in the treatment of heart failure. There are many vasodilators that may be used in the management of heart failure, and their haemodynamic effects depend on their ability to affect arterioles or venules. The most important agents are those targeting the RAAS.

Angiotensin-converting enzyme (ACE) inhibitors

The benefits from ACE inhibitors for patients with heart failure, in terms of mortality, morbidity and quality of life, are unequivocal (Flather et al, 2000). They should be introduced at a low dose early in CHF management, and titrated upward over several weeks to doses shown to be effective in clinical trials, and not just to the level that relieves symptoms. These are shown in Table 12.1.

The ACE inhibitors reduce the production of the potent vasoconstrictor angiotensin II, and increase bradykinin concentrations by inhibiting its breakdown. Although bradykinin is probably responsible for the common ACE inhibitor-associated dry cough, it has been shown to have beneficial effects on endothelial function. With vasodilatation, venous and arterial blood pressure falls, allowing an increase in cardiac output and renal blood flow. Aldosterone levels also fall, reducing fluid retention and enabling a reduction in the dose of diuretics.

The use of ACE inhibitors is often limited by side effects, including cough, renal impairment and symptomatic hypotension, but they should be prescribed in the maximum tolerated dose in all patients with CHF. Some ACE inhibitor is better than no ACE inhibitor, and more is better than less.

Blood biochemistry (urea, creatinine and electrolytes) should be checked after initiation of therapy and at each dose change. An increase in creatinine of up to 50% above baseline, or up to 200 μmol/L, is acceptable. In patients without fluid retention, a reduction in diuretic dose may be all that is required to improve renal function. If the rise in creatinine (or potassium) persists despite adjustment of concomitant medications [e.g. non-steroidal anti-inflammatory drugs (NSAIDs), diuretics], the dose of the ACE inhibitor should be halved and blood chemistry rechecked. A renal opinion may be needed, particularly if renal artery stenosis is suspected.

Angiotensin II receptor blockers (ARBs)

ARBs appear to have similar efficacy to ACE inhibitors in reducing morbidity and mortality in patients with heart failure. They probably should not be used first line, but as an alternative when ACE inhibitors are not tolerated (Jong et al, 2002). Best evidence currently exists for valsartan (80–320 mg/day) and candesartan (4–32 mg/day). ARBs may also be considered in combination with ACE inhibitors in patients who remain symptomatic despite ACE inhibitor and beta-blocker therapy, although there is an increased risk of hypotension, renal impairment and hyperkalaemia.

Beta-adrenergic blocking agents

Increased catecholamine concentrations in patients with heart failure result in hyperstimulation of the myocardium, with myocyte toxicity. Beta-blockers will protect the heart, and reduce total and cardiovascular mortality (ESC, 2004). All patients with chronic, stable heart failure already on ACE inhibitors and diuretics should be offered treatment with beta-blockers. Long-term treatment improves left ventricular function, reduces hospital admissions and associates with a reduction in all cause mortality of about 12%. Contraindications include asthma, hypotension (systolic blood pressure under 90 mmHg), bradycardia < 50 beats/minute or heart block. Therapy should be started with a very small dose, up-titrated very slowly to maximal dosage and then continued indefinitely.

Table 12.1   Recommended doses of ACE inhibitors.

	Starting dose	Maintenance dose
Captopril	6.25 mg tds	50 mg tds
Enalapril	2.5 mg od	20 mg twice daily
Lisinopril	2.5 mg od	30–40 mg daily
Ramipril	1.25 mg od	5 mg twice daily
Trandolapril	1 mg od	4 mg daily

tds, three times daily; od, every day.

Bisoprolol, nebivolol and carvedilol are the only beta-blockers currently licensed for heart failure in the UK. There are no randomised clinical trials of atenolol or many other commonly used beta-blockers in patients with heart failure. If patients develop heart failure and are already on treatment with a beta-blocker for angina or hypertension, there is no strong evidence to support a change to a licensed beta-blocker, although sotalol should not be used in CHF.

Initiation and uptitration of beta-blockers

Beta-blockade remains underutilised in heart failure because it is generally assumed that initiation and uptitration is difficult. This is not usually the case provided that the initial dose is low and subsequent dose increments are slow ('go low – go slow').

Initial doses are shown in Table 12.2. The dose should be doubled at a minimum of 2–4 weeks until the target dose is reached.

The heart rate, blood pressure, electrolytes, clinical status (especially signs of heart failure) and body weight should be monitored at each titration stage and for 4 weeks following the final titration. If there is transient worsening of heart failure symptoms, fluid retention, bradycardia or hypotension, the following are recommended:

- If *heart failure symptoms* worsen, the dose of diuretics should be increased with a temporary reduction in the dose of beta-blocker if needed.
- If there is *symptomatic hypotension*, the dose of the ACE inhibitor should be reduced, and the dose of beta-blocker should be reduced if required.
- If *symptomatic bradycardia* occurs, the dose of beta-blocker should be reduced.

Table 12.2 Initial doses of beta-blockers in CHF.

Drug	Starting dose	Target dose
Bisoprolol	1.25 mg od	10 mg od
Nebivolol	1.25 mg od	10 mg od
Carvedilol	3.125 mg bd	25 mg bd[a]

a 50 mg bd if body weight > 85 kg.

When the patient has stabilised, uptitration can be attempted again. It is important that the target dose is achieved if at all possible, but some beta-blocker is better than no beta-blocker. Often the patient is feeling well when beta-blocker therapy is started, and cannot see the need for yet another tablet, particularly when they may initially feel less well. Temporary symptomatic deterioration may occur in 20–30% of patients during initiation and/or uptitration, and it is important to explain that the treatment is given as much to prevent the worsening of heart failure as to improve symptoms. Further, their life expectancy will be increased. Symptomatic improvement may take up to 6 months to occur, so persistence is very important, and it is important to gain the confidence of the patient. Establishing beta-blocker therapy can be very labour intensive and is often better managed by a heart failure specialist nurse (Thompson et al, 2005).

The patients should be encouraged to weigh themselves daily and to seek medical advice if their weight is increasing. They should be advised not to stop beta-blocker therapy without advice. Tiredness, breathlessness and fatigue can usually be managed by adjustment of other medications.

Using beta-blockers as first-line therapy The use of ACE inhibitors as first-line therapy for CHF is usual, because the evidence supporting beta-blockade was not initially available. Using beta-blockade as first-line therapy may be preferable, because many patients with heart failure have, or have a predisposition to, abnormal heart rhythms. Atrial fibrillation is present in about a third of patients with heart failure, and many have complex ventricular dysrhythmias, which are not always symptomatic. Sudden death is the most common form of death in patients with heart failure (up to 70%), presumably secondary to sustained ventricular tachycardia or fibrillation. Some of the increased survival in chronic heart disease (CHD) associated with the use of beta-blockers may be due to antidysrhythmic actions. Initiating treatment of heart failure with a beta-blocker has been found to be as effective and as well tolerated as starting treatment with an ACE inhibitor (Willenheimer et al, 2005). Both drugs should be used in the long term, but should not be started simultaneously.

Calcium-channel blocking agents

These agents do not have a specific role in heart failure. While there may be a favourable acute response, long-term results have been disappointing, possibly because of negative inotropic activity. Nifedipine and verapamil are poorly tolerated in patients with heart failure, but the second-generation calcium antagonists, such as felodipine and amlodipine, have little cardiodepressant activity and may be used in heart failure patients with co-existing hypertension or angina.

Positive inotropic agents

Positive inotropic agents should be of value in the treatment of heart failure to promote cardiac output, but most are associated with decreased survival in the long term (Felker & O'Connor, 2001). Inotropic support may be of value in the short term in selected patients following acute myocardial infarction or cardiac surgery or in those awaiting cardiac transplantation.

Digoxin The role of digoxin in heart failure remains controversial, particularly when used following acute myocardial infarction (Spargias et al, 1999), and its main role is in patients with permanent atrial fibrillation and heart failure. The DIG trial in patients with an ejection fraction of under 45% showed that, if serum digoxin levels are maintained in the 0.5–0.9 ng/mL range, both mortality and hospitalisation for worsening heart failure are reduced (Ahmed et al, 2006). Maintaining higher serum levels also reduces hospitalisation, but does not affect mortality.

Beta–adrenergic agonists While short-term haemodynamic improvements may be seen in patients with heart failure, long-term use of beta-adrenergic agonists is limited by peripheral vasoconstriction. Dopamine and dobutamine are relatively cardioselective beta-1 stimulants, and may be useful in patients with heart failure and cardiogenic shock following myocardial infarction.

Preferential arterial vasodilatation with low-dose dopamine may help renal, coronary and cerebral hypoperfusion. Dobutamine is similar but does not seem to affect the pulse rate so much.

Phosphodiesterase inhibitors Selective phosphodiesterase inhibitors, such as enoximone and milrinone, have been used for severe heart failure, cardiogenic shock and other forms of shock unresponsive to catecholamine therapy alone. They strengthen cardiac contraction and dilate peripheral vessels, reducing ventricular preload and afterload with little effect on blood pressure. While they may be useful in the short term, there is no evidence that they improve survival. Optimal use requires invasive haemodynamic monitoring, preferably on an intensive care unit. These drugs are contraindicated if there is any valvular stenosis that limits cardiac output.

Calcium sensitisers Levosimendan is one of a new drug class that improves myocardial contractility without causing an increase in myocardial oxygen demand. In the LIDO trial (Follath et al, 2002), intravenous levosimendan improved haemodynamic performance more effectively than dobutamine in patients with severe, low-output heart failure. Mortality at 180 days was also reduced. Oral levosimendan may be considered in patients with symptomatic low cardiac output secondary to left ventricular systolic dysfunction without severe hypotension.

Antidysrhythmic agents

Antidysrhythmic agents should be of major value in CHF patients, to reduce sudden cardiac death. However, many agents are negatively inotropic and, in some cases, are proarrhythmic. Class II agents (beta-blockers) are the exception. Class I agents (e.g. flecainide, propafenone) increase mortality in patients with heart failure. The class III agent amiodarone can restore and maintain sinus rhythm in those with atrial fibrillation, maximising cardiac output, and might improve prognosis as a result (Amiodarone Trials Meta-Analysis Investigators, 1997). Sotalol increases mortality in patients with heart failure.

Non-drug therapy in heart failure

Salt and water restriction may be beneficial, reducing fluid intake to 1–1.5 L/24 hours and avoiding high-salt foods such as cheese, sausages, tinned soup and vegetables, chocolate, crisps and peanuts. Fresh fruit and vegetables, eggs and fish have a relatively low salt content. Prostaglandin inhibitors, such as NSAIDS, should be avoided. They inhibit the production of renal vasodilators and antagonise the effect of loop diuretics.

Non-invasive positive pressure ventilation (NIPPV), using continuous positive airway pressure (CPAP) or bilevel ventilation, reduces the need for invasive mechanical ventilation in patients with acute cardiogenic pulmonary oedema (Cooper & Jacob, 2002). It also improves oxygenation, corrects acidosis, improves left ventricular function and helps reduce mortality (Peter et al, 2006).

Effective education and counselling of patients is important and enhances long-term adherence to complex drug regimes, and there is an important role here for specialist heart failure nurses. Chronic heart failure predisposes to, and can be exacerbated by, pulmonary infections, so influenza and pneumococcal vaccination is advisable. While exercise training and rehabilitation may improve symptoms and quality of life, there has as yet been no effect shown on survival.

Surgical approaches

Although coronary disease is the commonest cause of heart failure in the UK, the benefits of revascularisation in patients without angina remain uncertain. A few small studies have suggested that coronary artery bypass surgery may be helpful in patients with heart failure if there are large areas of non-contractile but viable myocardium (hibernating myocardium). Specific imaging of these patients is required with nuclear scans, stress echocardiography and magnetic resonance imaging (MRI). Patients with ventricular dilatation often have clinically important mitral regurgitation, which might be amenable to mitral valve replacement or repair.

Cardiac transplantation, sometimes with prior ventricular support, is an established therapy for severe heart failure but, with the shortage of donor organs and the general level of co-morbidities in potential recipients, this is uncommon. Referral for transplantation should be considered in younger patients with severe refractory symptoms.

Cardiac resynchronisation therapy (CRT)

About 30% of patients with severe heart failure have intraventricular conduction defects that disturb the timing of right and left ventricular contraction. This may be suggested by a bundle branch block pattern or a QRS duration > 120 ms on the resting 12-lead ECG. Ventricular dys-synchrony results in decreased stroke volume, increased wall stress, delayed ventricular relaxation and a tendency to mitral regurgitation. This asynchronous contraction of the ventricles may be partially overcome with biventricular pacing. CRT depolarises the left ventricle earlier, and provides near-simultaneous contraction of the ventricular septum and the left ventricular free wall. Optimising the atrio-ventricular interval for patients in sinus rhythm may also help to improve cardiac haemodynamics by co-ordinating the timing of atrial systole relative to ventricular filling.

In some cases, both symptoms and prognosis may be improved by CRT (Cleland et al, 2005), although the selection of appropriate patients is difficult. Evidence suggests that the best results are obtained in those with the following features:

- sinus rhythm;
- ejection fraction less than 35%;
- QRS complex duration over 120 ms;
- NYHA functional class III or IV;
- maximal pharmacological therapy for heart failure.

While the resting ECG may be used to identify potential patients, detailed echocardiography is more accurate at demonstrating cardiac dys-synchrony and may define more exactly those patients who may benefit from pacing.

Automatic internal cardiac defibrillator implantation should be considered in CHF patients at particularly high risk of sudden death. This includes patients with previous myocardial infarction, cardiac arrest or episodes of sustained ventricular tachycardia. Combined biventricular pacemaker/defibrillator units are often chosen (Swedberg et al, 2005).

Treatment of diastolic heart failure

Optimal therapy for patients with heart failure and normal systolic left ventricular function is not known and, in general, the same pharmacological approach is used (Leite-Moreira, 2006). Beta-blockade may be especially helpful to slow the heart, prolonging diastole and thus allowing more time for the ventricles to fill. Diltiazem or vera-pamil would be alternatives in patients unable to take beta-blockers, and ivabradine may be partic-ularly beneficial here, as it does not affect myocar-dial contractility. ACE inhibitors may help with cardiac relaxation and, of course, may be needed to treat underlying hypertension, which is partic-ularly common in this group of patients. High doses of the angiotensin receptor blocker, candesar-tan, have been shown to be of particular value in patients with diastolic dysfunction (Yusuf et al, 2003). Diuretics should be used with caution, as even mild dehydration may reduce preload and worsen cardiac performance.

Reclassifying heart failure as a progressive disorder

Left ventricular dysfunction in CHF is generally progressive, with asymptomatic and symptomatic phases. Specific treatments targeted at each stage can reduce the morbidity and mortality (Hunt et al, 2005).

- *Stage A* (patients *at risk* of developing heart failure, but currently have no structural heart dis-ease). This includes patients with hypertension, diabetes mellitus, coronary artery disease and those with a family history of cardiomyopathy. Patients taking medication that may damage the heart (e.g. chemotherapy) are also in this group.
  - strategies to prevent ventricular remodelling, including ACE inhibitors and risk factor management are advised.
- *Stage B* (asymptomatic left ventricular dysfunc-tion):
  - ACE inhibitor and beta-blocker therapy is recommended.

- *Stage C* (symptomatic heart failure with left ventricular systolic dysfunction):
  - patients should be on beta-blockers and an ACE inhibitor;
  - diuretics, digoxin and aldosterone antago-nists may be added;
  - pacemaker resynchronisation therapy may benefit selected patients.
- *Stage D* (severe refractory heart failure):
  - all the above interventions;
  - cardiac transplantation;
  - end-of-life care.

Using guidelines and pathways for the man-agement of patients with heart failure, including specialised follow-up by a multidisciplinary team, will reduce readmission to hospital and mortality (McAlister et al, 2004). Disease management pro-grammes (DMPs) have evolved as an innovative clinical practice system to enhance the discharge outcomes of older people with heart failure (Yu et al, 2005).

HYPERTENSION

In adults, the normal systemic blood pressure is considered to be less than 140/90 mmHg, and blood pressures consistently above these levels are defined as hypertension. Higher blood pressures are more common in urban rather than rural pop-ulations, and in those with diabetes, obesity or a family history of hypertension. Most patients do not have an identifiable cause and are said to have *essential hypertension.*

Occasionally, patients may be admitted to hospital because of marked elevation in blood pressure. *Accelerated hypertension* is defined as a recent significant increase over baseline blood pressure that is associated with vascular damage, usually inferred by the presence of flame-shaped haemorrhages or soft exudates seen in the retina on fundoscopic examination. If there is papil-loedema, the term *malignant hypertension* is used. There are two groups of hypertensive emergencies often seen on coronary care:

1 *Those with hypertensive heart failure.* Pulmonary oedema and hypertension often co-exist, and the blood pressure usually falls with effective

treatment of left ventricular failure. Parenteral vasodilator therapy with nitrates is the first-line treatment, particularly if there is co-existent myocardial ischaemia. Nitrates dilate both arteries and veins, with a greater effect on the venous system. Sodium nitroprusside is an alternative, which dilates veins and arteries equally, thus reducing both preload and after-load, with minimal effect on cardiac output and myocardial blood flow. Its rapid onset and short duration of action reduce blood pressure immediately and allow minute-to-minute pressure regulation.

2 *Those with hypertension complicating an acute coronary syndrome.* Many patients with acute myocardial infarction will be hypertensive on admission to hospital, but this usually settles following pain relief with diamorphine. However, where the systolic blood pressure remains over 160 mmHg, it should be treated to reduce cardiac work and the risk of several cardiac complications, including cardiac rupture. Hypertension in the early stages of acute myocardial infarction also increases the risk of stroke following thrombolysis, and uncontrolled severe hypertension therefore provides a relative contraindication to thrombolytic therapy. Beta-blockers are first-line therapy because of their prognostic benefits. Intravenous nitrates can also be used acutely.

Emergency treatment of hypertension aims to lower the blood pressure as *safely* as possible, rather than as *quickly* as possible. A progressive, controlled reduction of the blood pressure will minimise the risk of hypoperfusion in cerebral, coronary and reno-vascular beds. Under normal conditions, blood flow to these organs remains relatively constant despite wide fluctuations in blood pressure. In the presence of severe hypertension, this process of autoregulation is disturbed, and the blood pressure range is shifted upwards so that higher pressures are tolerated, but organ perfusion may be put at risk with sudden reductions in blood pressure (Fig. 12.1). Hence, the initial reduction in mean arterial pressure should not exceed 20–25% below the pretreatment levels.

CHEST PAIN

Acute chest pain is a very common reason for emergency hospital admission, and many patients are admitted directly to the CCU The prevalence of central chest pain in the community in the 40- to 60-year-old age group is about 8%. Half these patients have 'typical' anginal pain, but only one-quarter will have coronary heart disease. The association of typical anginal symptoms and coronary artery disease is stronger in men than in women.

Figure 12.1   Cerebral autoregulation.

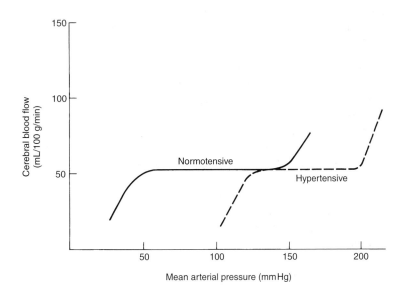

Formulating a diagnosis is sometimes very difficult given the number of possible sources of pain, including the heart, the pericardium, the lungs and pleura, the oesophagus, the spine and the chest wall. Many patients who arrive on the CCU subsequently prove not to have had a heart attack, and many do not even have cardiac disease. Patients with chest pain of unknown origin are a particular management problem.

Stable angina

> They who are afflicted with it, are seized while they are walking, (more especially if it be up hill, and soon after eating) with a painful and most disagreeable sensation in the breast, which seems as if it would extinguish life, if it were to increase or to continue; but the moment they stand still, all this uneasiness vanishes .... In all other respects, patients are, at the beginning of this disorder, perfectly well .... Males are most liable to this disease, especially such as have past their fiftieth year ....
>
> William Heberden, 1772

Angina is a common manifestation of coronary artery disease, with just under two million people affected in the UK (Allender et al, 2006). The history is the most important part of assessment. Typical angina pain is of short duration and is often expressed as a discomfort rather than a pain. 'Atypical chest pain' is a common term that is best avoided. It is important to separate non-cardiac pain (e.g. costochondritis, reflux pain) from atypical anginal symptoms, such as breathlessness.

Angina is regarded as stable if it has been present over several weeks without major change in symptom frequency or severity. The Canadian Cardiovascular Society (Campeau, 1976) has classified angina as shown in Table 12.3.

Causes of angina

Angina results from an imbalance of oxygen supply and demand to the myocardium. In most cases, this is due to fixed atheromatous deposits in the major epicardial arteries (stable angina). Myocardial ischaemia leads to left ventricular

Table 12.3 Canadian Cardiovascular Society (CCS) classification of angina.

CCS class	Description
I	No angina with normal physical activity. Angina with strenuous activity.
II	Slight limitation of ordinary activity.
III	Marked limitation of ordinary activity.
IV	Angina with minimal physical activity. Occasional rest pain.

dysfunction, which may further impair coronary blood flow and give rise to breathlessness as well as pain. Other non-specific symptoms include nausea, sweating and lethargy.

It is usually considered that a coronary artery must be narrowed by at least 70% at angiography before coronary blood flow is inadequate to meet the metabolic needs of the heart during exertion – but this may depend upon on the number and length of the individual stenoses. Additionally, some stenoses may alter with changes in coronary artery tone. Coronary arterial spasm most often occurs at the site of an atheromatous plaque, often waking the patient in the early morning. This is known as *Prinzmetal (variant) angina*. Ischaemic pain usually lasts longer than other types of angina, but almost always responds to glyceryl trinitrate (GTN). Spasm may be so severe as to result in myocardial infarction (1.2%/year) and sudden death (0.5%/year), but the precipitants are not fully understood. No single mechanism has been demonstrated, but a history of migraine or Raynaud's disease is common, suggesting that it may be part of a generalised vasospastic disorder. Cigarette smoking is an important risk factor. Symptoms wax and wane, with several attacks in a short space of time and then long periods of remission. About 0.5–1% of patients admitted to hospital with ischaemic chest pain have variant angina. ECGs taken during the pain typically show transient ST segment elevation, indicating transmural ischaemia, although ST depression may also occur in the same patient at different times, emphasising that regions of coronary spasm usually occur at the site of a fixed stenosis.

Syndrome X is a condition, usually of post-menopausal women, in which there is anginal pain, but angiographically normal epicardial arteries. Exclusion of other cardiac and non-cardiac causes is required for diagnosis. The cause of the syndrome is not known, and it is likely that there are many different underlying mechanisms. *Syndrome X* often associates with the metabolic syndrome (previously, and confusingly, known as syndrome X), suggesting that microvascular atheroma could be a cause (*microvascular angina*). In general, syndrome X has a good prognosis, with no increased incidence of adverse cardiac events but, in some patients, there may be progressive deterioration of left ventricular dysfunction, so echocardiographic surveillance is important, as is attention to cardiovascular risk factors.

Management is difficult, and symptoms may worsen over time. Recurrent hospital admissions and overinvestigation are common, and symptoms frequently interfere with work and home life. Traditional anti-ischaemic agents are used as first-line therapy (beta-blockers, diltiazem, nitrates), and statins can improve exercise tolerance, probably because of improvements in endothelial function. ACE inhibitors may similarly have a beneficial effect. Imipramine inhibits pain transmission from visceral tissues and might help to reduce the number of anginal episodes.

Investigation of patients with angina

Most patients with angina should be referred to a cardiologist for confirmation of the diagnosis, treatment of the symptoms and assessment of risk, although optimal management of individual patients is always a matter of clinical judgement, based on experience rather than flowcharts.

The ECG at rest is often normal, even in the presence of severe coronary artery disease, although half of these cases will develop an abnormal ECG during anginal pain. An abnormal ECG at rest both supports the diagnosis and identifies those with a poorer prognosis (Daly et al, 2006). Exercise stress testing is appropriate in most cases, but is of limited value in those with a low pretest probability of coronary heart disease (e.g. young women). Myocardial perfusion scintigraphy or stress echocardiography is an alternative.

Angiography is justifiable in all cases in which it would alter management, and may be considered in patients considered at high risk without prior functional testing. Such patients include those with severe symptoms, particularly of short duration (less than 6 months), patients with diabetes and those with left ventricular dysfunction.

A routine chest radiograph may show evidence of other non-cardiac causes of chest pain, but is not needed in all cases. A full blood count, renal and thyroid function tests, with fasting lipids and glucose, should be measured in all cases.

Management

General management includes risk factor intervention, with particular regard to cholesterol, smoking and hypertension. A GTN spray should be provided (with instructions on proper use) and first administered in the presence of medical supervision. Aspirin or clopidogrel should be administered in all cases unless contraindicated. Vasodilators such as nitrates and calcium channel blockers are effective in controlling symptoms, but there is no evidence of the superiority of either of these agents. When combined with other antianginal therapy, nicorandil reduces symptoms and may reduce coronary deaths and non-fatal myocardial infarcts.

Because most myocardial perfusion takes place during diastole, reducing the heart rate has important anti-ischaemic effects. Beta-blockade reduces both symptomatic and asymptomatic ischaemic episodes, and is highly effective in controlling exercise-induced angina, thus improving exercise capacity. Beta-blockers are the agents of first choice in patients with chronic angina in association with hypertension, previous myocardial infarction or poor ventricular function, where long-term treatment prevents myocardial infarction and improves survival (ESC, 2004). Diltiazem has a similar slowing effect on the heart, and should be considered where beta-blockers are contraindicated. Ivabradine is a novel agent, which inhibits pacemaker activity at the sino-atrial node, slowing the heart. It has anti-ischaemic efficacy similar to that of other usual antianginal therapies such as amlodipine and atenolol (Danchin & Aly, 2004). Because it does not influence myocardial contractility, it may be particularly valuable in the setting of myocardial stunning or acute left ventricular failure in the acute stage of myocardial infarction. It is not known whether isolated heart rate reduction will have the same protective efficacy as that of beta-blocking agents in secondary prevention after myocardial infarction.

Both coronary angioplasty and bypass surgery may be used to relieve symptoms, although those undergoing percutaneous coronary intervention (PCI) are more likely to need repeat procedures. In patients with moderate or poorly controlled angina, PCI is appropriate and is more effective than medical therapy (Bucher et al, 2000) and, in certain groups, coronary bypass surgery improves survival (Eagle et al, 2004).

Non-cardiac chest pain

Many patients admitted to coronary care do not have an acute cardiac problem, but may have other serious conditions requiring diagnosis and treatment. The most important of these are:

- pulmonary embolism;
- dissecting aortic aneurysm;
- pericarditis;
- oesophageal pain;
- pneumothorax;
- abdominal causes.

Pulmonary embolism

In the UK, there are an estimated 20 000 deaths per year from pulmonary embolism, as well as a further 40 000 non-fatal cases. The condition contributes to approximately 15–20% of all hospital deaths. Many cases of pulmonary embolism are not suspected prior to death. The commonest source of emboli is the deep veins of the legs, although clinical evidence of a deep vein thrombosis (DVT) is lacking in over half the patients (Goodacre et al, 2005). Most patients have clinical risk factors, including immobility, malignancy, recent surgery or recent myocardial infarction. Robust policies for inpatient DVT prophylaxis are vital if lives are to be saved, and simple scoring charts can quickly identify patients suitable for subcutaneous low-molecular-weight heparin (Table 12.4).

Occasionally, emboli may originate in the right ventricle following myocardial infarction, or from a pacing wire in those with pacemakers or implantable defibrillators. Septic emboli can complicate right-sided endocarditis.

Signs and symptoms Pulmonary emboli may cause varying degrees of symptoms and signs, depending upon their size, number and the presence of prior cardiorespiratory disease. Many episodes of pulmonary embolism may not be

---

Table 12.4 Assessment of patients for DVT prophylaxis – risk score chart.

Aged over 40 years	1	Anticipated bedrest over 72 h	2	HRT or combined oral contraceptive use within 4 weeks	2
Obesity	1	Severe chronic obstructive pulmonary disease	2	Malignancy	3
Major surgery (within 6 months)	1	Active inflammatory bowel disease	2	Heart failure	3
Severe varicose veins/leg ulcers	1	Severe infection, e.g. pneumonia	2	Myocardial infarction (within 3 months)	3

If the score is five or more, consider prophylactic treatment with enoxaparin 40 mg subcutaneously daily until patient fully mobile (14 days maximum).
Contraindications: active bleeding, cerebrovascular accident, clotting disorders, active gastric or duodenal ulceration, chronic liver disease, low platelet count.

detected clinically, even in patients with symptomatic DVT.

- *Acute minor pulmonary emboli* may cause pleuritic chest pain and some breathlessness, but little haemodynamic disturbance. There may be tachycardia, gallop rhythm and a raised jugular venous pressure.
- *Acute major pulmonary emboli* will obstruct the major pulmonary vessels and associate with sudden chest pain (pleuritic or cardiac), breathlessness, syncope, cyanosis and, sometimes, cardiac arrest, often marked by pulseless electrical activity (PEA) on the ECG.

Investigations The diagnosis of pulmonary emboli is not easy. Patients may present with non-specific signs and symptoms that mimic other clinical conditions. Many diagnostic tests are non-specific. Spontaneous endogenous thrombolysis starts within hours, and small emboli will not be detectable after a few days, making late diagnosis difficult.

Electrocardiography An ECG is needed to exclude myocardial infarction in patients presenting with acute chest pain, but there are no diagnostic changes of pulmonary embolism. The ECG is usually normal in acute minor pulmonary embolism. Non-specific findings include sinus tachycardia, widespread T wave inversion (especially in leads V1–V4), right axis deviation, right bundle branch block and the classical S_1, Q_3, T_3 pattern (i.e. an S wave in standard lead I, with a Q wave and inverted T wave in standard lead III). Atrial fibrillation is precipitated in about 5% of cases.

Arterial blood gases As pulmonary emboli can give rise to both vascular and airway changes, blood gas alterations are variable and may be within normal limits. The classic abnormalities are of type 1 respiratory failure (hypoxia and hypocapnia), but patients with heart failure or chronic lung disease may have pre-existing blood gas abnormalities.

Blood tests (D-dimer and troponin assays) D-Dimer concentrations are a measure of fibrinolytic activity, but assessment is only of value when thromboembolism is suspected. It should not be used as a screening test and is of no value postoperatively. The old agglutination assays are not very reliable, but newer second-generation rapid D-dimer tests using latex or enzyme-linked immunosorbent assay (ELISA) are much more sensitive, although non-specific (Kovacs et al, 2001). Hence, D-dimer assays are more useful in *excluding* rather than *confirming* venous thromboembolism, but may reduce the need for further investigation (British Thoracic Society, 2003). Because a negative result usually excludes pulmonary embolism in those considered to be at low to moderate probability of pulmonary embolism, definitive imaging can be reserved for patients with a positive result.

Measuring troponin concentrations can be used in patients with pulmonary embolism for prognostic reasons. Those with a positive result have higher morbidity and mortality rates (Kucher et al, 2003).

Radiology The chest radiograph is often normal, but occasionally reveals an alternative diagnosis, such as pneumothorax or pneumonia. Loss of lung volume (e.g. an elevated hemi-diaphragm) is the most common radiological sign of significant pulmonary embolism, and there may be pulmonary opacities (classically 'wedge' shaped) or linear atelectasis with a small pleural effusion. Larger emboli will produce an area of oligaemia with a 'plump' hilum.

Spiral computerised tomography pulmonary angiography (CTPA) is now the first-line imaging technique in diagnosing a pulmonary embolism. Lung scanning has largely been abandoned, as pulmonary emboli can only be diagnosed or excluded reliably in a minority of patients. The CTPA demonstrates emboli as filling defects within the proximal pulmonary arteries, or may identify alternative causes for chest pain and breathlessness. The CTPA may be superseded by multislice CT scanning (Perrier et al, 2005).

Bilateral leg ultrasonography or venography, even in the absence of leg symptoms, may be helpful in showing thrombus if other tests have been normal but where the degree of suspicion remains high. Computerised tomography of the leg veins immediately after spiral CT angiography can be used to identify thrombus without needing a separate examination.

Echocardiography Transthoracic echocardiography cannot identify thrombus in the pulmonary vessels, but may show thrombus in the right ventricle. The finding of right ventricular dysfunction is not specific, but a dilated right ventricle may be supportive of the diagnosis of large emboli. The echo may be normal, even in patients with large pulmonary emboli, but those with right ventricular overload are at high risk of death. Differential diagnoses, such as myocardial infarction, aortic dissection and pericardial tamponade, may be demonstrated by echocardiography.

Management   Treatment is determined by symptoms and the degree of haemodynamic upset. Most emboli will break up spontaneously, and management should be directed towards maintaining the circulation and preventing recurrent thromboembolism. Pain and anxiety are treated with diamorphine, and 100% oxygen should be given. Vasodilators are contraindicated, and a high central venous pressure should be maintained using plasma expanders and inotropic support if required.

There are then three treatment options:

- anticoagulation;
- thrombolysis;
- surgery.

Anticoagulation   Heparin accelerates the action of antithrombin III and prevents further fibrin deposition, allowing spontaneous endogenous thrombolysis.

For haemodynamically stable patients, low-molecular-weight heparins (LMWH) have revolutionised the early treatment of pulmonary embolism. Both dosing and administration are simple, and laboratory monitoring is not usually required. There is also a lower incidence of thrombocytopenia and no excess bleeding. Treatment with LMWH is also safe and effective in an outpatient setting (Kovacs et al, 2000) and may become more practicable with the introduction of two new anticoagulants:

- *Fondaparinux* is an engineered pentasaccharide, which binds antithrombin and enhances its activity towards factor Xa, with no activity against thrombin. This means that its action is more predictable and the half-life is prolonged (17 hours). It is as effective as unfractionated

heparin in treating pulmonary embolism, but much easier to administer (Buller et al, 2003).
- *Idraparinux* is similar with a much longer half-life (80 hours), so may be given once weekly (Weitz & Bates, 2005).

If patients are haemodynamically unstable and have poor tissue perfusion, intravenous heparin should be used, as LMWH may not be absorbed. A loading dose of unfractionated heparin 5000–10 000 units should be followed by a continuous intravenous infusion of 1000–2000 units/ hour. The infusion rate should vary to keep the activated partial thromboplastin time (APTT) at two or three times the control for at least 7 days.

Thrombolysis   Thrombolytic treatment should be the best treatment for pulmonary embolism, but it has not yet been shown to be superior to heparin with regard to mortality, despite allowing the patient to stabilise haemodynamically more quickly. Currently, thrombolysis is indicated in massive pulmonary embolism with right ventricular overload and hypotension (Hirsch et al, 2004). Streptokinase, urokinase, tissue plasminogen activator (tPA) and reteplase have all been used, and are equally effective if administered by either a pulmonary arterial catheter or peripherally. In contrast to coronary thrombolysis, treatment may be effective for up to 14 days after the acute event. The usual precautions and contraindications apply as for coronary thrombolysis, and complications are similar too.

Pulmonary embolism accounts for 10% of cardiac arrests, and over half of cases have a non-shockable rhythm (usually PEA). If a massive embolus is strongly suspected, an intravenous bolus of 50 mg of alteplase should be given during resuscitation. Most deaths from pulmonary emboli occur in the first hour, and the overall mortality is about 10%.

Surgery   Inferior vena cava filters may be inserted through the internal jugular or femoral vein when anticoagulation is contraindicated, or when there have been further pulmonary emboli despite adequate anticoagulation. Patients who continue to deteriorate despite thrombolytic therapy may be considered for surgical embolectomy. It requires cardiopulmonary bypass and is associated with a mortality of over 50%.

Dissecting thoracic aortic aneurysm

An acute dissecting aneurysm is the most frequent and most lethal disorder of the thoracic aorta. There is an incidence of 5–10 per million, and it is thus twice as common as rupture of abdominal aortic aneurysms. Patients are typically men over the age of 60 years, who have a previous history of hypertension (distal > proximal). A positive family history may be a useful diagnostic clue. Patients with a bicuspid aortic valve have a nine-fold risk of developing aortic dissection compared with those with normal aortic valves. Cocaine and amphetamine abuse associate with aneurysm formation, which may later present with dissection, leakage or rupture.

Dissection occurs as a result of disruption of the aortic wall, which allows blood to be driven into the aortic wall at high pressure. The dissection is usually spontaneous, initiated by a small tear in the aortic intima. This is typically 1–3 cm distal to the coronary sinuses, which is the site of maximal haemodynamic and torsional stress. The next most common site is distal to the origin of the left subclavian artery where the relatively mobile aortic arch is anchored to the chest wall by the *ligamentum arteriosum*. The aortic wall splits along the planes of least resistance to create a double lumen, with the aortic wall separating a true from a false lumen. Most dissections originate in the ascending aorta. The blood may then flow proximally into the pericardium causing tamponade, or distally to involve the aortic arch, descending and abdominal aorta and its branches. The Stanford classification divides dissections into type A and type B. Type A is any dissection involving the aortic arch, regardless of the site of the intimal tear. Type B dissections are those restricted to the aorta distal to the left subclavian artery.

Clinical features The presentation is usually dramatic and dominated by pain. There is sudden, sharp and excruciating pain felt anywhere from the epigastrium to the neck. The pain radiates to the back and sometimes into all four limbs. The patient is cold, clammy and paradoxically hypertensive, with systolic blood pressures often in excess of 200 mmHg, particularly if the dissection is distal. Shortness of breath may be due to left

ventricular failure, a haemothorax or pericardial tamponade. Blood in the pericardial sac may give rise to a pericardial friction rub, and aortic incompetence may develop secondary to dilatation of the aortic annulus. Slowly leaking aneurysms may present with pleuritic chest pain. Peripheral pulses may be absent, reduced or asymmetrical. Subsequent signs and symptoms depend upon which branches of the aorta are involved in the dissection process. Stroke and paraplegia may be the first manifestations of aortic dissection due to involvement of the carotid arteries. Visceral ischaemia may give rise to severe abdominal pain, and involvement of the renal arteries may lead to renal failure.

The ECG can show ST elevation, left ventricular hypertrophy or conduction defects. Inferior myocardial infarction may occur when the right coronary artery is involved, and thrombolytic therapy may be given in error (Blankenship & Almquist, 1989). Occlusion of the left coronary artery is usually rapidly fatal.

The chest radiograph supports the diagnosis in two-thirds of cases, showing a widened superior mediastinum, and sometimes a left-sided pleural effusion caused by extravasated blood. Care must be taken in interpreting the emergency antero-posterior (portable) chest film, as apparent mediastinal widening may be seen in a normal patient.

Echocardiography, particularly transoesophageal echocardiography (TOE), is useful in confirming the diagnosis, and will usually visualise any dissection flap in the descending aorta. Aortography is the standard technique for guiding interventions, but coronary angiography is not required in all cases. MRI or spiral CT scanning may also be used, but are often difficult in unstable patients. These techniques are helpful in monitoring chronic dissections.

Management The two leading problems are pain and shock. Large doses of diamorphine are often required to control the severe pain, and are best given by intravenous infusion. Shock is usually secondary to the severe pain, as there will only be slight blood loss unless there is aortic rupture.

After pain relief, the next vital step is to reduce the blood pressure. Beta-blockade is particularly useful, as it will reduce both systolic blood pressure and the pulse pressure. The reduced force of cardiac contraction may further limit intimal tearing. Atenolol and metoprolol are available for intravenous use, but esmolol may be preferable in the acute phase, as it has a short half-life, allowing optimal titration. If beta-blockade alone does not control the blood pressure, vasodilators are ideal additional agents (e.g. sodium nitroprusside), but will increase the force of ventricular contraction unless co-prescribed with a beta-blocker. Intravenous labetalol has the advantage of both alpha- and beta-blockade, with alpha-blocking activity helping to maintain peripheral vasodilatation. Antihypertensive therapy should be carefully titrated to keep the systolic blood pressure between 100 and 120 mmHg. With successful hypotensive treatment, up to half the patients can survive, particularly those with small, distal dissections. If complications emerge, or the blood pressure cannot be controlled, surgical intervention is required, and this is always needed if the ascending aorta is involved.

The aim of surgery is to prevent aortic rupture or cardiac tamponade (Erbel et al, 2001). For proximal dissections (type A), the intimal tear or whole flap is excised, and a composite Dacron graft is set in, with or without reimplantation of the coronary arteries. For type B dissections, medical treatment is preferred, unless there are clinical signs of aortic expansion, persistent chest pain or periaortic haematomas.

Aortic fenestration can be used if the intimal flap is occluding one of the abdominal, limb or renal arteries. A dilating balloon is passed into the aorta via the femoral artery and used to create a communication between the true and the false lumen.

Endovascular stent–graft placement is a new technique that involves inserting a metallic stent covered with graft material inside the aorta via the femoral artery. The aim is not to push the intimal flap against the aortic wall, but to gently cover the entry tear and induce thrombosis in the false lumen to stimulate the healing process.

Prognosis Untreated, the overall mortality from aortic dissection is 30% in the first day, increasing to 70% in 7 days and 90% by 3 months. With modern medical and surgical intervention, the 1-year survival is 52%.

Pericarditis

Acute pericardial disease has many causes (Box 12.3). The most common are acute viral pericarditis and post-infarction pericarditis, but frequently no cause is found. The pain may be severe, especially if the adjacent pleura is affected, when coughing and dyspnoea are common. Pericardial pain may radiate to the arms, back, upper abdomen, shoulder tip or neck. The diagnosis should be suspected if the pain is worse on inspiration or on lying flat, and may be confirmed by an audible pericardial friction rub, usually best heard at the left sternal edge. The rub is high pitched, superficial and scratchy, and is similar to the sound made by stroking the hair above the ear. It has a to-and-fro sound passing between diastole and systole as the ventricles fill. It may be missed as it is often soft, transient, localised and intermittent. Bronchial breathing at the left base can occur if a large pericardial effusion compresses the left

---

Box 12.3   Some causes of pericarditis.

Idiopathic
Infective
    Viral
    Bacterial
    Fungal
    Parasitic
Immunological
    Post myocardial infarction
    Dressler syndrome
    Post-cardiotomy syndrome
Connective tissue disorders
    Systemic lupus erythematosus (SLE)
    Polyarteritis nodosa (PAN)
    Rheumatoid arthritis
Rheumatic fever
Traumatic
Uraemia
Drug induced
    Cancer and radiotherapy

lower lobe (Ewart's sign). Shoulder tip pain is common if the inferior surface of the heart is involved. The ECG in acute pericarditis shows ST segment elevation, which is concave upwards (saddle shaped) in many leads (Fig. 12.2). Typical lead involvement is I, II, aVL, aVF and V3–V6. The ST segment is always depressed in aVR, frequently in V1 and occasionally in V2. ECG changes may be confused with those caused by acute myocardial infarction, although ECG changes in myocardial infarction are usually localised to a few leads within an anatomical distribution. As the inflammation improves, T wave inversion may develop.

Post-infarction pericarditis Up to 20% of transmural myocardial infarcts are complicated by pericarditis within the first week. Small effusions may be detectable on echocardiography.

Figure 12.2 ECG: acute viral pericarditis. Note widespread concave 'saddle-shaped' ST segment elevation.

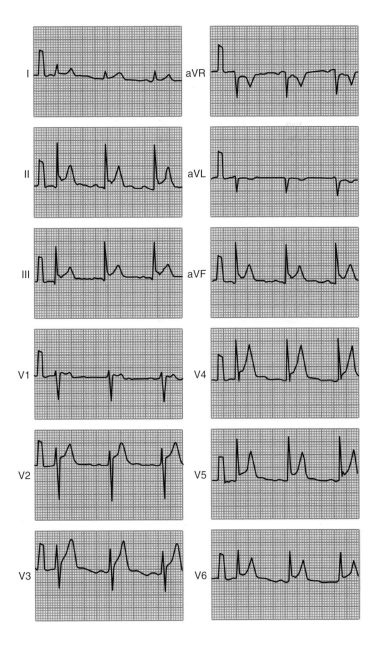

Pericarditis may recur within 3 months, in association with plural effusions and systemic symptoms, such as malaise and fever (Dressler syndrome). The mechanism is thought to be autoimmune, triggered by a response to the products of myocardial damage. Antimyocardial antibodies may be found in the blood. A similar condition may complicate cardiac surgery (post-cardiotomy syndrome).

Viral pericarditis Acute viral pericarditis affects young adults, and the usual viruses are from the Coxsackie B group, echoviruses, influenza and infectious mononucleosis. Following a 'flu-like illness, there is fever and chest pain, which is sharp, retrosternal and often radiates to the left shoulder. The pain may be mild or excruciating. Atrial dysrhythmias are common, possibly caused by inflammation of the superficially located sinus node. Pericardial manifestation of HIV infection can be due to infective, non-infective and neoplastic diseases.

Connective tissue disorders Pericarditis, with or without effusion, is a component of a multiple serositic process in systemic autoimmune diseases such as rheumatoid arthritis, systemic lupus erythematosus (SLE), polymyositis and sarcoidosis. Effusions may result from serous tissues around the lungs (pleural effusion), heart (pericardial effusion) and abdomen (ascites). Treatment should focus on pericardial symptoms, management of the pericardial effusion and the underlying systemic disease. Steroid therapy is usually indicated.

Treatment

Treatment depends on the severity of the symptoms. Admission to hospital is warranted for most patients to determine the aetiology, observe for tamponade and symptomatic treatment. Echocardiography should be carried out to look for an enlarging pericardial effusion and worsening left ventricular function due to an associated myocarditis.

In most cases, simple analgesia or NSAIDs are enough, although the latter should be avoided following myocardial infarction. NSAIDs may delay scar formation, and indomethacin has been shown to impair coronary blood flow by inducing coronary arterial spasm (Mori et al, 1997). Steroids will quickly control pain, fever and any resistant atrial dysrhythmias in more severe cases, but should not be used routinely, as they increase the risk of recurrence. If there is an associated myocarditis with raised cardiac markers, bedrest is important. A small number of patients will develop transient pericardial constriction or effusion following viral pericarditis. Anticoagulation therapy should be reduced or stopped to avoid haemorrhagic pericarditis.

In general, acute pericarditis is a benign disease with symptoms lasting under 2 weeks. Some cases become subacute, with continuing pyrexia and intermittent pain lasting several days. Recurrence of pericardial pain may return weeks or months after the initial attack, but the condition eventually settles within 12 months. Colchicine is the treatment of choice (0.5 mg twice a day), combined with NSAIDs if required, but therapy may be needed for many months. Pretreatment with steroids may impair the therapeutic effect of colchicine.

Oesophageal pain

Oesophageal pain has many patterns. It may be described as burning, gripping, pressing or stabbing. *Gastro-oesophageal reflux disease* (GORD) is very common, and can be demonstrated by barium studies or endoscopy in about 40% of the general adult population. Related pain is often confused with angina, because it often radiates to the jaw and arms and may be relieved by nitrates; hence the term 'heartburn'.

Endoscopic confirmation should not be performed until acute cardiac ischaemia has been excluded. Because it is so common, it frequently co-exists with ischaemic chest pain, and the diagnosis of reflux oesophagitis does not exclude co-existent myocardial ischaemia. Having oesophageal reflux lowers the threshold for anginal pain.

Oesophageal rupture is an uncommon disorder, which may easily be confused with myocardial infarction. The pain is severe, central and often radiates to the back, and the patient is often sweating, cyanosed or shocked. Chest pain follows, rather than precedes, the vomiting. If there is leakage of gastro-oesophageal contents into the mediastinum, the condition can be lethal.

Pneumothorax

The pain from a spontaneous pneumothorax is sudden, often severe and usually unilateral, although a mediastinal pneumothorax can present with central chest pain. Dyspnoea and hypotension may follow, sometime with cyanosis. Transient non-specific ECG changes may be seen. Diagnosis is by chest radiograph, and treatment is governed by the size of the pneumothorax and pre-existing respiratory function. Many cases can be treated conservatively but, for patients with previous respiratory disease or respiratory difficulty, aspiration or a chest drain will be required.

Intra-abdominal causes of chest pain

Peptic ulcer disease or *gallbladder disease* may present with lower chest/upper abdominal pain, which may be referred to the shoulders. Chronic cholecystitis may have many similarities to anginal pain. During acute cholecystitis, the ECG may show T wave inversion, especially in the inferior leads. A perforated peptic ulcer may mimic myocardial infarction.

Occult *gastrointestinal bleeding* may present with pain and shock and can easily be confused with acute myocardial infarction.

Acute pancreatitis may present with shock, hypoxia and severe upper abdominal/lower chest pain. Sitting forward may ease the pain forward, rather as in pericarditis. Common clues are alcohol misuse, hypertriglyceridaemia or gallstone disease.

PERICARDIAL EFFUSIONS AND CARDIAC TAMPONADE

Pericardial effusions are common. Often, the underlying cause is not clear but, in about two-thirds of cases, it is obviously related to an underlying general medical or cardiac disease (Box 12.4). The volume of fluid may vary from 150 mL to over 2000 mL. Larger effusions suggest a neoplastic, tuberculosis or uraemic pericarditis. In asymptomatic patients, small pericardial effusions (less than 10 mm on two-dimensional echo) may be an incidental finding, particularly in women.

Effusions that develop slowly are often asymptomatic, while rapidly accumulating smaller effusions can present with *cardiac tamponade* resulting

Box 12.4 Some causes of pericardial effusion.

Pericarditis (all causes)
Cardiac rupture following myocardial infarction
Following cardiac surgery
Chest trauma
Malignancy
Uraemia
Aortic dissection

from cardiac compression caused by the effusion and increased intrapericardial pressures. With large chronic effusions, patients may complain of dyspnoea, dull chest pain, swollen ankles or abdominal bloating. In acute cases, there may be threatened or actual circulatory collapse. Heart sounds are quiet, and the neck veins are elevated. There may be pulsus paradoxus. The chest radiograph may show globular cardiomegaly with sharp margins ('water bottle' silhouette). The ECG may show small complexes, and electrical alternans may be seen as the heart moves around the pericardial sac within a large effusion (Fig. 12.3). Electrical alternans is a broad term that describes alternate-beat variation in the direction, amplitude and duration of any part of the ECG waveform. Echocardiography is diagnostic. The size of effusions can be graded as small (echo-free space in diastole under 10 mm), moderate (more than 10 mm), large (over 20 mm) or very large (over 20 mm and compression of the heart). The effusions measured by CT or MRI may tend to be larger than those measured by echocardiography.

Tamponade may be suggested by early diastolic collapse of the right ventricular free wall. With colour Doppler, tricuspid flow increases and mitral flow increases on inspiration (and vice versa on expiration). Patients who are dehydrated may temporarily improve with intravenous fluids enhancing ventricular filling, but pericardiocentesis should be performed in more

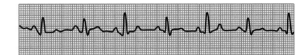

Figure 12.3 Electrical alternans – alternation of QRS complex amplitude (axis) between beats.

severe cases under ultrasound control, with appropriate resuscitation facilities. Echocardiography identifies the shortest route for the pericardium. Major complications during access (e.g. laceration of the myocardium and the coronary vessels) occur in about 2% of cases so, for non-urgent cases, pericardiocentesis should be guided by fluoroscopy and performed in the cardiac catheterisation laboratory with ECG monitoring. The subxiphoid approach is usual, with a long needle directed towards the left shoulder at a 30° angle to the skin. This route is extrapleural and avoids the coronary and internal mammary arteries, a hazard with anterior access (between the sixth or seventh rib space in the anterior axillary line). If fluid is aspirated freely, a small volume of contrast medium may be injected to check position, and then a soft J-tip guidewire is introduced to allow insertion of a multiholed pigtail catheter connected to an external drain. Fluid is removed in steps of less than a litre at a time to avoid sudden decompression syndrome associated with acute right ventricular dilatation. Pericardial fluid often recurs, when a surgical drain or a pericardial window may be needed.

DYSRHYTHMIAS

Dysrhythmias unassociated with an acute coronary syndrome are often sent to the CCU. Coronary artery disease may or may not be an underlying cause. The clinical importance is related to the ventricular rate, the presence of any underlying heart disease and the integrity of cardiovascular reflexes. Coronary blood flow occurs during diastole and, as the heart rate increases, diastole shortens. In the presence of coronary atherosclerosis, blood flow may become critical, and anginal-type chest pain may result. Reduced cardiac performance produces symptoms of faintness or syncope, and leads to increased sympathetic stimulation, which may increase the heart rate further. With any rhythm disturbance, it is important to consider:

- any associated cardiac disorder (e.g. coronary or valvular disease);
- any resting ECG abnormality (e.g. pre-excitation, long QT interval);
- any cardiotoxic drug therapy (e.g. tricyclic antidepressants, digoxin, L-dopa);

- metabolic derangement (e.g. hyperkalaemia, hypercalcaemia, hypoxia, acidosis);
- any precipitating factor (e.g. pyrexia, thyrotoxicosis, pneumonia, alcohol, illegal drugs).

Mechanisms of abnormal tachycardias

Most abnormal tachycardias are produced by one of two pathophysiological mechanisms: re-entry or enhanced automaticity.

Re-entry

Re-entry tachycardias may occur within the atria or the ventricles, or may involve the atrio-ventricular (AV) junction, and depend upon an electrical circuit created by the presence of two or more conduction pathways that have different electrical characteristics. Most commonly, this occurs at the AV junction, where the rapid passage of a circulating impulse between the atria and ventricles causes a *reciprocating tachycardia*. The re-entry circuit requires two separate connections between the atria and the ventricles, one part allowing forward (antegrade) conduction and the other allowing return (retrograde) conduction. In the minority of cases, this is due to an anatomically separate conduction pathway, such as occurs in the Wolff–Parkinson–White or Lown–Ganong–Levine syndrome (AV re-entry tachycardias). In most cases, the circuit is established within or around the AV node itself (AV nodal re-entry tachycardias), with part of the node becoming refractory, allowing a circuit to be established (Fig. 12.4).

Enhanced automaticity

Automaticity describes the inherent ability of specialised cardiac tissue to initiate electrical impulses. The cells responsible are known as pacemaker or automatic cells. In the sinus node, these will discharge spontaneously at about 80 times/minute but, elsewhere, automatic cells have a slower discharge rate. For example, in the AV node, this may be at about 60 times/minute and, within the ventricles, 30 times/minute. This back-up system of escape rhythms exists to prevent rhythm failure should the sinus node fail to discharge. In this instance, an alternative pacemaker usually takes

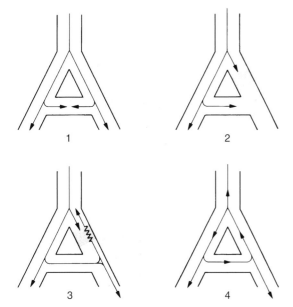

Figure 12.4   Reciprocating tachycardia mechanism.
(1) Normal electrical conduction through a common
proximal piece of tissue, which splits into two pathways.
(2) A unidirectional block develops in one limb of tissue
(possibly because of a slowing in the refractory period)
and this fails to conduct the impulse. The other pathway
conducts normally. (3) The normal conduction wave is
carried round to the proximal side of the block, which, if
it has recovered functionally, will transmit the impulse in
a retrograde direction. (4) If the normal limb of tissue
has recovered, it can be stimulated by the returning
impulse and a circus movement about the area of
conducting tissue is set up, which is self-propagating.
This gives rise to a re-entrant dysrhythmia.

over and, although the rate will initially be slow,
there is a tendency for the rate of this abnormal
pacemaker to speed up (enhanced automaticity).
When an ectopic site takes over pacemaker function, it is denoted by the prefix 'idio', as in idio-
ventricular tachycardia. Attempting to terminate
these dysrhythmias using drugs that suppress
re-entry circuits will usually be ineffective.

TYPES OF TACHYCARDIA

Tachycardia describes fast heart rhythms, and
abnormal rhythms are usually over 130 beats/
minute. The QRS complex may be either narrow
or broad.

Narrow–complex tachycardias

The main narrow-complex tachycardias are sinus
tachycardias, junctional tachycardias, atrial flutter and atrial fibrillation. With the exception
of atrial fibrillation, narrow-complex tachycardias are regular, and the P wave may or may not
be visible. If the P wave is seen, it is usually different from the normal sinus rhythm P wave and
is often inverted. Atrio-ventricular (AV) block
may occur during the tachycardia. Sometimes, it
is not possible to determine the exact atrial
rhythm during tachycardias unless specialised
ECG leads are used. The term supraventricular
tachycardia (SVT) is still used as a blanket term
for all narrow-complex tachycardias, but this is
anatomically incorrect as most tachycardias
incorporate both ventricular and atrial myocardial tissue within the circuit. It should also be
remembered that some SVTs might appear as
broad-complex tachycardias.

Differentiation between different types of SVT
may be difficult, particularly when ventricular
rates exceed 150 beats/minute. Increasing atrio-
ventricular block by manoeuvres such as carotid
sinus massage or administration of intravenous
adenosine may be of diagnostic value, as slowing
the ventricular rate allows more accurate visualisation of atrial activity. Such manoeuvres will not
usually stop the tachycardia, however, unless it is
due to re-entry involving the atrio-ventricular node.
In general, treatment is usually directed towards the
restoration of sinus rhythm, although in chronic or
unstable rhythms, treatment aims to control the
ventricular rate.

Sinus tachycardia

A sinus tachycardia is usually a physiological
response to sympathetic stimulation, but may be
precipitated by sympathomimetic drugs (e.g.
salbutamol) or endocrine disturbances (e.g. thyrotoxicosis).

The heart rate increases gradually and
may show beat-to-beat variation. A QRS complex
follows each P wave. P wave morphology and
axis are normal, although as the heart rate speeds
up, the height of the P wave increases, and the
PR interval will shorten. With a fast tachycardia, the

P wave may become lost in the preceding T wave. Recognition of the underlying cause usually makes diagnosis of sinus tachycardia easy. A persistent tachycardia in the absence of an obvious underlying cause (e.g. anxiety, pain, fever, anaemia, hypovolaemia or thyrotoxicosis) should prompt consideration of atrial flutter or atrial tachycardia.

Junctional tachycardias

A junctional tachycardia is characterised by the sudden onset of a tachycardia > 150 beats/minute (Fig. 12.5). In some patients, there may be no symptoms but, if there is coronary disease, there may be ischaemic pain, dyspnoea or syncope.

There are two forms of junctional tachycardia:

- AV nodal re-entry tachycardia (AVNRT);
- AV re-entry tachycardia (AVRT).

Atrio-ventricular nodal re-entry tachycardias
This is the most common type of regular narrow complex tachycardia, caused by a re-entry circuit in or around the AV node. It is relatively common, more often in women. It often presents in early adult life when maturation of the AV node associates with the development of two separate atrial pathways, one fast conducting and one slow conducting, predisposing to re-entry tachycardias. They share a final common pathway through the lower part of the AV node and bundle of His. The fast pathway has a long refractory period, and the slow pathway has a short refractory period. During normal sinus rhythm, the impulse travels preferentially to the ventricles via the fast pathway. Impulses also travel down the slow pathway, but terminate because the common pathway is refractory. Episodes of tachycardia may be provoked by a premature atrial beat that occurs when the fast pathway is refractory. It then travels via the slow pathway, and is returned through the fast pathway back up to the atria, and circuit

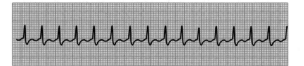

Figure 12.5 Junctional tachycardia.

movement through the AV node is initiated. This type of 'slow–fast' re-entry circuit is found in 90% of AVNRT patients. The rest have a 'fast–slow' circuit, in which the re-entrant tachycardia is initiated by a premature ventricular contraction, and the impulse travels back up the slow pathway. Atrial depolarisation is thus late and is seen as an inverted P wave between the QRS complexes in the inferior leads. The PR interval is therefore shorter than the RP interval, and the term 'long RP[1] tachycardia' is used. This may be difficult to distinguish from a true atrial tachycardia.

Episodes of AVNRT may begin at any age. The tachycardia starts and stops abruptly and can last a few seconds, several hours or days. The frequency of episodes can vary between several a day or one episode in a lifetime. Most patients have only mild symptoms, such as palpitations or the sensation that their heart is beating rapidly. Other symptoms include dizziness, dyspnoea, weakness, neck pulsation and central chest pain. Some patients report polyuria after the episode.

In sinus rhythm, the electrocardiogram is normal. During the tachycardia, the rhythm is regular, with narrow QRS complexes and a rate of 150–250 beats/minute. As atrial and ventricular depolarisation often occurs simultaneously, the P waves are frequently buried in the QRS complex and may be totally obscured. Where visible, P waves are inverted in leads II, III and aVF, because activation of the atria is backwards. Alternatively, the P wave may appear as a small positive deflection at the end of the QRS complex, giving rise to a 'pseudo' S wave in the inferior leads and a 'pseudo' R wave in V1. This may make the ECG pattern appear like incomplete right bundle branch block.

Atrio-ventricular re-entry tachycardias AVRTs are associated with the presence of an anatomically distinct accessory AV connection, such as the James or Mahaim bundles, which can be situated anywhere around the groove between the atria and the ventricles. Most are located within the free wall of the left ventricle and, in 10% of cases, more than one accessory bundle exists. These muscular connections are produced by a congenital abnormality of the AV rings that electrically connect atrial and ventricular tissue through breaks in the tricuspid or mitral annulus. The most frequent is the bundle of Kent in the Wolff–Parkinson–White syndrome (WPW). About 1 in 500 people have the WPW syndrome, although fewer than a quarter have sustained tachycardias, in part because the ability to conduct via the accessory pathway declines with age. Episodes of tachycardia tend to be more common in younger people, but may come and go through life. The condition sometimes occurs in association with mitral valve prolapse, Ebstein's anomaly or hypertrophic cardiomyopathy, so echocardiography is advisable.

In sinus rhythm, the atrial impulse conducts through the accessory pathway, avoiding the normal delay encountered with normal AV nodal conduction. Rapid AV transmission is reflected by a short PR interval on the ECG (< 0.12 seconds). The impulse enters the ventricles in non-specialised myocardial tissue, and ventricular depolarisation progresses slowly at first, distorting the early part of the R wave and producing the characteristic delta wave on the electrocardiogram (Fig. 12.6). This slow depolarisation is then rapidly overtaken by depolarisation propagated by the normal conduction system, and the rest of the QRS complex appears relatively normal.

The WPW syndrome has been classified into two types according to the ECG appearance in the precordial leads:

- In type A, there is a posterior left atrial or a paraseptal pathway, and the delta wave and QRS complex are predominantly upright in the precordial leads. The dominant R wave in lead V1 is sometimes misinterpreted as right bundle branch block or a posterior myocardial infarct.
- In type B, the pathway links the right atrium to the right ventricle. The delta wave and QRS complex are predominantly negative in leads V1 and V2 and positive in the other precordial leads, and may sometimes resemble anterior myocardial infarction or left bundle branch block.

In about 20% of cases, the accessory pathway is only able to conduct backwards, and the presence of the pathway is 'concealed'. Pre-excitation of the

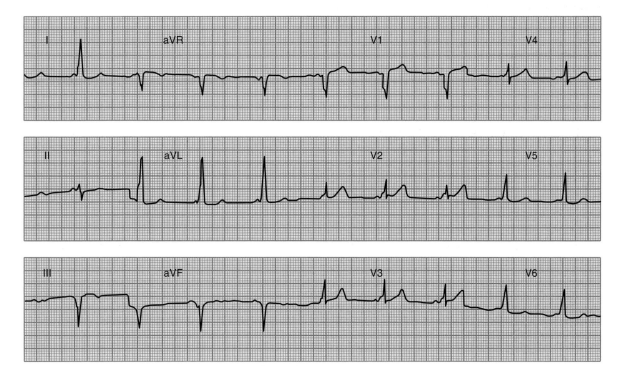

Figure 12.6 Wolff–Parkinson–White syndrome (type B).

ventricles does not occur, and the resting ECG is normal.

AVNT tachycardias

The presence of an accessory pathway allows the formation of a re-entry circuit, which predisposes to paroxysmal tachycardias. These may be either narrow- or broad-complex tachycardias, depending on whether the atrio-ventricular node or the accessory pathway is used for antegrade conduction.

Orthodromic conduction occurs during most tachycardias in the WPW syndrome, with normal forward conduction through the AV node that passes rapidly back up to the atria via the fast conducting accessory pathway ('slow forward–fast back'). The tachycardia is typically initiated by a premature atrial impulse that is conducted normally down through the AV node to the ventricles and then circles repeatedly between the atria and ventricles, through the bundle of Kent, producing a narrow-complex tachycardia. As atrial depolarisation lags behind ventricular depolarisation, P waves follow the QRS complexes. The P waves may be difficult to see, but brief interruptions of the tachycardia using carotid sinus massage or adenosine may be very helpful. The delta wave is not observed during the tachycardia because forward conduction is normal, and the QRS complex is of normal duration. The rate is usually 140–250 beats/minute with 1:1 conduction.

Antidromic conduction is less common (10%), and the impulse travels in the opposite direction ('fast forward–slow back'). Here, the rapidly conducting accessory pathway allows antegrade conduction from the atria to the ventricles, but arrives in non-specialised conducting tissues. Depolarisation is delayed, and the resulting QRS complex is broad and often bizarre in shape. The impulse returns to the atria via the AV node.

While AVRTs are usually well tolerated, a small number of patients have accessory pathways capable of very rapid conduction (in excess of 300 beats/minute). If the patient develops atrial fibrillation, fast AV conduction can precipitate ventricular fibrillation. The incidence of sudden death in WPW syndrome is estimated at 0.15% at 3 years rising to 0.39% at 10 years. Those with intermittent pre-excitation or whose abnormal conduction disappears on exercise are likely to have slow conducting (safe) accessory pathways.

If drugs are use to terminate an AVRT, agents that block the AV node should be avoided (e.g. digoxin, verapamil), as they can encourage rapid extranodal conduction, which may sometimes initiate ventricular fibrillation. Flecainide and amiodarone slow conduction in both the accessory pathway and the AV node, and are preferable. Electrophysiological studies are recommended in patients with pre-excitation syndromes with a view to ablation and cure.

Atrial tachycardia

Atrial tachycardia is a true SVT, as it does not involve the AV junction or the ventricular myocardium. The tachycardia is caused by the rapid discharge of an atrial pacemaker that arises from one or more foci in the atria (usually the interatrial septum) at a rate of 150–250/minute (i.e. slower than atrial flutter). The P waves may be abnormally shaped depending on the site of the ectopic pacemaker, and the ventricular rate depends on the degree of AV block. Second- or third-degree AV block is often present, so the ventricular response is usually not rapid and causes little systemic upset. *Atrial tachycardia with AV block* is described classically in relation to digoxin toxicity, although this is only the case in about 10% of episodes. The ventricular rhythm is usually regular but may be irregular if AV block is variable. Although often referred to as 'paroxysmal atrial tachycardia with block', the dysrhythmia is usually sustained. *Benign atrial tachycardia* is a common dysrhythmia in elderly people. It has an abrupt onset and cessation and is brief in duration, with an atrial rate of 80–140 beats/minute.

In most cases of atrial tachycardia, an intra-atrial re-entry circuit is present, but a *multifocal atrial tachycardia* may occur when multiple sites in the atria are discharging with increased automaticity. Because the atrial impulse arises from different sites, the P waves have varying morphologies and PR intervals. The ventricular rate is irregular, but can be distinguished from atrial fibrillation by an isoelectric baseline between the P waves. This type of atrial tachycardia is typically seen in association with chronic pulmonary disease or other causes of hypoxia.

Treatment of regular narrow-complex tachycardias

The urgency of treatment depends upon symptoms.

Vagal manoeuvres are a useful initial therapy, and may terminate the tachycardia in up to 25% of cases.

- *Valsalva manoeuvre* (forced expiration against a closed glottis). This manoeuvre is sometimes hard to explain, and even harder to get patients to perform. It thus has a low success rate in clinical practice. Asking patients to blow up a small balloon is an easier way to produce an involuntary Valsalva manoeuvre, and perhaps these should be kept on coronary care.
- *Muller manoeuvre* (inspiratory effort with the mouth and nose closed).
- *Gag reflex* (stimulation of the soft palate with a spatula).
- *Diving reflex* (cold water splashed on the face).
- *Carotid sinus massage*. The carotid sinus is located anterior to the sterno-mastoid muscle, at the upper level of, or just above, the thyroid cartilage. The carotid artery is massaged against the transverse process of the sixth vertebra for 10–20 seconds by direct pressure. The patient should be lying flat, and only one side should be massaged at a time. Following a case report in 1985, which speculated that carotid sinus massage might cause disruption of atheromatous carotid plaques (Bastulli & Orlowski, 1985), the UK Resuscitation Council advises caution in patients with carotid bruits. However, significant carotid stenoses may occur in the absence of a bruit, so caution is required in the elderly and those with known cerebrovascular disease. Interestingly, the patient described in the case report had no evidence of carotid disease at angiography! Carotid sinus massage should not be attempted by those unfamiliar with the procedure, as strong vagal manoeuvres may cause a sudden and profound bradycardia, which may in turn trigger ventricular fibrillation, particularly in the peri-infarction period.

Drug treatment is usually very effective, and long-term treatment should be considered for repeated and poorly tolerated attacks. The drug of choice for terminating acute narrow-complex tachycardias is adenosine, particularly if there is left ventricular dysfunction or hypotension. Intravenous adenosine may induce atrial fibrillation or even asystole, but this is usually short lived. Flushing or transient chest pain may occur. When given to patients in sinus rhythm, adenosine may be utilised to reveal otherwise latent pre-excitation (e.g. WPW syndrome). Verapamil (5–10 mg) may be preferable in patients with asthma, but should never be given for broad-complex tachycardias, as it may cause cardiovascular collapse. Beta-blockers are often successful, but should be avoided if there is uncontrolled cardiac failure or in patients who have been pretreated with verapamil. Refractory tachycardias usually respond to amiodarone. Overdrive pacing may be effective in selected cases.

Many recurrent, regular junctional tachycardias can be cured by catheter ablation, and this form of treatment should be considered for all patients in whom drug control is suboptimal or producing side effects (Schilling, 2002). The aim of ablation is to render one limb of the short circuit non-functional. Preferentially, the slow pathway is targeted, as this has a higher success rate (around 96%) and a lower risk of complete heart block (< 1%). About 5% require a further procedure. There is a small risk of death (under 0.2%), mostly from tamponade.

Atrial flutter and atrial fibrillation

Atrial flutter Atrial flutter usually associates with underlying cardiac disease. In typical atrial flutter, there is a re-entry circuit in the right atrium with secondary activation of the left atrium. Some forms of atrial flutter may use other pathways, such as around the mitral annulus or around surgical incisions. Usually, the circuit rotates in an anti-clockwise direction around the tricuspid annulus, travelling through the cavo-tricuspid *isthmus*, which is a narrow corridor of tissue that lies between the anterior lip of the inferior vena cava and the posterior part of the tricuspid annulus, at a rate of 300/minute (isthmus dependent atrial flutter). The normal AV node cannot conduct impulses at this rate, and 2:1 AV block usually occurs, giving rise to a regular narrow-complex tachycardia at a rate of 150 beats/minute.

Typical sawtooth waves may be visible on the ECG, especially in V1 and the inferior leads, with negative deflections in V6. The atrial rate is in the region of 220–320/minute. The non-conducting flutter waves are often mistaken for or merged with T waves and become apparent only if the block is increased. Adenosine or carotid sinus massage may be used to induce transient AV block to allow identification of flutter waves.

Treatment depends upon the clinical situation. Electrical cardioversion is usually the best therapy, because the rhythm is generally resistant to drug therapy. Class I antidysrhythmic agents may terminate the attack but, paradoxically, may permit 1:1 conduction by transiently slowing the flutter rate. Amiodarone is therefore the drug of choice; it helps to stabilise atrial activity, as well as blocking the AV node. Digoxin may produce atrial fibrillation that is easier to control. Radiofrequency ablation of the isthmus is usually possible in chronic or recurrent atrial flutter. Long-term success occurs in around 97% of cases, with fewer than 5% requiring a repeat procedure. About 30% of patients will later develop atrial fibrillation, particularly if this was present before ablation. Patients are at similar risk of thromboembolism to those with atrial fibrillation, and indications for anticoagulation are the same (see below).

Atrial fibrillation Atrial fibrillation (AF) is the most common cardiac dysrhythmia in adults, and many are admitted to the CCU to control symptoms or for cardioversion. The incidence of AF increases with age, affecting about 0.9% of the general population in the UK, 6% in those over 65 years of age, with prevalence rising to 17% in people over the age of 70 years (Psaty et al, 1997). It is twice as common in men as in women.

The dysrhythmia may be a marker for underlying cardiac pathology, or it may indicate a systemic abnormality that predisposes the individual to the dysrhythmia (Table 12.5). However, 50% of patients with paroxysmal AF and 20% with persistent or permanent AF have otherwise normal hearts ('lone' atrial fibrillation). In these people, autonomic dysfunction sometimes acts as a trigger.

- *Adrenergic AF* occurs in older people, and may relate to hypertensive changes in the heart.

Table 12.5 Some causes of atrial fibrillation.

Common	Less common
Coronary heart disease	Pulmonary embolism
Hypertension	Hypoxia
Mitral stenosis	Postoperative
Alcohol	Pregnancy
Pyrexial illness	Chest trauma
(especially pneumonia)	Thyrotoxicosis
After cardiac surgery	Cardiomyopathy
Chronic obstructive	Athletes (vagal atrial
pulmonary disease	fibrillation)
Heart failure	Herbal remedies (e.g. ephedra,
	ginseng)

Episodes of AF occur almost exclusively during daytime and are often preceded by meals, alcohol, exercise or emotional stress.

- *Vagal AF* is associated with an overactive parasympathetic nervous system (high vagal tone), and is often observed in athletic individuals, especially in men aged 40–50 years. Attacks occur in the evening or are nocturnal, lasting from a few minutes to several hours. Rest (particularly after heavy meals) and alcohol consumption are also predisposing factors. Many of these patients can abort an attack by exercising. If needing drug therapy, agents that slow the heart (e.g. beta-blockers, propafenone) may worsen the condition.

The development of AF requires both an underlying abnormality and a trigger (or triggers) to precipitate the onset. Triggers will vary between individuals and may include physical factors such as wall stress, ischaemia or metabolic factors. Ectopic foci originating from around the pulmonary veins may be responsible for the initiation of AF in many cases. Multiple wavelets of electrical activity propagate randomly in the atrial tissue, producing chaotic but continuous activation of the atrial tissue. Prolonged AF produces both structural and electrophysiological changes in the atria. Myocyte degeneration and fibrosis acts as a trigger for AF, and a vicious circle develops ('AF begets AF').

Atrial fibrillation may be classified as:

- first detected;
- paroxysmal (terminates spontaneously);
- persistent (reverts with electrical/pharmacological intervention);
- permanent (will not revert to sinus rhythm).

More than half of patients with first detected AF will spontaneously revert back to sinus rhythm, particularly if there is an obvious precipitant (e.g. alcohol, myocardial infarction, pyrexia) but, for those with paroxysmal AF, episodes usually become persistent and eventually permanent (Fig. 12.7).

Atrial fibrillation is easily recognised electrocardiographically, but management is often difficult. It is not a benign dysrhythmia, and associates with a doubling of mortality, mostly from stroke. The fast and irregular heart rate of AF can cause palpitations, dizziness, malaise, anxiety and may even precipitate heart failure from a tachycardia-induced cardiomyopathy (TAC), in which ventricular function deteriorates secondary to poorly controlled ventricular rate. Haemodynamic impairment in AF results principally from the rapid ventricular response, although the loss of synchronised atrial contraction may adversely affect cardiac efficiency in those with important underlying cardiac pathology.

Paroxysmal AF may disrupt the lives of patients, even if episodes are short and infrequent and may not require medical intervention. The need for long-term anticoagulation to reduce stroke may be unacceptable or contraindicated in many patients.

Short-term management   The approach to each patient must be individualised. Confirmation that an irregular pulse is due to AF must always be based on electrocardiographic findings (either a 12-lead ECG or Holter monitor). Baseline blood counts are needed to exclude underlying causes (e.g. anaemia or thyroid disease), and a chest radiograph will also be needed to exclude intrathoracic causes (e.g. infection or tumour). An echocardiogram is needed in most cases to define structural heart disease, left ventricular function and to refine risk stratification for antithrombotic therapy. It should not be used to decide which patients require warfarin, or where long-term management is not going to be affected (e.g. the very elderly, those with advanced cardiac disease or other major co-morbidities). Occasionally, trans-oesophageal echo is needed to define cardiac abnormalities or to exclude thrombus in the left atrial appendage prior to cardioversion.

In general, four issues must be addressed.

1 Is there an underlying cause? Treating the underlying cause will often take away the trigger (Table 12.5). If this is removed fast enough, AF it is not likely to become a chronic or recurring disorder.
2 Is the heart rate controlled? In the absence of AV nodal dysfunction, the ventricular rate of acute onset AF will be rapid, and control of the ventricular response is needed for symptom reduction and to prevent cardiac failure. Digoxin will usually control the resting ventricular rate, but will seldom control the heart rate during exercise. Consequently, a beta-blocker or a rate-limiting calcium channel blocker (e.g. diltiazem, verapamil) should be considered as first-line treatment, particularly in patients with co-existing hypertension or coronary disease. If monotherapy is ineffective, digoxin may then be added in. When verapamil is prescribed, less digoxin is required. Beta-blockers should not be given in combination with verapamil.

Development of a tachycardia-induced dilated cardiomyopathy is more likely to occur with chronic fast ventricular rates. The efficacy of

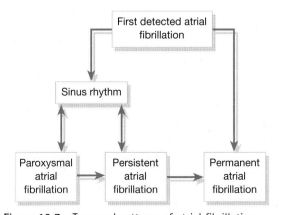

Figure 12.7 Temporal patterns of atrial fibrillation.

drug therapy is best determined with a 24-hour ambulatory recorder, ensuring that the average heart rate is under 100 beats/minute.

3 Should cardioversion be attempted? A patient with recent onset AF requires early assessment as therapy to restore sinus rhythm is most successful when given early. Where AF has been present for over 3 months or where the duration is uncertain, relapse is frequent even if cardioversion is attempted. Higher risk of recurrence is also seen in patients with previous episodes of AF, patients with structural heart disease or where there is a history of failed cardioversion.

4 Anticoagulation. If it is certain that AF has been present for 48 hours or less, heparin should be started, and electrical or pharmacological cardioversion should be attempted as soon as possible. Anticoagulation following successful cardioversion is not required. If AF has been present for longer, warfarin should be given to achieve an international normalised ratio (INR) target of 2.5 for 3–4 weeks before cardioversion, and continued for at least 4 weeks after cardioversion, and perhaps indefinitely. With this strategy, the risk of thromboembolism early after cardioversion is reduced from 5–7% to 1–2%.

RESTORATION AND MAINTENANCE OF SINUS RHYTHM

Cardioversion with drugs Digoxin will not convert AF to sinus rhythm, and will not help to maintain sinus rhythm. If there is no underlying cardiac disease (valvular or coronary disease or left ventricular dysfunction), intravenous flecainide 2 mg/kg over 10 minutes is the drug of choice. Disopyramide is an alternative (50–150 mg intravenously over 5 minutes). Supplemental magnesium sulphate enhances rate control and conversion to sinus rhythm in patients with rapid AF (Davey & Teubner, 2005). Dofetilide and ibutilide are also very effective for acute cardioversion, but are not currently available in the UK.

Where there is underlying cardiac disease, class III drugs are effective in converting AF to sinus rhythm and for the maintenance of sinus rhythm after conversion. Amiodarone and sotalol are equally efficacious in converting AF to sinus rhythm, and amiodarone is superior for maintaining sinus rhythm (Singh et al, 2005). Sotalol is not

better than other beta-blockers for the prevention of relapse where, at low doses, class II effects predominate over the class III activity. A study comparing sotalol (80 mg twice a day) and atenolol (50 mg every day) in the treatment of symptomatic paroxysmal AF found no significant difference between the two agents in preventing recurrences (Steeds et al, 1999).

Other class III agents under investigation include tedisamil and azimilide. Piboserod is a selective 5-HT receptor antagonist that is being used for irritable bowel syndrome, and may also become useful in the management of AF.

The main concern over long-term drug therapy for AF is the potential for inducing dysrhythmias, particularly polymorphic ventricular tachycardia (torsades-de-pointes). The reason for this occurring is not clear, but it often occurs when there is prolongation of the QT interval on the resting ECG (denoting prolongation of action potential). The risk is higher in those with structural heart disease, left ventricular dysfunction, a resting bradycardia or hypokalaemia. Amiodarone is usually safe in this respect, but flecainide, propafenone and sotalol can predispose to ventricular tachycardia in 2% of all patients treated (Lafuente-Lafuente et al, 2006). A 1- to 3-day period of inpatient monitoring is recommended for at-risk patients starting antidysrhythmic medication.

Electrical cardioversion Elective direct current (DC) cardioversion is described in Chapter 10, and is successful in over 80% of cases. A starting energy of at least 150 J (biphasic) should be selected, and energies lower than this are unlikely to be successful. There is no difference in success rates between the antero-posterior and antero-apical electrode positions when modern impedance-compensated biphasic defibrillators are used. Starting antidysrhythmic treatment (sotalol or amiodarone for at least 4 weeks) prior to cardioversion may help to prevent relapse (NICE, 2006).

LONG-TERM MANAGEMENT

Anticoagulation Patients with AF are at two- to sevenfold risk of thromboembolism compared with age-matched control subjects. The absolute risk for stroke is between 1% and 5% per annum, but it varies according to clinical characteristics. Atrial fibrillation is found in 15% of patients presenting with established stroke, and in 2–8% of patients with transient cerebral ischaemia (TIA).

There is strong evidence to support the use of warfarin in patients at moderate and high risk of stroke. In those at lower risk of stroke, the increased risk of major bleeding offsets the benefits, and aspirin is preferable. In general, all patients over 75 years, those with previous stroke and those with cardiovascular risk factors (diabetes, hypertension and heart failure) should be on warfarin (Box 12.5). Isolated left atrial enlargement is not an independent risk factor for thromboembolism, and echocardiography is not essential to decide who to anticoagulate. In patients with paroxysmal AF, the decision to anticoagulate should be based upon risk stratification, and not on the frequency or duration of the paroxysms (Hart et al, 2000). Warfarin remains underprescribed in clinical practice.

Contraindications to warfarin include risk of bleeding due to co-existent medical conditions and any tendency to falls or other exposure to trauma. Another consideration is the likelihood of poor compliance, which will be influenced not only by the patient's ability to manage medications but also by the local facilities available for control of the INR.

Rate control or rhythm control Optimal cardiovascular function is best achieved by the restoration and maintenance of normal sinus rhythm. For many, if not most, patients, this is not achievable, and the goal of treatment is then to limit the ventricular rate to under 90 beats/minute at rest and no more than 180 beats/minute on strenuous exercise to prevent any tachycardia-induced cardiomyopathy.

The decision as to whether simply to control ventricular rate or to try and restore sinus rhythm is difficult. Restoring sinus rhythm holds the theoretical advantage of reducing the risk of thromboembolism, improved haemodynamics and quality of life. However, most current antiarrhythmic drugs have limited efficacy and several side effects and, even when combined with serial electrical cardioversion for early relapse, only half of patients are in sinus rhythm at 1 year, falling to 25% at 5 years.

Recent trials have specifically looked at whether it is better simply to control the ventricular rate

---

Box 12.5 Selection of antithrombotic therapy in atrial fibrillation based on risk reduction.

High risk (stroke rate = 12% per annum)
Rheumatic heart disease (especially mitral stenosis)
Previous cardiac thromboembolism
Age > 75 years
Age > 65 years with diabetes or hypertension
Previous myocardial infarction with poor left ventricular function
Heart failure
Aspirin will reduce the stroke rate to 10% per annum.
Warfarin will reduce the stroke rate to 5% per annum.
TREAT WITH WARFARIN

Moderate risk (stroke rate = 8% per annum)
Age > 65 years
Age < 65 years with risk factors
Aspirin will reduce the stroke rate to 4% per annum.
Warfarin will reduce the stroke rate to under 2% per annum.
TREAT MOST WITH WARFARIN

Low risk (stroke rate = 1% per annum)
Age < 65 years with no risk factors
Both aspirin and warfarin will reduce the stroke rate to under 1% per annum.
TREAT WITH ASPIRIN

Notes: risk assessment should be repeated annually. Clopidogrel 75 mg may be substituted for aspirin. A target INR of 2.5 gives satisfactory protection while minimising the risks of major haemorrhage. The risk–benefits of full anticoagulation must be discussed with the patient. Elderly patients have much to gain, but may be more prone to falls and poor compliance with therapy. In patients over 75 years of age, a target ratio of 2 may represent a better balance between risk and benefit.

(rate control) or whether strenuous steps need to be taken to restore and maintain sinus rhythm (rhythm control). Although these studies compared heterogeneous groups of patients, several consistent messages have emerged (Boos et al, 2003).

First, a rhythm control approach does not lead to an improvement in symptom control or quality of life or a reduction in clinical events in the short to medium term. In fact, in the longer term, mortality may increase (Wyse et al, 2002).

Second, maintenance of sinus rhythm remains poor, even with an aggressive strategy combining electrical cardioversion and current drug therapy. Overall, the rhythm control strategy associates with more hospitalisations, greater cost, minimally improved symptoms, more strokes and greater total mortality.

Finally, an important lesson from the AFFIRM and RACE trials is that anticoagulation often needs to be continued, even if sinus rhythm is restored, as patients remain at risk from thromboembolism (Van Gelder et al, 2002; Wyse et al, 2002). Without adequate thromboprophylaxis, patients may well return with stroke secondary to a relapse of AF. Relapse rates as great as 88% may occur even in those 'optimal' for antidysrhythmic treatment (Israel et al, 2004).

In the light of these findings, aggressive pursuit of sinus rhythm can no longer be justified in asymptomatic AF, and a strategy of rate control with anticoagulation is as effective as rate control in the majority of patients (McNamara et al, 2003). Digoxin should only be considered as monotherapy in sedentary patients, and beta-blockers or rate-limiting calcium antagonists should be used as first-line therapy.

Rhythm control is still an important treatment option for patients with symptomatic AF, many of whom complain of lethargy or poor exercise capacity despite good heart rate control. Rhythm control should be considered in the young and in those with heart failure. Where drug control to prevent relapse is ineffective, invasive treatments, such as pulmonary vein isolation, atrial pacemaker therapy or AV nodal ablation, may be considered.

Implantable atrial defibrillators can be programmed to restore sinus rhythm in paroxysmal AF. Cardioversion is synchronised to the R wave, and shocks are given between the coronary sinus and the right ventricular leads. The problem is that most patients cannot tolerate multiple shocks (Doaud et al, 2000). An 'ablate and pace' strategy involving AV nodal ablation with pacemaker implantation is sometimes used, which may improve ventricular function and quality of life (Wood et al, 2000). It is destructive, and most would regard it as a last resort.

Triggered atrial pacemakers continually scan the sinus rate and monitor atrial extrasystoles. Intermittent right atrial overdrive pacing suppresses the frequency of extrasystoles that are thought to initiate each paroxysm of fibrillation. The pacing rate then slows to allow sinus activity to take over, provided no further extrasystoles are sensed. *Atrial resynchronisation* (simultaneous pacing at two different atrial sites) in patients with intra-atrial conduction delay may also be beneficial.

Pulmonary vein isolation The pulmonary veins form as a bud that grows from the heart towards the lungs, carrying a sleeve of cardiac muscle fibres with them. These are an important source of ectopic beats capable of triggering AF. To prevent this, attempts were made to ablate these ectopic foci, but this approach has been superseded by a more selective technique referred to as *ostial segmental pulmonary vein isolation*. Although the atrial muscle covers a large area around the pulmonary veins, there are specific electrical breakthrough points from the left atrium that allow pulmonary vein isolation with minimal ablation and fewer complications (e.g. pulmonary stenosis, tamponade). Although curative treatment is possible, there are limitations, including failure rates of around 25%, recurrences in 40% with the need for repeat procedures and the potential for serious complications. It takes around 6 hours and demands high levels of expertise for trans-septal puncture and catheter manipulation in the left atrium. The technique is still being refined and cannot yet be recommended for routine intervention (Haywood, 2006).

Treatment of paroxysmal AF (PAF) Treatment of PAF is often difficult, and much depends on the frequency, duration and inconvenience of the attacks. Management strategies should be discussed with the patient.

Where a precipitant can be identified, or when attacks are infrequent and well tolerated, no treatment may be appropriate. The 'pill in the pocket' strategy may be considered for those with a structurally normal heart and a good understanding of when and how to use the chosen drug.

Flecainide 50 mg is often used, but this should first be tried in hospital. Beta-blockade is an alternative. The decision on antithrombotic therapy should be based on risk stratification (Box 12.5) and not on frequency, duration or symptoms of each attack.

If antidysrhythmic therapy is required, beta-blockers are the first choice. If this is ineffective or contraindicated, class Ic agents (propafenone, flecainide) may be used if the heart is structurally normal. Where there is heart disease, amiodarone is the only safe drug if beta-blockers cannot be tolerated. Non-pharmacological therapies should be considered.

Broad–complex tachycardias

Almost any dysrhythmia can present as a broad-complex tachycardia, and determining the origin may be difficult. The majority will be (and should be assumed to be) of ventricular origin (80%), but broad-complex supraventricular tachycardias may occur if there is rate-related or pre-existing bundle branch block. Age is a useful clue to the origin of a broad-complex tachycardia and, if the patient is over 35 years, the tachycardia is more likely to be ventricular in origin. A history that includes ischaemic heart disease or chronic heart failure is 90% predictive of ventricular tachycardia (VT). Symptoms of broad-complex tachycardia may include dizziness, palpitations, syncope, chest pain or heart failure, but it is wrong to assume that a patient with ventricular tachycardia will inevitably be in a state of collapse. Some patients with VT look surprisingly well, while those with a supraventricular tachycardia and poor ventricular function may present with haemodynamic collapse.

The most important diagnostic tool is the 12-lead ECG, and access to a previous ECG in sinus rhythm is very helpful. Clinical signs of atrioventricular dissociation, such as variation in the venous pulse, loudness of the first heart sound and changes in the systolic blood pressure, are usually too subtle, and the absence of these findings does not exclude the diagnosis.

The diagnosis of VT is supported by an ECG that shows:

- AV dissociation;
- QRS duration more than 160 ms;

- axis deviation (often gross);
- concordance of the QRS complexes in the chest leads (either predominantly positive or predominantly negative);
- capture and fusion beats (uncommon).

If the tachycardia has a right bundle branch block morphology (a predominantly positive QRS complex in lead V1), the origin is likely to be left ventricular, and there will be concordance throughout the chest leads (all deflections positive). If the tachycardia has a left bundle branch block morphology (a predominantly negative deflection in lead V1), a right ventricular origin is likely, with negative concordance throughout the chest leads.

Episodes of ventricular tachycardia are unlikely to be isolated, and recurrence may be anticipated unless a precipitant can be identified and eliminated. Further investigation is always necessary, and most should undergo coronary angiography. Where there is no easily remediable cause, electrophysiological studies are usual, with ablation or implantation of automatic defibrillators in selected cases.

Polymorphic ventricular tachycardia

Torsades-de-pointes ('twisting of points') is a polymorphic ventricular tachycardia in which the cardiac axis rotates over a sequence of 5–20 beats, changing from one direction to another and back again. The QRS amplitude varies similarly, such that the complexes appear to twist around the baseline. Prominent U waves may be seen. This form of VT is not usually sustained, but it will recur unless the underlying cause is corrected. Prolonged episodes may degenerate into ventricular fibrillation.

Torsades-de-pointes is usually associated with conditions that prolong the QT interval on the resting ECG, such as coronary disease, chronic heart failure and metabolic abnormalities (e.g. hypokalaemia and hypomagnesaemia). Many antidysrhythmic drugs are known to prolong ventricular repolarisation (as reflected in the QT interval) and provoke torsades-de-pointes. In addition, an increasing number of non-cardiac drugs have also been reported to have the same effects. The non-sedating antihistamine, terfenadine, was one of the first drugs to attract regulatory attention because of its association with QT prolongation, torsades-de-pointes and sudden death, but many other drugs have been implicated. Tricyclic antidepressants are particularly cardiotoxic, and some antibiotics (such as macrolides and fluoroquinolones), antimalarials and imidazole antifungal agents can cause QT prolongation. Drugs that prolong the QT interval and thereby predispose to torsades-de-pointes are listed at www.qtdrugs.org. Avoiding these drugs, or restricting the dose, is recommended in patients with pre-existing heart disease, with avoidance of hypokalaemia.

The long QT syndrome (LQTS) is a congenital condition characterised by a prolonged QT interval on the resting ECG, with recurrent syncope or sudden death resulting from torsades-de-pointes. The incidence of LQTS has been estimated as 1:7000 to 1:10 000 live births, and more than 250 mutations in seven genes have been described. High-risk LQTS patients are treated prophylactically with beta-blockers. Implantable cardioverter defibrillators (ICDs) are usually considered in patients with syncope despite beta-blocker treatment, or in patients with syncope and a family history of sudden death.

The short QT syndrome (SQTS) associates with sudden cardiac death in otherwise healthy patients with structurally normal hearts (Gussak et al, 2000). Patients have a QT interval of < 270 ms on the 12-lead ECG, and suffer from palpitations, syncope or sudden cardiac arrest due to a fast polymorphic VT. Currently, ICD implantation is the only therapeutic option.

Benign ventricular tachycardias

Ventricular tachycardia in a structurally normal heart usually originates from the right ventricular outflow under the pulmonary valve or from the left posterior branch of the left bundle. Less commonly, it originates from the left ventricular outflow tract below the aortic valve.

Right ventricular outflow tachycardias produce ventricular complexes similar to those seen in left bundle branch block. The impulse travels inferiorly, and produces right axis deviation on the ECG. The VT is non-sustained, and usually exertion or stress related. Most settle with beta-blockade.

Some cases may be amenable to ablation therapy, which is usually preferable to lifelong antidysrhythmic therapy. In most cases, a cardiac MRI should be performed to exclude *arrhythmogenic right ventricular dysplasia*, a cardiomyopathy in which there is structural and functional deterioration of the right ventricle. Associated VT can be life threatening and requires implantation of a defibrillator.

Fascicular tachycardias usually arise from around the posterior hemi-fascicle of the left bundle. The complexes are of a right bundle branch block appearance, and there is left axis deviation. When the tachycardia originates from the anterior fascicle, right axis deviation is seen. The complexes are often only slightly widened to between 0.12 and 0.14 seconds, and may appear as a SVT. Patients are usually young males. The VT is often unresponsive to beta-blockers, but frequently responds to verapamil. The prognosis is generally good, but these patients may be highly symptomatic. Catheter ablation offers curative therapy and should be considered early in the management of symptomatic patients.

Bradycardias

Symptomatic bradycardias are common, and are usually secondary to age-related degenerative disease affecting the conducting tissues, often exacerbated by institution of AV nodal blocking drugs. In patients without myocardial infarction, fibrosis of the AV junction is the most common cause of complete heart block. It is probably a degenerative process and predominantly affects men. Cardiac pacing is often required (see Chapter 13).

RECREATIONAL DRUGS AND THE CORONARY CARE UNIT

> One of the first duties of the physician is to educate the masses not to take medicine.
> Sir William Osler (1849–1919)

While the adverse effects of alcohol and tobacco on the cardiovascular system are well known, easy access to a number of illegal 'recreational' drugs that may have profound effects on the cardiovascular system is resulting in escalating numbers of admissions to the CCU. Drug abuse has reached epidemic proportions, with an estimated three million people in the UK using illegal drugs every month. Polysubstance misuse is a worrying trend. Simultaneous administration of cocaine or amphetamines with heroin ('speedballs') on a background of alcohol and cannabis is now common in nightclubs (Cole et al, 2005), while adolescents favour inhalation of volatile substances while under the influence of alcohol and cannabis. Such drug cocktails may produce a synergistic and detrimental effect on cardiovascular function, irreversible damage to the heart and sudden death (Ghuran et al, 2001). Intravenous drug addicts may also present with chronic bacterial endocarditis, often affecting the tricuspid valve and associated with pulmonary abscess formation.

Amphetamines, ecstasy, cocaine and khat

These drugs activate the sympathetic nervous system and produce similar effects.

Cocaine and its free base 'crack cocaine' can be smoked, inhaled or injected. It has a short serum half-life of about 1 hour. Cocaine both stimulates catecholamine release from the adrenal medulla and inhibits uptake at sympathetic nerve endings. As a result, catecholamine concentrations rise dramatically, an effect enhanced by simultaneous cannabis use.

Amphetamine and its derivative, ecstasy (MDMA), can be ingested orally, inhaled or, less commonly, injected. It is readily absorbed from both the nasal mucosa and the gut, and freely penetrates the blood–brain barrier. The plasma half-life varies from as little as 5 hours to as much as 30 hours depending on urine flow and pH. Some patients deliberately take bicarbonate to delay excretion and enhance the drug effect. Catecholamines and serotonin are released from both the central and the autonomic nervous systems.

Fresh leaves from khat trees (*Catha edulis celestrasae*) are chewed for their euphoric properties, particularly by those from Yemeni, Somali and East African communities living in the UK (Al-Motarreb et al, 2002). The active ingredient is cathinone, which causes release of noradrenaline from peripheral neurones.

Cardiovascular effects of sympathetic stimulants

Sympathetic activation by this group of drugs leads to varying degrees of tachycardia, vasoconstriction, hypertension and dysrhythmias, depending on the dose given and the presence of co-existing cardiovascular disease. Acute and chronic cardiovascular effects include myocardial infarction, myocardial ischaemia (both silent and symptomatic), premature atherosclerosis, myocarditis, cardiomyopathy, dysrhythmias, hypertension and aortic dissection (Costa et al, 2001). Severe hypotension can follow catecholamine exhaustion. Cocaine and amphetamine have been associated with non-cardiogenic pulmonary oedema and a dilated cardiomyopathy.

Cocaine and myocardial infarction

Cocaine has become the second commonest illicit drug used in the UK, and the most frequent cause of drug-related death. Reports from the United States suggest that as many as one in four myocardial infarctions in people aged 18–45 years are linked to cocaine abuse (Quesheri et al, 2001), and the lifetime risk of a heart attack is seven times that of the normal population. In the hour after cocaine use, the risk of myocardial infarction rises 24-fold, and most users have no idea of the dangers (Egred & Davis, 2005). Myocardial infarction appears to be an idiosyncratic response to the drug, unrelated to dose, duration of use or route of administration. There is no way of identifying those who may have life-threatening cardiac effects after taking cocaine, but those who experience myocardial ischaemia once are at risk of recurrence.

Management

Sedation with benzodiazepines is helpful to attenuate the cardiac and central nervous system toxicity of sympathetic stimulation. Beta-blockers should be avoided, as they may be associated with unopposed alpha-receptor-mediated vasoconstriction. This in turn associates with a sudden and severe increase in blood pressure and coronary artery vasoconstriction. Hypertension can be managed safely with directly acting vasodilators such as nitrates or sodium nitroprusside.

An otherwise healthy young person presenting with symptoms of myocardial ischaemia should be asked about substance abuse, especially cocaine. Regular cocaine users as young as 25–30 years without any other cardiovascular risk factors may have triple-vessel coronary artery disease. Where a related acute coronary syndrome is suspected, benzodiazepines should be given early with usual treatment of oxygen, aspirin, heparin and nitrates. ST elevation on the ECG may indicate coronary spasm but, if there is persistent ST segment elevation following the administration of nitrates, reperfusion should be considered. Primary angioplasty is particularly advantageous to determine the relative contribution of coronary atherosclerosis, spasm and thrombus.

Other commonly misused drugs

The other four groups of recreation drugs with potential cardiovascular side effects are the opiates, volatile substances, cannabis and LSD (lysergic acid diethylamide). In general, these patients seldom reach coronary care, because adverse effects are transient, require intensive care management with ventilatory support or are rapidly fatal.

Opiates

The most commonly misused narcotic analgesics are heroin and morphine, which are injected, smoked or ingested orally. Heroin is a semi-synthetic analogue of morphine that acts more rapidly. The duration of effect is highly variable, being affected by the dose given, the purity of the preparation and previous drug habits.

Heroin acts centrally to increase parasympathetic activity, reduce sympathetic activity and cause release of histamine from mast cells, leading to bradycardia and hypotension. The induced bradycardia along with enhanced automaticity can precipitate an increase in ectopic activity, atrial fibrillation, idio-ventricular rhythm or potentially lethal ventricular rhythms.

The most serious effect of heroin is respiratory depression, which may lead to respiratory failure and cardiac arrest. This is the commonest cause of death in heroin users. Respiratory depression, cardiovascular collapse, dysrhythmias and an acute non-cardiac pulmonary oedema may relate to an anaphylactic reaction to the drug. Pulmonary oedema may not develop until 24 hours after admission, and may require invasive monitoring to guide fluid and inotropic administration. Diuretics are contraindicated in this form of pulmonary oedema, which is best treated by mechanical ventilation.

In the presence of severe hypotension and bradycardia, however, repeated boluses or an infusion of narcan will be required, but this drug should be avoided in an otherwise stable patient, as it may occasionally precipitate pulmonary oedema. Cardiac dysrhythmias should be treated in the usual way. Hypoxic, metabolic and electrolyte deficits should be corrected.

Volatile substance abuse

Most inhaled volatile substances are legal, cheap and easily obtained. Solvents from adhesives, dry cleaning fluids and aerosol propellants are commonly abused. Deep breathing techniques are used to maximise the inhaled concentration with the volatile substances contained in a plastic bag or bottle. Some misusers may spray the compound directly into the mouth. In the UK, up to 10% of young people have at least experimented with volatile substances, and there are over 100 related deaths every year.

These agents sensitise the heart to circulating catecholamines, such that sudden noise, anxiety or exercise may precipitate sudden death from ventricular tachycardia. Resuscitation is rare, as the majority of deaths are unwitnessed. Deaths from cardiac arrest during or soon after volatile substance exposure are unpredictable, and previous uneventful sessions of abuse provide no protection from death (Williams & Cole, 1998). Some volatile substances can reduce sino-atrial node automaticity and suppress cardiac conduction. Myocardial ischaemia and infarction can be caused by coronary vasospasm, and chronic misuse can cause cardiomyopathy. Hypoxia is common owing to direct respiratory depression, aspiration and asphyxia (polythene bags stuck over the head).

Cannabis

Cannabis is usually smoked, with effects lasting from 4 to 6 hours. At low doses, the drug leads to an increase in sympathetic activity and a reduction in parasympathetic activity, producing tachycardia with a rise in cardiac output. In patients with coronary heart disease, this may precipitate angina or an increase in supraventricular and ventricular ectopic activity. Serious dysrhythmias are rare. There may be reversible ECG abnormalities affecting the P and T waves and the ST segment. Paradoxically, at higher doses, sympathetic activity is inhibited and parasympathetic activity increased, leading to bradycardia, hypotension and sometimes presyncope in patients with poor left ventricular function. Sudden death has been reported in cannabis users with no prior evidence of coronary heart disease. Death from a heart attack is fourfold higher in the hour following cannabis use (Mittleman et al, 2001).

LSD (lysergic acid diethylamide)

LSD and 'magic mushrooms' (psilocybin) are hallucinogenic agents. Psilocybin is derived from a common wild mushroom, whereas LSD (which was also originally extracted from a fungus) is usually manufactured synthetically. These drugs are structurally related and have similar physiological, pharmacological and clinical effects. Both drugs are usually ingested orally, with LSD being 100 times more potent than psilocybin. Their mechanisms of action are complex with effects at various serotonin, dopaminergic and adrenergic receptors. Following ingestion, symptoms of general sympathetic arousal (dilated pupils, tachycardia, hypertension, euphoria) begin within 15–45 minutes and usually last for 4–6 hours, although anxiety and paranoia, with visual and auditory hallucinations, can occur days, months or even years later. Cardiovascular complications are uncommon, but dysrhythmias and myocardial infarction have been reported (Choi & Pearl, 1989).

References

Ahmed A, Rich MW, Love TE et al (2006) Digoxin and reduction in mortality and hospitalisation in heart failure: a comprehensive post-hoc analysis of the DIG trial. *European Heart Journal* 27: 178–186.

Allender S, Peto V, Scarborough P et al (2006) *Coronary Heart Disease Statistics*. London: British Heart Foundation Statistics database. www.heartstats.org.

Al-Motarreb A, Al-Kebsi M, Al-Adhi B et al (2002) Khat chewing and acute myocardial infarction. *Heart* 87: 279–280.

Amiodarone Trials Meta-Analysis Investigators (1997) Effect of prophylactic amiodarone on mortality after acute myocardial infarction and in congestive heart failure: meta-analysis of individual data from 6500 patients in randomised trials. *Lancet* 350: 1417–1424.

Bastuli JA, Orlowski JP (1985) Stroke as a complication of carotid sinus massage. *Critical Care Medicine* 13: 869.

Blankenship JC, Almquist AK (1989) Cardiovascular complications of thrombolytic therapy in patients with a mistaken diagnosis of acute myocardial infarction. *Journal of the American College of Cardiology* 14: 1579–1582.

Boos CJ, More RS, Carlsson J (2003) Persistent atrial fibrillation: rate control or rhythm control. *New England Journal of Medicine* 326: 1411–1412.

British Thoracic Society (2003) Guidelines for management of suspected acute pulmonary embolism. *Thorax* 58: 1–14.

Bucher HC, Hengstler P, Schindler C et al (2000) Percutaneous transluminal coronary angioplasty versus medical treatment for non-acute coronary heart disease: meta-analysis of randomised controlled trials. *British Medical Journal* 321: 73–77.

Buller HR, Davidson BL, Decousus H et al (2003) Subcutaneous fondaparinux versus intravenous unfractionated heparin in the initial treatment of pulmonary embolism. *New England Journal of Medicine* 349: 1695–1702.

Campeau L (1976) Grading of angina pectoris. *Circulation* 54: 522–523.

Choi YS, Pearl WR (1989) Cardiovascular effects of adolescent drug abuse. *Journal of Adolescent Health Care* 10: 332–337.

Cooper N, Jacob B (2002) Biphasic positive pressure ventilation in acute cardiogenic pulmonary oedema. *British Journal of Cardiology* 9: 38–41.

Cleland JGF, Clark A, Caplin JL (2000) Taking heart failure seriously. *British Medical Journal* 321: 1095–1096.

Cleland JGF, Daubert JC, Erdmann E et al for the Cardiac Resynchronization – Heart Failure (CARE-HF) Study Investigators (2005) The effect of cardiac resynchronization on morbidity and mortality in heart failure. *New England Journal of Medicine* 352: 1539–1549.

Cole JC, Sumnall HR, Smith GW et al (2005) Preliminary evidence of the cardiovascular effects of polysubstance misuse in nightclubs. *Journal of Psychopharmacology* 19: 67–70.

Costa GM, Pizzi C, Bresciani B et al (2001) Acute myocardial infarction caused by amphetamines: a case report and review of the literature. *Italian Heart Journal* 2: 478–480.

Cowie MR (2004) B type natriuretic peptide testing: where are we now? *Heart* 90: 725–726.

Daly CA, De Stavola B, Fox KM on behalf of the Euro Heart Survey investigators (2006) Predicting prognosis in stable angina – results from the Euro heart survey of stable angina: prospective observational study. *British Medical Journal* 332: 262–265.

Danchin N, Aly S (2004) Heart rate reduction: a potential target for the treatment of myocardial ischaemia. *Therapie* 59: 511–555.

Davey MJ, Teubner D (2005) A randomised controlled trial of magnesium sulfate, in addition to usual care, for rate control in atrial fibrillation. *Annals of Emergency Medicine* 45: 347–353.

Doaud EG, Timmermans C, Fellows C for the Metrix Investigators (2000) Initial clinical experience with ambulatory use of an implantable atrial defibrillator for cardioversion of atrial fibrillation. *Circulation* 102: 1407–1413.

Eagle KA, Guyton RA, Davidoff R (2004) ACC/AHA guideline update for coronary artery bypass graft surgery. *Circulation* 110: e340–437.

Egred M, Davis GK (2005) Cocaine and the heart. *Postgraduate Medical Journal* 81: 568–571.

Erbel R, Alfonso F, Boileau C et al (2001) Diagnosis and management of aortic dissection. *European Heart Journal* 22: 1642–1681.

ESC (2004) European Society of Cardiology expert consensus document on beta-adrenergic receptor blockers. *European Heart Journal* 25: 1341–1362.

Felker GM, O'Connor CM (2001) Inotropic therapy for heart failure: an evidence-based approach. *American Heart Journal* 142: 393–401.

Flather MD, Yusuf S, Kober L et al (2000) Long term ACE-inhibitor therapy for patients with heart failure or left ventricular dysfunction: a systematic overview of data from individual patients. *Lancet* 355: 1575–1581.

Follath F, Cleland JG, Just H et al (2002) Efficacy and safety of intravenous levosimendan compared with dobutamine in severe low-output heart failure (the LIDO study): a randomised double-blind trial. *Lancet* 360: 196–202.

Ghuran A, van der Wieken LR, Nolan J (2001) Cardiovascular complications of recreational drugs. *British Medical Journal* 323: 464–466.

Goodacre S, Sutton AJ, Sampson FC (2005) Meta-analysis: the value of clinical assessment in the diagnosis of deep venous thrombosis. *Annals of Internal Medicine* 143: 129–139.

Gussak I, Brugada P, Brugada J et al (2000) Idiopathic short QT interval: a new clinical syndrome? *Cardiology* 94: 99–102.

Hart RG, Pearce LA, Rothbart RM et al (2000) Stroke with intermittent atrial fibrillation: incidence and predictors during aspirin therapy. Stroke Prevention in Atrial Fibrillation Investigators. *Journal of the American College of Cardiology* 35: 183–187.

Haywood G (2006) Can we ablate permanent atrial fibrillation? *Heart* 92: 152–154.

Heberden W (1772) Some account of a disorder of the breast. *Medical Transactions of the Royal College of Physicians of London* 2: 59.

Hirsch J, Guyatt G, Albers G et al (2004) Seventh ACCP conference on anti-thrombotic and thromboembolic therapy. *Chest* 126: S172–696.

Hunt SA, Abraham WT, Chin MH (2005) ACC/AHA guideline update for the diagnosis and management of chronic heart failure in the adult. *Circulation* 112: e154–235.

Israel CW, Gronefeld G, Ehrlich JR et al (2004) Long-term risk of recurrent atrial fibrillation as documented by an implantable monitoring device: implications for optimal patient care. *Journal of the American College of Cardiology* 43: 47–52.

Januzzi JL, van Kimmenade R, Lainchbury J et al (2006) NT-proBNP testing for diagnosis and short-term prognosis in acute destabilized heart failure: an international pooled analysis of 1256 patients. *European Heart Journal* 27: 330–337.

Jong P, Demers C, McKelvie RS et al (2002) Angiotensin receptor blockers in heart failure: meta-analysis of randomised controlled trials. *Journal of the American College of Cardiology* 39: 463–470.

Kovacs MJ, Anderson D, Morrow B et al (2000) Outpatient treatment of pulmonary embolism with dalteparin. *Thrombosis and Haemostasis* 83: 209–211.

Kovacs MJ, MacKinnon KM, Anderson D et al (2001) A comparison of three rapid D-dimer methods for the diagnosis of venous thrombo-embolism. *British Journal of Haematology* 115: 140–144.

Kramer K, Kirkman P, Kitzman D et al (2000) Flash pulmonary edema: association with hypertension and re-occurrence despite coronary revascularisation. *American Heart Journal* 140: 451–455.

Kucher N, Wallmann D, Carone A et al (2003) Incremental prognostic value of troponin I and echocardiography in patients with acute pulmonary embolism. *European Heart Journal* 24: 1651–1656.

Lafuente-Lafuente C, Mouly S, Longas-Tejero MA et al (2006) Antiarrhythmic drugs for maintaining sinus rhythm after cardioversion of atrial fibrillation: a systematic review of randomized controlled trials. *Archives of Internal Medicine* 166: 719–728.

Latini R, Maggioni AP, Masson S (2001) What does the future hold for BNP in cardiology? *Heart* 86: 601–602.

Leite-Moreira AF (2006) Current perspectives in diastolic dysfunction and diastolic heart failure. *Heart* 92: 712–718.

Levy WC, Mozaffarian D, Linker DT et al (2006) The Seattle Heart Failure Model: prediction of survival in heart failure. *Circulation* 113: 1424–1433.

McAlister FA, Stewart S, Ferrua S et al (2004) Multi-disciplinary strategies for the management of heart failure patients at high risk for admission: a systematic review of randomized trials. *Journal of the American College of Cardiology* 44: 810–819.

McMurray JJ, Stewart S (2000) Epidemiology, aetiology and progress of heart failure. *Heart* 83: 596–602.

McNamara RL, Tamariz LJ, Segal JB et al (2003) Management of atrial fibrillation: review of the evidence for the role of pharmacologic therapy, electrical cardioversion and echocardiography. *Annals of Internal Medicine* 139: 1018–1033.

Mittleman MA, Lewis RA, Maclure M et al (2001) Triggering myocardial infarction by marijuana. *Circulation* 103: 2805–2809.

Mori E, Ikeda H, Ueno T et al (1997) Vasospastic angina induced by non-steroidal anti-inflammatory drugs. *Clinical Cardiology* 20: 656–658.

NICE (2003) *Chronic Heart Failure. National Clinical Guidelines for Diagnosis and Management in Primary and Secondary Care*. Clinical guideline 5. London: NICE. www.nice.org.uk.

NICE (2006) *The Management of Atrial Fibrillation*. Clinical guideline 36. London: NICE. www.nice.org.uk.

Northridge D (1996) Furosemide or nitrates for acute heart failure? *Lancet* 347: 667–668.

O'Dochartaigh CS, Kelly B, Riley MS et al (2005) Lung water content is not increased in chronic cardiac failure. *Heart* 91: 1473–1474.

Perrier A, Roy P-M, Sanchez O et al (2005) Multi-detector-row computed tomography in suspected pulmonary embolism. *New England Journal of Medicine* 352: 1760–1768.

Peter JV, Moran JL, Phillips-Hughes J et al (2006) Effect of non-invasive positive pressure ventilation (NIPPV) on mortality in patients with acute cardiogenic pulmonary oedema: a meta-analysis. *Lancet* 367: 1155–1163.

Pitt B (2003) Aldosterone blockade in patients with systolic left ventricular dysfunction. *Circulation* 108: 1790–1794.

Pitt B, Zannad, Remme WJ et al for the RALES investigators (1999) The effects of spironolactone on morbidity and mortality in patients with severe heart failure. *New England Journal of Medicine* 341: 709–717.

Psaty BM, Manolio TA, Kuller LH et al (1997) Incidence and risk factors or atrial fibrillation in older adults. *Circulation* 96: 2455–2461.

Quesheri AI, Suri MFK, Gutermann LR et al (2001) Cocaine use and the likelihood of non-fatal myocardial infarction and stroke; data from the third national health and nutrition examination survey. *Circulation* 103: 502–506.

Schilling RJ (2002) Which patients should be referred to an electrophysiologist: supraventricular tachycardia. *Heart* 87: 299–304.

Singh BN, Singh SN, Reda DJ for the Sotalol Amiodarone Atrial Fibrillation Efficacy Trial (SAFE-T) Investigators (2005) Amiodarone versus sotalol for atrial fibrillation. *New England Journal of Medicine* 352: 1861–1872.

Spargias KS, Hall AS, Ball SG (1999) Safety concerns about digoxin after acute myocardial infarction. *Lancet* 354: 391–392.

Steeds RP, Birchall AS, Smith M et al (1999) An open label, randomised, crossover study comparing sotalol and atenolol in the treatment of symptomatic paroxysmal atrial fibrillation. *Heart* 82: 170–175.

Swedberg K, Cleland JC, Dargie H (2005) Guidelines for the diagnosis and treatment of chronic heart failure: executive summary (update 2005). *European Heart Journal* 26: 1115–1140.

Thompson DR, Roebuck A, Stewart S (2005) Effects of a nurse-led, clinic and home-based intervention on recurrent hospital use in chronic heart failure. *European Journal of Heart Failure* 7: 377–384.

Van Gelder IC, Hagens VE, Bosker HA et al (2002) A comparison of rate control and rhythm control in patients with recurrent persistent atrial fibrillation. *New England Journal of Medicine* 377: 1834–1840.

Wang TJ, Evans JC, Benjamin EJ (2003) Natural history of left ventricular systolic dysfunction in the community. *Circulation* 108: 977–982.

Weitz JI, Bates SM (2005) New anticoagulants. *Journal of Thrombosis and Haemostasis* 3: 1843–1853.

Willenheimer R, van Veldhuisen DJ, Silke B for the CIBIS III Investigators (2005) Effect on survival and hospitalization of initiating treatment for chronic heart failure with bisoprolol followed by enalapril, as compared with the opposite sequence. Results of the Randomized Cardiac Insufficiency Bisoprolol Study (CIBIS) III. *Circulation* 112: 2426–2435.

Williams DR, Cole SJ (1998) Ventricular fibrillation following butane gas inhalation. *Resuscitation* 37: 43–45.

Wood MA, Brown-Maloney C, Kay GN et al (2000) Clinical outcomes after ablation and pacing therapy for atrial fibrillation. A meta-analysis. *Circulation* 101: 1138–1144.

Wu EB, Yu CM (2005) Management of diastolic heart failure – a practical review of pathophysiology and treatment trial data. *International Journal of Clinical Practice* 59: 1239–1246.

Wyse DG, Waldo AL, DiMarco JP et al (2002) The Atrial Fibrillation Follow-up Investigation of Rhythm Management (AFFIRM) Investigators. A comparison of rate control and rhythm control in patients with atrial fibrillation. *New England Journal of Medicine* 347: 1825–1833.

Yu DS, Thompson DR, Lee DT (2005) Disease management programmes for older people with heart failure: crucial characteristics which improve post-discharge outcomes. *European Heart Journal* 27: 596–612.

Yusuf S, Pfeffer MA, Swedberg K et al (2003) Effect of candesartan in patients with chronic heart failure and preserved left ventricular ejection fraction; the CHARM-preserved trial. *Lancet* 362: 777–781.

Chapter 13

Cardiac pacing and implantable defibrillators

CHAPTER CONTENTS

Control over the electrical activity of the heart may be made by means of an artificial pacemaker. Temporary cardiac pacing is often used in coronary care and intensive care units to treat transient conduction problems, or sometimes to terminate abnormal tachycardias. If pacing is for a short time only, an external power source is used to deliver electricity to the heart, internally (endocardial pacing), via the skin (transcutaneous pacing) or via the oesophagus (oesophageal pacing). However, when long-term control is required, a permanent pacemaker is implanted. The first pacemaker implant was reported in 1958, and now over 26 000 permanent pacemakers are implanted every year in the UK alone.

INDICATIONS FOR PACING

The two main indications for pacing are where there is failure of impulse generation or where there is failure of atrio-ventricular conduction. The American College of Cardiology and the American Heart Association have produced pacing guidelines (ACC/AHA/NAPSE, 2002), and a summary of some of the indications for temporary and permanent pacing is shown in Boxes 13.1 and 13.2.

Stokes–Adams attacks

The Stokes–Adams syndrome describes sudden collapse, usually with loss of consciousness, caused by a disorder of cardiac rhythm. This is most often secondary to paroxysmal or chronic atrio-ventricular (AV) block (50–60%) or sino-atrial (SA) block (30–40%). Infrequently, it is caused by a paroxysmal tachycardia (less than 5%). In between attacks, the electrocardiogram (ECG) is usually in sinus rhythm, but is very rarely normal. Patients with second- and third-degree heart block require pacing without the need for further investigation. The underlying disease in most of these cases is *Lev's disease* (or Lenegre–Lev syndrome), an acquired disorder caused by idiopathic fibrosis of the conducting tissue. Lev's disease is most commonly seen in the elderly, and is often ascribed to senile degeneration of the conduction system. Only a small number of cases are due to ischaemic damage, so left ventricular function is usually normal, and the outcome following pacing is good with a 1-year survival of 95%. Without pacing, the 1-year survival is under 50%.

Box 13.1   Some indications for temporary cardiac pacing.

Emergency

Acute myocardial infarction with:

- Asystole
- Mobitz type II heart block
- Symptomatic bradycardia not responsive to atropine
- Bilateral bundle branch block (alternating BBB or RBBB with alternating LAHB/LPHB)
- New bifascicular block with first-degree AV block

Bradycardia (unassociated with acute myocardial infarction) with:

- Asystole
- Second- or third-degree AV block with haemodynamic compromise or syncope at rest
- Ventricular tachy-dysrrhythmias secondary to bradycardia

Elective

Patients undergoing general anaesthesia with:

- Second- or third-degree AV block
- Intermittent AV block
- First-degree AV block with bifascicular block
- First-degree AV block and LBBB

During cardiac surgery for:

- Aortic surgery
- Tricuspid surgery
- Ventricular septal defect closure
- Ostium primum repair

Overdrive pacing of tachycardias

Box 13.2   Some indications for permanent pacing.

Acquired atrio-ventricular block (Mobitz type 2 or complete heart block)
Intermittent complete heart block
Pauses > 3 s (if awake)
Alternating right and left bundle branch block
After acute phase of myocardial infarction

- Persistent second-/third-degree heart block
- Persistent second-degree heart block with bundle branch block

Sinus node dysfunction with symptomatic bradycardia
Neuromuscular diseases with AV block (e.g. muscular dystrophy)
Antitachycardia pacing
Carotid sinus syndrome
Biventricular pacing for heart failure

Sick sinus syndrome

The sick sinus syndrome is a collection of conditions relating to sinus node dysfunction that may also present with Stokes–Adams attacks. While the syndrome can have many causes, it is usually idiopathic and, like Lev's disease, may be associated with degenerative fibrosis of nodal tissue. Coronary artery disease may co-exist with sick sinus syndrome, although this is not considered to be a major cause. Sinus node dysfunction may follow an acute myocardial infarction, but is usually a temporary phenomenon. Drug therapy is another important cause (beta-blockers, digoxin and calcium channel blockers).

Most of the symptoms are caused by decreased cerebral perfusion (syncope, presyncope, dizziness), although some individuals may be asymptomatic or have non-specific symptoms. The 24-hour tape may show sinus bradycardia, sinus arrest, sino-atrial block or alternating patterns of bradycardia and tachycardia ('brady–tachy syndrome'). Sixty per cent of patients have abnormal tachycardias.

With the exception of those patients with chronic atrial fibrillation, atrial pacemakers are recommended. Compared with ventricular pacing, atrial pacing is associated with a lower incidence of atrial fibrillation, thromboembolism, heart failure, cardiovascular and total mortality. Pacing with a dual-chamber demand pacemaker with automatic mode-switching function is appropriate in patients with sick sinus syndrome who have intermittent tachycardias. Permanent pacing does not prolong life.

Conduction defects following acute myocardial infarction

Pacing is not usually indicated for heart block following inferior myocardial infarction, unless there are symptoms or signs attributable to low-output cardiac failure. Most bradycardias are responsive to atropine. The prognosis for conduction defects following anterior myocardial infarction is poor, with mortality relating to the extent of myocardial damage rather than the conduction defects. Temporary pacing is often carried out, but it seldom influences outcome. Prognosis is influenced not only by the complications of the procedure (dysrhythmias, cardiac perforation and septicaemia), but also by the degree of underlying myocardial damage that originally led to the conduction defect. Many patients effectively treated acutely by temporary pacing die later while still in hospital from heart failure due to extensive myocardial infarction. For those who survive, permanent pacing is usually delayed for 3–4 weeks to allow cardiac stabilisation.

Refractory tachycardias

Where tachy-dysrhythmias are not controlled by medical therapy, pacing may have a beneficial role, although implantation of devices for terminating supraventricular tachycardias is now rarely required because of the high success rate of radiofrequency ablative procedures. *Underdrive pacing* using slow fixed rate pacing in short bursts was used by early pacemakers to treat tachycardias, but is no longer used. *Overdrive pacing*, however, is often effective, and is associated with low battery drain of the pacemaker. Overdrive pacing for ventricular tachycardia is frequently successful, but may induce ventricular fibrillation, so devices must also have defibrillatory capability.

Perioperative heart block

Patients with sino-atrial disease or incomplete heart block may be at risk of developing complete heart block during drug therapy or surgery. General anaesthesia with fluorinated hydrocarbons (e.g. halothane) may adversely affect atrioventricular conduction. A pacing wire may need to be inserted perioperatively for prophylactic reasons.

Carotid sinus syndrome

Carotid sinus hypersensitivity (CSH) is an exaggerated response to carotid sinus baroreceptor stimulation, leading to dizziness or syncope from transient diminished cerebral perfusion. Although baroreceptor function usually diminishes with age, some people experience hypersensitive carotid baroreflexes, and even mild stimulation to the neck results in marked bradycardia and a drop in blood pressure. CSH predominantly affects older males, and is a potentially treatable cause of unexplained falls and syncopal episodes in elderly people, although is often not considered.

In most cases, carotid sinus stimulation results in sinus bradycardia, atrio-ventricular block or asystole due to vagal action on the sinus and atrio-ventricular nodes (cardioinhibition). Around 5–10% of cases experience a decrease in vasomotor tone without a change in heart rate, resulting in a significant drop in blood pressure. About a quarter of cases have a mixture of these two effects.

Diagnosis may be made by observing the ECG and blood pressure during carotid sinus massage. The diagnosis is confirmed if there is:

- asystole exceeding 3 seconds;
- a fall in systolic blood pressure > 50 mmHg (independent of heart rate slowing);
- a combination of both the above.

Management is based on the frequency and severity of the symptoms. Most patients can be treated with avoidance of carotid stimulation (e.g. neckties, neck movements). A few individuals who have incapacitating and recurrent symptoms will need dual-chamber pacemaker therapy. Cardiac pacing has little or no effect on the pure vasodepressor type.

Miscellaneous

Temporary pacing may be required in cases of permanent pacemaker failure or for extreme bradycardias caused by drugs (e.g. digoxin or beta-adrenergic blocking agents) or electrolyte disturbances.

TEMPORARY CARDIAC PACING

There are three main forms of temporary pacing:

Transcutaneous pacing

External temporary cardiac pacing was first introduced by Zoll in 1952, and was used widely as a temporary measure for the treatment of profound bradycardia and asystole until superseded by transvenous pacing in 1959. Contemporary temporary pacing guidelines place more emphasis on transcutaneous pacing, as invasive techniques involved in endocardial pacing may be hazardous, particularly following thrombolysis (AHA/ACC, 2004). External pacing devices should be available in all coronary care and emergency units, and may be effective for up to 12 hours, or to act as a 'bridge' to transvenous pacing when the patient cannot be moved, or transvenous pacing experience is not immediately available. Prophylactic pacing electrodes can also be applied to those patients who do not require immediate pacing, but are at risk of progression to atrio-ventricular block (Box 13.3). The two large pad electrodes are attached to the chest (preferably in the antero-posterior position), and allow monitoring, pacing and defibrillation if required. When temporary pacing is required, the output from the unit is increased, until the pacing impulse 'captures' the heart. Modern units use longer pulse duration, allowing lower pulse amplitude, so that pacing is usually well tolerated with little more than slight cutaneous discomfort (tingling or tapping) and occasional muscle twitching.

Transoesophageal pacing

Transoesophageal atrial pacing is feasible because of the proximity of the oesophagus to the posterior aspect of the atria, and it was originally described in the late 1960s (Burack & Furman, 1969). Unfortunately, the method is not very reliable, but it may act as a holding measure until a percutaneous wire can be inserted. The pacing electrode is passed transnasally into the oesophagus (rather like a nasogastric tube) and then connected to a dedicated high-output pacing box. The current is switched on, initially at about 30 V. When the diaphragm is reached (producing diaphragmatic twitching), the electrode is slowly withdrawn until ventricular capture is seen on the ECG monitor. Pacing usually produces a burning sensation in the chest, but most patients seem to tolerate this in the short term. Ventricular stimulation by positioning the electrode in the fundus of the stomach and pacing through the diaphragm has also been described.

Transoesophageal pacing is effective in the treatment of atrial flutter and can convert to sinus rhythm in more than 50% of cases (Vincenti et al, 2001).

Transvenous pacing

Temporary endocardial pacing has been used since the early 1960s to maintain cardiac output during episodes of extreme bradycardia, heart block and asystole, particularly in association with acute myocardial infarction. Before the advent of cardiac pacemakers, the combination of acute myocardial infarction and complete heart block was usually fatal, but pacing electrodes are now easily passed into the right ventricle under local anaesthesia and, in experienced hands, this is a safe and simple procedure (Gammage, 2000). The wire is best positioned with the aid of fluoroscopy, but may be located 'blindly' using a balloon-tipped flotation pacing wire when radiograph facilities are not immediately available. Wires positioned in this way are often unstable, and transthoracic (external) pacing is probably a better emergency alternative. Use of balloon catheters with fluoroscopy helps to reduce screening time and aids positioning of the wire (Ferguson et al, 1997). It is usual for a special room to be set aside for pacing, so that there are facilities for sterility, fluoroscopy and resuscitation. The use of fluoroscopy is governed by a European Economic Community Directive (EEC, 1988). Those operating such equipment are

---

Box 13.3 Some indications for placement of transcutaneous pacing patches following acute myocardial infarction.

Sinus bradycardia < 50 beats/minute, with hypotension
Mobitz type II heart block
Inferior myocardial infarction with complete heart block
Newly acquired bifascicular block
Bundle branch block with first-degree heart block

required to be certified for proficiency, with an awareness of the safety aspects of radiation to the patient, the operator and others present.

Thrombolysis and other acute reperfusional strategies have resulted in a decline in the number of patients requiring temporary pacing, so experience of the procedure is much less widespread than in the past, which may increase morbidity of the procedure (Rajappan & Fox, 2003).

Choice of route for insertion of temporary pacing wires

The choice of site of insertion depends upon the expertise of the operator and the problems with the wire in the chosen location. Of the usual insertion sites (internal jugular, subclavian, femoral, brachial), the least skill is required for the femoral and brachial approaches, while the subclavian route is the most hazardous, largely because of the dangers of pneumothorax and subclavian arterial puncture. The jugular line is much more stable, is the most comfortable for the patient and does not inhibit mobility.

The right internal jugular approach is the most direct to the right ventricle, and the British Cardiac Society recommends this approach, particularly for those with limited experience of central venous catheterisation (Parker & Cleland, 1993).

Methods of catheterisation

Catheterisation methods include:

- percutaneous needle and sheath techniques;
- percutaneous Seldinger technique, using a guidewire;
- cut-down (suitable for the arm veins).

The method of choice is the Seldinger technique, which allows a long cannula to be passed into the superior vena cava and helps the passage of the pacing wire into the heart. In addition, unlike shorter cannulae, it will not become displaced if external cardiac massage is required during the insertion procedure. If there is a cardiac arrest, it can be occluded and pacing resumed following resuscitation. The cannula can also be used for infusing drugs and other fluids as required.

The pacing wire becomes more pliable as it warms to body temperature, so should be inserted

as quickly as possible. Sometimes, there is difficulty in passing the electrode into the superior vena cava from the subclavian vein, which may be made easier by moving the patient's arm across the body. Passage through the heart requires experience and the ability to judge position from the fluoroscopic image. Traversing the tricuspid valve is a frequent problem, particularly if the heart rate is fast or if the myocardium is irritable. Occasionally, it is necessary to loop the wire in the right atrium and allow it to prolapse into the right ventricle. Gentle withdrawal then allows the tip to flick through the valve. Passage into the right ventricle can be confirmed by observing the characteristic 'bucking' of the catheter by the tricuspid valve. Wedging the electrode is sometimes made easier by passing it directly into the pulmonary artery (especially if a balloon flotation-type catheter has been used) and then letting it fall back into the apex. This can be seen just medial to the apex on the cardiac silhouette, and the tip of the electrode should point slightly inferiorly. Once wedged, verification of pacing and threshold measurements are necessary. The former is judged from the appearance of a pacing 'spike' preceding the QRS complex on the ECG. Each spike should capture a QRS complex (Fig. 13.1). The pacing threshold is obtained by determining the lowest pacing voltage that produces a paced beat. This threshold should be less than 1 V and preferably below 0.5 V. The wire can then be fixed to the skin with a suture. Pacing should be performed at an output of at least twice the voltage or current threshold. If pacing output needs to

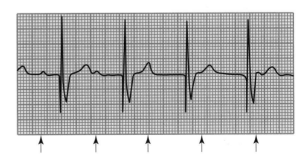

Figure 13.1   ECG: trace obtained when the cardiac pacing wire is correctly positioned. The pacing spike can be seen preceding each QRS complex. Independent atrial P waves are indicated.

exceed 5.0 V, repositioning of the lead should be considered.

The external generator

The external generator allows adjustment of pacing output, rate, mode and sensitivity to ventricular activity. Some generators may also offer high rate pacing (usually three times the normal upper pacing rate) to allow overdrive pacing of abnormal tachycardias. The generator batteries must be checked daily, and the generator should be sited so that it cannot fall and exert traction on the pacing lead. Mobility will necessarily be restricted but, if the jugular insertion site has been used, this will be minimal. Modern pacing boxes are sufficiently small and portable, allowing early mobilisation. Generator covers should be locked after checking and adjustment to prevent inadvertent changes in programming.

Problems during transvenous pacing

Complications and other problems are reported in up to half of all cases, and inexperience is often a major factor (Murphy, 2001). Failure to gain venous access itself is very common (up to 20% of cases) and may also result in local trauma or pneumothorax. The use of a two-dimensional imaging ultrasound-guided approach to central venous cannulation and greater collaboration with anaesthetists may be beneficial (NICE, 2002).

Dysrhythmias

Ventricular tachycardia and fibrillation may result from mechanical irritation of the endocardium. The appearance of ventricular ectopics is usually a good sign that the catheter has entered the right ventricle, but the wire should be moved if these are frequent or occur in runs. This complication may also be caused electrically if the 'fixed' rather than the 'demand' mode is selected on the pacing box or if an inappropriately high pacing threshold is used. Standard resuscitation is required during ventricular fibrillation, although overpacing can sometimes be used to terminate ventricular tachycardia. Recurrent ventricular dysrhythmias may require repositioning or even removal of the wire.

Perforation of the heart or septum

This may be an early or a late complication, and may be indicated by:

- failure to pace despite good radiological position;
- signs of pericarditis or tamponade (pericardial pain or a friction rub);
- diaphragmatic twitching.

The lead can usually be withdrawn back into the ventricle and repositioned without any problem. Tamponade is very uncommon.

A change in the ECG pacing pattern from the usual left bundle branch block to right bundle branch block indicates that the wire has perforated the septum. This is usually insignificant, but the wire should be moved.

Failure to pace

Pacing failure may be evident from the absence of a pacing spike (implying failure of pulse generation) or the spikes failing to capture (implying a displaced electrode or change in threshold). Failure to sense or capture is more common after 48 hours, and the wire will then need to be replaced or repositioned.

Pacemaker dependence

Pacing wires often need repositioning because they have moved, because of increasing pacing thresholds or because of dysrhythmias. Unfortunately, pre-existing rhythms are often abolished after pacing for a while, leaving complete asystole as the underlying 'rhythm' (seen if the pacing box is momentarily turned off). Movement of the wire may then be associated with Stokes–Adams attacks, because the heart has become 'pacemaker dependent'. This problem may need the passage of a second pacing wire to take over while the other is relocated or removed.

Effects on cardiac function

Temporary transvenous pacing from the right ventricle is associated with detrimental effects on cardiac function. Loss of atrio-ventricular synchrony results in a reduced cardiac output that may be no better than that produced by the underlying bradycardia (Murphy et al, 1992). Higher pacing rates can partially compensate for reduced cardiac output.

Infection

Infection is more common when the temporary wire is left in for several days or has been introduced via the femoral vein, when antibiotic prophylaxis should be considered. Most infections are with *Staphylococcus epidermidis*, but coliforms may complicate the femoral approach. Deep vein thrombosis is more common with femoral lines.

Because of the problem of infection, temporary pacing should be avoided if permanent pacing is going to be required (Hickling-Smith & Petch, 1999). Where temporary wires have been inserted for over 48 hours, there is a sixfold increased risk of permanent pacemaker infection. A cycle of infected temporary wires delaying permanent pacing, requiring temporary wire replacement that may again become infected, is particularly distressing for patient and carers alike.

ACUTE MYOCARDIAL INFARCTION, HEART BLOCK AND PACING

Pathophysiology (Table 13.1)

Inferior myocardial infarction is usually caused by occlusion of the right coronary artery, which supplies the inferior wall of the heart. The AV node is supplied by the right coronary artery in 90% of cases, and by the circumflex artery in the remainder. As a result, conduction disturbances commonly occur following acute inferior myocardial infarction, caused by ischaemia or oedema of the AV node. For unknown reasons, ischaemic injury to the AV node following inferior myocardial infarction is rarely permanent. Complete heart block usually develops slowly, and the escape rhythm usually has a high junctional origin at 40–60 beats/minute. This is generally haemodynamically stable, and pacing is not usually necessary, providing blood pressure and renal perfusion are maintained (Jowett et al, 1989). Conduction disturbances can occur at any time in the first 2 weeks, but are usually transient with normal conduction returning in hours or days.

Anterior myocardial infarction is caused by occlusion of the left anterior descending coronary artery, which provides the major blood supply to the bundle of His and bundle branches. Proximal occlusion of the left coronary artery leads to extensive myocardial damage, often resulting in heart failure and cardiogenic shock. Heart block is a sinister and sudden complication, and is due to ischaemic destruction of the conducting tissues below the AV node. Emergent ventricular escape rhythms are unreliable, slow and irregular; there is a marked tendency to develop asystole. These patients often have severe left ventricular damage and a poor prognosis. The insertion of a temporary pacing wire under these circumstances probably has little influence on the outcome, although it is

Table 13.1   Characteristics of complete heart block complicating inferior and anterior myocardial infarction.

	Anterior infarction	Inferior infarction
Incidence	25–40%	60–75%
Pathology	Septal necrosis and infarction of the AV node and bundle branches	Ischaemia of the bundle branches
Timing	Usually sudden, following sinus rhythm or second-degree heart block	Normally slow, following first- and second-degree heart block
Ventricular response	30–40, unstable	40–60, stable
QRS morphology	Widened	Narrow
Risk of asystole	High	Low
Mortality	60–75%	25–40%
Prognosis	Often permanent	Most reverse within 14 days

usual practice. Dual-chamber pacing can be used to maximise cardiac output. Mortality is high and late deaths are common.

Hypertension, pre-existing diabetes mellitus and high blood glucose concentrations on admission to hospital are common risk factors for those requiring temporary pacing following acute myocardial infarction. Disorders of atrio-ventricular and intraventricular conduction are significantly more common in diabetic patients with acute myocardial infarction than in those who are not diabetic, and may be due to pre-existing microangiopathic damage to the conducting system (Blandford & Burden, 1984). The higher incidence of previous myocardial infarctions and hypertension in those patients requiring pacing is probably an indication of underlying myocardial damage.

The presence of complete heart block following acute myocardial infarction should not provide a contraindication to thrombolysis. As in other cases of myocardial infarction, thrombolysis should be given immediately, along with atropine. In the majority of cases, AV conduction improves, and many cases of complete heart block may be tolerated without the need to insert a temporary pacemaker. If pacing is required, an insertion site should be chosen that may be easily compressed, and thus the femoral or brachial routes are preferred.

Prophylactic pacing following myocardial infarction

The potential complications of temporary pacing (especially bleeding following thrombolysis) should be considered before prophylactic wires are inserted following acute myocardial infarction. While transvenous pacing may be unavoidable, transcutaneous pacing pads should be applied in high-risk groups in case of conduction failure (Box 13.3).

When to stop temporary pacing

Following acute myocardial infarction, it is usual to leave pacing wires *in situ* for 24–48 hours after reliable atrio-ventricular conduction has recovered.

Removal of the pacing wire is a simple and straightforward procedure carried out at the patient's bedside. The unit should be turned off and the dressing and retaining sutures removed. While observing the ECG monitor for ectopic activity, the wire should be slowly withdrawn and a sterile pad held firmly over the puncture site for a few minutes to prevent bleeding. If the patient has been pyrexial, the tip of the disposable pacing wire should be removed aseptically and sent to the bacteriology laboratory for culture.

Care of patients with temporary pacing wires

Patients often feel much better following temporary pacing, and are in a much better physical and psychological state for discussion about the pacemaker and its implications. There is usually not much pain at the site of wire insertion, but this should be observed for signs of bleeding and infection. Routine checks are also required on the equipment, with attention to connections and performance. The threshold and underlying rhythm need to be charted on a twice-daily basis, and settings should be discussed for the following 12-hour period. This should be documented in the patient's notes and the nursing notes, as well as on the charts beside the bed.

PERMANENT PACEMAKERS

Permanent pacing may be considered for symptomatic benefit or to improve prognosis. For example, untreated complete heart block has a mortality of up to 30% per year, even in asymptomatic patients, and pacing restores normal life expectancy.

The modern permanent pacemaker is a small metal box measuring about 4 cm in diameter and less than 1 cm thick, weighing 30–130 g and powered by a lithium battery that lasts between 8 and 10 years. Single-chamber pacemakers have the electrode placed in either the atrium or the ventricle, and dual-chamber pacemakers have electrodes situated in both chambers. Pacemaker function (e.g. rate, output, sensitivity and inhibitory functions) can be altered to meet the specific requirements of the individual patient. The essential elements are that the ventricle should be paced if there is threatened or actual AV block, and the atrium should be sensed and/or paced unless contraindicated. Wherever possible, a pacing mode that produces the best equivalent of sinus rhythm should be adopted and, for most purposes, this is best produced by dual-chamber systems.

Pacemaker codes

A five-letter code (the NBG code) provides a standardised means of identifying the functional operation of a cardiac pacemaker, regardless of its make or model (Bernstein et al, 2002), and is shown in Table 13.2. The minimum code length is three letters (I–III), and positions IV and V are often omitted.

The first two letters indicate the chambers in which the pacemaker operates. *Position I* represents the chamber paced, and *position II* indicates the chamber sensed. If the pacemaker can sense and pace the same chamber, it is designated D (dual). *Position III* describes the mode of response to sensing, such as I for 'inhibited' (when the presence of sensed electrical activity from the heart inhibits the pacemaker) or T for pacemakers that are 'triggered' by spontaneous cardiac electrical activity. D in position III indicates a double response – an atrial-triggered and a ventricular-inhibited pacemaker. Position IV specifies only the presence or absence of rate modulation, and position V specifies the location or absence of multisite pacing. Some pacemaker generators have a code that can be seen on a standard chest radiograph.

In most patients, the most appropriate pacemaker system is the DDD, where atria and ventricles may be activated sequentially despite AV block, optimising cardiac output. This may not be appropriate in some old or frail patients or in those in permanent atrial fibrillation, when ventricular pacing would be more appropriate (NICE, 2005). DDD pacemakers should not be used in patients with sick sinus syndrome, as the AV node is normal. Atrial pacing is therefore adequate.

Pacemaker magnets

In most programmable generators, applying a magnet over the generator opens a telemetry channel, but its action is dependent on the programmed status of the *magnet-mode* within the device. Usually, the magnet activates reed switches that temporarily turn off demand function, and the pacemaker functions in asynchronous mode (A00, V00, D00). Magnets can be used during diathermy or electrocautery to prevent inhibition of pacing (Salukhe et al, 2004). Concealed magnets in clothing and fashion accessories as alternatives to buttons may accidentally deactivate the reed switches in pacemakers (and implantable defibrillators), so patients should be warned. While the effect of asynchronous pacing may be well tolerated in most patients, a sustained increase in pacing rate may cause symptoms. Removing the magnet returns the generator to normal function.

The situation may be more serious in those with implantable defibrillators. Some may be temporarily toggled to 'monitor only', but this is often permanent if the magnet is operated for more than half a minute.

Other devices with risk include anti-theft systems in shops and metal detectors. They are

Table 13.2 NASPE/BPEG generic pacemaker codes (NBG).

Position I Chamber(s) paced	II Chamber(s) sensed	III Response to sensing	IV Rate modulation	V Multisite pacing
V = Ventricle	V = Ventricle	T = Triggered	R = Rate modulated	0 = None
A = Atrium	A = Atrium	I = Inhibited	0 = None	
				A = Atrium
D = Dual	D = Dual	D = Dual		
				V = Ventricle
0 = None	0 = None	0 = None		D = Dual

NAPSE, North American Society for Pacing and Electrophysiology; BPEG, British Pacing and Electrophysiology Group.

unlikely to cause clinically significant symptoms in most patients, but patients should not stay nearby for longer than is necessary. Any handheld metal detector should not be held near the pacemaker any longer than is necessary. The stainless steel metal casing and some of the internal components will trigger the security screening devices at airports. Patients should carry their pacemaker identity card.

Permanent pacing following acute myocardial infarction

The long-term prognosis of survivors of acute myocardial infarction who develop heart block is mostly related to the extent of myocardial damage, rather than the effects of the heart block itself. Permanent pacing is seldom required following inferior myocardial infarction, as those patients who do not regain normal conduction usually do not survive the acute infarct. The prognosis in terms of conduction is excellent for those who survive.

Most patients who develop heart block following anterior myocardial infarction die, but serious conduction defects are often permanent in those who survive. It is likely that all these patients are at risk of further symptomatic rhythm disturbances, and indications for permanent pacing do not necessarily depend upon symptoms. Possible indications for permanent pacing in this group are shown in Table 13.3.

Table 13.3 Possible indications for permanent pacing in patients with heart block following acute myocardial infarction.

Infarct/block	Pace?
Inferior with transient AV block	No
Inferior with permanent second-/third-degree block	Yes
Anterior with fascicular block	No?
Anterior with transient second-/third-degree block	Yes?
Anterior with permanent second-/third-degree block	Yes

IMPLANTABLE CARDIOVERTER DEFIBRILLATORS

Sudden cardiac death (SCD) is common, representing 25–30% of all cardiovascular deaths and responsible for up to 100 000 deaths in the UK each year. About 80% of episodes of SCD are due to ventricular tachycardia or ventricular fibrillation, usually associated with coronary heart disease. In some cases, SCD will be a presentation of acute ischaemia, which may need reperfusion (thrombolysis or primary angioplasty). In the absence of an acute myocardial infarction, patients who survive SCD have a 15% risk of further episodes, which may be fatal. Although it is usual for patients with malignant ventricular dysrhythmias to be initiated on drugs, recurrence of SCD may still affect half these patients within 5 years. Alternative prophylaxis is often required and may now be provided by an automatic implantable cardioverter defibrillator (AICD). A meta-analysis involving 934 patients treated with an AICD and 932 treated with amiodarone showed a relative risk reduction of 27% in total mortality and 52% in dysrhythmic deaths in those treated with an AICD (Connolly et al, 2000). This equates with one death averted per 10 patients treated by implanting an AICD.

Dr Michel Mirowski developed the AICD in the 1970s, and the first human implant was undertaken in 1980 (Mirowski et al, 1980). There are now over 50 000 new units implanted throughout the world each year. The total cost of the hardware for an implant is about £20 000 and, although expensive, it may be more cost-effective than lifelong treatment with drug therapy (Wever et al, 1996). Compared with drug treatment, patients with an ejection fraction of less than 30% after a heart attack would get an extra 1.8 years of life from an implantable defibrillator, at a cost of £28 000 per life year gained (Al-Khatib et al, 2005).

The equipment

The original AICDs were implanted in the abdomen, and a thoracotomy was needed so that the defibrillation electrode patches could be sewn on to the myocardium. This major operation had a 3–5% mortality. With advances in technology, the units have become smaller, so they resemble and can be inserted like normal cardiac pacemakers, with the result that implantation mortality is now only 0.5%. The device is implanted either subcutaneously, in the left or right delto-pectoral area, or subpectorally in thin patients to prevent the device eroding the skin. All current AICD functions can be mediated through a single ventricular lead, although atrial sensing wires may sometimes be needed. Changing the shock to a biphasic waveform has been the major improvement that allows a reduction in the strength of the defibrillatory shock to 20 J or less in most cases. This has also helped to extend battery life to about 4–7 years, depending upon defibrillator use.

In addition to high-energy defibrillation shocks, modern devices now have many other programmable functions as indicated by the international NBD code. This code is summarised in Table 13.4. Different units have the capability of low-energy synchronised cardioversion, bradycardia and antitachycardia pacing. Normal back-up pacemaker function is important, as some patients require antidysrhythmic medication to suppress the development of VT/VF, which may induce clinically significant bradycardia. Holter function by the units can be used to capture long rhythm strips. The information may be useful diagnostically or to provide evidence of correct and efficient device functioning. Dynamic electrocardiography has the great advantage of being able to show what happened to the heart rhythm before and after administration of the shock, and greater storage facilities are being developed. Atrial defibrillation is not likely to gain widespread application unless acceptable methods of lowering pain associated with defibrillation shocks are implemented.

Implantation

An incision is made below the left clavicle, and a pocket is made either subcutaneously or deep to the pectoralis major muscle. The ventricular lead is then inserted into the right ventricle via the subclavian vein, and standard tests of pacing and sensing are performed. The unit is then tested by delivering a small shock synchronous with the T wave on the ECG to induce ventricular fibrillation. The device should be able to sense the abnormal rhythm and deliver a defibrillatory shock on three occasions before implantation is viewed as complete. The device may also be programmed to detect and treat episodes of ventricular tachycardia by antitachycardia pacing, low-energy cardioversion or high-energy defibrillation.

Predischarge management

Most patients are in hospital for 2–4 days, with pacing and sensing functions of the device being retested before discharge home. The patient should be provided with an AICD identity card that should be carried at all times and shown to relevant people as appropriate (e.g. hospital personnel, airline security).

Lifting should be avoided for the first 4–6 weeks, and the arm on the implant side should not be elevated above shoulder height. Patients are usually followed up at 3- to 6-monthly intervals, when the

Table 13.4 The NASPE/BPEG implantable defibrillator (NBD) code.

I Shock chamber	II Antitachycardia pacing chamber	III Tachycardia detection[a]	IV Antibradycardia pacing chamber
0 = None	0 = None		0 = None
A = Atrium	A = Atrium	E = ECG	A = Atrium
V = Ventricle	V = Ventricle	H = Haemodynamic	V = Ventricle
D = Dual (A + V)	D = Dual (A + V)		D = Dual (A + V)

NAPSE, North American Society for Pacing and Electrophysiology; BPEG, British Pacing and Electrophysiology Group.
a Detection of tachycardias is either by means of an ECG (E) alone or by one or more haemodynamic (H) related variables, such as blood pressure.

device memory is interrogated and standard pacing and sensing tests are performed. Any stored dysrhythmic events may be correlated with the patient's symptoms, and appropriate programming changes or alterations in the patient's medication can be made. Many of the patients have coronary heart disease and heart failure, and need usual treatment and follow-up as for other similar cardiac patients (Stevenson et al, 2004).

Pre- and post-implantation counselling is important. Syncopal or presyncopal attacks may still occur, if only for a few seconds before a shock is delivered, so many patients face significant lifestyle restrictions with particular reference to driving and occupation. Current regulations in the UK allow driving provided the device has been implanted for at least 6 months and has not delivered a therapeutic shock in that time. Driving is also permitted if previous discharges have not been accompanied by incapacity, and provided that there has not been any symptomatic antitachycardia pacing therapy for 6 months. Patients must stop driving for 1 month if the lead or generator has been revised, or if any change is made in antiarrhythmic treatment. Licensing is reviewed annually. Patients with AICDs lose any class 2 driving privileges (vocational licences).

Fears also arise from living with the device, including practical aspects of efficacy, malfunction and battery failure, as well as the shock itself. Many patients tolerate defibrillation shocks very poorly, particularly multiple shocks. Although recipients are generally happy to have the device, and feel more optimistic and confident, fear, anxiety and depression are common and are worsened by the unpredictability of the shocks (Gallagher et al, 1997). For this reason, antidysrhythmic drugs may have a role in reducing the incidence of both ventricular and supraventricular arrhythmias in patients with AICDs.

Some patients have had to have their units removed because of worry. Adjustment disorders include anxiety with panic, and imaginary shocks are not uncommonly experienced (Prudente, 2005). Recipients are also affected by intellectual changes. Adverse psychological reaction to AICD implantation often improves with time as they become accustomed to having the device and adapt to their physical and social limitations. Although professional support tends to focus on the patient, family involvement is important, as both recipient and families may be affected by these psychological problems (Mars et al, 2001). Preparation and rehearsed responses to AICD shocks may limit and adversely affect quality of life (Sears et al, 2005).

AICDs are sensitive to electromagnet interference produced by surgical cautery, which is sensed as VF and leads to the delivery of a shock.

Box 13.4 Patient groups recommended for implantation of AICDs (excluding non-ischaemic dilated cardiomyopathy).

Primary prevention

1 Patients with a history of previous myocardial infarction (> 4 weeks) and:
- Left ventricular dysfunction (ejection fraction < 35%) and
- Non-sustained ventricular tachycardia of Holter monitoring and
- Inducible ventricular tachycardia on electrophysiological testing
2 Patients with a history of previous myocardial infarction (> 4 weeks) and:
- Left ventricular dysfunction (ejection fraction < 30%) and
- QRS duration > 120 ms
3 Family history of sudden cardiac death
- Hypertrophic obstructive cardiomyopathy (HOCM)
- Other patients at high risk of sudden death (e.g. long QT syndrome, Brugada syndrome)
- Arrhythmogenic right ventricular dysplasia
4 After surgical repair of congenital heart disease

Secondary prevention

1 Cardiac arrest due to ventricular tachycardia or ventricular fibrillation
2 Spontaneous ventricular tachycardia producing syncope or significant haemodynamic compromise
3 Sustained ventricular tachycardia with left ventricular dysfunction (ejection fraction < 35%)

AICD function can be temporarily suspended by taping a magnet over the device. Should VF occur during the operation, the magnet can be removed, and the device will recognise and treat the dysrhythmias provided the unit has not been programmed to change to 'monitor-only' function in response to magnet placement.

Complications of AICDs

All the common complications of cardiac pacing may complicate AICD implantation, and many of these complications may require operative revision or even replacement of the system (Kumar & Jowett, 1999). Inappropriate shocking, usually provoked by atrial fibrillation, may be problematical. Patients require evaluation and the unit should be reprogrammed if inappropriate firing is documented.

Which patients should be offered an AICD?

A cardiologist trained in electrophysiology will need to make the assessment for AICD therapy and will be involved in implantation, programming and follow-up. The National Institute for Health and Clinical Excellence has published guidance on who should be considered for AICDs (NICE, 2006). These patients are either at high risk of sudden cardiac death or have been resuscitated from a sudden cardiac death, but further investigation has not found any treatable cause (Box 13.4).

Patients with chronic heart failure are at high risk of sudden death, and AICD may be indicated in patients with low ejection fractions following myocardial infarction, particularly if the QRS is prolonged or there are episodes of ventricular tachycardia. The addition of a third pacing lead in the coronary sinus allows left ventricular pacing and resynchronisation of ventricular contraction, which associates with significant mortality benefit (Pires, 2006). There are also significant improvements in indexes of left ventricular function, symptoms and quality of life. Resynchronisation alone prolongs survival and improves symptoms in patients with advanced congestive heart failure (Cleland et al, 2005).

References

ACC/AHA/NAPSE (2002) Guideline update for implantation of cardiac pacemakers and anti-arrhythmia devices: Executive Summary. *Circulation* 106: 2145–2161.

AHA/ACC (2004) American College of Cardiology/ American Heart Association Guidelines for the Management of Patients with ST-elevation Myocardial Infarction. *Circulation* 110: e82–e293.

Al-Khatib SM, Anstrom KJ, Eisenstein EL et al (2005) Clinical and economic implications of the Multicenter Automatic Defibrillator Implantation Trial-II. *Annals of Internal Medicine* 142: 593–600.

Bernstein AD, Daubert JC, Fletcher RD et al (2002) The revised NASPE/BPEG generic code for antibradycardia, adaptive-rate, and multi-site pacing. North American Society of Pacing and Electrophysiology/British Pacing and Electrophysiology Group. *Pacing and Clinical Electrophysiology* 25: 260–264.

Blandford RL, Burden AC (1984) Abnormalities of cardiac conduction in diabetics. *British Medical Journal* 289: 1659.

Burack B, Furman S (1969) Trans-oesophageal cardiac pacing. *American Journal of Cardiology* 23: 469–472.

Cleland JGF, Daubert J-C, Erdmann E for the Heart Failure (CARE-HF) Study Investigators (2005) The effect of cardiac resynchronization on morbidity and mortality in heart failure. *New England Journal of Medicine* 352: 1539–1549.

Connolly SJ, Hallstrom AP, Cappato R et al (2000) Meta-analysis of the implantable cardioverter defibrillator secondary prevention trials. AVID, CASH and CIDS studies. *European Heart Journal* 21: 2071–2078.

EEC (1988) *Ionising Radiation Regulations*. Brussels: EEC.

Ferguson JD, Banning AP, Bashir Y (1997) Randomised trial of temporary cardiac pacing with semi-rigid and balloon-flotation electrode catheters. *Lancet* 349: 1883.

Gallagher RD, McKinley S, Mangan B et al (1997) The impact of the implantable defibrillator on quality of life. *American Journal of Critical Care* 6: 16–24.

Gammage MD (2000) Temporary cardiac pacing. *Heart* 83: 715–720.

Hickling-Smith DJR, Petch MC (1999) Temporary pacing before permanent pacing should be avoided unless essential. *British Medical Journal* 317: 79–80.

Jowett NI, Thompson DR, Pohl JEF (1989) Temporary transvenous endocardial pacing: six years experience in one coronary care unit. *Postgraduate Medical Journal* 65: 211–215.

Kumar S, Jowett NI (1999) Twiddler's twitch: symptomatic failure of an automatic implantable cardio-defibrillator. *British Journal of Cardiology* 6: 42–44.

Mars A, Bollmann A, Dunbar SB et al (2001) Psychological reactions among family members of patients with implantable defibrillators. *International Journal of Psychiatry Medicine* 31: 375–387.

Mirowski M, Reid PR, Mower MM et al (1980) Termination of malignant ventricular arrhythmias with an implanted automatic defibrillator in human beings. *New England Journal of Medicine* 303: 322–324.

Murphy JJ (2001) Problems with temporary cardiac pacing. *British Medical Journal* 323: 527.

Murphy P, Morton P, Murtagh JG et al (1992) Haemodynamic effects of different temporary pacing modes for the management of bradycardias complicating acute myocardial infarction. *Pacing and Clinical Electrophysiology* 15: 391–396.

NICE (2002) *Central Venous Catheters – Ultrasound-locating Devices*. Technology appraisal guidance no. 49. London: NICE. www.nice.org.uk.

NICE (2005) *Dual Chamber Pacemakers for the Treatment of Symptomatic Bradycardia*. Technology appraisal no. 88. London: NICE. www.nice.org.uk.

NICE (2006) *Arrhythmia – Implantable Cardioverter Defibrillators (ICDs)*. Technology appraisal no. 95. London: NICE. www.nice.org.uk.

Parker J, Cleland JGF (1993) Choice of route for insertion of temporary pacing wires: recommendations of the medical practice committee and council of the British Cardiac Society. *British Heart Journal* 70: 294–296.

Pires LA (2006) Implantable devices for management of chronic heart failure: defibrillators and biventricular pacing therapy. *Current Opinion in Anaesthesiology* 19: 69–74.

Prudente LA (2005) Psychological disturbances, adjustment, and the development of phantom shocks in patients with an implantable cardioverter defibrillator. *Journal of Cardiovascular Nursing* 20: 288–293.

Rajappan K, Fox KF (2003) Temporary cardiac pacing in district general hospitals – sustainable resource or training liability? *Quarterly Journal of Medicine* 96: 783–785.

Salukhe TV, Dob D, Sutton R (2004) Pacemakers and defibrillators: anaesthetic considerations. *British Journal of Anaesthesia* 93: 95–104.

Sears SF, Shea JB, Conti JB (2005) How to respond to an implantable cardioverter-defibrillator shock. *Circulation* 111: 380–382.

Stevenson WG, Chaitman BR, Ellenbogen KA et al (2004) Clinical assessment and management of patients with implanted cardio-defibrillators presenting to non-electrophysiologists. *Circulation* 110: 3866–3869.

Vincenti A, Ciro A, De Ceglia S et al (2001) Predictors of failure of transoesophageal cardioversion of common atrial flutter. *Europace* 3: 10–15.

Wever EFD, Hauer RNW, Schrivers G et al (1996) Cost-effectiveness of implantable defibrillators as first-choice therapy versus electrophysiologically guided, tiered strategy in post-infarction sudden death survivors. *Circulation* 93: 489–496.

Zoll PM (1952) Resuscitation of the heart in ventricular standstill by external electrical stimulation. *New England Journal of Medicine* 247: 768–771.

Chapter **14**

Cardiac rehabilitation/secondary prevention programmes

CHAPTER CONTENTS

The World Health Organization has defined cardiac rehabilitation as '… the sum of activities required to influence favourably the underlying cause of the disease, as well as to ensure the patients best possible physical, mental and social conditions so that they may, by their own efforts preserve or resume when lost, as normal a place in the life of the community' (World Health Organization, 1993). It is thus a process by which patients with coronary heart disease are helped to achieve their optimal physical, psychological, social, vocational and economic status. In addition, it aims to stabilise, slow or even reverse the progression of atherosclerosis, thereby reducing morbidity and mortality.

Rehabilitation cannot be regarded as an isolated form of therapy, but must be integrated with the whole management plan. Modern practice is therefore moving away from pure exercise-based intervention towards programmes promoting long-term lifestyle adaptation and change. While exercise training remains fundamental to recovery from cardiac illness, comprehensive cardiac rehabilitation programmes now provide a focus for secondary prevention through nutritional counselling, weight management and promoting adherence to prescribed drug therapy, bringing together medical treatment, education, exercise, sexual and vocational counselling and behaviour change (Ades, 2001), and initiating an evolving process for helping people to address risk factors and thereby lessen the impact of the disease on the quality and quantity of life (American Association of Cardiovascular and Pulmonary Rehabilitation, 2004). Rehabilitation should be regarded as an integral part of cardiac care, a process that should start at the time of the cardiac event, continue through the hospital stay and transfer seamlessly to aftercare in the community.

Although standards for cardiac rehabilitation are documented in the National Service Framework (NSF) for Coronary Heart Disease (Department of Health, 2000), rehabilitation is not always seen as an important component of contemporary comprehensive cardiac care, often resulting in a fragmented, mechanistic and haphazard approach (Thompson & Oldridge, 2004). The NSF target is for more than 85% of eligible patients to be offered cardiac rehabilitation, and that, at 1 year after hospital discharge, at least 50% of people will be non-smokers, exercise regularly and have a body mass index (BMI) under 30 kg/m². A review of progress with the NSF shows that movement has been made towards developing rehabilitation services; progress is varied and there is little evidence that it has resulted in a significant increase in uptake of these services (Healthcare Commission, 2005). Indeed, a recent survey concluded that the current cardiac rehabilitation service in England could barely cope with the 30% of eligible patients who take up the service because of inadequate staffing, facilities, space and underfunding (Brodie et al, 2006). If the recommended 85% of eligible patients were included, the service could not cope.

THE BENEFITS OF REHABILITATION

There is good evidence supporting the benefits of cardiac rehabilitation, including significant reductions in mortality and morbidity and improvements in health-related quality of life (Taylor et al, 2004; Clark et al, 2005). Exercise tolerance increases, and there are improvements in psychosocial well-being and risk factors (improved blood lipid profiles, less stress, less smoking). The intervention appears to be cost effective (Papadakis et al, 2005), at less than £500 per patient depending upon the scale of the programme, location, components and staff mix (Beswick et al, 2004). The application of cardiac rehabilitation/secondary prevention programmes to other chronic conditions, such as patients with the metabolic syndrome, warrants consideration. Preventing these conditions from following their natural course into acute and chronic vascular disease would be life saving and economically beneficial.

Originally, cardiac rehabilitation services were developed for patients who had recently suffered a myocardial infarction, but were later expanded to those who had undergone coronary artery bypass surgery. Evidence for the efficacy of rehabilitation came initially from observations in white, middle-aged men following acute transmural myocardial infarction, and the elderly, women and high-risk subgroups were excluded (e.g. those with angina

or heart failure). Evidence of benefit in patients with hypertension, heart failure and following cardiac surgery now exists (Leon et al, 2005), although many centres still restrict access to patients with acute coronary syndromes, and certain groups remain under-represented, including women, elderly people, ethnic minority groups and individuals who live in rural areas (Beswick et al, 2005). Uptake of schemes is generally poor, with reports of fewer than one in four post-infarction patients participating (Bethel et al, 2001). In some centres, only half of the patients complete the programme (Dalal & Evans, 2003), and barriers to participation such as distance and lack of transport often have to be addressed (Daly et al, 2002).

PHASES OF REHABILITATION

A systematic and structured framework can be useful to guide service provision at the right time and in the right place. Many programmes use a framework consisting of four phases.

Phase one – before discharge from hospital

This is started as soon as is practical as an integral part of acute cardiac care. An early assessment of physical, psychological and social needs should be established so that a written individual plan for meeting these needs can be developed. The patient should receive initial advice on important lifestyle interventions (smoking cessation, physical activity, diet). Involvement of the pharmacy is very helpful during the inpatient phase with education on medication, benefits and side effects. Early involvement of relevant carers is recommended. Written information about local cardiac support groups and the cardiac rehabilitation programme should be provided at this early stage.

Phase two – early post–discharge period

Phase two rehabilitation occurs at a time when patients feel isolated and insecure. Maintenance of contact is important (by phone, home visits), and the role of the British Heart Foundation cardiac liaison nurse has been found to be invaluable. Self-help manuals may reduce anxiety, depression and reduce hospital readmission rates following acute myocardial infarction. The assessment of cardiac risk, including physical, psychological and social needs for cardiac rehabilitation, is completed with a review of the initial plan for meeting these needs.

Phase three – 4–6 weeks after the acute event

Phase three rehabilitation provides structured exercise sessions with counselling to meet the assessed needs of individual patients. Access to relevant advice and support from appropriately trained individuals on topics such as exercise, relaxation, psychological interventions, health promotion and vocational advice is maintained. Traditionally, this has taken place in the hospital, but community-based schemes are becoming more common. The ratio of patients to trained staff at exercise-based sessions should be no more than 10:1. Supervisors must be trained in basic life support and have easy access to a defibrillator. High-risk patients should be exercised in hospital where advanced cardiac life support is available. Exercise intensity should be monitored by pulse monitoring, and electronic devices are preferable to patients taking their own pulse. Some programmes monitor patients with the Borg scale (Borg, 1998), a perceived exertion scale that actually correlates quite well with oxygen uptake and heart rate. The Borg scale has 15 points (6–20), with point 6 being the equivalent of sitting down doing nothing, point 9 walking gently, point 13 a steady exercising pace and 19/20 the hardest exercise ever undertaken. Many patients like using this scale to help them exercise to a point of 'comfortable breathlessness'.

Phase four – long-term maintenance of behavioural change

Phase four rehabilitation is that of chronic disease management, with monitoring of secondary prevention interventions, maintenance of lifestyle and behavioural change. Exercise-based rehabilitation offers most benefit when continued beyond 12 weeks. Unfortunately, participation dwindles when supervision is withdrawn. Formal classes in community centres, sports clubs and leisure centres have been found to be helpful. Self-help groups should be encouraged, but are often limited to small numbers of enthusiastic participants. Some patients prefer to make their own arrangements rather than attend class-based activities. Referral to specialist cardiac, behavioural (e.g. exercise, smoking cessation) or psychological services may be indicated in individual cases.

Organising rehabilitation

Cardiac rehabilitation/secondary prevention programmes should start with a baseline assessment, followed by instruction on aggressive risk factor management (including the appropriate use of cardioprotective drugs for secondary prevention), psychosocial support with counselling on diet, physical activity and exercise training. The rehabilitation process should include the following elements (Thompson et al, 1997):

- explanation and understanding;
- specific rehabilitation interventions;
- methods to assist readaptation.

Programmes are moving towards a modular system, to allow the patient and their relatives to access the individual components appropriate for them (a rehabilitation 'menu'). Patients can attend the programme for as little as 2 weeks to a maximum of 8 weeks, followed by referral to a recognised phase four class. The phases and the elements contained within them should be flexible and tailored to suit the individual needs of the patient and his/her partner and family. This means that the timing and location of sessions need to be adaptable and the length of participation in a programme sufficient to cater for the patient. Patient (and family/carers) expectations should also be taken into account (Lau-Walker, 2004).

Cardiac rehabilitation involves the use of a wide range of skills from different health professionals, including the nurse, doctor, physiotherapist, occupational therapist, clinical psychologist, dietician and social worker. Nursing staff usually assume the central role by being responsible, directly or indirectly, for controlling the many factors that influence the patient's recovery, and are usually in the most frequent contact with the patient and family. The nurse can assist the patient and family to understand, accept and adapt to the illness, and may be able to stimulate them to take an active part in recovery and rehabilitation. In addition, the nurse can assist them in making realistic plans for the future. Attainable goals need to be defined, plans being jointly agreed by the patient, the family and other members of the healthcare team. An attitude of optimism should be adopted by staff, remembering that most patients who are going to die from acute myocardial infarction do so before reaching hospital.

From early convalescence in hospital, the patient and partner should understand that a return to normality within a matter of a few weeks is not only expected, but also safe and beneficial, given that the patient's condition warrants it. It is the success of coping and support that often ultimately determines the outcome of the patient's illness; the heart may recover more rapidly than the patient's often depressed mental state. Individualised cardiac rehabilitation that starts early leads to improvements in quality of life, more confidence about returning to activities and fewer further treatment needs (Mayou et al, 2000, 2002).

EDUCATION

Education and counselling involve teaching patients and their families to understand the illness and its management. Education initiated on the coronary care unit (CCU) helps the patient to understand what has happened, what is immediately being done and what is likely to happen over the ensuing days. Teaching needs to be relevant to the individual concerned; vagueness and ambiguity will only result in increased fear and anxiety. A programme centred upon these principles is likely to improve the patient's attitudes, behaviour and understanding of the illness and improve his or her recovery.

At an early stage, brief explanations of the staff, equipment, procedures and routines of the CCU will reduce anxiety and misunderstanding. Bombarding patients with too much information during the early phase should be avoided, as they invariably retain very few facts during this acute stage. Capacity for learning is impaired by fear, anxiety, pain and fatigue. Patients will, however, benefit from answers to specific questions, and answers should be clear, simple and repeated frequently. Understanding the factors that may have caused their condition may also help them to assume a large degree of responsibility for their care. Information provided to patients and their partners during their stay in hospital is often poor and, although patient teaching is recognised as an important nursing function, there is little evidence to show that it is being effectively and consistently accomplished (Scott & Thompson, 2003). It is the responsibility of the healthcare team to ensure that the patient and family understand the illness, the purpose of treatment and how to cope both within and outside the hospital. Nurses are in an ideal position to teach, because they frequently become the most familiar person to the patient, and are thus often in the best position to communicate with the patient and family.

Teaching programmes during the patient's stay in hospital are designed to decrease the patient's feeling of helplessness, to help restore self-esteem and to bolster the patient's confidence in terms of a successful outcome. Those who understand the cause and significance of their illness and its management are likely to have improved motivation to comply with therapy and cope with the consequences of their illness. Patients particularly need information about potential events that may occur after their return home, when professional help is not immediately available. Teaching and learning is a two-way process, and the individual patient's requirements will vary with his or her general educational background and intellectual capabilities. Demographic variables need consideration, such as family composition, ethnic, cultural and religious background. There may be prior knowledge or even misconceptions of coronary heart disease. Simple language should be used, and earlier communication is remembered better than that given later on. Repetition increases recall, as does specific rather than general advice. *Cognitive behavioural therapy* is a structured therapy that addresses these core beliefs and assumptions. It helps to manage changes in behaviour, and deals with anxiety and depressive symptoms in cardiac patients (Lewin et al, 1995).

The *Heart Manual* is a 6-week, facilitated self-help rehabilitation programme for people recovering from a heart attack based on a cognitive behavioural model (Lewin et al, 1992). The manual is introduced to the patient as soon as possible after their heart attack. A facilitator spends 20–45 minutes showing the manual and checking that they can understand and complete the simple exercise programme. The patient keeps a workbook that consists of a phased programme of health education, home-based exercises and stress management that the patient works through over 6 weeks. It also contains answers to specific problems or worries about medication and sex. There are also two audiotapes, one a scripted interview between a doctor and a patient targeted at the family to help them understand what has happened, and a second being a programme of relaxation training. After discharge, contact is made with the patient, by either a home visit or a phone call, to check progress. At the end of the programme, the patient can complete a questionnaire pack to check that their needs have been met.

It can be seen that contemporary approaches to patient teaching are numerous and varied, and information should be tailored to individual needs and given in a consistent and structured fashion. The comprehension of new information will be at its best when the patient is motivated and when the information is presented clearly, concisely and in small doses. There is no substitute for personal advice, and its value depends upon the attending medical and nursing staff adopting an informed, committed and uniform approach. Similar education of the patient's family is equally important, and giving this at the bedside (when the patient is surrounded by high technology and obvious intensive care) may reinforce the importance of such advice.

Instructional aids, such as the *Heart Manual*, are very useful as part of the educational process, and there are a range of interactive media such as CDs and DVDs that can be used or loaned to the patient. Vocabulary, sentence length, illustrations, type size and style, as well as readability and accuracy of the information presented should be carefully considered. Visual information is usually assimilated better than the spoken word, so illustrations, pamphlets and models are a helpful and useful adjunct. A model of the heart can be used to demonstrate cardiac anatomy and the coronary arteries, and explain about the blood supply to the heart. It is important to stress that coronary heart disease is a chronic health problem and that there is no 'cure', but that some medical intervention and modification in lifestyle may be necessary to alleviate symptoms and reduce the risk of further problems.

Topics that should be included for discussion include the recognition of signs and symptoms of myocardial infarction, the names, dosages and side effects of medications, and knowledge of personal risk factors and how to modify them. Other aspects that need to be covered are the nature of the disease, emergency treatment, resumption of activities and physical, psychosocial and financial problems encountered on return to home and work. Aspects frequently neglected include how to take the pulse, sexual activity and instruction on the normal convalescence. Advice should be realistic, practical and accurate, based on evidence and imparted in clear, unambiguous ways, such as 'eat five portions of fresh fruit and vegetables every day', instead of 'try and eat more fruit' (Thompson & Lewin, 2000).

The technique of *motivational interviewing* has a potentially useful application to cardiac rehabilitation in terms of facilitating health behaviour change and thus gains in secondary prevention (Miller & Rollnick, 2002). The interviewer helps the patient to explore the importance of, readiness for and confidence (or ambivalence) to change. This increases the patient's motivation for and commitment to making a change in behaviour in the interests of their own health. This is important as the patient's individual perspective is needed to ensure that long-term health behaviour is sustained. This will include how the illness is perceived and fosters self-efficacy (Lau-Walker, 2006).

As half the advice in a 5-minute consultation is forgotten within the next 5 minutes, it is helpful if written or tape-recorded advice is provided. Written information should be produced following the empirically determined guidelines for maximising comprehension and adherence.

Questionnaires may be useful for evaluating the patient's needs and level of comprehension. However, when assessing the efficacy of the education programme, it is important to differentiate between what patients learn and what they are actually going to do about it; the acquisition of new information does not necessarily result in a change in behaviour.

The family can have a direct influence on the education process by understanding the illness and helping the patient to adapt. They can also assist in lifestyle modification, and should therefore be included in most, if not all, teaching. Partner involvement has been minimal in rehabilitation, despite the widespread opinion that success generally depends upon their support (Thompson, 2002). A programme that involves both patients and partners provides an ideal opportunity for giving information, instilling hope and redefining health. The rest of the family also need information in order to feel useful to the patient and to understand that he or she is receiving appropriate care.

It is not uncommon for the patient and family to be left to cope by themselves with only vague instructions about discharge and rehabilitation, which results in uncertainty, distress and failure to adjust. A well-planned programme is desirable, to anticipate the patient's homecoming and return to work. Patients and spouses often have specific questions about convalescence, medication, diet, drinking, driving and smoking, as well as resumption of leisure and sexual and work activities. Because the transition from hospital to home is frequently a traumatic and neglected aspect of post-myocardial infarction management, it may be appropriate to make arrangements that will ensure continuity of care. Periodic checks (e.g. telephoning the patient and partner or home visits) may be useful, in some instances, to bridge this gap, and this is probably best achieved by close liaison between the hospital and the community team. The community nurse can play an important role in teaching, counselling and evaluating the care that has been initiated within the hospital, and is also ideally placed for informing the patient and partner about community resources, including counselling services, home help and rehabilitation facilities.

EXERCISE

Structured exercise as a therapeutic intervention is central to cardiac rehabilitation, as physical deconditioning occurs following myocardial infarction, and regular exercise will restore muscular strength and protect against cardiovascular disease. Exercise training involves a graduated programme to avoid the complications of bedrest and to encourage a positive approach to recovery, passive and low-level activities and aiming for a full return to normal activities.

Emphasising physical exercise following an acute coronary event usually represents a major change to the typical patient's sedentary lifestyle, involving the car, labour-saving devices and long hours in front of the television. However, exercise improves mood and morale, and physical fitness allows an earlier return to normal lifestyle and work. Regular exercise also helps cardiovascular performance, keeps the body supple and helps to control body weight. To produce the maximum benefit, the activity needs to be regular and aerobic. This involves using the large muscle groups in the arms, legs and back steadily and rhythmically so that breathing and heart rate are significantly increased.

Regular moderate exercise (30 minutes on 5 or more days per week) at a level of 75–85% of maximal capacity is an ideal way of achieving physical fitness. Vigorous physical activity may be employed later and is recognised as an important factor in protection against the development of coronary heart disease. However, care is required in those with pre-existing heart disease; exercise is not without hazard, and low-level activities are preferable in older and less fit patients.

Formal exercise programmes are very useful following acute myocardial infarction. Early graduated physical activity, starting with gentle passive exertion, has been designed to avert or minimise the risk of venous stasis, deep vein thrombosis and pulmonary emboli. When the patient is first allowed out of bed, they are often shocked by the feeling of physical weakness, which is usually not expected or easily explicable in terms of the short period of bedrest and inactivity. The patient will need reassuring and encouragement to gradually increase the level of activity.

Any restrictions thought necessary should be carefully explained in a positive fashion, so that the patient does not become frustrated.

Information regarding physical activity will depend on the stage of recovery the patient has reached. Initially, the reasons for temporary restriction of activity will need to be explained, and that the resumption of activity will be gradual to allow the myocardium to heal. Advice about specific activities should be individualised, and take into account the extent and severity of the myocardial infarction, the patient's previous level of activity, the extent of recovery and the stability of the current condition. Encouraging cardiac patients to engage in regular physical activity is more likely to be successful if they are offered action plans on when, where and how to act, and coping plans on how to deal with anticipated barriers (Sniehotta et al, 2006).

Physical activity in hospital

Early ambulation in uncomplicated myocardial infarction is essential to avert or minimise the deleterious effects of prolonged bedrest, including decreased physical work capacity. It also reduces the anxiety and depression that often follow acute myocardial infarction. In some CCUs, patients are encouraged to sit out of bed on the day of admission, provided they are free from pain and significant dysrhythmias. If there has been a prolonged period of bedrest, resumption of activity often results in a moderate tachycardia and orthostatic hypotension. Physical activities should, therefore, be at a low level of intensity, such as eating, dressing and undressing, washing the hands and face, use of a bedside commode, simple arm and leg exercises. Observation of patients as they perform these activities is useful to ensure that they can cope and that inappropriate symptoms (chest pain, dyspnoea, sweating) are not provoked. Patients are usually the best judge of how much they can do, but they should be warned of the feelings of weakness that may accompany increases in activity.

Once patients leave the CCU, the aim is for them to attain a level of activity that permits personal care and independence (or at least semi-independence) by the time of discharge

from hospital. Walking with a gradual and progressive increase in speed and distance should be the major component of the activity plan. It is advisable for most patients who will have to climb stairs at home to try stairs in hospital under supervision. This results in increased confidence and reduced worry for the patient and family. At the time of discharge from hospital, patients should be able to perform activities at peak levels of up to five metabolic equivalents (METs) for short periods to simulate usual activities at home (Table 14.1).

Predischarge exercise stress testing

The current practice of early ambulation after myocardial infarction has resulted in the more widespread use of exercise testing earlier in the course of the illness, and often before discharge home. Exercise stress testing after myocardial infarction is helpful not only for risk stratification and assessment of prognosis, but also in assessing functional capacity after hospital discharge, including domestic and occupational work evaluation. A normal response to an early exercise test reliably identifies patients at low risk of future cardiac events. The exercise protocols can be either submaximal or symptom limited.

Submaximal tests have a predetermined endpoint, often defined as a peak heart rate of 120 beats/minute, attaining 70% of the predicted maximum heart rate, or a peak level of 5 METs; failure to achieve this level associates with a poor prognosis.

Symptom-limited tests are designed to continue until the patient demonstrates signs or symptoms that necessitate termination of exercise (i.e. angina, fatigue) or the production of an abnormal haemodynamic or electrocardiogram (ECG) response.

Symptom-limited protocols at 4–7 days after myocardial infarction are twice as likely to produce an ischaemic response as a submaximal test. It is thus a better estimate of peak functional capacity, but is more hazardous, being associated with an adverse event rate nearly twice that of submaximal tests (e.g. severe angina, ventricular tachycardia, cardiac arrest, reinfarction).

Performing a submaximal stress test prior to hospital discharge is useful for counselling patients and their families about domestic, recreational

Table 14.1   Energy levels required to perform everyday activities (METs).[a]

Under 3 METs	3–5 METs	5–7 METs	7–9 METs	Over 9 METs
		Common activities		
Washing/dressing	Cycling (slow)	Gardening	Heavy shovelling	Carrying loads upstairs
Desk work	Housework	Lawn mowing	Climbing stairs (moderate	Running up stairs
Washing dishes	Carrying light objects	Climbing stairs (slowly)	speed)	
Driving car	Walking the dog	Level walking	Carrying heavy objects	
Walking at 2 mph	Unloading the car	(4.5–5.0 mph)		
Lying in bed		Digging		
		Work		
Typing	Shelf filling	Light physical	Moderate manual	Heavy manual
Clerical	Light manual	Operating tools		
Sales staff				
		Play		
Sewing	Dancing	Badminton	Swimming (crawl)	Squash
Stationary bike	Golf (with cart)	Tennis (singles)	Bicycling (12 mph)	Running (> 6 mph)
Computer games	Tennis	Swimming, breast	Jogging (5 mph)	Bicycling (> 13 mph)
Piano playing	(doubles)	stroke	Football	
		Bicycling (9–10 mph)	Climbing hills	

a The MET represents a simple and practical expression of the energy cost of physical activities as a multiple of the resting metabolic rate. One metabolic equivalent (MET) is defined as the amount of oxygen consumed while sitting at rest and is equal to 3.5 mL of O_2 per kg body weight per minute.

and occupational activities that can be safely undertaken after going home, as most domestic activities require fewer than 5 METs. Partners who observe stress testing are likely to gain more confidence in the patient's physical and cardiac capability.

A follow-up symptom-limited stress test can be performed 4–6 weeks after the myocardial infarction to assess the need for angiography, and to assess the safety of exercise-based cardiac rehabilitation. A symptom-limited stress test is also advised before rehabilitation in those with recent coronary artery bypass surgery, recent coronary angioplasty, chronic stable angina or controlled heart failure.

Physical activity during convalescence

When the patient returns home, progressive increases in physical activity are used to achieve a level of activity that allows normal daily activities

and will later permit a return to work. The activity plan within hospital will usually have helped to allay fears of a further heart attack or sudden death resulting from physical exertion. Patients should be encouraged to exercise daily, and it should be stressed that a lack of exercise may be harmful rather than beneficial. The best form of exercise is walking, but golf, swimming, jogging and cycling can be encouraged when the patient feels well enough. Exercises that use less than half of the patient's working capacity will not help to increase fitness.

The benefits of exercise, including weight control, improvement in respiratory function and a general feeling of well-being, should be stressed. Practical advice is helpful too, such as only exercising in warm environments and not after heavy meals, by the fireside in winter or in the midday sun in summer. Competitive sports are not advisable in the early months following myocardial infarction.

The levels of activity performed at the end of the hospital stay should be maintained and gradually increased. Walking speed and distance should be increased, so that, by the end of 4–6 weeks, the patient may walk up to 5 miles per day. The patient and family will usually gain confidence, and the patient more independence, when accomplishing each objective. Improved fitness will also allow those patients who ordinarily experience angina to perform activities at a higher intensity level before reaching their anginal threshold.

Formal exercise programmes for outpatients

The main emphasis for rehabilitation has been early programmes of hospital-based exercise training, but it is now widely accepted that there is need for a wider and more flexible range of methods, greater individual prescription of care and closer co-operation with ongoing medical care. Exercise is popular with many patients and appears to be effective in the early stages in improving exercise capacity, reducing anxiety and encouraging a rapid return to activities. Both light and heavy exercise have been shown to be of benefit in improving physical conditioning and, although these can easily be provided in a hospital gym, they can be provided just as successfully in the community.

Exercise-based cardiac rehabilitation also appears to be very safe, with a risk of death of one per 0.75 million hours (Leon et al, 2005). Treadmill testing and echocardiography are recommended to assess residual ischaemia and ventricular function, respectively, in all patients following myocardial infarction, but are not necessarily a prerequisite to cardiac rehabilitation except for high-risk patients. For most patients, clinical risk stratification based on history, examination and resting ECG, combined with a functional capacity test such as a shuttle walking test or a 6-minute walking test, will be sufficient (Tobin & Thow, 1999; Demers et al, 2001). The shuttle walking test was originally developed for patients with respiratory disease, but is often used to assess functional capacity before cardiac rehabilitation. It is an easier alternative to formal exercise testing that

allows the assessment of suitability and progress during cardiac rehabilitation without the need for cardiac physiologists, doctors or expensive equipment. The incremental shuttle walking test protocol is shown in Box 14.1. Briefly, this test requires the patient to walk at gradually increasing speeds up and down a 10-minutes course identified by two cones until they reach a symptom-limited maximum, or 12 minutes, whichever occurs first.

Exercise sessions usually have a 15-minute warm-up period before the aerobic conditioning phase of the exercise session (20–30 minutes). Maintaining a target heart rate on a pulse monitor is a useful guide for achieving the correct intensity of exertion. The level of activity is altered until the desired heart rate is achieved, and the exercise is maintained for the duration of the session (continuous training) or interspersed with brief rest periods (intermittent training). At the conclusion of the exercise session, it is important to taper the activity down gradually (a 'cool down') rather than to stop it abruptly.

Relaxation is as important as exercise and is an important component of cardiac rehabilitation, as it enhances recovery from an ischaemic cardiac event and contributes to secondary prevention (van Dixhoorn & White, 2005). Regular relaxation techniques produce a reduction in resting heart rate, a reduction in anxiety and in the frequency of angina, increased return to work and reduced risk of death.

The formal exercise component of cardiac rehabilitation should be offered at least twice a week for a minimum of 8 weeks. Low- to moderate-intensity resistance training may be incorporated after 4 weeks of supervised aerobic training, which improves muscular strength, cardiovascular function, coronary risk factors and psychological well-being. Home-based exercise programmes are probably as effective as group training, although a rehabilitation programme that is community based may be more beneficial in terms of social contact and support (Arthur et al, 2002; Smith et al, 2004). Once-weekly, hospital-based exercise plus two equivalent home-based exercise sessions is as effective in improving physical work capacity as thrice-weekly hospital-based exercise.

Box 14.1   The incremental shuttle walking test.

Equipment

Compact disc (CD) player and shuttle walk test instruction CD

Two markers and a flat walking surface of at least 10 metres

Heart rate monitor

Method

The two markers are placed 9 metres apart, allowing the subjects to walk 10 metres when they go round the cone at the end of each shuttle

Subjects walk around the course in time with an audio signal from the CD

There are 12 levels each of 1-minute duration with walking speeds that rise incrementally from 1.2 mph to 5.3 mph (0.5–2.37 m/second)

Walking speeds and progression to the next level of exercise are externally paced and controlled by a series of beeps played by the CD

Number of shuttles range from 3 at level one to 14 at level twelve

The test is completed at 12 minutes or if one of the endpoint criteria is met

Endpoint criteria

Symptoms (angina, dyspnoea, fatigue)

Desirable heart rate achieved (220 – the patient's age × 85%)

Failure to meet the speed requirements of the test (being more than 0.5 metres away from the cone when the beep sounded)

Post-test assessment

Subjects should continue to walk slowly around the course to avoid any symptoms associated with abrupt cessation of exercise

Record total number of shuttles, total distance walked, peak heart rate and reason for test termination

If patients have ongoing symptoms after 10 minutes, they may need sublingual nitrates or a medical opinion, as appropriate

The benefits of exercise

Exercise training and regular daily physical activities are essential for improving physical fitness, and may even help older adults to live independently (Stewart et al, 2003). Improvement in cardiorespiratory endurance on exercise testing is associated with a significant reduction in major adverse cardiovascular events independent of other risk factors (Mark & Lauer, 2003). A Cochrane review found that exercise-only cardiac rehabilitation reduced all-cause mortality by 27%, cardiac death by 31% and a combined endpoint of mortality, non-fatal myocardial infarction and revascularisation by 19% (Jolliffe et al, 2006). However, there appeared to be no effect on non-fatal myocardial infarction alone, and there was no apparent additional benefit from comprehensive cardiac rehabilitation (exercise in addition to psychological and educational interventions). On the other hand, a comprehensive rehabilitation programme has been shown to slow the progression of coronary atherosclerosis (Niebauer et al, 1997), with an accompanying reduction in body weight and central adiposity. While exercise-only programmes considered in the trials documented improvement in physical performance, muscle strength and symptoms, the benefits of group exercise in preventing social isolation and aiding psychological function and social recovery were not specifically considered if they were administered in a non-structured fashion. Comprehensive cardiac rehabilitation aids psychological function, social recovery and return to work, and the exercise component leads to improvements in insulin sensitivity, helping to reduce blood pressure and serum triglycerides, with increases in high-density lipoprotein cholesterol. Concomitant improvement in glucose homeostasis reduces the risk of type 2 diabetes mellitus in patients with impaired glucose tolerance (Tuomilehto et al, 2001).

PSYCHOSOCIAL CARE

Psychosocial dysfunction is common in patients attending cardiac rehabilitation programmes, with symptoms of depression, anger and anxiety disorders. Such patients are at risk of recurrent cardiovascular events. Cardiac patients who are distressed in hospital are at high risk of adverse psychological and quality of life outcomes during the ensuing year (Mayou et al, 2000). Many of these patients are confronted by fear and uncertainty when they arrive back home, which, when combined with minor physical symptoms, result in increased anxiety and depression, thus compounding the situation.

The prevalence of major depressive disorders among patients with coronary heart disease ranges from 16% to 27% with an additional 20–30% of cardiac patients exhibiting minor depression or elevated depressive symptoms (Davidson et al, 2004). A substantial number of patients enrolled in rehabilitation report depression (Todaro et al, 2005), which influences adherence and improvements (Glazer et al, 2002). Formal screening needs to be considered as part of routine practice (Martin & Thompson, 2006), and those patients identified with clinically significant depression need to be referred to appropriate specialist services as soon as possible after the cardiac event. While intervention may not alter the cardiac outcome, intervention will improve the psychological well-being and quality of life of cardiac patients (Berkman et al, 2003). The recommended instrument for routine use is the Hospital Anxiety and Depression (HAD) scale, which is quick and easy to use, and provides a reliable and valid measure for detecting anxiety and depression (Zigmond & Snaith, 1983).

Predischarge counselling is useful in improving morale and aiding a successful return to home and work, including discussions of potential problems, such as anxiety, depression, poor concentration, irritability, sleeplessness and fear of complications (especially death). 'Homecoming blues' are almost universal, and patients and partners should be warned that it is likely to happen. The partner often experiences a greater degree of anxiety than the patient and may need careful and supportive counselling (Thompson, 2002). The family particularly needs to be cautioned against overprotectiveness towards the patient. Ultimately, each individual is responsible for his or her own health and must be encouraged to assume overall responsibility and control. Impressive improvements in mood have been

claimed for a self-help home-based behavioural programme, which is especially suitable for low-risk patients (Lacey et al, 2004). It is estimated that up to 30% of subjects might benefit from individually planned help in later convalescence, even if they have attended early rehabilitation programmes (Lewin et al, 1992).

SEXUAL COUNSELLING

The subject of sex should be approached as a matter of routine in the rehabilitation of all coronary patients and their partners. Although discussion of this intimate aspect of the patient's life is difficult for both patient and healthcare staff, sexual counselling should be viewed as an integral part of the cardiac rehabilitation programme. Sexual problems are common, and many patients have concerns about erectile dysfunction and about resumption of sexual activity (Taylor, 1999). The complicated association between psychological distress, sexual adjustment, organic factors and existing family support should be considered in cardiac rehabilitation (Friedman, 2000).

The energy expenditure during intercourse is not as great as is popularly believed, being equivalent to that of climbing about two flights of stairs (4 METs). The peak heart rate occurs during orgasm, and adequate foreplay will allow the pulse rate to increase gradually from resting levels to a transient peak. Blood pressure also rises gradually, with an increase in the respiratory rate. These physiological variables rapidly return to resting levels after orgasm. Extramarital and other illicit encounters may, however, expend much more energy, and are often associated with faster heart rates, higher blood pressures and an increased risk of sudden death.

Patients recovering from acute myocardial infarction often suffer from a depressed libido, which may result in sexual disharmony. The partner is often more concerned than the patient and may be frightened of resuming sexual activity because of precipitating a heart attack or sudden death. The severity of the infarct and the extent of cardiac decompensation are much less important causes of sexual debility than is the psychological condition of the patient. Many factors, including normal age-related changes in sexual response, medication-induced dysfunction, diabetes and the emotional impact of heart disease, may influence sexual function in these patients.

If psychological problems remain unresolved, it may be necessary to refer the patient for specialised sexual counselling by a clinical psychologist, often within a sexual dysfunction clinic; intensive therapy may be indicated in resistant cases. There are detailed guidelines available for the management of sexual dysfunction in cardiac patients (Jackson et al, 2006), and the British Heart Foundation (pamphlet no. 2/2000, available at www.bhf.org.uk) have produced a fact file for patients.

MEDICATION

Mortality can be reduced in patients with heart disease by treating individual risk factors with evidence-based pharmacological interventions (Mukherjee et al, 2004). Adherence to drug therapy varies from patient to patient, but is often poor. Difficulty in understanding and complying with drug therapy may occur for a variety of reasons, including fear of dependency or of side effects. Multiple drugs are prescribed routinely following a cardiac event, and a typical patient will leave the CCU with aspirin, clopidogrel, a beta-blocker, an angiotensin-converting enzyme (ACE) inhibitor and a statin. The situation is even more complicated if warfarin is needed. The more complex the drug regimen, the less likely compliance seems to be, and careful review of the patient's medication is necessary before discharge. Many patients will not have taken tablets before their heart attack, and the habit of taking regular medication will be unfamiliar and difficult.

Information should include correct identification of the drug, what it is for, the dosage and other special instructions (e.g. the storage and limited life of glyceryl trinitrate). Reissue of prescriptions needs to be covered, as many stop what is intended to be continuous therapy when they have finished 'the course'. In addition, they should be warned that they should not allow themselves to run out of tablets or go away on holiday with insufficient supplies. Sudden withdrawal of certain drugs (e.g. beta-blockers) may be associated with sudden cardiac events, including unstable angina, myocardial infarction and sudden death. Patients should enquire about whether or

not it would be cheaper to obtain an annual prescription ('season ticket'), rather than paying for individual medications.

It may be useful to issue a small record card listing the patient's medications, with dose, time to be taken, action and possible side effects written on the card. This may be kept with the medication at home, thus serving as a reminder and providing important information about the drugs. The cards are also useful to summarise therapy when the patient's family doctor is reissuing prescriptions, and they can be taken to hospital appointments so that all concerned know what medication is actually being taken.

Family participation in teaching about drugs may exert a strong influence on the patient's understanding and thus improve compliance with therapy.

DRIVING

Patients can usually resume driving 4 weeks after uncomplicated myocardial infarction, coronary artery bypass grafting or unstable angina. They should initially avoid rush-hour traffic and long journeys, as well as aggressive or competitive driving. If recovery is satisfactory, driving is permitted without notifying the licensing authority, although motor insurance companies normally require formal notification about changes in health circumstances. Patients are advised not to drive for 1 week after coronary angioplasty, and patients with vocational (class 2) driving licences may be precluded from holding licences to drive large goods vehicles or passenger-carrying vehicles after they have had a myocardial infarction. Full guidance can be obtained from the driver and vehicle licensing agency (www.dvla.gov.uk/at_a_glance).

FLYING

All flights, whether long or short distances, impose stresses on passengers from complicated check-in procedures, tight schedules, noise, turbulence, jet lag and often cramped seating. There is always the potential for cardiac passengers to become ill during or after the flight due to these stresses (Aerospace Medical Association, 2003).

The major problem for cardiac patients is hypoxia. Modern aircraft cabins are not pressurised to sea level equivalent, but an altitude of between 5000 and 8000 feet. This results in reduced barometric pressure and a decrease in partial pressure of oxygen (pO_2). This is known as *hypobaric hypoxia*. The primary cardiac response of the body to hypoxia is tachycardia, which results in increased myocardial oxygen demand that may result in symptoms requiring oxygen therapy. High-risk patient groups are shown in Box 14.2, for whom flying may be inadvisable.

Most patients with angina can travel safely as long as they remember their medications. Patients with recent uncomplicated percutaneous coronary interventions (PCI) are at low risk. Patients with a recent uncomplicated myocardial infarction should not fly until at least 2–3 weeks after the event, and they are back to usual daily activities. A symptom-limited treadmill test may be considered in some cases to estimate their ability to tolerate air travel. Patients with complicated infarcts or with poor exercise tolerance should wait until they are medically stable.

Coronary artery bypass grafting poses no intrinsic risk as long as the patient has fully recovered without complications. However, because air is transiently introduced into the chest cavity perioperatively, there is a risk of barotrauma when trapped gas expands at altitude. Consequently, patients should wait about 1–2 weeks before air travel.

Box 14.2 Contraindications to commercial flying.

Uncomplicated myocardial infarction within 2–3 weeks

Complicated myocardial infarction within 6 weeks

Unstable angina

Uncontrolled, severe chronic heart failure

Uncontrolled hypertension

Coronary artery bypass surgery within 2 weeks

Uncontrolled dysrhythmias

Severe symptomatic valvular heart disease

Box 14.3 Advice to cardiac patients flying in commercial airlines.

Ensure sufficient quantities of cardiac medications are kept in hand luggage

Keep a list of medications in case medications are lost

Adjust dosing intervals if crossing time zones

Carry a copy of the most recent ECG

Pacemaker (or defibrillator) patients should carry a pacemaker card

Contact the airline before travel if there are special needs (diet, wheelchair, etc.)

Consider the need for in-flight medical oxygen (CCS class III–IV angina or concomitant pulmonary disease)

CCS, Canadian Cardiovascular Society; ECG, electrocardiogram.

Specific travel recommendations for cardiovascular patients are shown in Box 14.3.

RETURN TO WORK

The importance of vocational assessment and counselling cannot be overestimated. For many individuals, return to work usually increases self-satisfaction, restores self-respect and relieves financial worries. Many consider return to work to be the goal of cardiac rehabilitation although, in the current employment climate, the use of return to work as a valid outcome of post-infarction rehabilitation is questionable. In addition, return to work can be influenced by demographic, clinical, psychosocial and workplace-related factors.

At about 6 weeks after acute myocardial infarction, the greater part of the affected heart muscle should be healed by the formation of a firm scar, and any collateral circulation should also be well developed. As a consequence, most patients should be ready to resume work, provided it is not physically or mentally too demanding. It is important that the myocardial infarction is not seen as an absolute deterrent to returning to work. Although exercise training improves functional capacity and reduces cardiorespiratory symptoms, it is usually factors unrelated to physical fitness that have a greater influence on when or if a patient returns to work. The rates of return to work for post-infarction patients are not as good as might be anticipated. Only about one-half to three-quarters of patients return to their former employment. Several factors influence the return to work, including:

- the severity of myocardial infarction;
- complications and symptoms (especially breathlessness and angina);
- advanced working age;
- stressful work environment;
- a sporadic work record before illness.

Discouragement by the family is a major cause of the patient not returning to work. This may be because of shared fear of further cardiac problems, although the possibility of early retirement and social security payments may sometimes create a disincentive to return. Ill-considered advice from the patient's medical advisor to 'lay off work and take things easy for a few months' will not help, and some employers seem to believe that coronary patients cannot, or should not, work at all.

Non-cardiac causes of invalidity are just as important as cardiac causes in failure to return to work. It is important, therefore, for rehabilitation staff to explore the physical and psychosocial dimensions of the job, the receptivity of the employer and other issues needed to promote a safe and timely return to work (Shrey & Mital, 2000). There is some evidence that a low-intensity cardiac rehabilitation programme that simulates elements of work results in better return to work rates (Mital et al, 2000).

The patients likely to do best are those given encouragement from the start of the illness, particularly from their family. The better a patient perceives their health to be, the more likely they are to return to work. A multidisciplinary approach is often required, involving the social worker, disability employment advisor and employer. Initially, the patient may be advised to return to work on a part-time basis, occasionally with lighter work. A few patients involved in heavy manual work may need to change their occupation, although this is not always acceptable or practical. When patients do return to work, their level of

activity may need to be closely monitored. Many manual workers continue to try to carry out heavy duties, which may be harmful. The patient may dispute this and feel fully capable or not wish to show weakness.

The daily workload of the female patient who is a housewife also needs careful consideration. She has often played a central role in home life and usually feels a tremendous responsibility to her family, both while she is in hospital and on her return home. Such patients often feel that the house has been neglected, shopping for essential items has been forgotten and the house has not been cleaned adequately. They worry about being unable to look after their family, including cleaning, shopping and cooking. The family will need careful counselling about the psychological stresses on such women and must provide both moral and physical support. Patients should not initially be left at home alone and will need help in performing the household chores, particularly physically taxing jobs such as making the beds and hanging out the washing. Careful consideration should be given to those individuals who live alone.

SICKNESS BENEFIT

Many patients and partners are anxious about how and when to claim sickness benefit. It is helpful to provide them with brief details. In the UK, sickness benefit is paid by the employer, providing that sufficient national insurance contributions have been paid during the relevant tax year. Sickness benefit will be paid for up to 28 weeks and, thereafter, an invalidity benefit may be paid. Supplementary benefit (for items such as the mortgage) may additionally be payable from the Department of Social Security. The old-age pension is payable at the age of 65 years for men and 60 years for women, the amount being dependent on the length of working life and the contributions paid.

QUALITY OF LIFE

Cardiac rehabilitation aims to prolong life, relieve symptoms and improve function in patients. Measurement of quality of life is important in evaluating the efficacy of cardiac interventions and treatments, including rehabilitation (Dempster & Donnelly, 2000). Despite the widespread use of the phrase, there is vagueness and little agreement as to the precise definition of quality of life, although health, defined as physical, mental and social well-being, is an important aspect. The assessment of physical outcomes alone is not sufficient and, as a consequence, assessment of well-being and health-related quality of life is considered to be important. There has been a rapid and significant growth in the measurement of quality of life as an indicator of health outcome. A number of measures have evolved that provide an assessment of the patient's experience of his or her health problems in areas such as physical function, emotional function, social function, role performance, pain and fatigue (Thompson & Roebuck, 2001).

AUDIT AND EVALUATION

UK national guidelines have been developed to ensure that cardiac rehabilitation is offered to all who are likely to benefit, based on an individual assessment of need, and followed by other options, including exercise, risk intervention and education and counselling (Thompson et al, 1997). It should be accompanied by audit and individual monitoring of progress (Mayou et al, 2002). The routine audit and evaluation of cardiac rehabilitation provision has generally been poor, in part because of the lack of common audit data. An audit tool was developed for use alongside the clinical guidelines for cardiac rehabilitation and has been included in the National Service Framework (Thompson et al, 1997).

The British Association of Cardiac Rehabilitation, the British Heart Foundation, the Healthcare Commission, the Central Cardiac Audit Dataset (CCAD) project, the Royal College of Physicians, the Department of Health Heart Team, the CHD Collaborative, clinicians and patients have worked together to develop a *National Audit of Cardiac Rehabilitation Project*. The audit consists of a minimum data set and a computer database.

The minimum data set collects all the NSF data and relevant medical, lifestyle and psychological data (anxiety, depression, quality of life). The patients complete most of the information themselves. The computer database is linked to the computers at CCAD, and the data automatically goes on to that system. It is then possible to see individual unit performance (no one else can) compared with the other rehabilitation programmes in the country in real time online.

At present, the CCAD database covers six clinical 'domains':

- *MINAP*: Myocardial Infarction National Audit Project (all patients admitted to UK hospitals with a suspected or actual heart attack);
- *BCIS*: British Cardiac Intervention Society (all patients in UK hospitals undergoing coronary angioplasty);
- *NPDB/ICD*: National Pacing/Implantable Cardiac Defibrillators DataBase (all patients in UK/Eire hospitals receiving implanted pacemakers/implantable cardiac defibrillators);
- *PAEDS*: Paediatrics (all children in UK hospitals undergoing surgery or catheter-based intervention for heart disease);
- *SCTS*: Society of CardioThoracic Surgeons (all adults in UK hospitals undergoing cardiac surgery);
- *EPS*: Cardiac ablation procedures (all patients in the UK receiving ablation treatment for arrhythmias).

A new data set for each clinical domain is collected when a patient undergoes an event or procedure and, eventually, the whole patient journey will be available online.

References

Ades PA (2001) Cardiac rehabilitation and secondary prevention of coronary heart disease. *New England Journal of Medicine* 345: 892–902.

Aerospace Medical Association Medical Guidelines Task Force (2003) Medical guidelines for airline travel. *Aviation, Space, and Environmental Medicine* 74: A1–A19.

American Association of Cardiovascular and Pulmonary Rehabilitation (2004) *Guidelines for Cardiac Rehabilitation and Secondary Prevention Programs*, 4th edn. Champaign, IL: Human Kinetics.

Arthur HM, Smith KM, Kodis J et al (2002) A controlled trial of hospital versus home-based exercise in cardiac patients. *Medicine & Science in Sports and Exercise* 34: 1544–1550.

Berkman LF, Blumenthal J, Burg M et al (2003) Effects of treating depression and low perceived social support on clinical events after myocardial infarction: the Enhancing Recovery in Coronary Heart Disease Patients (ENRICHD) randomized trial. *Journal of the American Medical Association* 289: 3106–3116.

Beswick AD, Rees K, Griebsch I et al (2004) Provision, uptake and cost of cardiac rehabilitation programmes: improving services to under-represented groups. *Health Technology Assessment* 8: 1–152.

Beswick AD, Rees K, West RR et al (2005) Improving uptake and adherence in cardiac rehabilitation: literature review. *Journal of Advanced Nursing* 49: 538–555.

Bethel HJ, Turner SC, Evans JA et al (2001) Cardiac rehabilitation in the United Kingdom. How complete is the provision? *Journal of Cardiopulmonary Rehabilitation* 21: 111–115.

Borg G (1998) *Borg's Perceived Exertion and Pain Scales*. Champaign, IL: Human Kinetics.

Brodie D, Bethell H, Breen S (2006) Cardiac rehabilitation in England: a detailed national survey. *European Journal of Cardiovascular Prevention and Rehabilitation* 13: 122–128.

Clark AM, Hartling L, Vandermeer B et al (2005) Meta-analysis: secondary prevention programs for patients with coronary artery disease. *Annals of Internal Medicine* 143: 659–672.

Dalal HM, Evans PH (2003) Achieving national service framework standards for cardiac rehabilitation and secondary prevention. *British Medical Journal* 326: 481–484.

Daly J, Sindone AP, Thompson DR et al (2002) Barriers to participation in and adherence to cardiac rehabilitation programs: a critical literature review. *Progress in Cardiovascular Nursing* 17: 8–17.

Davidson KW, Rieckmann N, Lesperance F (2004) Psychological theories of depression: potential application to the prevention of acute coronary syndrome recurrence. *Psychosomatic Medicine* 66: 165–173.

Demers C, McKelvie RS, Negassa A et al (2001) Reliability, validity and responsiveness of the six minute walk test in patients with heart failure. *American Heart Journal* 142: 698–703.

Dempster M, Donnelly M (2000) Measuring the health related quality of life of people with ischaemic heart disease. *Heart* 83: 641–644.

Department of Health (2000) *National Service Framework for Coronary Heart Disease*. London: The Stationery Office.

van Dixhoorn J, White A (2005) Relaxation therapy for rehabilitation and prevention in ischaemic heart disease: a systematic review and meta-analysis. *European Journal of Cardiovascular Prevention and Rehabilitation* 12: 193–202.

Friedman S (2000) Cardiac disease, anxiety, and sexual functioning. *American Journal of Cardiology* 86(suppl F): 46F–50F.

Glazer KM, Emery CF, Frid DJ et al (2002) Psychological predictors of adherence and outcomes among patients in cardiac rehabilitation. *Journal of Cardiopulmonary Rehabilitation* 22: 40–46.

Healthcare Commission (2005) *Getting to the Heart of it. Coronary Heart Disease in England: a Review of Progress towards the National Standards*. London: Healthcare Commission.

Jackson G, Rosen RC, Kloner RA et al (2006) The second Princeton consensus on sexual dysfunction and cardiac risk: new guidelines for sexual medicine. *Journal of Sexual Medicine* 3: 28–36.

Jolliffe JA, Rees K, Taylor RS et al (2006) *Exercise-based Rehabilitation for Coronary Heart Disease* (Cochrane Review). The Cochrane Library 2. Chichester: Wiley, pp. 1–44.

Lacey EA, Musgrave RJ, Freeman JV et al (2004) Psychological morbidity after myocardial infarction in an area of deprivation in the UK: evaluation of a self-help package. *European Journal of Cardiovascular Nursing* 3: 219–224.

Lau-Walker M (2004) Cardiac rehabilitation: the importance of patient expectations – a practitioner survey. *Journal of Clinical Nursing* 13: 177–184.

Lau-Walker M (2006) A conceptual care model for individualized care approach in cardiac rehabilitation – combining both illness representation and self-efficacy. *British Journal of Health Psychology* 11: 103–107.

Leon AS, Franklin BA, Costa F et al (2005) Cardiac rehabilitation and secondary prevention of coronary heart disease. *Circulation* 111: 369–376.

Lewin B, Robertson IH, Cay EL et al (1992) Effects of self-help post-myocardial-infarction rehabilitation on psychological adjustment and use of health services. *Lancet* 339: 1036–1040.

Lewin B, Cay EL, Todd I et al (1995) The angina management programme: a rehabilitation treatment. *British Journal of Cardiology* 2: 221–226.

Mark DB, Lauer MS (2003) Exercise capacity: the prognostic variable that doesn't get enough respect. *Circulation* 108: 1534–1536.

Martin CR, Thompson DR (2006) Depression in coronary heart disease patients: etiological and screening issues. *Current Psychiatry Reviews* 2: 245–254.

Mayou RA, Gill D, Thompson DR et al (2000) Depression and anxiety as predictors of outcome after myocardial infarction. *Psychosomatic Medicine* 62: 212–219.

Mayou RA, Thompson DR, Clements A et al (2002) Guideline-based early rehabilitation after myocardial infarction. A pragmatic randomized controlled trial. *Journal of Psychosomatic Research* 52: 89–95.

Miller WR, Rollnick S (2002) *Motivational Interviewing. Preparing People for Change*, 2nd edn. New York: Guilford.

Mital A, Shrey DE, Govindaraja M et al (2000) Accelerating the return to work (RTW) chances of coronary heart disease (CHD) patients. Part 1: Development and validation of a training programme. *Disability and Rehabilitation* 22: 604–620.

Mukherjee D, Fang J, Chetcuti S et al (2004) Impact of combination evidence-based medical therapy on mortality in patients with acute coronary syndromes. *Circulation* 109: 745–749.

Niebauer J, Hambrecht R, Velich T et al (1997) Attenuated progression of coronary artery disease after 6 years of multifactorial risk intervention: role of physical exercise. *Circulation* 96: 2534–2541.

Papadakis S, Oldridge NB, Coyle D et al (2005) Economic evaluation of cardiac rehabilitation: a systematic review. *European Journal of Cardiovascular Prevention and Rehabilitation* 12: 513–520.

Scott JT, Thompson DR (2003) Assessing the information needs of post-myocardial infarction patients: a systematic review. *Patient Education and Counselling* 50: 167–177.

Shrey DE, Mital A (2000) Accelerating the return to work (RTW) chances of coronary heart disease (CHD) patients. Part 2: Development and validation of a vocational rehabilitation programme. *Disability and Rehabilitation* 22: 621–626.

Smith KM, Arthur HM, McKelvie RS et al (2004) Differences in sustainability of exercise and health-related quality of life outcomes following home or hospital-based cardiac rehabilitation. *European Journal of Cardiovascular Prevention and Rehabilitation* 11: 313–319.

Sniehotta FF, Scholz U, Schwarzer R (2006) Action plans and coping plans for physical exercise: a longitudinal intervention study in cardiac rehabilitation. *British Journal of Health Psychology* 11: 23–37.

Stewart KJ, Turner KL, Bacher AC et al (2003) Are fitness, activity, and fatness associated with health related quality of life and mood in older persons? *Journal of Cardiopulmonary Rehabilitation* 23: 115–121.

Taylor HA Jr (1999) Sexual activity and the cardiovascular patient: guidelines. *American Journal of Cardiology* 84(5B): 6N–10N.

Taylor RS, Brown A, Ebrahim S et al (2004) Exercise-based rehabilitation for patients with coronary heart disease: systematic review and meta-analysis of randomized trials. *American Journal of Medicine* 116: 682–697.

Thompson DR (2002) Involvement of the partner in rehabilitation. In: Jobin J, Maltais F, Poirier P et al (eds) *Advancing the Frontiers of Cardiopulmonary Rehabilitation.* Champaign, IL: Human Kinetics.

Thompson DR, Lewin RJP (2000) Management of the post-myocardial infarction patient: rehabilitation and cardiac neurosis. *Heart* 84: 101–105.

Thompson DR, Oldridge N (2004) Secondary prevention and cardiac rehabilitation: have we got the terms right? *European Journal of Cardiovascular Prevention and Rehabilitation* 11: 183–184.

Thompson DR, Roebuck A (2001) The measurement of health-related quality of life in patients with coronary heart disease. *Journal of Cardiovascular Nursing* 16: 28–33.

Thompson DR, Bowman GS, de Bono DP et al (1997) *Cardiac Rehabilitation: Guidelines and Audit Standards.* London: Royal College of Physicians.

Tobin D, Thow MK (1999) The 10-m shuttle walk test with Holter monitoring: an objective outcome measure for cardiac rehabilitation. *Coronary Health Care* 3: 3–17.

Todaro JF, Shen BJ, Niaura R et al (2005) Prevalence of depressive disorders in men and women enrolled in cardiac rehabilitation. *Journal of Cardiopulmonary Rehabilitation* 25: 71–75.

Tuomilehto J, Lindström J, Eriksson JG et al (2001) Finnish Diabetes Prevention Study Group. Prevention of type 2 diabetes mellitus by change in lifestyle among subjects with impaired glucose tolerance. *New England Journal of Medicine* 344: 1343–1350.

World Health Organization (1993) *Needs and Action Priorities in Cardiac Rehabilitation and Secondary Prevention in Patients with Coronary Heart Disease.* Copenhagen: WHO Regional Office for Europe.

Zigmond AS, Snaith RP (1983) The hospital anxiety and depression scale. *Acta Psychiatrica Scandinavica* 67: 361–370.

Chapter 15

Assessing prognosis and reducing risk in patients with acute coronary syndromes

Approximately half of all cases of myocardial infarction and three-quarters of sudden cardiac deaths occur in patients already known to have cardiovascular disease (CVD). In the UK, there are about 1.3 million survivors of myocardial infarction who remain at increased risk of angina, another myocardial infarct or sudden death (Allender et al, 2006).

Episodes of unstable angina and reinfarction are most likely to occur in the early post-infarction period, and more than half the deaths occur within 3 months of the original myocardial infarction. The 12-month mortality for those leaving hospital is 10%, after which the annual mortality falls to 5%.

Women have twice the rate of mortality compared with men, and all diabetic patients have a poor prognosis. There is a strong relationship between age and prognosis that seems to be independent of the extent of coronary disease, and may be because the ageing myocardium is less able to withstand the effects of chronic ischaemia and cardiac damage. Even with thrombolysis, mortality is about 4% for patients under 55 years of age, but 25% for those over 75 years.

The results of various clinical trials support an intensified approach to secondary prevention and rehabilitation following an acute coronary syndrome. This usually involves a major change in the patient's lifestyle with specific drug treatments that will reduce any further adverse cardiac events. These lifestyle changes include stopping smoking, making healthier food choices and increasing aerobic exercise to increase physical fitness and reduce obesity. Unfortunately, modifying behaviour and lifelong habits is often a difficult and long-term process. Rehabilitation programmes need to be personalised, fostering changes that are relevant to the patient and allowing time for the patient to consider and reappraise the situation. Although the hospital setting provides an ideal environment for discussion and motivation towards a healthier way of life, educational opportunities are often constrained by the acute illness and rapid hospital discharge. Nevertheless, in-patient counselling provides an ideal foundation for patient and family education, while the severity of the illness is still in their minds.

ASSESSING PROGNOSIS FOLLOWING MYOCARDIAL INFARCTION

Risk stratification is a continuous process and should not be based upon a single assessment, as prognosis may change with various interventions. Overall, the most important determinants of prognosis seem to be:

- the extent of myocardial damage (and thus residual left ventricular function);
- the extent of coronary arterial disease (and thus how much residual myocardium is in jeopardy).

The extent of myocardial damage

The size of the myocardial infarction influences outcome, and loss of more than 40% of the left ventricular myocardium usually associates with cardiogenic shock and death. This may be the result of a single extensive infarct, or may accumulate with several episodes of myocardial infarction. Hence, a history of a previous myocardial infarction has a major adverse influence on outcome.

The degree of damage may be assessed clinically, electrocardiographically or by imaging techniques, such as echocardiography or myocardial scintigraphy. The prognosis is best in patients with left ventricular ejection fractions of 50% or more at rest. Those with ejection fractions of less than 35% are at greatest risk. Early indications of infarct size and, thus, risk may come from cardiac marker concentrations in the blood. Increasing troponin concentrations have been shown to correlate with outcome following an acute coronary syndrome (Antman et al, 1996).

The location of the infarct is also of prognostic importance. Mortality is lower with inferior, as opposed to anterior, infarction, even when estimates of infarct size are identical, and this may be because infarct extension, mural thrombus, left ventricular aneurysm and cardiac rupture are all more common with anterior myocardial infarction. Following thrombolysis, fatality at 28 days is 1.5 times greater with anterior compared with inferior infarctions (Lee et al, 1995).

Short-term prognosis is better with non-transmural, as opposed to full-thickness, infarcts, although non-transmural infarcts do not seem to have such a good outcome in the long term, probably because of residual myocardial ischaemia (de Wood et al, 1986). As reperfusional therapy is now usual, the degree of myocardial damage following acute coronary thrombosis is usually limited, and it is the extent of the underlying coronary disease that greatly affects outcome.

The extent of co-existing coronary arterial disease

Most patients who present with acute myocardial infarction have multivessel coronary disease and, if there is poor perfusion of the surviving myocardium following the infarct, not only will left ventricular function be impaired, but the surviving myocardium will also be placed in jeopardy from further coronary events. An initial clue to the presence of extensive coronary arterial disease is ST segment depression on the first electrocardiogram (ECG). Others patients likely to have prognostically important coronary disease include those with heart failure or previous myocardial infarction, the elderly and those with diabetes. Peri-infarction angina is a marker of extensive coronary artery disease and associates with a poor prognosis. It is often easy to recognise patients at high risk without exercise testing (Box 15.1), and these patients should undergo coronary angiography without any further assessment.

For all others, submaximal treadmill stress test can be performed before hospital discharge (70% predicted heart rate or a maximum of 120 beats/minute) to determine those needing angiography prior to discharge. Early stress testing following myocardial infarction is safe, provided there is no heart failure, hypotension, recurrent ventricular dysrhythmia or post-infarct angina. The response to exercise stress testing is of particular value in determining those at low risk who require less intensive evaluation and who are candidates for early rehabilitation and return to work (Bigi et al, 2003). If patients will be returning

Box 15.1   Factors associated with a poor prognosis following acute myocardial infarction.

Age over 60 years
Male sex
Poor left ventricular function (heart failure, hypotension)
Post-infarction angina
Cardiomegaly on the chest radiograph
Previous evidence of coronary heart disease
ECG:
- Persistent ST/T wave changes
- Ventricular ectopic activity
- Atrial fibrillation
- Conduction defects
- Left ventricular hypertrophy
Other co-existing diseases:
- Hypertension
- Diabetes

patients may be risk stratified at this time with a Bruce protocol exercise stress test as follows:

- *low risk*: able to exercise to stage III with < 1 mm ST depression;
- *moderate risk*: able to exercise to stage II or III, but with > 1 mm ST depression;
- *high risk*: unable to exercise beyond stage I with > 1 mm ST depression.

All high-risk and most moderate-risk patients will need coronary angiography to define coronary anatomy (Fig. 15.1).

Myocardial perfusion scintigraphy should be used in those in whom the baseline ECG makes exercise-induced changes difficult to interpret, as may occur with bundle branch block, left ventricular hypertrophy or in those taking digoxin. It may also be helpful in the 20% of patients who are unable to exercise on a treadmill and in younger women. Stress echocardiography is an alternative, but is labour-intensive and requires expertise.

to work in strenuous occupations, or will engage in strenuous leisure activities, a further symptom-limited stress test should be carried out at 4 weeks. Data from the Coronary Artery Surgery Study (CASS) registry (Weiner et al, 1995) suggests that

REDUCING GLOBAL RISK

European surveys show a high prevalence of ongoing adverse lifestyles and modifiable risk factors in patients known to have coronary artery disease

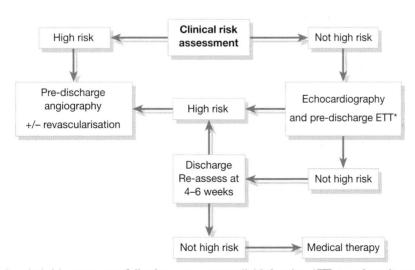

Figure 15.1   In-hospital risk assessment following acute myocardial infarction. *ETT, exercise tolerance test, stress echo or myocardial perfusion scan.

(EUROASPIRE I and II Groups, 2001). Risk factor status is worse in diabetic patients (Pyorala et al, 2004). Risk modification targets include:

- lifestyle changes;
- blood pressure control;
- modification of serum lipids;
- control of dysglycaemia;
- use of cardioprotective drugs [aspirin, beta-blockers, angiotensin-converting enzyme (ACE) inhibitors, etc.].

The therapeutic goals defined by the Joint British Societies (JBS-2, 2005) emphasise that individual cardiovascular risk factors should not be considered in isolation, and an integrated approach should be adopted to help prevent further major adverse cardiac events in patients who have recovered from an acute coronary syndrome. The use of statins, beta-blockers and ACE inhibitors is recommended for patients with symptomatic CVD, regardless of cholesterol or blood pressure levels. Some of these patients may already be below recommended target levels before treatment, and it may be more appropriate to recommend drug dosages rather than risk factor targets.

LIFESTYLE CHANGES

There is considerable scope for lifestyle modification in most patients following myocardial infarction. Two-thirds of patients with symptomatic atherosclerotic disease are overweight, half take little or no exercise, and most ingest large quantities of dietary fat. The major lifestyle targets are:

- stopping smoking;
- controlling body weight and avoiding central obesity;
- improving the diet;
- increasing aerobic physical activity.

For married couples, there is concordance for these modifiable risk factors, so encouraging the whole family rather than the individual to change is more likely to be effective.

Advice on diet

Apart from providing essential nutrients to the body, eating and drinking are pleasurable experiences, a fact that seems to be forgotten by many of those giving proscriptive advice. Misconceptions regarding diet clutter the popular press, compounded by conflicting and unsubstantiated information given by friends, relatives, advertising and even some health professionals. Dietary modifications often require major changes in the patient's normal eating habits, and it is important that factual information is presented objectively and consistently in a way that can be readily understood by the patient and his family. For most, it is better to emphasise an alteration in general eating habits, rather than the necessity of adhering to a specific 'diet sheet'. Patients are not going to change the habits of a lifetime based on a 10-minute chat with a doctor, nurse or dietician. Involvement of the patient's family is very important. Eating is usually a family or communal activity, and it is important to educate not only those who eat the food, but also those who buy and prepare it.

Population data confirm that a diet high in saturated fat, low in fruit and vegetables and high in salt associates with an increased risk of atherosclerotic disease (Kromhout et al, 2002). Accordingly, the Committee on Medical Aspects of Food Policy (COMA, 1994) recommend less fat in the diet (particularly saturated fat), at least five portions of fruit and vegetables per day, reduced salt and at least two portions of fish (one oily) each week (Table 15.1). Sugar should be avoided, and foods high in starch and fibre are to be encouraged. In general, individuals should eat a wide variety of foods and in the right amounts to prevent obesity.

In addition to these usual recommendations on diet, there is much interest in the health properties of so-called *functional foods*. These foods are believed to have positive benefits to overall health and an ability to reduce the risk of chronic diseases beyond their basic nutritional function. They include a large range of products, such as sterol-enriched spreads, fortified breads and cereals and substances that introduce and promote the growth of specific bacteria (probiotics and prebiotics). While some of these foodstuffs may have health benefits, functional foods are generally expensive and only play a small part in lifestyle changes. An exception to this may be plant sterols

Table 15.1   Dietary goals for a healthy population.

Food type	Total calories (%)
Total fat	Less than 30% (but more monounsaturated and polyunsaturated)
Carbohydrate	Over 50%
Protein	10–20%
Fibre	Over 35 mg/day
Cholesterol	Under 300 mg/day
At least five portions of fruit and vegetables per day	
Less salt (under 6 g/day)	
Less alcohol (21 units for men, 14 units for women per week)	
Two or more portions of fish each week (preferably oily)	

and stanols, which may help to control serum cholesterol.

Plant sterols and stanols (saturated plant sterols) are found naturally in a range of plant sources such as vegetable oils, nuts, grains and seeds. They have a chemical structure similar to cholesterol, but differing side chains mean they are minimally absorbed from the gut. Intake of 2 g/day will achieve reductions in total serum cholesterol of 5–10%, and could be expected to reduce the risk of coronary disease by 25% if maintained for more than 2 years (Law, 2000). Unfortunately, the typical daily intake ranges from 160 to 400 mg/day, which is thought to have little effect on cholesterol absorption, and even strict vegetarians will only consume between 600 and 800 mg of plant sterols/stanols each day.

Esterification of natural plant sterols/stanols (by the attachment of a fatty acid) has increased their solubility in fat and has now allowed them to be incorporated into spreading fats and other fat-based products such as mayonnaise. In the UK, these are marketed under the names *Benecol* and *Flora proactive* in various food products including margarine, yoghurt and cereal bars. While these products are not very powerful in their ability to reduce blood fats, any reduction in blood cholesterol will be additional to that achieved by diet and lipid-lowering drugs. Foods containing high levels of plant-derived sterol/stanol esters should be considered as an additional option for risk reduction in adults with coronary heart disease (CHD) (Cater, 2000).

Weight control

The most important goal of dietary modification is to achieve and maintain normal body weight, with specific reduction in abdominal obesity. Being overweight [body mass index (BMI) of more than 25 kg/m^2] is associated with elevated plasma lipids, glucose intolerance and hypertension. Weight loss reduces triglyceride concentrations, blood pressure, insulin levels and increased high-density lipoprotein (HDL) cholesterol concentrations (James et al, 2000).

The factors leading to excess body fat exist on many levels, which may reflect societal and cultural attitudes towards food, economic factors (such as the cost of different food) but, most importantly, individual choice. Body weight is essentially controlled by food intake, but long-established western dietary habits are hard to break. We generally eat and drink more than is good for us, particularly saturated fats, simple sugars and alcohol. As each kilogram of fat equates to about 7500 calories, a weight loss of 1 kg/week means that either calorie intake needs to be reduced by at least 1000 calories/day or a combination of reduced intake and increased energy expenditure is needed. Attending 'Weight Watchers' or other slimming clubs may be helpful, but it will be more difficult to influence the individual if other family members and those counselling the patient are overweight. A mutually agreed goal for weight reduction should be established and a record kept, such as a graph that gives a quick visual indication of how the patient is progressing. Weight loss of around 0.5 kg/week is a realistic objective until target weight is achieved. Practical advice should include an explanation of calorific intake vs. expenditure, the regular and slow eating of smaller amounts of food and the participation in regular physical activity. The ultimate goal is to achieve a body weight appropriate for age, height and sex (Fig. 15.2). The potential health benefits of

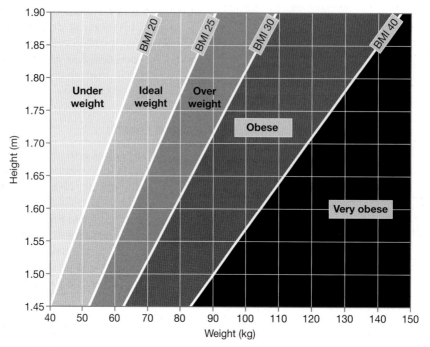

Figure 15.2 Desirable body weights based on body mass index.

a 10% body weight reduction for secondary prevention have been summarised by Jung (1997) as shown in Box 15.2.

Making a direct relationship between BMI and associated health hazards is probably too simplistic, and the regional distribution of body fat is well recognised as a very important consideration. Abdominal obesity is a better predictor of type 2 diabetes and CVD, although the point at which abdominal circumference begins to confer risk is not the same in all groups and is age, sex and race dependent (IDF, 2005; see Table 15.2). Epidemiologically, it is better to use ethnic origin rather than country of residence.

The simple assessment of waist circumference is quicker and easier than other more complex assessments of obesity, such as BMI, waist/hip ratio (WHR) and skin fold thickness, although the WHR is the best for assessing risk (Yusuf et al, 2005). Simple advice on controlling the waistline may prove a very useful strategy for reducing cardiovascular risk (Lamarche, 1998). In general, waist measurement for Caucasians should not exceed 102 cm in men and 88 cm for women (JBS-2, 2005).

Box 15.2 Potential health benefits of a 10% body weight reduction.

Mortality
- 20–25% reduction in total mortality
- 40–50% fall in obesity-related cancer deaths

Lipids
- 10% reduction in total cholesterol
- 15% reduction in LDL cholesterol
- 30% reduction in triglycerides
- 8% increase in HDL cholesterol

Blood pressure
- 10-mmHg reduction in systolic and diastolic blood pressures

Glucose tolerance
- Over 50% reduction in the risk of developing diabetes
- Fasting blood glucose reduced by 30–50%
- HbA1c reduced by 15%

Table 15.2 Abdominal circumference as a risk factor for type 2 diabetes and cardiovascular disease by race and sex.

	Europeans/ Africans	South Asians/ Chinese	Japanese
Men	> 94 cm	> 90 cm	> 85 cm
Women	> 80 cm	> 80 cm	> 90 cm

While sedentary living associates with increased abdominal fat deposition, dietary factors may also be important, and higher intakes of protein and fibre are associated with reduced central adiposity.

Exercise, drugs and surgery

Obesity is usually managed within primary care with advice on weight control, diet, physical exercise and lifestyle. Powerful and complex biological factors are involved in the long-term regulation of body weight, making it difficult for individuals to maintain weight loss, so other interventions such as drug therapy, referral to specialist weight loss clinics, behavioural therapy and low-calorie and very-low-calorie diets may be considered. Even patients with a BMI as low as 23 kg/m^2 and a WHR of 0.95 may benefit from anti-obesity treatments if this helps to reduce their abdominal adiposity.

Dieting alone is largely ineffective in maintaining any initial weight loss, with most individuals regaining their original weight within 3–5 years. Regular exercise has been shown to be one of the best interventions for successful weight maintenance, and cardiovascular morbidity and mortality are reduced, even without weight loss. It is better to be fat and active than thin and inactive (Press et al, 2003).

Prescribing exercise rather than issuing a simple instruction to 'diet' is likely to be the key to ensuring long-term weight loss and improved health (McInnis, 2000). For many obese people, their excessive weight is a disincentive to physical activity (Swinburn & Egger, 2004). Their reduced levels of activity tend to promote further weight gain associated with arthritis, low back pain and shortness of breath. Consequently, overweight and obese people are less likely to take opportunities to become active. Supportive exercise, such as swimming pool-based activities, can overcome some of their mechanical problems. For others, physical activity that can be incorporated into everyday life (brisk walking, cycling to work) will improve the chances of success. Physical activity tends to become easier with time, thereby promoting a virtuous cycle in which physical activity increases further. In addition, those people who persist with regular physical activity are more likely to maintain their weight loss. The greatest health gains are achieved in previously sedentary individuals.

On its own, increased physical activity results in only modest changes in weight (0.5–1 kg reduction each month), but regular physical activity has important effects on the distribution of body fat away from abdominal adiposity, and thus removes one of the features of the metabolic syndrome. The *metabolic syndrome* is a proinflammatory and prothrombotic condition associated with abdominal obesity and insulin resistance. Affected individuals have impaired glucose tolerance, hypertension, dyslipidaemia and an excess cardiovascular risk above and beyond the contribution of the individual risk factors (Zarich, 2005). Reducing the waist circumference favourably influences the adverse risk profile of the metabolic syndrome, reducing the risk of CHD and of type 2 diabetes.

Drug therapy

Combining exercise with behavioural therapy or drug treatment appears to help in maintaining weight loss rather than diet alone, but weight gain is frequent on cessation of therapy (Despres, 2001).

Sibutramine promotes a sense of satiety through its central action as a serotonin and noradrenaline reuptake inhibitor. There is often an elevation in blood pressure that may be counterproductive in terms of global risk. It is not licensed for continuous use for more than 1 year.

Orlistat inhibits pancreatic and gastric lipase, thereby decreasing fat absorption. Some of the weight loss probably results from individuals reducing their fat intake to avoid severe gastrointestinal effects, including steatorrhoea. Fat-soluble vitamin supplementation (especially of vitamin D) should be considered. The drug is licensed for 2 years of continuous therapy.

Randomised controlled trials of orlistat and sibutramine suggest that approximately 60% of patients will achieve and maintain a 5% loss from their starting weight after 12 months of treatment, and 40% of patients will experience a 10% weight loss. The National Institute for Health and Clinical Excellence has provided guidance for the use of orlistat and sibutramine (NICE, 2001, 2002a).

Rimonabant is the first in a new class of anti-obesity drug, which targets cannabinoid receptors in adipose tissue, the gut and skeletal muscle. The RIO-Europe study showed that rimonabant had beneficial effects on waist circumference, HDL cholesterol, triglycerides, insulin resistance and the prevalence of the metabolic syndrome (Van Gaal et al, 2005). Some of these improvements are independent of weight loss.

Surgical treatment of obesity

Surgery to aid weight reduction (bariatric surgery) may be considered when all other measures have failed, but is not commonly undertaken, with perhaps only 200–300 such operations carried out in the UK every year, mostly outside the NHS. Surgical techniques are usually reserved for those with a BMI ≥ 40 in the presence of significant co-morbidity. There are two main types of surgical intervention:

- malabsorptive surgery (e.g. jejuno-ileal, gastric bypass) limits absorption of food by surgically bypassing large amounts of the gut;
- restrictive surgery (e.g. gastroplasty and gastric banding) reduces the size of the stomach, so the patient feels full with less food.

Bypass operations are more successful in terms of weight loss, but have more complications, some of which may be serious.

NICE (2002b) has recommended surgery as a treatment option for people with morbid obesity provided that they meet all the following criteria:

- They are aged 18 years or over.
- They have been receiving treatment in a specialist obesity clinic at a hospital.

- They have tried all other appropriate non-surgical treatments to lose weight but have not been able to lose weight or maintain weight loss.
- There are no specific medical or psychological reasons why they should not have this type of surgery.
- They are generally fit enough to have an anaesthetic and surgery.
- They should understand that they will need to be followed up by a doctor and other healthcare professionals such as dieticians or psychologists over the long term.

Postoperatively, patients should receive dietary and, where appropriate, psychological advice to help them to modify their eating habits to promote weight loss and to prevent complications such as nutrition imbalance, vomiting, dumping syndrome and diarrhoea.

EXERCISE

Modern lifestyles are associated with reduced energy expenditure; in recent years, the number of cars has doubled while levels of walking and cycling have fallen by 26%. Currently, only one-third of men and a quarter of women achieve the recommended target of 30 minutes of physical activity five times a week.

Exercise training programmes aid recovery from myocardial infarction, although these need not be of very high intensity (Worcester et al, 1993). Approximately 30 minutes of moderate aerobic exercise on alternate days, or 20 minutes daily, is sufficient, although this should be related to individual capacity. For those with physical impairment, light physical activities, such as walking, gardening and swimming, are beneficial too. Men who become inactive following myocardial infarction have the highest all-cause and cardiovascular mortality (Wannamethee et al, 1998). A meta-analysis of cardiac rehabilitation trials based on exercise showed a 20% reduction in all-cause mortality and a 26% reduction in cardiac mortality (Taylor et al, 2004). Physical fitness is also psychologically beneficial, and exercise favourably influences lipid profiles, glucose tolerance, fibrinolytic activity and blood pressure, as well as helping to combat obesity (Box 15.3).

DYSLIPIDAEMIA

There is a strong, positive, graded relationship between serum cholesterol and death from CHD (Neaton & Wentworth, 1992), and a raised low-density lipoprotein (LDL) cholesterol and low HDL cholesterol continue to be risk factors for recurrent cardiac events after acute myocardial infarction. The evidence for reducing cholesterol, particularly LDL cholesterol, in patients with CHD is exceptionally strong, and has been demonstrated in many clinical trials using diet, drugs and surgery. The greater the reduction in LDL cholesterol, and the longer the duration of treatment, the greater was the reduction in coronary events (Law et al, 2003).

The most compelling evidence to support cholesterol reduction has come from large clinical trials using 3-hydroxy-3-methylglutaryl co-enzyme A (HMGCoA) reductase inhibitors (statins). These trials have demonstrated unequivocally that reducing the serum cholesterol with statin therapy reduces cardiovascular morbidity and mortality in patients either with or without established CHD (Cholesterol Treatment Trialists' Collaboration, 2005). These benefits are independent of gender and other treatments such as aspirin or antihypertensive agents. The efficacy and safety of intensive LDL cholesterol reduction to levels well below 2.6 mmol/L was shown in the TNT study (La Rosa et al, 2005), and a quantitative relationship between reduced LDL cholesterol levels and reduced CVD remains true even at these very low levels of LDL cholesterol.

Lipid assessment

Blood lipid concentrations should be measured in all patients with atherosclerotic disease at first contact and then at least annually thereafter. It must be remembered that, after an acute vascular event, such as an acute coronary syndrome or stroke, total cholesterol, LDL cholesterol and HDL cholesterol concentrations fall, and triglycerides may rise. These induced changes may last up to 8 weeks, and obtaining a full profile too early may give misleading results. While a random total cholesterol and HDL cholesterol on admission to hospital will give a reasonable guide to baseline concentrations, a full fasting lipoprotein profile should be obtained at about 8–12 weeks following the acute event, even though most patients will already be taking a statin. At this time, a full profile may be helpful to:

- exclude a familial dyslipidaemia;
- ensure attainment of total and LDL cholesterol targets;
- give clues to a secondary hyperlipidaemia.

It is often helpful to measure baseline creatine phosphokinase (CK) and liver function tests before starting treatment with a statin, as some people may have high values that are physiological, not pathological. If the CK and liver function are normal, repeating these tests is not indicated unless the person develops related symptoms. In asymptomatic individuals, a threefold transaminase rise or even a 5- to 10-fold rise in CK of the upper limit of normal level may be acceptable for those on statin therapy.

Treatment targets

For people with established CVD, the total cholesterol and LDL cholesterol targets are under 4.0 mmol/L and under 2.0 mmol/L respectively.

Alternatively, there should be a 25% reduction in total cholesterol and a 30% reduction in LDL cholesterol, whichever results in the lowest absolute level (JBS-2, 2005). This is important for those patients who have a cholesterol concentration already below target when first seen.

Treatment of dyslipidaemia

The main dietary influence on plasma cholesterol levels is ingestion of saturated fats rather than eating cholesterol. The average daily British diet contains only about 500 mg of cholesterol, and reducing this to the recommended level of less than 300 mg/day will have only a small effect on the serum cholesterol. The general dietary recommendations shown in Table 15.1 are appropriate, but will probably only reduce the total serum cholesterol by 5–10%, and few will achieve currently recommended target cholesterol concentrations with diet alone (Jowett & Galton, 1987). In the past, it has been normal practice when treating hypercholesterolaemia to start with dietary advice and then consider lipid-lowering therapy some months after an acute vascular event. However, evidence supports the view that statin therapy should be started early (in hospital), regardless of the initial cholesterol level. This aids compliance with treatment and helps to reduce the risk of further cardiovascular events (Schwartz et al, 2001; Cannon et al, 2004).

The statins are first-line drugs for reducing total and LDL cholesterol, although they also raise HDL cholesterol and lower triglycerides to some extent (NICE, 2006). There seems to be increased efficacy of statins if taken in the evening, as most cholesterol synthesis takes place when dietary intake is at its lowest. The newer synthetic statins (atorvastatin, rosuvastatin) have longer half-lives and may be taken at any time of the day. Other lipid-lowering drugs will be needed if there is intolerance of all statins, or plasma lipids remain abnormal despite optimal statin therapy.

Fibrates are effective in controlling hypertriglyceridaemia and in raising HDL cholesterol, but vary in their ability to reduce LDL cholesterol. Cardiovascular trials using fibrates have found a reduction in the risk of major coronary events, but no reduction in total mortality (Birjmohun et al, 2005) so, while filtrates are more suitable for patients with both raised cholesterol and triglycerides, statins should still be used first and will be effective in most cases. There have been no large randomised clinical trials with statin–fibrate combinations to demonstrate benefit. Gemfibrozil should not be used in combination with a statin, and other combinations should be used only following specialist advice. Monitoring of CK and liver function tests is important with combination therapy.

There may be a particular role for fibrates in patients with the metabolic syndrome who have low HDL cholesterol and hypertriglyceridaemia, where lifestyle interventions (particularly weight reduction and increased exercise) have not raised HDL cholesterol concentrations to over 1 mmol/L (UK HDL-C Consensus Group, 2004). However, the FIELD trial (Keech et al, 2005), the largest cardiovascular prevention trial using fibrates in type 2 diabetes, did not give conclusive results supporting benefit in at-risk patients, and did not provide evidence on efficacy or long-term safety when co-prescribed with statins (Jowett, 2006).

SMOKING

Smoking is a complex addiction with strong dependence. It exerts its addictive influence by satisfying a physical need, providing stimulation and pleasure as well as relieving anxiety and tension. Smoking is the most important risk factor for first and subsequent heart attacks, and even passive smoking increases this risk by as much as 20% (Doll & Peto, 1976; Law et al, 1997).

Stopping smoking after myocardial infarction is associated with a substantial reduction in major adverse cardiovascular events and death in both the long and the short term (Wilhelmsen, 1998), and reduces death from other causes too (Critchley & Capewell, 2003). Observational studies suggest that, for every 1000 patients who stop smoking, there will be 15 deaths and 46 reinfarctions prevented. A 20% reduction in the number of cigarette smokers could result in 8000 fewer deaths in the UK every year.

Surveys show that about 70% of smokers say they want to stop, but only a minority succeed.

One in five patients will continue to smoke following an acute coronary syndrome (Campbell et al, 1998), and fewer than half give up smoking as a result of suffering an acute myocardial infarction (Reimer et al, 2005). Others will try, and many will need support. Only 2–3% of those who try by themselves will still be abstinent 1 year later (Royal College of Physicians, 2000). On the other hand, brief, opportunistic advice from the medical profession can prompt attempts to stop in up to 40% of patients and can increase 1-year abstinence rates by 2.5% (Silagy & Stead, 2001).

Advice on smoking should start on the coronary care unit, and non-smokers are more credible role models. Like all rehabilitation advice, its value depends heavily upon an informed, committed and uniform approach. Similar education of the patient's family is equally important, and giving such information in coronary care reinforces the importance of such advice. Current smokers substantially underestimate their excess risk over non-smokers, and more than half believe myths such as that exercise can reverse the ill-effects of smoking. They usually believe that their risk of lung cancer is lower than that of other smokers, and anyway that cure is usual (Weinstein et al, 2005).

Withdrawal-oriented therapy is the predominant form of treatment used within the UK's smoking cessation clinics, with the aim of complete cessation of smoking. Cutting down is not the answer, nor is switching to low-tar cigarettes, cigars or a pipe, because the smoking pattern will change to extract the same amount of nicotine from weaker or fewer cigarettes by automatically puffing harder (Woodward & Tunstall-Pedoe, 1993). With this come other harmful constituents of tobacco smoke including carbon monoxide, thiocyanates and tar. For many smokers, particularly heavy smokers, nicotine addiction is a major factor in the persistence of the habit and the high relapse rate on attempts to stop.

Treatment at smoking cessation clinics focuses on preventing early relapse in smokers and assists them through the first 4 weeks when withdrawal symptoms are strongest (Table 15.3). The benefits of smoking cessation include improved health and finances, improvement of the senses of taste and smell and a greater physical attraction when freed from the smell of smoke, and these should

Table 15.3 Tobacco withdrawal symptoms.

In first 2 weeks	In first 4 weeks	In first 12 weeks
Difficulty concentrating	Depression	Increased appetite/weight
Sleep disturbance	Irritability	Bradycardia
	Restlessness	
	Mouth ulcers	
	Constipation	

be stressed. Many smokers advance the excuse that they will put on weight if they stop smoking. This is not an inevitable consequence, and a weight gain of 10–15 kg would be required to nullify the benefits of stopping smoking.

Nicotine replacement therapy doubles sustained cessation rates and can achieve success rates of about 10% in a medical care setting provided the smoker is sufficiently motivated (McRobbie & Hajek, 2001). Although particular caution is advised in the peri-infarction period, it seems unlikely that the effects of nicotine replacement could be any worse than a return to smoking. There are currently six different nicotine replacement products available in the UK, comprising transdermal nicotine patches, four oral products (gum, lozenge, sublingual tablet and inhalator) and a nasal spray. Products differ in their strength, speed of absorption, ease of use and ability of dose titration. None can compete with the speed or dose delivered by smoking, but nicotine replacement therapy does reduce the severity of withdrawal symptoms. All these products are available on prescription or can be purchased in pharmacies.

Other smoking cessation interventions (e.g. acupuncture, hypnotherapy) have not been shown to be of benefit in most cases, but the antidepressant bupropion (Zyban) is an effective aid to smoking cessation (Jorenby et al, 1999), and may double the chance of long-term abstinence when combined with behavioural support.

Varenicline is a partial nicotine receptor agonist in development. It is not addictive, and may reduce symptoms of withdrawal, making quitting easier.

Rimonabant is a selective cannabinoid receptor antagonist that has been shown to help in smoking cessation. In addition, it helps to reduce body weight (particularly from the waist), and also reduces insulin resistance, blood glucose and triglycerides. It may thus become an ideal treatment for smokers with cardiac disease.

HYPERTENSION

While hypertension remains the most important treatable risk factor for the prevention of stroke, the most common cause of death in patients with hypertension is myocardial infarction. Nearly a quarter of patients with hypertension have a past history of CHD, and a raised blood pressure continues to be a risk factor for subsequent cardiovascular events in patients following acute myocardial infarction.

In patients with established CVD, diabetes or renal failure, optimal blood pressure goals are for a systolic blood pressure of < 130 mmHg and diastolic blood pressure of < 80 mmHg. Most people will require at least two blood pressure-lowering drugs to achieve this (Williams et al, 2004). Non-pharmacological intervention is helpful regardless of the need for medication, including advice on exercise and weight reduction with dietary restriction of salt and alcohol. Vegetarian diets and foods high in potassium may also help to reduce blood pressure.

If drug therapy is required, it must be made clear that it is usually permanent. Patients should not just complete the 'course' of tablets, and doses may also need titration to achieve target blood pressure reductions. In the ASPIRE trial (Bowker et al, 1996), when the blood pressure was measured in patients 6 months after myocardial infarction, 56% of patients still had blood pressures > 140/85 mmHg.

Many classes of drugs are available for treatment, and debate continues regarding whether the benefits of treatment are purely a function of the quality of blood pressure control or whether the type of drug used might also be a powerful determinant of outcome. Overviews suggest that the main benefits from antihypertensive therapy are derived from blood pressure lowering, and that the various drug classes are about as effective

as each other in reducing cardiovascular morbidity and mortality for the same reduction in blood pressure (Blood Pressure Lowering Treatment Trialists' Collaboration, 2003).

The ASCOT trial results (Dahlof et al, 2005) may have weakened the role of beta-blockers in the management of uncomplicated hypertension, but indications for patients with established cardiac disease remain the same. In people with raised blood pressure and symptomatic angina, a beta-blocker is the preferred treatment choice, although calcium channel blockers may also be effective in improving symptoms of angina and reducing the risk of myocardial infarction (Pepine et al, 2003). For those who have suffered a myocardial infarction, beta-blockers and ACE inhibitors (or angiotensin II receptor blockers) will already have been prescribed for cardioprotection, and doses should be optimised. If the blood pressure remains off target, diuretics are the next logical choice. Amlodipine and felodipine may then be added, but verapamil and diltiazem should be avoided if there is evidence of left ventricular dysfunction (Turnbull, 2003).

Whether ACE inhibitors are of particular value in those with CHD (but without left ventricular dysfunction) above and beyond that of blood pressure reduction remains debatable (ALLHAT Collaborative Research Group, 2002; EUROPA, 2003).

DYSGLYCAEMIA

Dysglycaemia is a qualitative term used to describe blood glucose that is abnormal, without defining a threshold. The term reflects uncertainty about optimal blood glucose ranges given that cardiovascular risk and mortality risk exist in people with even slightly elevated blood glucose levels. The response to an oral glucose tolerance test (OGTT) is often used to categorise individuals into four main groups:

1 normal glucose tolerance;
2 impaired fasting glycaemia (IFG);
3 impaired glucose tolerance (IGT);
4 diabetes mellitus.

The OGTT is of course very inconvenient, time-consuming and expensive, but it is still required for the accurate diagnosis of diabetes and impaired glucose regulation. Clinically, it is easier to measure a random glucose followed, where necessary, by a fasting blood glucose to detect dysglycaemia. This approach will detect most, though not all, cases.

IGT is associated with an increased risk of death, particularly from atherosclerotic disease, and patients with IFG or IGT may worsen to develop type 2 diabetes. This progression can be prevented or postponed by lifestyle intervention, particularly weight control (Tuomilehto et al, 2001).

A fasting glucose should be measured on at least one occasion in patients presenting with an acute coronary syndrome or any other vascular disease. Where there is a suggestion of impaired fasting levels (6.0–7.0 mmol/L) or of diabetes (over 7.0 mmol/L), the measurement should be repeated at least twice more in the convalescent period, usually with a formal OGTT at 8–12 weeks following discharge from hospital. If diabetes is excluded, a fasting glucose should be checked annually.

In patients with dysglycaemia, both beta-blockers and diuretics should be used with care, as there is an increased risk of precipitating diabetes.

STRESS

Stress (including type A behaviour) may be reduced in patients undergoing regular counselling, at least in the short term, which may reduce cardiovascular mortality (Friedman et al, 1986). Some would suggest that counselling should be a routine component of post-infarction rehabilitation for all patients (Lloyd, 1991). Polyphasic activities during everyday life (e.g. watching television, eating and reading simultaneously) must be avoided. The role of frequent, moderate exercise is often underplayed. Jogging, for example, is ideal for reducing muscular tension and giving the patient an opportunity for privacy and self-appraisal while running. The risk of developing persistent psychological disturbance is greater for those patients who were psychiatrically ill before their myocardial infarction. Drug therapy needs careful consideration in view of the frequent cardiovascular side effects of antidepressant medication. Serotonin uptake inhibitors (SSRIs) are safer than traditional tricyclic drugs.

CARDIOPROTECTIVE DRUG THERAPY

In addition to medication that may be needed to control cardiovascular symptoms and reach blood pressure, lipid and glucose targets, there are several cardioprotective drugs that may be needed to reduce morbidity and mortality.

Aspirin

Administration of aspirin to patients with coronary disease acutely and long term greatly reduces subsequent vascular events and death (Anti-thrombotic Trialists' Collaboration, 2002). There is an absolute reduction of 12 deaths for every 1000 patients treated over a 15-month period. The beneficial dose of aspirin is unknown, but is probably in the range of 75–325 mg daily. Higher doses (500–1500 mg daily) are no more effective and are associated with gastrotoxicity. Treatment is recommended for life.

Clopidogrel should be substituted where aspirin is contraindicated (CAPRIE Steering Group, 1996), and the addition of clopidogrel to aspirin for patients with unstable acute coronary syndromes for 12 months protects against further additional cardiovascular events (CURE Trial Investigators, 2001).

Beta-blockers

Beta-blockers are used extensively in patients with coronary disease to control blood pressure and angina and, more recently, in the treatment of cardiac failure. Beta-blockers are considered to be cardioprotective, although most evidence arises from trials in the prethrombolytic era. Timolol, metoprolol or propranolol reduces the risk of sudden death, non-fatal reinfarction and all-cause mortality by 20–30% (Yusuf et al, 1985), and it seems that reduction in heart rate is an important factor, as those with intrinsic sympathomimetic activity (e.g. pindolol and oxprenolol) do not confer benefit. A meta-analysis of beta-blockade use following myocardial infarction confirms a significant reduction in all-cause mortality, cardiovascular death (especially sudden death) and reinfarction (Freemantle et al, 1999). Patients at highest risk benefit most from beta-blockade, particularly the elderly (> 60 years), diabetics, those with large and anterior infarcts and those with heart failure. These patients are often denied beta-blocker therapy. Beta-blockers reduce all-cause mortality in people with heart failure caused by ischaemic heart disease (Heidenreich et al, 1997).

Treatment should be started when the patient is haemodynamically stable, and continued for at least 2–3 years if tolerated (Freemantle et al, 1999). Most physicians would continue the drug indefinitely unless there were problems.

Use of beta-blockers following myocardial infarction remains suboptimal because of perceived rather than actual side effects. There is no significantly increased risk of depression and only small increases in the risks of fatigue and sexual dysfunction in patients taking beta-blockers (Ko et al, 2002). In addition, beta-blockers have little effect on the peripheral circulation in most patients with peripheral vascular disease. Importantly, beta-blockers do not produce major adverse respiratory effects, even in patients with mild to moderate obstructive airway disease. A study of 46 000 survivors of myocardial infarction with asthma and chronic obstructive pulmonary disease reported a 40% reduction in total mortality in patients treated with beta-blockers, including benefits for patients aged over 80 years and those with heart failure.

Calcium antagonists

In general, these agents have not been shown to have any benefit following myocardial infarction and, in patients with heart failure, their use may be hazardous. Verapamil and diltiazem slow the pulse, and have been used where beta-blockers are contraindicated.

Verapamil reduces the reinfarction rate in patients with good left ventricular function (DAVIT II, 1990), and diltiazem helps to prevent reinfarction in the 6 months following non-transmural myocardial infarction (Gibson et al, 1986), although late reinfarction rates are similar to those treated with placebo.

ACE inhibitors

The benefits of ACE inhibitors in unselected patients following acute myocardial infarction have been confirmed in a large meta-analysis of over 100 000 patients (ACE Inhibitor Myocardial Infarction Collaborative Group, 1998). ACE inhibition not only reduces the risk of death, but also helps to prevent progression of left ventricular dysfunction and recurrent myocardial infarction. A greater reduction effect is seen in those patients with asymptomatic left ventricular dysfunction or overt heart failure. The Heart Outcomes Prevention Evaluation (HOPE) (2000) and EUROPA (2003) studies support the indefinite use of ACE inhibitors to reduce the risk of myocardial infarction and cardiovascular mortality in high-risk people, even in the absence of left ventricular dysfunction or uncontrolled blood pressure. However, the PEACE trial (2004) in patients with stable coronary disease and normal left ventricular function found that there were no additional benefit in terms of death from cardiovascular causes, myocardial infarction or coronary revascularisation from adding in trandolapril to usual therapy. This is probably explained by the fact that the PEACE trial patients were at lower risk because other interventions were in place (Pitt, 2004). For example, only 29% of the HOPE patients were on a statin, and many had low ejection fractions.

ACE inhibitors should always be used for the treatment of symptomatic or asymptomatic left ventricular dysfunction. In patients with stable coronary disease, where secondary interventions are in place, the addition of an ACE inhibitor is likely only to make a marginal further reduction in overall risk and cannot therefore be considered cost effective in most cases. The exception to this is in those with diabetes, in whom ACE inhibitors have multiple actions that improve both cardiovascular and non-cardiovascular outcomes.

Angiotensin II receptor blockers (ARBs) are recommended for heart failure when patients are intolerant of ACE inhibitors (Demers et al, 2005). Trials comparing ACE inhibitors and ARBs in chronic heart failure (as opposed to post-myocardial left ventricular dysfunction) suggest that ARBs are as effective in reducing mortality as the ACE inhibitors, but no trial has yet shown superiority.

The doses of ACE inhibitors currently prescribed in the UK are significantly lower than those shown to improve survival, and there is no evidence that lower doses are of prognostic benefit. Larger doses are not associated with increased toxicity, and asymptomatic hypotension or a modest creatinine change should not prevent titration to target dose:

- captopril 50 mg tid;
- enalapril 20 mg bd;
- ramipril 5 mg bd;
- lisinopril 40 mg od;
- trandolapril 4 mg od;
- perindopril 8 mg od.

The dosage schedule as shown above is necessary to cover the full 24-hour period because, if the renin–angiotensin system kicks in during the early morning, the diseased left ventricle will not be able to cope with the extra burden and fails (early morning heart failure).

ANTICOAGULANTS

Studies of anticoagulant treatment after myocardial infarction indicate reduction in death, recurrent infarction and thromboembolic complications, but there is no major difference between aspirin and warfarin, and no benefit from using both. Warfarin is indicated for those who are aspirin intolerant and for those at high risk of cardiac thromboembolism (e.g. large left ventricle, ventricular aneurysm, atrial fibrillation). The suggested target international normalised ratio (INR) is 2.5.

The incidence of left ventricular thrombus is now much lower than previously because of routine treatment with heparin, thrombolysis and ACE inhibitors that attenuate ventricular dilatation and aneurysm formation. High-risk patients can be identified by predischarge echocardiography, and those with large anterior dyskinetic areas should receive warfarin. The SOLVD and SAVE trials (Pfeffer et al, 1992) showed the benefits of long-term anticoagulation in those with ejection fractions under 35% (Wiegers & St John Sutton, 2000).

Risk/benefits must be assessed and discussed with the patient. In some patients, particularly the elderly, the risks of bleeding, compliance and poor anticoagulant control may make warfarin dangerous.

Benefits of secondary prevention

The relative benefits of treatment following acute myocardial infarctions are shown in Table 15.4. Despite the clear benefits of secondary prevention, many patients in Europe remain on inadequate therapy (Table 15.5). The ASPIRE study demonstrated failure to achieve targets in those recently discharged from hospital (Bowker et al, 1996). At 6-month review following a coronary event:

- 27% of patients were still smoking;
- 75% were still overweight;
- 25% were still hypertensive;
- 75% had a cholesterol over 5.2 mmol/L;
- 20% were not taking aspirin;
- 66% were not taking a beta-blocker.

Supervision and follow-up often fail because of breakdown in the link between primary and secondary care, and there is considerable scope for risk factor clinics and nurse-led intervention (Brady et al, 2001). Interventional targets are shown in Box 15.4.

Table 15.4 Relative benefits of secondary intervention following myocardial infarction.

Treatment	Events prevented per 1000 treated
Aspirin	16 deaths/myocardial infarcts/strokes
Stopping smoking	27 deaths
Beta-blockers	13 deaths 5 myocardial infarctions
Reducing cholesterol by 10%	7 deaths/myocardial infarcts
ACE inhibitors	12 deaths 9 myocardial infarcts 16 cases of heart failure

Table 15.5 Percentage of patients receiving adequate therapy for secondary prevention in Europe.

Study[a]	Where/when	Percentage of patients treated			
		Aspirin	Statin	B-blocker	ACE inhibitor
ASPIRE	UK, 1994	86	16	36	18
EUROASPIRE I	Europe, 1995	81	32	54	30
HEALTHWISE	UK, 1997–98	50	16	21	13
PRAIS-UK	UK, 1998	78	44	41	–
PREVENIRE	France, 1998	90	52	68	42
EUROASPIRE II	Europe, 1999	84	63	66	43

a References: Bowker et al (1996), Collinson et al (2000), EUROASPIRE I and II Groups (2001), Marques-Vidal et al (2001).

Box 15.4 Medical interventions for all patients following an acute coronary syndrome.

Lifestyle targets

Advice on smoking cessation and the use of nicotine replacement therapy
Advice on weight control, diet, alcohol and exercise

- Maintain ideal body weight (BMI 20–25 kg/m^2) and avoid central obesity
- Maintain total dietary intake of fat at < 30% of total energy intake
- Saturated fats to < 10% of total fat intake
- Cholesterol intake < 300 mg/day
- Increased intake of monounsaturated fats to replace saturated fats
- Increase the intake of fresh fruit and vegetables (> five portions/day)
- Regular intake of fish and other sources of omega-3 fatty acids (> two servings of fish/week)
- Alcohol intake < 21 units/week for men and < 14 units/week for women
- Limit the intake of salt to < 100 mmol/L day

Regular aerobic physical activity (> 30 min/day on most days)

Drug therapy

Treat blood pressure to target of under 140/85 mmHg (especially with beta-blockers/ACE inhibitors)
Aspirin (and/or clopidogrel)
Statin therapy to reduce total cholesterol concentrations EITHER to < 4 mmol/L (LDL-C to below 2 mmol/L) OR a 25% reduction in total cholesterol and a 30% reduction in LDL-C, whichever gets the person
    to the lowest level
ACE inhibitors
Beta-blockade
Warfarin or aspirin for those in atrial fibrillation
Meticulous blood pressure and glycaemic control in those with diabetes (HbA1c < 6.5%;
    blood pressure < 130/80 mmHg)

SURGICAL THERAPY

The role of cardiac surgery and other reperfusional strategies following myocardial infarction is discussed in Chapter 16. Both coronary by pass surgery (CABG) and percutaneous coronary intervention (PCI) are widely utilised to relieve symptoms and prolong survival following myocardial infarction. In the absence of diabetes, the benefits are now almost identical among patients with multivessel disease assigned to PCI vs. those assigned to CABG, although additional intervention is two to four times more likely in those initially treated by PCI (Bourassa, 2000).

Motivating lifestyle change

Health-threatening behaviours are the commonest cause of premature and recurrent CVD in the western world. Motivating behavioural change to reduce cardiovascular risk is challenging unless it is precisely defined and the patient acknowledges the existence of a problem. Simply informing people that they are at risk of worsening disease is rarely sufficient to change behaviour. This will usually only occur when the individual believes that it is both of value and achievable.

The role of the health professional is to clarify the potential problems with the patient, and then use interventions such as motivational interviewing or behaviour change counselling techniques (Rollnick et al, 1993). Motivational interviewing is a directive, patient-centred counselling style to affect behaviour change by helping the patient to explore and resolve ambivalence towards adverse behaviours, including smoking, long-term dietary change to reduce weight and improve lipid profile and increasing exercise to a therapeutic level. By setting realistic, achievable goals and offering support to reinforce and progress the changes, benefits can be achieved and maintained. Reflective listening and using open questions will allow the patient to determine their own goals rather than being expected to pursue unachievable targets.

Guidelines present an oversimplified view of lifestyle change. Maintaining change is not easy, and a successful outcome often requires multiple attempts. Intervention with appropriate medication for those at high risk of CVD may be inevitable, but these cannot be independent of intensive lifestyle modification.

References

ACE Inhibitor Myocardial Infarction Collaborative Group (1998) Indications for ACE inhibitors in the early treatment of acute myocardial infarction: systematic overview of individual data from 100,000 patients in randomised trials. *Circulation* 97: 2202–2212.

Allender S, Peto V, Scarborough P et al (2006) *Coronary Heart Disease Statistics*. London: British Heart Foundation Statistics database. www.heartstats.org.

ALLHAT Collaborative Research Group (2002) Major outcomes in high-risk hypertensive patients randomized to angiotensin-converting enzyme inhibitor or calcium channel blocker vs. diuretic: the antihypertensive and lipid lowering treatment to prevent heart attack trial (ALLHAT). *Journal of the American Medical Association* 288: 2981–2997.

Anti-thrombotic Trialists' Collaboration (2002) Collaborative meta-analysis of randomised trials of anti-platelet therapy for prevention of death, myocardial infarction, and stroke in high risk patients. *British Medical Journal* 324: 71–86.

Antman EM, Tanasijevic MJ, Thompson B et al (1996) Cardiac specific troponin I levels to predict the risk of mortality in patients with acute coronary syndromes. *New England Journal of Medicine* 335: 1342–1349.

Bigi R, Cortigiani L, Desideri A (2003) Exercise electrocardiography after acute coronary syndromes: still the first testing modality? *Clinical Cardiology* 26: 390–395.

Birjmohun RS, Hutten BA, Kastelein JJP et al (2005) Efficacy and safety of high-density lipoprotein cholesterol increasing compounds. A meta-analysis of randomized controlled trials. *Journal of the American College of Cardiology* 45: 185–197.

Blood Pressure Lowering Treatment Trialists' Collaboration (2003) Effects of different blood-pressure-lowering regimens on major cardiovascular events: results of prospectively designed overviews of randomised trials. *Lancet* 362: 1527–1545.

Bourassa MG (2000) Clinical trials of coronary revascularisation: coronary angioplasty versus coronary bypass grafting. *Current Opinions in Cardiology* 15: 281–286.

Bowker TJ, Clayton TC, Ingham J (1996) A British Cardiac Society survey of potential for the secondary prevention of coronary disease ASPIRE (Action on Secondary Prevention through Intervention to Reduce Events). *Heart* 4: 334–342.

Brady AJB, Oliver MA, Pittard JB (2001) Secondary prevention in 24,431 patients with coronary heart disease. Survey in primary care. *British Medical Journal* 322: 1463.

Campbell NC, Thain J, Deans HG et al (1998) Secondary prevention in coronary heart disease: baseline survey of provision in general practice. *British Medical Journal* 316: 1430–1434.

Cannon CP, Braunwald E, McCabe CH for the Pravastatin or Atorvastatin Evaluation and Infection Therapy – Thrombolysis In Myocardial Infarction 22 Investigators (2004) Intensive versus moderate lipid lowering with statins after acute coronary syndromes (PROVE-IT). *New England Journal of Medicine* 350: 494–504.

CAPRIE Steering Group (1996) A randomised blinded trial of clopidogrel versus aspirin in patients at risk of ischaemic events (CAPRIE). *Lancet* 348: 1329–1339.

Cater NB (2000) Plant stanol ester: review of cholesterol-lowering efficacy and implications for coronary heart disease risk reduction. *Preventive Cardiology* 3: 121–130.

Cholesterol Treatment Trialists' Collaboration (2005) Efficacy and safety of cholesterol-lowering treatment: prospective meta-analysis of data from 90,056 participants in 14 randomised trials of statins. *Lancet* 366: 1267–1278.

Collinson J, Flather M, Fox KA et al (2000) Clinical outcomes, risk stratification and practice patterns of unstable angina and myocardial infarction without ST elevation: Prospective Registry of Acute Ischaemic Syndromes in the UK (PRAIS-UK). *European Heart Journal* 21: 1450–1457.

COMA (1994) *Diet and Risk*. Report of the Committee on Medical Aspects of Food Policy, Department of Health. London: HMSO.

Critchley JA, Capewell S (2003) Mortality risk reduction associated with smoking cessation in patients with coronary heart disease: a systematic review. *Journal of the American Medical Association* 290: 86–97.

CURE Trial Investigators (2001) Effects of clopidogrel in addition to aspirin inpatients with acute coronary syndromes without ST-segment elevation. *New England Journal of Medicine* 345: 494–502.

Dahlof B, Severs PS, Poulter NR et al (2005) Prevention of cardiovascular events with an anti-hypertensive regimen of amlodipine adding perindopril as required versus atenolol adding bendroflumethaside as required in the Anglo-Scandinavian Cardiac Outcomes Trial blood pressure lowering arm (ASCOT-BPLA). *Lancet*, 366: 895–906.

DAVIT II (1990) The Danish Study Group on Verapamil in Myocardial Infarction. Effect of verapamil on mortality and major events after acute myocardial infarction. *American Journal of Cardiology* 66: 779.

Demers C, McMurray JJV, Swedberg K for the CHARM Investigators (2005) Impact of candesartan on nonfatal myocardial infarction and cardiovascular death in patients with heart failure. *Journal of the American Medical Association* 294: 1794–1798.

Despres J-P (2001) Drug treatment for obesity. *British Medical Journal* 322: 1379–1380.

Doll R, Peto R (1976) Mortality in relation to smoking: 20 years' observations on male British doctors. *British Medical Journal* ii: 1525–1536.

EUROASPIRE I and II Groups (2001) Clinical reality of coronary prevention guidelines. A comparison of EUROASPIRE I and II in nine countries. *Lancet* 357: 995–1001.

EUROPA (2003) Efficacy of perindopril in reduction of cardiovascular events among people with stable coronary artery disease: randomized, double blind, placebo-controlled trial (the EUROPA study). *Lancet* 362: 782–788.

Freemantle N, Cleland J, Young P et al (1999) Beta-blockade after myocardial infarction: systematic review and meta-regression analysis. *British Medical Journal* 318: 1730–1737.

Friedman M, Thorensen CE, Gill JJ (1986) Alteration of type A behavior and its effect on cardiac recurrences in post-myocardial infarct patients: summary results in the Recurrent Coronary Prevention Project. *American Heart Journal* 112: 653–665.

Gibson R S, Boden W E, Theroux P et al (1986) Diltiazem and re-infarction in patients with non-Q-wave myocardial infarction. *New England Journal of Medicine* 315: 423–429.

Heart Outcomes Prevention Evaluation Study (HOPE) Investigators (2000) Effects of angiotensin-converting-enzyme inhibitor, ramipril, on cardiovascular events in high-risk patients. *New England Journal of Medicine* 342: 145–153.

Heidenreich PA, Lee TT, Massie BM (1997) Effect of beta-blockade on mortality in people with heart failure: a meta-analysis of randomized clinical trials. *Journal of the American College of Cardiology* 30: 27–34.

IDF (2005) Consensus worldwide definition of the metabolic syndrome. www.idf.org/webdata/docs/ DF_Metasyndrome_definition.pdf.

James WPT, Astrup A, Finer H et al (2000) Effect of sibutramine on weight maintenance after weight loss: a randomised trial. *Lancet* 356: 119–125.

JBS-2 (2005) Joint British Societies' guidelines on prevention of cardiovascular disease in clinical practice. Prepared by: British Cardiac Society, British Hypertension Society, Diabetes UK, HEART UK, Primary Care Cardiovascular Society, The Stroke Association. *Heart* 91: 1–52.

Jorenby DE, Leischow SJ, Nides MA et al (1999) A controlled trial of sustained-release bupropion, a nicotine patch, or both for smoking cessation. *New England Journal of Medicine* 340: 685–691.

Jowett NI (2006) Use of fibrates in diabetes: what does the FIELD trial tell us? *Practical Diabetes International* 23: 135–137.

Jowett NI, Galton DJ (1987) The management of the hyper-lipidaemias. In: Hamer J (ed.) *Drugs for Heart Disease*, 2nd edn. London: Chapman and Hall.

Jung RT (1997) Obesity as a disease. *British Medical Bulletin* 53: 307–321.

Keech A, Simes RJ, Barter P and the FIELD study investigators (2005) Effects of long-term fenofibrate therapy on cardiovascular events in 9795 people with type 2 diabetes mellitus (the FIELD study): randomised controlled trial. *Lancet* 366: 1849–1861.

Ko DT, Hebert PR, Coffey CS et al (2002) Beta-blocker therapy and symptoms of depression, fatigue, and sexual dysfunction. *Journal of the American Medical Association* 288: 351–357.

Kromhout D, Menotti A, Blackburn H (2002) *Prevention of Coronary Heart Disease. Diet, Lifestyle and Risk Factors in the Seven Countries Study.* Dordrecht: Kluwer Academic Publishers.

Lamarche B (1998) Abdominal obesity and its metabolic complications: implications for the risk of ischaemic heart disease. *Coronary Artery Disease* 9: 473–481.

La Rosa, JC, Grundy, SM, Waters, DD for the TNT Investigators (2005) Intensive lipid lowering with atorvastatin in patients with stable coronary disease. *New England Journal of Medicine* 352: 2389–2397.

Law MR (2000) Plant sterol and stanol margarines and health. *British Medical Journal* 320: 861–864.

Law MR, Morris JK, Wald N (1997) Environmental tobacco smoke exposure and ischaemic heart disease: an evaluation of the evidence. *British Medical Journal* 315: 937–980.

Law MR, Wald NJ, Rudnicka AR (2003) Quantifying effect of statins on low-density lipoprotein cholesterol, ischaemic heart disease, and stroke: systematic review and meta-analysis. *British Medical Journal* 326: 1423–1429.

Lee KL, Woodlieff LH, Topol EJ et al (1995) Predictors of 30-day mortality in the era of reperfusion for acute myocardial infarction. Results from an International trial of 41,021 patients. *Circulation* 91: 1659–1668.

Lloyd GG (1991) Myocardial infarction and the mind. *Hospital Update* 12: 943–944.

McInnis KJ (2000) Exercise and obesity. *Coronary Artery Disease* 11: 111–116.

McRobbie H, Hajek P (2001) Nicotine replacement therapy in patients with cardiovascular disease: guidelines for health professionals. *Addiction* 96: 1547–1551.

Marques-Vidal P, Cambou JP, Ferrieres J et al (2001) Distribution and treatment of cardiovascular risk factors in coronary patients: the PREVENIR study. *Archives des Maladies du Coeur et des Vaisseaux* 94: 673–680.

Neaton JD, Wentworth D (1992) Serum cholesterol, blood pressure, cigarette smoking and death from coronary heart disease. Overall findings and differences by age for 316,099 white men. Multiple Risk Factor Intervention Trial (MRFIT) Research Group. *Archives of Internal Medicine* 152: 56–64.

NICE (2001) *Guidance on the Use of Orlistat for the Treatment of Obesity in Adults.* Technology appraisal no. 22. London: NICE. www.nice.org.uk.

NICE (2002a) *Guidance on the Use of Sibutramine for the Treatment of Obesity in Adults.* Technology appraisal no. 31. London: NICE. www.nice.org.uk.

NICE (2002b) *Guidance on the Use of Surgery to aid Weight Reduction for People with Morbid Obesity.* Technology appraisal no. 46. London: NICE. www.nice.org.uk.

NICE (2006) *Statins for the Prevention of Cardiovascular Events.* Technology appraisal no. 94. London: NICE. www.nice.org.uk.

PEACE Trial Investigators (2004) Angiotensin-converting-enzyme inhibition in stable coronary artery disease. *New England Journal of Medicine* 351: 2058–2068.

Pepine CJ, Handberg EM, Cooper-DeHoff RM for the INVEST investigators (2003) A calcium antagonist vs a non-calcium antagonist hypertension treatment strategy for patients with coronary artery disease: the international verapamil-trandolapril study (INVEST): a randomized controlled trial. *Journal of the American Medical Association* 290: 2805–2816.

Pfeffer MA, Braunwald E, Moyle LA et al (1992) Effect of captopril on mortality and morbidity in patients with left ventricular dysfunction after myocardial infarction: results of the survival and ventricular enlargement trial (SAVE). *New England Journal of Medicine* 327: 669–677.

Pitt B (2004) Ace inhibitors for patients with vascular disease without left ventricular dysfunction – may they rest in PEACE. *New England Journal of Medicine* 351: 2115–2117.

Press V, Freestone I, George CF (2003) Physical activity: the evidence of benefit in the prevention of coronary heart disease. *Quarterly Journal of Medicine* 96: 245–251.

Pyorala K, Lehto S, De Bacquer D et al for the EUROASPIRE I Group and the EUROASPIRE II Group (2004) Risk factor management in diabetic and non-diabetic patients with coronary heart disease. Findings from the EUROASPIRE I and II surveys. *Diabetologia* 47: 1257–1265.

Reimer WS, Swart E, De Bacquer D et al for the EUROASPIRE Investigators (2005) Smoking behaviour in European patients with established coronary heart disease. *European Heart Journal* 27: 35–41.

Rollnick S, Kinnersley P, Stott N (1993) Methods of helping patients with behaviour change. *British Medical Journal* 307: 188–190.

Royal College of Physicians (2000) *Nicotine Addiction in Britain.* A report of the tobacco advisory group of the Royal College of Physicians. London: Royal College of Physicians.

Schwartz GG, Olsson AG, Ezekowitz MD et al (2001) Effects of atorvastatin on early recurrent ischemic events in acute coronary syndromes. The MIRACL study: a randomized controlled trial. *Journal of the American Medical Association* 285: 1711–1718.

Silagy C, Stead LF (2001) Physician advice for smoking cessation. In: *Tobacco Addiction Module of Cochrane Database of Systematic Reviews.* Cochrane Library Issue 1. Oxford: Update Software.

Swinburn B, Egger G (2004) The runaway weight gain train: too many accelerators, not enough brakes. *British Medical Journal* 329: 736–739.

Taylor RS, Brown A, Ebrahim S et al (2004) Exercise-based rehabilitation for people with coronary heart disease: systematic review and meta-analysis of randomized controlled trials. *American Journal of Medicine* 116: 682–692.

Tuomilehto J, Lindstrom J, Eriksson JG for the Finnish Diabetes Prevention Study Group (2001) Prevention of type 2 diabetes mellitus by changes in lifestyle among subjects with impaired glucose tolerance. *New England Journal of Medicine* 344: 1343–1350.

Turnbull F (2003) Blood pressure lowering treatment trialists' collaboration. Effects of different blood pressure lowering regimens on major cardiovascular events: results of prospective designed overviews of randomized trials. *Lancet* 362: 1527–1535.

UK HDL-C Consensus Group (2004) Role of fibrates in reducing coronary risk: a UK consensus. *Current Medical Research and Opinion* 20: 241–247.

Van Gaal LF, Rissanen AM, Scheen AJ et al (2005) Effects of the cannabinoid-1 receptor blocker rimonabant on weight reduction and cardiovascular risk factors in overweight patients: 1-year experience from the RIO-Europe study. *Lancet* 365: 1389–1397.

Wannamethee SG, Shaper AG, Walker M (1998) Changes in physical activity, mortality and incidence of coronary heart disease in older men. *Lancet* 351: 1603–1608.

Weiner DA, Ryan TJ, Parsons L et al (1995) Long-term prognostic value of exercise testing in men and women from the Coronary Artery Surgery Study (CASS) registry. *American Journal of Cardiology* 75: 865–870.

Weinstein ND, Marcus SE, Moser RP (2005) Smokers' unrealistic optimism about their risk. *Tobacco Control* 14: 55–59.

Wiegers SE, St John Sutton M (2000) When should ACE inhibitors or warfarin be discontinued after myocardial infarction? *Heart* 84: 361–362.

Wilhelmsen L (1998) Effects of cessation of smoking after myocardial infarction. *Journal of Cardiovascular Risk* 5: 173–176.

Williams B, Poulter NR, Brown MJ (2004) Guidelines for management of hypertension: report of the fourth working party of the British Hypertension Society, 2004 – BHS IV. *Journal of Human Hypertension* 18: 139–185.

de Wood M, Stifter WF, Simpson CS et al (1986) Coronary angiographic findings soon after non-Q-wave myocardial infarction. *New England Journal of Medicine* 315: 412–422.

Woodward M, Tunstall-Pedoe H (1993) Self-titration of nicotine: evidence from the Scottish Heart Health Study. *Addiction* 88: 821–830.

Worcester MC, Hare DL, Oliver RG et al (1993) Early programmes of high and low intensity exercise and quality of life after acute myocardial infarction. *British Medical Journal* 307: 1244–1247.

Yusuf S, Peto R, Lewis J et al (1985) Beta-blockade during and after myocardial infarction: an overview of randomised trials. *Progress in Cardiovascular Diseases* 27: 335–371.

Yusuf S, Hawken S, Ôunpuu S on behalf of the INTER-HEART Study Investigators (2005) Obesity and the risk of myocardial infarction in 27000 participants from 52 countries: a case-control study. *Lancet* 366: 1640–49.

Zarich SW (2005) Cardiovascular risk factors in the metabolic syndrome: impact of insulin resistance on lipids, hypertension, and the development of diabetes and cardiac events. *Reviews in Cardiovascular Medicine* 6: 194–205.

Chapter 16

Percutaneous coronary intervention and cardiac surgery in patients with coronary artery disease

Coronary artery bypass grafting (CABG) and percutaneous transluminal coronary angioplasty (PTCA) are well-established methods of myocardial revascularisation that are used to alleviate symptoms and improve prognosis. Percutaneous coronary intervention (PCI) is now the modern term used to describe a group of techniques including PTCA, coronary stenting and athero-ablation. Other novel approaches to revascularisation, such as transmyocardial laser revascularisation and angiogenesis with growth factors and cell transplantation, may prove useful in the future (Mukherjee, 2004; Goldberg et al, 2005). The number of coronary artery bypass operations has increased sixfold in the UK since 1980, and the number of percutaneous coronary interventions has increased at an even faster rate, with the current ratio of PCI to CABG procedures being about 3:1. Both treatments have hazards as well as benefits, and revascularisation is only part of a multi-interventional strategy that includes risk factor modification, adjunctive drug therapy and rehabilitation.

WHAT IS THE BEST METHOD OF REVASCULARISATION?

Evidence supporting the best method of revascularisation is limited, because the major randomised trials were carried out before the routine use of arterial grafts and improved medical therapy (Opie et al, 2006). Reocclusion following PTCA has also become less frequent since the introduction of new antithrombotic agents and the routine deployment of coronary arterial stents.

PCI has obvious clinical and financial advantages over bypass surgery, as it is performed under local anaesthesia and allows early discharge from hospital. However, it has important limitations, including the likelihood of restenosis and the potential for incomplete revascularisation compared with surgery. Trials comparing CABG with PCI in patients with multivessel disease have shown similar outcomes in terms of morbidity and mortality, although repeat revascularisation procedures are required more often in those undergoing PCI (Stables, 2002). Conventional coronary artery bypass surgery enables a more thorough revascularisation with longlasting symptom relief and need for reintervention, probably because, while PCI usually addresses culprit lesions, CABG bypasses both culprit and future culprit lesions (Gersh & Frye, 2005). As such, CABG is particularly suited to those with left main stem coronary disease and those with three-vessel disease (Taggart, 2005), whereas patients with single-vessel disease (excluding the left main stem) do not benefit prognostically from CABG (Hannan et al, 2005). Diabetic patients with multivessel disease do not do so well with percutaneous intervention, with a twofold increase in 5-year mortality compared with those who undergo bypass grafting (Niles et al, 2001). For most other patient groups, there is usually little difference between CABG and PCI in terms of symptom relief (Bourassa, 2000). However, patients undergoing PCI do not get an arterial graft to the left anterior descending coronary artery, an intervention that improves both symptoms and survival, with freedom from infarction and angina for over 10 years (Cameron et al, 1996).

PERCUTANEOUS CORONARY INTERVENTION

Grüntzig first described a procedure for dilating coronary arteries in 1977, and PTCA quickly became an established and effective way of treating many serious arterial stenoses around the body (Grüntzig, 1984). Simple balloon angioplasty of occluded coronary arteries became prevalent until 1987, when adjunctive atherectomy and laser-assisted angioplasty were introduced. Provided there was no immediate complication (especially acute vessel closure), results from PTCA were very good, with patency of coronary arteries continuing to improve in the early weeks due to healing and remodelling. However, vessel wall recoil, neointimal proliferation and early thrombus formation each contributed towards restenosis and affected up to 50% of procedures. Recoil of the artery was common, either when the balloon was deflated or within the first 24 hours. About 3–7% of cases needed emergency coronary artery bypass surgery, and a further 3–5% of patients sustained a myocardial infarction. Since 1993, improvements in technique and the widespread use of intracoronary stents have helped to prevent acute vessel recoil and minimise the vessel wall trauma that leads to late negative remodelling of the coronary artery. In the

UK, stent usage rose steeply between 1993 and 1999, from below 10% to nearly 80% of procedures, and the British Cardiovascular Intervention Society (BCIS) audit figures for 2004 indicate that stents are now being used in 93% of PCI procedures. Immediate complications such as acute myocardial infarction and the need for emergency CABG have been reduced to less than 1% (Yang et al, 2005).

Stents

Coronary artery stents are small mesh cylinders cut by laser from stainless steel or cobalt–chrome alloy tubes into a variety of designs, each with different radial strength and flexibility. They are chemically etched or electropolished to a fine finish and sometimes coated. According to design, they may offer differing flexibility, strength, trackability and reduced risks of in-stent stenosis.

Following balloon angioplasty, improvement in coronary patency is produced by a combination of plaque splitting, plaque compression and stretching of the arterial media, sometimes leading to coronary artery dissection. Using a stent helps to increase the vessel lumen diameter, prevents acute elastic recoil and seals any dissection by tagging the intimal flap between the stent and the arterial wall. Most stents are self-expanding, but others require a balloon to ensure full stent expansion and better apposition of the stent around the circumference of the vessel.

While stent deployment successfully addressed the problem of abrupt vessel closure, it soon became clear that perfectly deployed stents were becoming occluded later by a proliferative tissue response to the vessel wall injury – in-stent stenosis (ISS). This seemed to be more frequent where long stenoses had been tackled, and particularly where the post-procedural luminal diameter was small. Although ISS rates initially affected 10–20% of patients, with increasingly complex lesions now being attempted (total occlusions, saphenous vein bypass grafts, small vessels, etc.), ISS rates may be well over 50% (Bennett, 2003). Late stenosis (weeks–months) is caused by many factors, such as organisation of thrombus, cell proliferation, matrix synthesis and remodelling. Sudden occlusion can occur at 4 weeks after deployment of bare metal stents caused by platelet aggregation (subacute thrombosis) but, after this time, new endothelial cells cover the stent and thrombosis is rare. Adequate antiplatelet therapy is essential during and after stent implantation. The next critical period is up to 6 months when the dilated segment heals. After this period, the artery usually remains patent for very long periods.

Until recently, the only effective treatment for ISS was *vascular brachytherapy* (Kandzari & Mark, 2002), and strontium-90/yttrium and phosphorus-32 radionuclides have both been used following in-stent angioplasty to deliver radiation at 2 mm inside the vessel wall to reduce in-stent recurrence. Although effective, this has not been widely applied for logistical reasons, such as the presence of a radiopharmacy and the ability to comply with statutory radiation regulations. In contrast, *drug-eluting stents* have been shown to be of major value in the prevention and treatment of ISS. Sirolimus (rapamycin) is one of several agents that have powerful antimitotic and anti-inflammatory effects that inhibit new tissue growth inside the stent. The first drug-eluting stent was the sirolimus-coated *Cypher* stent, which remains very popular and effective. The *Taxus* paclitaxel-eluting stent is also in common use now, and numerous other types are under development. The decision to utilise a bare metal stent or a drug-eluting stent is usually based on the anatomy of the target vessel and individual patient factors (NICE, 2003). Drug-eluting stents are of particular value where the internal diameter of the target artery is less than 3 mm or the lesion is longer than 15 mm, and in patients with diabetes. Overall, there is a very significant reduction in restenosis (and cardiac events) in patients who receive drug-eluting rather than bare metal stents, and possibly a higher efficacy with sirolimus-eluting stents (Roiron et al, 2006). Oral rapamycin taken for 14 days after bare metal stent implantation significantly reduces angiographic and clinical parameters of restenosis.

Despite drug-eluting stents costing three times more than bare metal stents, the need for repeat procedures is halved. By reducing the incidence of restenosis (and therefore recurrent symptoms), antiproliferative stents will probably alter the balance of treating coronary artery disease in favour of percutaneous intervention rather than coronary artery bypass surgery in many cases. There is still underuse of drug-eluting stents in the UK because of cost.

Biodegradable stents such as the Japanese Igaki–Tamai stent are being investigated. These are made of poly-L-lactic acid that takes 18–24 months to biodegrade. The scaffolding prevents abrupt vessel closure in the acute phase, but then disappears, taking away the stimulus for occlusion.

Indications for PCI

The relative advantages and disadvantages of surgery and PCI continue to change as improvements in both surgical and medical treatments evolve. Some indications for PCI are shown in Box 16.1. Twenty years ago, a typical PTCA procedure treated one proximally located lesion in a young patient with good left ventricular function. Now, patients may have two- or even three-vessel disease, perhaps with multiple complex lesions, impaired left ventricular function, advanced age and co-morbidities. Even the left main stem coronary artery, a target always considered to be exclusively surgical, is sometimes being tackled (McGowan et al, 2005).

Major complications of PCI are uncommon but include death (0.2%), acute myocardial infarction (1%), embolic stroke (0.5%), cardiac tamponade (0.5%) and systemic bleeding (0.5%). Minor complications are more common and include allergy and nephropathy (from the contrast medium) and complications of the access site (bleeding, haematoma and pseudo-aneurysm). Anxiety and depression are not uncommon before and after PCI, and it is important to identify those at risk of sustained psychological distress (Astin et al, 2005).

Box 16.1 Some clinical indications for percutaneous coronary intervention (PCI).

Stable angina with single- or two-vessel disease
Primary angioplasty following acute myocardial infarction
Rescue PCI for failed thrombolysis
Cardiogenic shock
Post-infarction angina
Graft occlusion following bypass surgery
Unstable coronary syndromes

The procedure

Most operators undertake angioplasty and stenting via the femoral artery using small catheters of 6 or 7 French diameter or less, although the radial artery approach has become increasingly popular as it allows earlier hospital discharge.

A sedative is sometimes given before the procedure, as well as aspirin, clopidogrel and the patient's usual anti-anginal drugs. In high-risk cases, an intra-aortic balloon pump or a prophylactic temporary transvenous pacemaker may be required. Using fluoroscopy, a soft-tipped, steerable guidewire is passed up into the ascending aorta. The proximal end of the catheter is attached to a Y connector to allow continuous monitoring of arterial blood pressure, which can indicate reduced coronary flow because of overengagement of the guide catheter, catheter tip spasm or a previously unrecognised ostial lesion.

Following intracoronary injections of contrast medium down the chosen coronary artery, the guidewire is passed across the stenosis. A balloon or stent catheter is then passed over the guidewire and positioned at the stenosis. Stents are usually directly engaged without predilatation, which reduces vessel trauma and equipment cost. Alternatively, a PTCA balloon is inflated for about 60–120 seconds and repeated several times, depending upon results. This is very prothrombotic, but the use of glycoprotein IIb/IIIa antagonists such as abciximab during PCI reduces the incidence of thrombosis, myocardial infarction and death without causing excess bleeding. Heparin therapy is usual, and subacute thrombosis is now usually less than 2% under elective conditions. Long-term antiplatelet therapy substantially reduces the risk of reocclusion.

Balloon inflation inevitably stops coronary blood flow, which may induce angina. Patients usually tolerate this quite well, especially if they have been warned beforehand. If it becomes severe or prolonged, however, an intravenous opiate may be given. Ischaemic electrocardiographic changes are often seen at this time, although they are usually transient and return to baseline once the balloon is deflated.

For an uncomplicated single lesion, a percutaneous procedure may take as little as 30 minutes, but the duration of the procedure and radiation exposure will vary according to the number and complexity of the treated stenoses and vessels. After the procedure, the patient is monitored for signs of ischaemia and haemodynamic instability. If a femoral arterial sheath was used, it may be removed when the heparin effect has declined to an acceptable level, followed by manual compression. Arterial sealing devices (AngioSeal, VasoSeal, Perclose) permit immediate sheath removal and haemostasis, are more comfortable for patients and allow earlier mobilisation and discharge.

Other percutaneous interventions

Coronary atherectomy

These can be used to debulk arteries that have large or calcific atheromatous stenoses, or to modify plaques in preparation for PTCA and stenting.

- *Direction atherectomy* removes atherosclerotic plaques with a cylindrical, rotating, cup-shaped blade. The catheter has a soft tapering nose cone that provides a collecting chamber for ablated tissue. The cutter is applied to different parts of the vessel wall in sequence, and PTCA is then applied to achieve a satisfactory result. Complications include side branch occlusion, perforation, abrupt vessel closure and distal embolisation.
- *Rotational atherectomy* debulks heavily calcified plaques by drilling, using a diamond-tipped elliptical burr. This results in a larger vessel diameter than that achieved by PTCA. Complications relate to perforation of the vessel wall, embolisation of plaque and dissections.
- *Laser atherectomy* uses ultraviolet, pulsed excimer light laser energy that ablates the plaque by providing thermomechanical shock waves that disrupt the plaque and vaporise the tissue. This has proved useful in chronically occluded vessels or in debulking occluded stents that cannot initially be treated by traditional PTCA (Topaz et al, 2001). The laser is utilised to clear a path for passage of the balloon catheter. Unfortunately, vessel perforation and dissections may complicate this technique.
- *Cutting balloon atherectomy* utilises a standard balloon catheter with three or four microblades folded within the balloon. It is particularly

useful for in-stent stenosis. When the balloon is inflated, the blades cut into the neointima, helping plaque compression by the balloon.

Aspiration and capture devices

These devices are used to protect the distal circulation from atheromatous debris that is dislodged into the microcirculation during angioplasty, which may be accompanied by the 'no reflow' phenomenon or significant elevation of cardiac markers. Particles may be either directly aspirated or filtered distally. Both systems appear to be equally effective.

The *Angiojet* uses a high-velocity saline stream to break up and aspirate soft thrombus, and the *Acolysis* device uses high-frequency sound waves rather than fluid. Distal *capture devices* (PercuSurge, Angioguard and Filterwire) are of particular advantage during PCI to degenerate vein grafts.

Pressure wires

Passing pressure wires across stenotic lesions of intermediate severity may be useful if there is doubt about the benefits of intervention. Pressures are measured proximally and distally to the lesion before and after vasodilator therapy (usually adenosine).

Surgical cover

Since the introduction of coronary stents, glycoprotein IIb/IIIa receptor blockers and other technical refinements, the need for emergency surgical cover during PCI has diminished, although the current ACC/AHA guidelines do not support elective PCI being undertaken in centres without on-site surgery (Smith et al, 2001). Nevertheless, in the UK, increasing numbers of patients are treated in non-surgical centres, as the need for emergency surgical intervention has fallen 10-fold from 2.6% of cases in 1991 to only 0.29% in 2003. Such centres must be able to managing haemodynamically unstable patients, with expertise in inotropic support, invasive haemodynamic monitoring, temporary pacing, intra-aortic balloon pumping and assisted ventilation. High-dependency facilities

with fully trained nursing, technical and radiographic staff should also be available (Dawkins et al, 2005). In 2004, PCI was being undertaken at 20 UK centres without any on-site surgical facilities.

PRIMARY ANGIOPLASTY FOLLOWING ACUTE MYOCARDIAL INFARCTION

Despite the introduction of more effective thrombolytic agents, only around 60% of patients treated with fibrinolytic therapy achieve normal thrombolysis in myocardial infarction (TIMI) grade III flow in the infarct-related artery (GUSTO Angiographic Investigators, 1993). Even if the coronary artery has been opened, there may be suboptimal tissue perfusion as a result of distal embolisation and microvascular spasm. Reocclusion may also affect up to 30% of patients in whom fibrinolysis was initially successful. Outcome after acute coronary occlusion depends upon whether the artery remains fully open or partially or totally obstructed. Attainment of TIMI grade III flow has been shown to reduce short- and medium-term mortality by up to 50% compared with other grades of TIMI patency, and the only treatment better than thrombolysis in this regard is primary PCI.

Primary angioplasty uses balloon dilatation to disrupt the thrombus as well as the underlying plaque, and usually restores normal antegrade flow. The procedure was first carried out nearly 25 years ago (Hartzler et al, 1983), and some of the advantages and disadvantages are shown in Box 16.2. Direct stenting allows mechanical stabilisation of the unstable plaque and reduces the incidence of angiographic 'no reflow', thus increasing myocardial reperfusion (Grines et al, 1999). A meta-analysis of trials has confirmed the clear benefit of primary angioplasty compared with in-hospital thrombolysis, with improvements in mortality, non-fatal myocardial infarction and stroke (Keeley et al, 2003).

Primary angioplasty is of particular value in patients who have had previous bypass surgery, the elderly and those in cardiogenic shock. In most cases of primary angioplasty, only the culprit lesion is attacked but, in cardiogenic shock, all diseased vessels with accessible lesions are tackled. Elderly patients (who constitute almost one-third of all patients with acute myocardial infarction) are

Box 16.2 Comparative advantages of primary angioplasty and thrombolysis.

Primary angioplasty

Advantages

Coronary anatomy defined; prognosis may
  be established
Up to 98% of vessels recanalise immediately
Residual stenosis cleared and stented
Left ventricular function improves
Intraplaque haemorrhage minimised
Less post-infarction angina and reinfarction

Disadvantages

Expensive
Specialised (requires catheter laboratory
  and expertise 24/7)
Slower to institute
Poor availability

Thrombolysis

Advantages

Cheap
Quick and simple to administer
Avoids risks of invasive study
Infarct-related artery opened in over half of cases

Disadvantages

Systemic and plaque haemorrhage may occur
Slow and unpredictable restoration of coronary
  blood flow
Residual stenoses remain; post-infarction
  ischaemia likely
Coronary anatomy unknown; angiography may
  be required later

Intra-aortic balloon pumps (IABP) must be available during primary angioplasty and can improve overall clinical outcomes in some patients undergoing emergency PCI, particularly those with right coronary artery lesions where intervention is sometimes accompanied by heart block and hypotension. An IABP is of course essential during PCI in patients with cardiogenic shock (Bates et al, 1998).

Despite these advantages of primary angioplasty, the main drawback is lack of facilities, with adequate staffing of sufficient skill and experience to cover the 24-hour period (Rogers et al, 2000). Expansion of facilities in the UK to permit primary stenting in acute myocardial infarction to deal with the 200 000 myocardial infarction admissions each year would require considerable investment. What is important now is that, where fibrinolysis is contraindicated (or where thrombolysis fails), there are strategies in place for rapid transfer to an intervention centre for mechanical reperfusion by primary or rescue angioplasty (Montalescot et al, 2004).

SURGERY FOR CORONARY ARTERY DISEASE

The main application of surgery for coronary heart disease is to improve the blood supply to the ischaemic myocardium. However, operations may also be required to repair mechanical defects that have arisen as a consequence of a myocardial infarction (e.g. mitral incompetence or ruptured interventricular septum). Surgery is most often and most safely performed electively, but is sometimes required urgently when these complications occur suddenly (Box 16.3).

CORONARY ARTERY BYPASS GRAFTING (CABG)

Surgical revascularisation was first attempted on the beating heart, and it was not until the introduction of cardiopulmonary bypass in 1967, allowing the heart to be stopped, that modern coronary bypass surgery emerged (Garrett et al, 1973). As experience of this operation has improved, there has been a progressive fall in operative mortality and morbidity, attributed to better patient selection,

generally good candidates for primary angioplasty as they often have contraindications to thrombolysis and are more likely to suffer haemorrhagic complications (particularly stroke). Primary angioplasty may also have a role in the treatment of patients who present too late for thrombolysis. Even in the absence of ongoing symptoms, PCI may reduce infarct size, (and thus potentially prevent remodelling) in those presenting up to 48 hours after the onset of symptoms (Schomig et al, 2005).

Box 16.3 Some indications for surgery in coronary heart disease.

Elective surgery

Poorly controlled stable angina
Significant left main stem coronary artery stenosis
Three-vessel coronary artery disease
Left main stem equivalent disease
Left ventricular aneurysm producing symptoms

Emergency surgery

Repair of mechanical defects
    Mitral valve dysfunction
    Ventriculo-septal defect
    Cardiac rupture
Cardiogenic shock
Following unsuccessful percutaneous intervention

with improved preoperative assessment and surgical techniques. In the early 1980s, cardiac surgeons attempted to attain a greater degree of revascularisation by bypassing most of the diseased vessels. The original 'triple bypass' then became a much longer affair, often involving five or six separate bypass vein grafts, but results did not improve, and the typical bypass operation these days involves between two and four grafts.

The usual bypass conduits are saphenous veins, but progressive intimal hyperplasia and accelerated atherosclerosis frequently cause graft failure, which is particularly evident beyond the fifth year, with about 90% of vein grafts being occluded at 10 years. Arterial grafts are now employed routinely to promote long-term graft patency and, provided there are no technical errors during implantation that result in early graft failure, the internal mammary artery appears to remain patent almost indefinitely, with a 10-year patency rate of around 95%. More importantly, patient survival is greater in those receiving arterial grafts to the left anterior descending coronary artery (LAD), either alone or in association with saphenous vein grafts (Cameron et al, 1996). This survival benefit is almost certainly due to resistance of arterial grafts to atherosclerosis, which continues to progress in both native coronary vessels and vein grafts.

In the UK, over 90% of CABG patients now receive an arterial graft to graft the LAD, with supplemental saphenous vein grafts to other coronary lesions. The radial artery has also been used as a free graft, with 5-year patency rates of about 85% (Buxton et al, 1997).

Using both the left and the right internal mammary arteries may offer additional clinical and survival benefits. Bilateral grafting is a more demanding procedure, but significantly reduces the need for redo surgery, without increasing perioperative mortality or morbidity (Patil et al, 2001). The right gastro-epiploic and inferior epigastric arteries can also be used in association with double internal mammary grafts to completely revascularise the heart arterially (Suma, 1999).

Indications for CABG

Expected survival rates following surgery rely on data acquired before many advances in medical, surgical and catheter-based treatments (Table 16.1). Early randomised trials comparing bypass surgery with medical therapy demonstrate that the greater the amount of at-risk myocardium from extensive or proximal coronary disease, the greater the improvements in prognosis following CABG, even in asymptomatic patients (Yusuf et al, 1994). Whether achieving this objective with modern multivessel PCI has a similar effect on long-term prognosis is currently not clear. Continuing advances in PCI and stent designs, the use of brachytherapy and drug-eluting stents will change current opinions on the best method of revascularisation. At present, patients with single or double artery disease can usually be managed by PCI in the first instance. Surgery is recommended for prognostic reasons if there is significant stenosis

Table 16.1 Five-year survival in the European Coronary Surgery Study (1980).

Group	Medical	Surgical
Left main stem disease	62%	93%
Three-vessel disease	85%	95%
Two-vessel disease	88%	92%

of the left main stem, 'left main equivalent' disease (i.e. over 70% stenoses in the proximal LAD and proximal left circumflex arteries) or triple artery disease, even if there is little or no angina (Eagle et al, 2004).

Patient selection

Patients vary in their reaction to anginal symptoms, and the decision to proceed to coronary artery bypass surgery needs careful consideration. Coronary artery surgery is palliative, and should be postponed in those with mild to moderate coronary heart disease and good left ventricular function. CABG should still be viewed as a one-off intervention, sometimes described as a 'get out of jail free' card that may only be played once! Young men are often urgently referred for bypass surgery, but buying time with angioplasty is preferable, as most will live long enough to develop clinically important graft atheroma if they are operated on prematurely. Repeat operations are sometimes indicated following graft failure, but these are technically more difficult to perform and carry a greater risk to the patient than the initial operation. Operative risk is also greater in the elderly and for female patients, presumably because the smaller vessels and compact anatomy compromise surgical techniques and graft patency. Co-existent diabetes and hypertension also increase perioperative risk. Poor operative risk factors need to be balanced against poor prognostic features of the disease itself, including low exercise tolerance and arterial stenoses at dangerous sites. Poor left ventricular function is an important preoperative risk, but survival of such patients following surgery is superior compared with treatment with medical therapy, and it may be justified to take the risk. Occasionally, a severely reduced ejection fraction is related to hibernating myocardium rather than scarring, and cardiac function improves with surgery.

Many surgeons resist operating on patients who have not stopped smoking, because of the higher perioperative risk and poorer outcome. Ten-year survival in patients following coronary artery bypass surgery is 84% in those who stopped smoking and 68% in those who continue to smoke (Cavender et al, 1992). Postoperatively, chronic smokers are more likely to develop angina, are more often unable to return to work, usually have more hospital admissions and have a 5-year mortality of nearly 20%.

The European System for Cardiac Operative Risk Evaluation (Euro-SCORE) uses a number of risk factors to predict mortality from cardiac surgery (Roques et al, 2003). It includes patient factors (e.g. age, sex, co-morbidities), cardiac-related factors (e.g. recent unstable coronary syndrome, left ventricular dysfunction) and type of cardiac procedure (e.g. CABG, mechanical complications). A risk calculator can be used or downloaded easily from the EuroSCORE website (http://www. euroscore.org).

Operative procedure

Most CABG patients require grafting of the three main native coronary arteries, and the 'standard' operation uses the left internal mammary artery (LIMA) to the left anterior descending coronary artery with supplemental saphenous vein grafts to the other vessels.

The heart is exposed through a median sternotomy and, in most cases, the left internal mammary artery is dissected down. Limited grafting procedures may be carried out on the beating heart, but most cases require cardioplegia with extracorporeal cardiopulmonary bypass. Myocardial damage is limited by reducing the body temperature to below 32°C before cardiac arrest is induced with a potassium-rich cardioplegic solution. Cannulae are inserted in the right atrium and ascending aorta, with blood passing outside the body for oxygenation. While this is going on, the long saphenous vein is stripped from the leg, flushed with heparinised blood and checked for leaks. The radial artery may also be dissected from the forearm as a free graft.

The aorta is cross-clamped, and the proximal ends of the grafts are sutured to the ascending aorta. The period of ischaemia is kept as short as possible, and the heart can be reperfused while the proximal ends are sewn in.

The patient is then rewarmed, normal cardiac rhythm established by defibrillation and the chest closed. Inotropes are not usually needed, but the patient is normally ventilated for 3–4 hours postoperatively.

Postoperative management

Catheters are used to monitor intracardiac pressures for the first 24 hours, after which time the majority of patients can leave the intensive care unit. Patients are mobilised quickly, and are often fit for discharge from hospital within a week. The majority of patients are able to return to work between 2 and 6 months after the operation, although many patients are beyond the retirement age. Aspirin must be started within 6 hours of the operation, because benefits on graft patency are lost when begun later. Aspirin should be continued for at least 12 months, and probably indefinitely to reduce the risk of graft occlusion and help to prevent other major clinical vascular events, such as myocardial infarction or stroke (Anti-platelet Trialists' Collaboration, 1994). Graft patency is not prolonged by the addition of dipyridamole or by using warfarin instead. If patients have contraindications to aspirin, clopidogrel 300 mg should be used within 6 hours, continuing at 75 mg daily.

Problems following surgery

Early effects

Morbidity and mortality following coronary artery surgery have fallen as surgical expertise has improved. In most centres, the overall mortality is less than 3%, but much depends upon the patient group and the number of emergency operations that are undertaken. Certain variables, such as age, diabetes, left ventricular function and other co-morbidities, can be used to predict the risk of death, stroke or mediastinitis in individual cases (Eagle et al, 2004).

The commonest problem following bypass surgery is disturbance of heart rhythm, affecting up to one-third of all patients in the first few days. Most are benign supraventricular dysrhythmias. New onset atrial fibrillation occurs in 30% of patients, and increases the risk of stroke. Temporary heart block occurs in 5–10% of patients.

Perioperative myocardial infarction is a risk factor for premature death, but frequency is down to under 2.5%. Careful attention to perioperative ischaemia is important, particularly during induction of anaesthesia and extracorporeal bypass. Global left ventricular damage is more difficult to diagnose, but is probably common. A low-output period may follow, particularly if the left ventricular function was poor to start with. Some patients need to be supported by extracorporeal bypass while the ventricular myocardium recovers.

Renal dysfunction may occur in about 8% of patients, and a fifth of these may require dialysis. This is more common in the elderly and those with heart failure, diabetes or prior renal disease. If the creatinine is more than 130 mmol/L preoperatively, the risk of acute renal failure is doubled. There may also be temporary haematological dysfunction, pulmonary disease and immunological suppression.

Pain from the sternotomy and cracked ribs can cause discomfort for a few weeks, as can pain around the long incision made for removing the saphenous vein. Mediastinitis from deep wound infections is more frequent where arterial grafts are used, and occurs in 1–4% of cases. It carries a high mortality (25%). Patients are more prone to this complication if they are obese or have diabetes.

The most important complications are neurological, caused by haemorrhage, metabolic problems or cardiopulmonary bypass itself. Cardiopulmonary bypass requires the cannulation of the heart and the ascending aorta, which may dislodge atherosclerotic microemboli, especially during aortic manipulation. Air emboli may also be a problem, and the use of membrane as opposed to bubble oxygenators helps to reduce this complication. The risk of stroke is approximately 0.7% for a 50-year-old man, rising to 8% in an 80-year-old, and is thus a sufficiently common complication that it should be discussed preoperatively. Many of the embolic complications may not be so obvious. Temporary impairment of concentration or memory is common, affecting up to half of patients in the first 6 weeks, but it may persist for several months following surgery (Pandit & Pigott, 2001).

Anxiety and depression are common following cardiac surgery, with women being more often affected. This is a natural reaction to the stress surrounding open-heart surgery, and family support with visits from the district nurse or cardiac liaison nurse is very helpful. Younger women, those with more perioperative complications and those with a history of depression are at risk of clinical depression (Doering et al, 2006). All patients should be monitored for signs of clinical depression before discharge home, with referral for specialist assessment and treatment as appropriate.

Long-term effects

It takes about 2–3 months to recover fully after bypass surgery, and patients are often easily fatigued during this period. Chest pain related to the sternotomy is common, but immediate and complete relief from angina is reported in most patients, and most of the remainder have marked improvement in their symptoms. Numbness is frequent around the scars, particularly where the vein grafts were obtained. Ankle swelling is common, and elevating the legs and compression hosiery may be helpful.

The long-term benefits of coronary artery bypass surgery are determined by changes in left ventricular function, patency of the grafts and progression of generalised atherosclerosis. The 1-year survival is 95%, and the 5-year survival is 88%. An early return of angina is due to either incomplete revascularisation or premature graft occlusion. More than 90% of patients are free from angina at 1 year, declining to 60% at 10 years. During the first month after bypass surgery, vein graft failure results from thrombotic occlusion, whereas later, the dominant process is atherosclerotic obstruction. Failure of at least one vein graft is quite common within 12–18 months after CABG surgery. Failure of at least one vein graft is quite common within 12 to 18 months but, by 10 years, this has gone up to 50–60%.

The pathology underlying graft occlusion varies. Immediately following anastomosis, endothelial cells become oedematous and damaged, and early occlusion is usually due to platelet aggregation and thrombosis. Fibro-intimal hyperplasia of grafts first appears at 2 weeks, characterised by proliferation of vascular smooth muscle cells and synthesis of matrix. It is usually self-limiting, but underlies most cases of occlusion within the first year. Grafts over 3 years old show plaque formation and, beyond 5 years, rupturing of atheromatous plaques is the commonest initiator of graft stenosis. Preventing, retarding or reversing graft atheroma requires attention to classical risk factors, including hypertension, smoking and hypercholesterolaemia. Failure to control lipid levels results in an increased rate of graft occlusion, as well as progression of atheroma in native vessels. The low-density lipoprotein (LDL) cholesterol should be reduced and maintained at less than 2 mmol/L.

One-third of patients experience recurrent stable angina after 10 years, although it will not necessarily be so severe. PCI with stenting is the favoured method of revascularisation if possible because, although reoperation will produce nearly as good results (60% angina free at 1 year), operative mortality is higher and surgery is technically more difficult. Conduits to perform bypass grafts may be lacking, and candidates are usually older, with advanced coronary and non-coronary atherosclerosis. Despite a higher initial morbidity and mortality, survival rates after reoperation are about of 90–95% at 5 years, and more than 75% at 10 years. The use of arterial grafts, antiplatelet agents and statins has reduced the need for repeat operations.

MINIMALLY INVASIVE AND OFF-PUMP CORONARY ARTERY BYPASS

Avoiding cardiopulmonary bypass may help to reduce morbidity, given that many perioperative complications are actually due to extracorporeal bypass, rather than CABG itself (Al-Ruzzeh et al, 2006). Off-pump coronary artery bypass (OPCAB) is coronary arterial surgery performed on the beating heart, with anastomoses being carried out using stabilisers that sit astride the artery being operated on, holding the heart relatively steady. The heart rate is slowed with beta-blockers or diltiazem to help stability. As there is no cardiopulmonary bypass, OPCAB may reduce the incidence of stroke and atrial fibrillation, but the operation takes longer (Sellke et al, 2005). Although OPCAB was used first for easily accessible single-vessel disease, it is increasingly being used in elderly patients with multivessel disease and in patients with significant co-morbidity. Advantages and disadvantages are shown in Box 16.4. Off-pump bypass surgery can be performed with or without sternotomy, but is more often used with minimally invasive direct coronary artery bypass surgery (MIDCAB) using a mini-thoracotomy.

MIDCAB can be used in patients with disease confined to the left anterior descending and/or the right coronary arteries, using the two internal

> **Box 16.4** Potential advantages and disadvantages of off-pump coronary artery bypass surgery (OPCAB).
>
> **Advantages of OPCAB**
>
> Less bleeding
> Less cardiac damage
> Less renal dysfunction
> Less neurocognitive dysfunction
> Shorter hospital stay
> Fewer postoperative chest infections
>
> **Disadvantages of OPCAB**
>
> Technically demanding
> Longer operation time
> Difficulty in grafting posterior vessels
> Incomplete revascularisation more frequent

mammary arteries as bypass grafts. A 10-cm-long transverse incision is made on the front of the chest towards the left side, and a small portion of rib is removed. The internal mammary arteries are dissected from the chest wall using either direct vision or video endoscopic guidance and sutured directly to the LAD or right coronary artery without needing to stop the heart. MIDCAB is less expensive than traditional CABG, but urgent conversion to conventional open-chest methods has occasionally been necessary (Kettering et al, 2004). The hybrid procedure of MIDCAB to the LAD with angioplasty to the other vessels in those with multivessel disease may be safer and more effective than either modality alone, particularly in those with multiple co-morbidities.

Totally endoscopic robotically assisted coronary artery bypass (TECAB) involves grafting through small port incisions in three intercostal spaces through which one robotic arm carrying an endoscope and two arms through which surgical attachments are introduced. The surgeons work from a viewing and control console using handles to control the robotic arms that position and precisely manoeuvre the instruments within the patient. Some equipment uses voice-controlled robotic arms. Operating time is about 4 hours for single-vessel surgery and 6 hours for multivessel surgery. Conversion rates to open procedures (either mini-thoracotomy or full sternotomy) are very frequent, and evidence on the safety and efficacy of TECAB is not yet compelling (NICE, 2005).

Percutaneous transmyocardial laser revascularisation

Percutaneous transmyocardial revascularisation is of value in selected cases of medical refractory angina where PCI or bypass surgery cannot be performed. It involves application of laser energy via a cardiac catheter to create channels in the ischaemic myocardium from the endocardial side of the left ventricular wall to allow direct perfusion of the subendocardium by oxygenated blood within the left ventricle. These channels appeared to remain open and endothelialised at 8 weeks, but may close within several months due to fibrosis. Nevertheless, longlasting effects may be derived from secondary stimulation of vascular growth factors and denervation of the myocardium (Patil et al, 2001). Initially, the procedure required surgical thoracotomy, which limited patient selection because of associated morbidity and mortality, but several different catheter-based approaches are now used, meaning that many more patients may benefit. Procedural mortality, myocardial infarction and haemopericardium are very uncommon. Compared with medical therapy, there is a sustained improvement in angina class for at least the first year, although these beneficial effects tend decline thereafter (Salem et al, 2006). Nevertheless, the procedure does offer some help to the 'no-option' patient with refractory angina.

Bypass surgery following acute myocardial infarction

While the results of elective CABG have improved markedly over the last 20 years, emergency surgery for acute coronary syndromes is still associated with an approximate fivefold mortality and morbidity rate. The recently infarcted heart is more susceptible to global ischaemia induced by CABG, and it may be preferable to utilise PCI in the short term. Operative mortality is not influenced if the infarct was sustained more than 30 days prior to isolated CABG surgery, but is most significantly increased in the first week after myocardial infarction, especially in older patients. This critical period should be avoided whenever possible (Voisine et al, 2006). If patients are taking clopidogrel, this should be stopped for at least 5 days preoperatively.

OPERATIONS FOR THE COMPLICATIONS OF MYOCARDIAL INFARCTION

There are three commonly performed operations for patients who have developed mechanical post-infarction complications. These are resection of left ventricular aneurysms, repair or replacement of the mitral valve and repair of the interventricular septum.

Resection of left ventricular aneurysms

After myocardial infarction, parts of the damaged left ventricle may be akinetic (i.e. do not move) or dyskinetic (i.e. moves paradoxically). The latter areas, if sufficiently large, will act as a chamber that fills during diastole, but does not contribute to ejection of blood during systole, because the area bulges outwards. This situation will usually improve as the infarct heals. Left ventricular aneurysms usually produce symptoms several weeks or even months after acute myocardial infarction, presenting with angina, heart failure, dysrhythmias or thromboembolic events. Surgery will usually help overall left ventricular function, but prognosis is dependent upon how well the left ventricle performs postoperatively, as well as on the overall perfusion of the remaining myocardium. Hence, CABG is often performed at the same time as resection of the aneurysm. Using endoventricular patches rather than performing a simple linear repair may allow better retention of ventricular geometry to maintain physiological function, and hence reduce morbidity and mortality.

Mitral valve surgery

Left ventricular dilatation following acute myocardial infarction often associates with mitral incompetence, which resolves with medical therapy. Surgery may be required if there has been acquired mitral regurgitation due to partial or complete papillary muscle rupture or major ischaemic dysfunction. The degree of valvular incompetence can vary from slight to massive. Total rupture of a papillary muscle complicates about 1% of myocardial infarctions, usually in the first week. Medical treatment of this condition is associated with 50% mortality within the first 24 hours, and 94% within 8 weeks, so urgent operative intervention is required. Although operation carries a high mortality (around 30%), normal valve function may be restored with a prosthetic valve. While emergency surgery is being arranged, a sodium nitroprusside infusion can be used to help lower pulmonary capillary pressures and improve peripheral perfusion.

Where technically possible, repairing rather than replacing the mitral valve may be beneficial in preserving long-term cardiac function, as the supporting structure of the mitral valve is retained.

Repair of a ruptured interventricular septum

Rupture of the interventricular septum occurs in about 1–2% of all transmural myocardial infarcts, usually within the first week. Rupture usually associates with anterior infarction and, if untreated, will be lethal in nearly all patients within a few days. An increased frequency of acute rupture of the interventricular septum with earlier presentation has been noted in patients receiving thrombolytic therapy. The clinical picture varies considerably, but patients usually present within the first 4 days with severe heart failure and the presence of a loud pan-systolic murmur at the left sternal edge. The diagnosis is confirmed by echocardiography and right heart catheterisation.

Immediate surgical repair is indicated when pulmonary oedema or cardiogenic shock is present, although mortality in this group is high. Initial therapy is with diuretics and vasodilators, such as sodium nitroprusside, with insertion of an intra-aortic balloon pump to augment coronary, cerebral and renal blood flow. Early surgical intervention is also important in haemodynamically stable patients because the rupture site can expand abruptly, resulting in sudden haemodynamic collapse. Delaying for a short while may still be beneficial, as mortality is about 34% in the first week after infarction compared with 11% after the first week. Patients usually have associated multivessel disease, and will need concomitant bypass surgery (Pellerin & Bourassa, 1996).

Left ventricular free wall rupture (cardiac rupture)

The incidence of cardiac rupture has increased since the introduction of routine thrombolysis, and usually occurs suddenly in the first week. Routine treatment with beta-blockade may help to reduce this complication. Most cases present with cardiac arrest, usually with pulseless electrical activity (PEA). About 25% of cases have a subacute course because pericardial adhesions limit the speed of leakage. The presentation is then of cardiac tamponade, which can be diagnosed by echocardiography. Pericardial aspiration may be required to relieve the haemopericardium, followed by emergency cardiac surgery irrespective of the clinical status, as complete rupture may occur at any time. Repair of the ventricle is by direct suture or using cyanoacrylate glue to hold a Teflon patch over the necrotic myocardium (Bates et al, 1997). Patching and simple closure of a tear on the antero-lateral surface of the heart can be undertaken on the beating heart without the need for cardiopulmonary bypass, although many surgeons may wish to undertake coronary bypass of palpable or clinically evident disease, as patients usually have multivessel coronary disease.

SURGERY FOR HEART FAILURE

Despite the fall in mortality from cardiovascular disease, the incidence and prevalence of heart failure is increasing, particularly in those aged over 65 years. While thrombolysis and angioplasty save lives acutely, late or incomplete reperfusion associates with more left ventricle damage and dysfunction. Modern treatment with angiotensin-converting enzyme (ACE) inhibitors and beta-blockers has improved the outlook for patients with cardiac failure, but the natural course of the disorder is progressive and associates with a high mortality.

The only surgical option for many patients with severe cardiac failure has been heart transplantation, but donor hearts are a rare commodity. Revascularisation may help hibernating myocardium to recover contractile performance, but sufficient resuscitatable myocardium must be present. Dobutamine stress testing or positron emission tomography (PET) scanning may assess the presence of myocardium hibernation. Surgical management of mitral regurgitation that occurs secondary to left ventricular dilation needs consideration. Mitral regurgitation increases volume overload of the left ventricle, worsening heart failure. Mitral valve repair with preservation of the subvalvular apparatus can be carried out with good symptomatic results.

Left ventricular restoration surgery aims to reshape the left ventricle from a globular to a more elliptical shape, reducing left ventricular cavity volume and improving function (Tonnessen & Knudsen, 2005).

HEART TRANSPLANTATION

The first human heart transplant was carried out in 1967, and cardiac transplantation is now sufficiently commonplace not to attract public attention. More than 55 000 heart transplants have now been performed worldwide (www.ishlt.org), and there are currently seven centres in the UK performing the operation.

Heart transplantation is usually carried out in patients with endstage heart failure caused by coronary artery disease and, in the last 20 years, it has become the gold standard treatment in selected cases (Dreng, 2002). Despite improved medical and surgical treatments in advanced heart failure, transplantation offers the best survival in those at highest risk of dying. Less commonly, transplantation has been performed for non-ischaemic cardiomyopathies caused by alcohol, chemotherapy or other drugs. Transplantation may also be performed following failed valvular surgery, for intractable angina or for certain forms of congenital heart disease.

The donor heart can be implanted to replace (orthotopic) or support (heterotopic) the recipient heart. Heterotopic ('piggy-back') transplantation places the new heart in the right pleural cavity and can be used to overcome size mismatch. There are more complications with this approach, and partial (excising at the mid-atrial level) or total orthotopic transplantation is more usual.

One of the greatest advances in transplant surgery has been the development of drugs that suppress rejection. The introduction of ciclosporin A (Sandimmune) in 1982 led to improved results by permitting a reduction in the high-dose steroid therapy that compromised surgical healing. Immunosuppression is now based on a triple drug regime of ciclosporin A, azathioprine and prednisolone. Tacrolimus can be used as a substitute for ciclosporin. Daclizumab, a humanised monoclonal antibody against the interleukin-2 receptor, has been found to be efficacious as prophylaxis against acute cellular rejection after cardiac transplantation.

For routine first transplants, the 1-year survival is around 83% and 5-year survival is 66% (NHS UK Transplant, 2005). Mortality is higher in females, patients over the age of 40 years, those patients being transplanted for valvular disease, or where the donor heart is older than 30 years. Early morbidity is due to graft failure, acute rejection and infection. Opportunistic infections after transplantation continue to constitute a challenge for management. Cytomegalovirus (CMV) remains the most important infection affecting heart transplant recipients, but *Pneumocystis carinii* pneumonia, tuberculosis, toxoplasmosis, pulmonary aspergillosis and other fungal infections continue to constitute challenges for the immunocompromised heart transplant recipient.

After the first year, the commonest cause of death is from an unusual form of accelerated coronary artery disease, called *cardiac allograft vasculopathy* (CAV). It is seen particularly in smokers and those with hypertension and, because of the diffuse nature of the disease, percutaneous and surgical revascularisation procedures have a limited role. Annual coronary angiography is performed for diagnostic and surveillance purposes, and diltiazem and statins have been shown to be effective in retarding CAV. Retransplantation may need to be considered in extreme cases. Malignancies, particularly lymphoma and skin cancers, are another major cause of death after cardiac transplantation (1–2% per year).

Despite these complications, there seems to be little doubt of the value of cardiac transplantation in prolonging the quantity and quality of patients' lives. Cost–benefit studies show significant improvement in key aspects of lifestyle, and most patients are able to resume normal lives. The cost of a heart transplant and the first 5 years of follow-up is approximately half the cost of 5 years of renal dialysis.

The main constraint on cardiac transplantation is the lack of donors. In 2004, 290 heart transplants were carried out in the UK, a decrease of 10% from the previous year. Of the 832 patients on the transplant list for a cardiothoracic organ in 2004, over half were still waiting at the end of the year, a third had received a transplant, and the rest had either died or been removed from the transplant list. The annual transplantation rate is likely to remain under 4500 worldwide, so the impact on the treatment of advanced heart failure will remain limited. Nevertheless, it is important that transplantation programmes survive to provide an option for patients with endstage heart disease, while new therapies evolve, including novel transplantation strategies such as xenotransplantation and regrowth of heart muscle.

Left ventricular assist devices (LVADs)

Although transplantation remains the 'gold standard' for the treatment of patients with endstage heart failure, left ventricular assist devices (LVADs) can be used to support patients until transplantation. Early artificial hearts and ventricular assist devices were usually driven by external pneumatic pumps, but the current generation of assist devices are electrically powered, ultracompact and totally implantable and may allow patients to return to their daily activities. Successful bridging to recovery with ventricular support systems has been reported in post-cardiotomy cardiogenic shock, acute myocarditis and in the peri-infarction period. The REMATCH trial demonstrated a survival benefit from mechanical circulatory support therapy compared with all other options in non-transplant candidates (Rose et al, 2001), and we are likely to see an increasing usage of these devices in potential cardiac transplantation candidates.

References

Al-Ruzzeh S, George S, Bustami M et al (2006) Effect of off-pump coronary artery bypass surgery on clinical, angiographic, neurocognitive, and quality of life outcomes: randomised controlled trial. *British Medical Journal* 332: 1365–1368.

Anti-platelet Trialists' Collaboration (1994) Overview II. Maintenance of vascular graft or arterial patency by anti-platelet therapy. *British Medical Journal* 308: 159–168.

Astin F, Jones K, Thompson DR (2005) Prevalence and patterns of anxiety and depression in patients undergoing elective percutaneous trans-luminal coronary angioplasty. *Heart and Lung* 34: 393–401.

Bates RJ, Beutler S, Resnekov L et al (1997) Cardiac rupture: challenge in diagnosis and management. *American Journal of Cardiology* 42: 429–437.

Bates ER, Stomel RJ, Hochman JS et al (1998) The use of intra-aortic balloon counterpulsation as an adjunct to reperfusion therapy in cardiogenic shock. *International Journal of Cardiology* 65(suppl 1): S37–42.

Bennett MR (2003) In-stent stenosis: pathology and implications for the development of drug eluting stents. *Heart* 89: 218–224.

Bourassa MG (2000) Clinical trials of coronary revascularisation: coronary angioplasty vs. coronary bypass grafting. *Current Opinion in Cardiology* 15: 281–286.

Buxton B, Windsor M, Komeda M et al (1997) How good is the radial artery as a bypass graft? *Coronary Artery Disease* 8: 225–233.

Cameron A, Davis KB, Green G et al (1996) Coronary bypass surgery with internal-thoracic-artery grafts – effects on survival over a 15-year period. *New England Journal of Medicine* 334: 216–219.

Cavender JB, Rodgers WJ, Fisher LD (1992) Effects of smoking on survival and morbidity in patients randomised to medical or surgical therapy in the Coronary Artery Surgery Study (CASS). *Journal of the American College of Cardiology* 20: 287–294.

Dawkins KD, Gershlick T, de Belder M et al (2005) Percutaneous coronary intervention: recommendations for good practice and training. *Heart* 91(suppl VI): v1–v27.

Doering LV, Magsarali MC, Howitt LY et al (2006) Clinical depression in women after cardiac surgery. *Journal of Cardiovascular Nursing* 21: 132–139.

Dreng MC (2002) Cardiac transplantation. *Heart* 87: 177–184.

Eagle KA, Guyton RA, Davidoff R et al (2004) ACC/AHA 2004 guideline update for coronary artery bypass graft surgery: a report of the American College of Cardiology/American Heart Association Task Force on Practice Guidelines. *Circulation* 110: e340–437.

European Coronary Surgery Study Group (1980) Second interim report. *Lancet* ii: 491–495.

Garrett HE, Dennis EW, DeBakey ME (1973) Aortocoronary bypass with saphenous vein graft. Seven-year follow up. *Journal of the American Medical Association* 223: 792–794.

Gersh BJ, Frye RL (2005) Methods of coronary revascularization – things may not be as they seem. *New England Journal of Medicine* 352: 2235–2237.

Goldberg RF, Fass AE, Frishman WH (2005) Transmyocardial revascularization: defining its role. *Cardiology in Review* 13: 52–55.

Grines CL, Cox DA, Stone GW et al (1999) Coronary angioplasty with or without stent implantation for acute myocardial infarction. Stent-PAMI Group. *New England Journal of Medicine* 341: 1949–1956.

Grüntzig AR (1984) Percutaneous transluminal angioplasty: six years' experience. *American Heart Journal* 107: 818–819.

GUSTO Angiographic Investigators (1993) The effect of tissue plasminogen activator, streptokinase, or both on coronary artery patency, ventricular function and survival after acute myocardial infarction. *New England Journal of Medicine* 329: 1615–1622.

Hannan EL, Racz MJ, Walford G et al (2005) Long-term outcomes of coronary artery bypass grafting versus stent implantation. *New England Journal of Medicine* 352: 2174–2183.

Hartzler GO, Rutherford BD, McConahay DR (1983) PTCA with and without thrombolytic therapy for treatment of acute myocardial infarction. *American Heart Journal* 106: 965–973.

Kandzari DE, Mark DB (2002) Intra-coronary brachytherapy: time to sell short? *Circulation* 106: 646–648.

Keeley EC, Boura JA, Grines C (2003) Primary angioplasty versus intravenous thrombolytic therapy: a quantitative review of 23 randomised trials. *Lancet* 361: 13–20.

Kettering K, Dapunt O, Baer FM (2004) Minimally invasive direct coronary artery bypass grafting: a systematic review. *Journal of Cardiovascular Surgery* 45: 255–264.

McGowan JH, Begley DA, Sutton AG (2005) Stenting of left main stem thrombosis. *Heart* 91: 483

Montalescot G, Andersen HR, Antoniucci D et al (2004) Recommendations on percutaneous coronary intervention for the perfusion of acute ST elevation myocardial infarction. *Heart* 90: 676–677.

Mukherjee D (2004) Current clinical perspectives on myocardial angiogenesis. *Molecular & Cellular Biochemistry* 264: 157–167.

NHS UK Transplant (2005) Transplant Activity Report 2004. Bristol: NHS UK Transplant. www.uktransplant.org.uk.

NICE (2003) *Guidance on the Use of Coronary Artery Stents.* Technology appraisal guidance no. 71. London: NICE. www.nice.org.uk.

NICE (2005) *Totally Endoscopic Robotically Assisted Coronary Artery Bypass (TECAB).* Interventional procedure guidance no. 128. London: NICE. www.nice.org.uk.

Niles NW, McGrath PD, Malenka D et al (2001) Survival of patients with diabetes and multi-vessel coronary artery disease after surgical or percutaneous revascularization: results of a large regional prospective study. *Journal of the American College of Cardiology* 37: 1008–1015.

Opie LH, Commerford PJ, Gersh BJ (2006) Controversies in stable angina. *Lancet* 367: 69–78.

Pandit J, Pigott D (2001) Cognitive dysfunction after cardiac surgery: strategies for prevention. *British Journal of Cardiology* 8: 613–616.

Patil CV, Nikolsky E, Boulos M et al (2001) Multi-vessel coronary artery disease: current revascularisation strategies. *European Heart Journal* 22: 1183–1197.

Pellerin M, Bourassa MG (1996) Post-infarction ventriculo-septal rupture. *European Heart Journal* 17: 1778–1779.

Rogers WJ, Canto JG, Barron HV et al (2000) Treatment and outcome of myocardial infarction in hospitals with and without invasive capabilities. *Journal of the American College of Cardiology* 35: 371–379.

Roiron C, Sanchez P, Bouzamondo A et al (2006) Drug eluting stents: an updated meta-analysis of randomised controlled trials. *Heart* 92: 641–649.

Roques F, Michel P, Goldstone AR et al (2003) The logistic EuroSCORE. *European Heart Journal* 24: 882–883.

Rose EA, Gelijns AC, Moskowitz AJ for the REMATCH Study Group (2001) Long-term mechanical left ventricular assistance for end-stage heart failure. *New England Journal of Medicine* 345: 1435–1443.

Salem M, Rotevatn S, Nordrehaug JE (2006) Long-term results following percutaneous myocardial laser therapy. *Coronary Artery Disease* 17: 385–390.

Schomig A. Mehilli J, Antoniucci D et al (2005) Mechanical reperfusion in patients with acute myocardial infarction presenting more than 12 hours from symptom onset: a randomized controlled trial. *Journal of the American Medical Association* 293: 2865–2872.

Sellke FW, DiMaio JM, Caplan LR et al (2005) Comparing on-pump and off-pump coronary artery bypass grafting. *Circulation* 111: 2858–2864.

Smith SC Jr, Dove JT, Jacobs AK et al (2001) ACC/AHA guidelines for percutaneous coronary intervention (revision of the 1993 PTCA guidelines). *Circulation* 103: 3019–3041.

Stables R (2002) Coronary artery bypass surgery versus percutaneous coronary intervention with stent implantation in patients with multi-vessel coronary artery disease (the Stent or Surgery trial): a randomized controlled trial. *Lancet* 360: 965–970

Suma H (1999) Arterial grafts in coronary bypass surgery. *Annals of Thoracic and Cardiovascular Surgery* 5: 141–145.

Taggart DP (2005) Surgery is the best intervention for severe coronary artery disease. *British Medical Journal* 330: 785–786.

Tonnessen T, Knudsen CW (2005) Surgical left ventricular remodelling in heart failure. *European Journal of Heart Failure* 7: 704–709.

Topaz O, Das T, Dahm J et al (2001) Excimer laser revascularisation: current indications, applications and techniques. *Lasers in Medical Science* 16: 72–77.

Voisine P, Mathieu P, Doyle D et al (2006) Influence of time elapsed between myocardial infarction and coronary artery bypass grafting surgery on operative mortality. *European Journal of Cardio-Thoracic Surgery* 29: 319–323.

Yang EH, Gumina RJ, Lennon RJ et al (2005) Emergency coronary artery bypass surgery for percutaneous coronary interventions. Changes in the incidence, clinical characteristics, and indications from 1979 to 2003. *Journal of the American College of Cardiology* 46: 2004–2009.

Yusuf S, Zucker D, Peduzzi P et al (1994) Effect of coronary artery bypass graft surgery on survival: overview of 10-year results from randomised trials by the Coronary Artery Bypass Graft Surgery Trialists' Collaboration. *Lancet* 344: 563–570.

Chapter 17

Therapeutics

CHAPTER CONTENTS

The following is a summary of drug groups and some individual agents commonly used on the coronary care unit (CCU). Usual doses and common side effects are detailed, but this is not fully comprehensive and serves only as a guide. Further information should always be sought from the hospital pharmacy department, manufacturers' data sheets, the *Monthly Index of Medical Specialities* (MIMS) or the *British National Formulary* (BNF), particularly if the drug is unfamiliar. The BNF is a joint publication from the British Medical Association and the Pharmaceutical Society of Great Britain and, apart from providing a comprehensive drugs list, it also has useful sections on drug interactions, intravenous additives, prescribing for the elderly, cardiovascular risk factor calculation and resuscitation guidelines. For a small number of cardiovascular drugs [e.g. angiotensin-converting enzyme (ACE) inhibitors and thrombolytic drugs], there is differing susceptibility to adverse reactions between ethnic groups, which may also need to be considered. For example, the relative risk of cough from ACE inhibitors in East Asian patients is nearly three times higher than in white patients, and the relative risk of intracranial haemorrhage with thrombolytic therapy is 1.5 in black compared with non-black patients (McDowell et al, 2006).

Some patients with cardiovascular disease use complementary treatments, which they perceive as being 'natural' and therefore safe. In the USA, herbal medicines are used by 10% of adults, especially women and those from higher socioeconomic groups (De Smet, 2002). Apart from dubious efficacy, certain herbs are cardiotoxic, while others can interact to either accentuate or reduce the effectiveness of conventional medicines used to treat cardiac problems. For example, St John's Wort affects the metabolism of digoxin, warfarin and simvastatin, reducing efficacy. It is important to ask directly about herbal and other complementary medicines, as these are seldom reported when obtaining a drug history.

European law now requires drugs to be prescribed by the recommended International Non-proprietary Names (rINNs) for medicinal substances when trade names are not used. In most cases, the previous British Approved Name (BAN) is identical, but several commonly used drugs have had their BAN modified to accord with the rINN. A complete list is available at www.mhra.gov.uk.

ADENOSINE (ADENOCOR)

Adenosine is an endogenous nucleoside that produces transient atrio-ventricular (AV) nodal block when injected intravenously. Because it has a brief half-life of around 5 seconds, it is very safe, but needs a bolus injection for effect. Adenosine is the treatment of choice to terminate re-entry tachycardias and may also have a diagnostic role in determining the origin of regular broad-complex tachycardias.

Dose

The dose is 6 mg by rapid intravenous injection into a fast-running intravenous infusion or followed by 5–10 mL of saline flush. If ineffective, a second and third bolus of 12 mg can be tried.

Side effects

Transient chest pain, dyspnoea and flushing (warn the patient – it is unpleasant but very transient). It may cause bronchospasm, and should not be used in patients with severe asthma. If pre-excitation is suspected, adenosine should be avoided as AV blockade causes a relative increase in pre-excitation and may precipitate atrial fibrillation associated with a dangerously rapid ventricular response. Electrical cardioversion is usually the safest treatment option.

Adenosine should also not be given to patients taking dipyridamole (Persantin), as significant hypotension may result. Heart transplant patients are very sensitive to adenosine.

ADRENALINE (EPINEPHRINE)

Adrenaline is the first drug intervention for cardiac arrest. It has strong alpha- and beta-adrenergic agonist activity. Alpha-activity causes peripheral vasoconstriction that augments the effect of chest compression, leading to increased cerebral and coronary perfusion. The beta-agonist properties (positive chronotropic and inotropic effects) help myocardial function following attainment of sinus rhythm. Adrenaline is also used in the treatment of anaphylaxis.

Adrenaline remains the approved name utilised in the European Pharmacopoeia.

Dose

For cardiac arrest: regardless of the arrest rhythm, 1 mg of adrenaline should be given intravenously (10 mL of a 1:10 000 solution) every 3–5 minutes until recovery.
For anaphylaxis: 0.5 mL of 1:1000 solution (500 µg) intramuscularly (*not* intravenously), repeated after about 5 minutes if required (some cases may need several doses if improvement is transient).

For symptomatic bradycardia: add 1 mg (1 mL of a 1:1000 solution) to 500 mL of normal saline, and infuse at 1 µg/minute, titrated to the desired haemodynamic response.

ALPHA-BLOCKERS

Doxazosin, indoramin, terazosin and prazosin have post-synaptic alpha-blocking and vasodilator properties, and may be used with other antihypertensive drugs in the treatment of hypertension. A rapid reduction in blood pressure may be seen after the first dose. Used alone, they may cause tachycardia.

Side effects

Postural hypotension and dizziness are common, as well as headache and oedema.

AMIODARONE (CORDARONE X)

Amiodarone is a potent class III antidysrhythmic agent that exhibits some class II (beta-blocking) properties when given intravenously. It prolongs the duration of the action potential and increases the effective refractory period of both the atria and the ventricles, reflected in QT prolongation. Amiodarone is of value in many different atrial and ventricular dysrhythmias, including re-entry tachycardias. In the UK, amiodarone is licensed for treatment of severe cardiac rhythm disorders where other agents have failed or cannot be used. It should be initiated and monitored under hospital supervision.

During cardiac arrest, amiodarone is indicated in refractory VF/VT following the three initial shocks, and improves short-term survival. It may also be effective in haemodynamically stable ventricular tachycardia and other resistant tachy-dysrhythmias.

Doses

Slow intravenous administration

Amiodarone (150–300 mg) diluted in 10–20 mL of 5% glucose given by slow intravenous injection, over at least 3 minutes. Cardiac monitoring is required as acute haemodynamic effects may occur.

Repeat bolus administration should not be undertaken for at least 15 minutes.

Amiodarone 300 mg should be considered after adrenaline to treat VT/VF cardiac arrest refractory to defibrillation. A further dose of 150 mg followed by infusion can be used.

Infusions

The dose is usually 150–300 mg intravenously (5 mg/kg over 20–120 minutes), followed by intravenous infusion of 900 mg over 24 hours (in 5% dextrose, not saline), to a maximum dose of 2 g/day. Amiodarone may reduce the drop size in certain infusion devices, and the calculated infusion rate may be too slow. Repeated boluses or continuous infusions associate with thrombophlebitis which may be severe. Administration by a central venous line is desirable.

Oral therapy

Oral therapy is usually started at the same time as intravenous treatment, because the half-life of the drug is very long (30–45 days), and oral amiodarone takes about a week for maximal effect. The usual oral loading dose is 200 mg three times daily for 1 week, 200 mg twice daily for 1 week and then 200 mg/day. Normal maintenance is 100–200 mg/day. Some patients require a faster loading rate and higher maintenance doses.

Side effects

Acutely, the drug may be proarrhythmic. Chronic use is limited by side effects that are mostly dose related and time dependent (Shukla et al, 1994). Virtually all are extracardiac:

- Reversible corneal deposits are universal, but are usually asymptomatic. They occasionally produce visual haloes. Optic neuritis is a very rare complication. Patients with visual symptoms should be referred to an ophthalmologist.
- Photosensitivity is very common and, rarely, a bluish discoloration of the skin develops.
- Thyroid dysfunction occurs in 3–4% of patients, and there may also be problems with biochemical analysis of serum thyroid hormone levels.

Thyroid function tests should be carried out before treatment and then every 6 months during therapy. Patients with abnormal thyroid function tests should be referred to hospital for evaluation.

- Interstitial pulmonary fibrosis or pneumonitis may develop insidiously, and can be fatal. Symptoms are similar to those of heart failure, and may be missed. Respiratory side effects are commoner in the elderly and those with prior respiratory disorders. If suspected, the patient should be referred to a chest physician.
- Abnormal liver function tests are common and often transient. Hepatic dysfunction is rare. If abnormalities are severe or persistent, the drug may need to be discontinued.
- Neurological complications may occur in 4–5% of patients. Tremor, ataxia and peripheral neuropathy may occur during the loading phase, but usually disappear at lower doses. A chronic peripheral neuropathy may develop with higher maintenance doses, which may not disappear on stopping the drug. Patients should be referred to a neurologist to exclude other causes of neuropathy.
- Miscellaneous effects include constipation, headache, nausea, fatigue, tremor and nightmares.

Monitoring for toxicity

It should be made clear who is going to monitor for chronic toxicity (primary care or hospital). The patient should also be made aware, and this should be documented in the clinical notes. Thyroid liver and renal function tests should be carried out prior to therapy, as well as a chest radiograph and an electrocardiogram (ECG). Blood tests should be repeated 6-monthly, and a repeat chest radiograph with pulmonary function tests should be carried out if respiratory symptoms develop or worsen.

Interactions

Blood levels of digoxin may be doubled by concurrent use of amiodarone and, if co-prescribed, the dose of digoxin should be halved. The international normalised ratio (INR) should be monitored carefully after starting therapy because of enhanced anti-coagulant activity.

Amiodarone should not be used with other drugs that increase the QT interval, as there is a risk of torsades-de-points.

Drugs that use the cytochrome P450 (CYP3A4) pathway will increase blood levels of amiodarone, predisposing to toxicity. Statins are commonly co-prescribed, and both atorvastatin and simvastatin are metabolised through the same metabolic pathway. In contrast, pravastatin and rosuvastatin are not, and are less likely to cause toxicity.

ANGIOTENSIN–CONVERTING ENZYME (ACE) INHIBITORS

The major product of the renin–angiotensin–aldosterone system (RAAS) is angiotensin II, a potent vasoconstrictor that also stimulates salt and water retention through aldosterone release from the adrenal glands. Angiotensin II is synthesised by the action of angiotensin-converting enzyme (ACE) on angiotensin-I, which in turn derives from a precursor, angiotensinogen, under the influence of renin, a protease enzyme secreted by the kidneys. The major stimulus for renin release is renal hypoperfusion, as may be caused by volume depletion or low cardiac output. Vasoconstriction, mediated by angiotensin-II, helps to maintain blood pressure, while salt and water retention restore plasma volume.

The ACE inhibitors are competitive inhibitors of the angiotensin-converting enzyme, and block the conversion of angiotensin-I to angiotensin-II, relieving vasoconstriction in arteries and veins and producing a fall in blood pressure. In addition, the ACE inhibitors reduce the breakdown of bradykinin (by inhibiting kininase II), another potent vasodilator. In the short term, there are decreased angiotensin-II and aldosterone levels (Fig. 17.1), with decreased secretion of catecholamines at nerve endings and from the adrenal medulla.

With chronic use, there is 'aldosterone escape', and angiotensin-II and aldosterone levels return to pretreatment values, due to activation of alternative synthetic pathways, so the benefits of chronic therapy must be explained by other mechanisms. Inhibition of plasma ACE seems to be less important during chronic therapy, when tissue ACE (in the heart, kidneys and blood vessels)

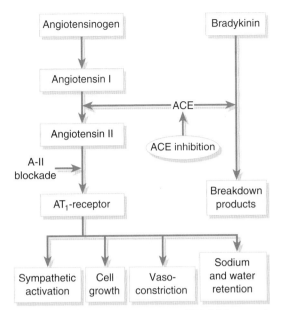

Figure 17.1 Sites of action of the ACE inhibitors and angiotensin-II blockers.

appears to determine the sustained pharmacological effect. The relative affinity for binding to tissue ACE differs with different ACE inhibitors, but no clinical advantage has yet been seen.

Although the ACE inhibitors were originally introduced for the treatment of hypertension, their major role is in the treatment of chronic heart failure (CHF), where they improve symptoms and reduce mortality. In patients with CHF, the RAAS is extremely active, resulting in angiotensin-mediated vasoconstriction with increased sodium and water retention secondary to increased aldosterone secretion, which the ACE inhibitors oppose. The inhibitors also antagonise angiotensin-induced left ventricular hypertrophy, and slow the progression of left ventricular dysfunction. ACE inhibitors started early after myocardial infarction (< 36 hours) will limit left ventricular remodelling and reduce mortality and other serious cardiovascular events, mostly in the first few weeks (ACE Inhibitor Myocardial Infarction Collaborative Group, 1998). In patients with coronary disease and *normal* left ventricular function, treatment with an ACE inhibitor for an average duration of 4.4 years will only prevent one cardiovascular death, one non-fatal infarction or one coronary revascularisation procedure (Al-Mallah et al, 2006).

About 80% of the angiotensin-II is not derived from the circulating RAAS, but from a tissue-bound autocrine/paracrine RAAS, whose primary physiological role appears to be modulation of vascular function and proliferative effects affecting ventricular hypertrophy and remodelling. ACE inhibition helps to improve endothelial function, opposes ventricular hypertrophy and reduces the progression of atherosclerosis. As a result, ACE inhibitors should be used first line when hypertension is associated with high-risk co-morbidities such as heart failure, diabetes or coronary artery disease to reduce the risk of cardiovascular events, even if left ventricular function is normal (Brown & Hall, 2005).

There are nine different ACE inhibitors available in the UK, of which five (captopril, enalapril, lisinopril, trandolapril and ramipril) have good evidence bases for the treatment of heart failure. Despite claims of potential advantages of one compound over another, no clinically significant differences have yet been shown in the treatment of either hypertension or heart failure.

Doses

- Captopril (Capoten, Acepril): 50 mg three times daily.
- Enalapril (Innovace): 20 mg twice daily.
- Lisinopril (Zestril, Carace): 10–20 mg twice daily.
- Ramipril (Tritace): 5 mg twice daily.
- Trandolapril (Gopten, Odrik): 4 mg daily.

Side effects

Rash and cough are frequent (particularly in women), and are the most common reason for stopping therapy. These symptoms probably relate to increased bradykinin levels, and affect up to 10% of patients. Iron supplements may be a simple remedy for the dry cough, and should work within a week. The mechanism is not known. First-dose hypotension is rarely a problem in mild to moderate heart failure, and hospital admission for initiation of therapy is seldom required. A transient (metallic) taste disturbance may occur in 5% of patients. Renal failure and hyperkalaemia are important complications of therapy, particularly in patients treated with concomitant spironolactone.

Some side effects occur with one ACE inhibitor but not another. Patients of African origin appear to be less responsive to ACE inhibitors, and higher doses may be necessary. In hypertension, efficacy is enhanced by co-prescription with diuretics.

ANGIOTENSIN–II RECEPTOR BLOCKERS (ARBs)

The deleterious effects that angiotensin-II produces on blood pressure and cardiovascular remodelling are actually through stimulation of the angiotensin type 1 (AT_1) receptor. Angiotensin receptor blockers selectively block AT_1 receptors and, unlike the ACE inhibitors, block the actions of angiotensin-II, irrespective of the synthetic pathway. In addition, they do not associate with raised bradykinin concentrations, and thereby avoid bradykinin-related cough and angioneurotic oedema (Fig. 17.1). Non-AT_1 receptors remain unblocked, although the benefits of this are not yet clear.

Losartan was licensed for treating hypertension in 1994, and six other members in this class have now been introduced. Individual agents have been used for a wide range of cardiovascular disorders, such as hypertension, stroke, diabetic nephropathy and heart failure. In theory, ARBs should be better than ACE inhibitors, because they block the action of all angiotensin-II produced but, in practice, this has not been confirmed. ARBs differ from other classes of antihypertensive agents, in that no specific side effects have been identified in placebo-controlled trials, and increasing dosages do not appear to increase the likelihood of side effects occurring.

The ARBs have not been shown to be superior to the ACE inhibitors in the treatment of heart failure. Improvements in morbidity (although not mortality) have been seen when candesartan was added to an ACE inhibitor for CHF.

Doses

- Candesarten cilexitil (Amias): 4–16 mg daily.
- Eprosartan (Teveten): 300–600 mg daily.
- Irbesartan (Aprovel): 150–300 mg daily.
- Losartan potassium (Cozaar): 25–100 mg daily.
- Olmesartan medoxomil (Olmetec): 10–40 mg daily.

- Telmisartan (Micardis): 20–40 mg daily.
- Valsartan (Diovan): 40–160 mg daily.

Side effects

These are very few, but include rhinitis, urticaria and myalgia.

ANTIDYSRHYTHMIC AGENTS

Despite great advances in our understanding of the pathogenesis and pharmacological treatment of cardiac dysrhythmias, management is still largely unsatisfactory, and many patients are treated empirically.

Classification of the antidysrhythmic agents

There are many ways of classifying antidysrhythmic drugs, such as the type of rhythm disturbance, the anatomical site of action or their electrophysiological action. This last classification was devised by Vaughan Williams in 1969, based on the actions on isolated myocardium, but it is still used today (Vaughan Williams, 1984). It has many limitations, but does provide many theoretical and practical benefits for a rational approach to the treatment of dysrhythmias. Initial selection of a drug can often be simplified and, should a second agent be required, selection from a different action group is frequently more successful than if an agent from the same group is employed.

There are four classes of drug in the Vaughan Williams classification, based on their *in vitro* effects on the action potentials of normal cardiac cells.

Class I: Membrane-stabilising (local anaesthetic) effect

These agents depress membrane responsiveness and slow myocardial conduction by inhibiting the fast sodium current responsible for phase 0 of the action potential (see Chapter 2). Some drugs depress the rate of depolarisation (phase 4), which reduces automaticity.

The group is subdivided into classes Ia, Ib and Ic on the basis of the overall effect on the action potential. Class Ia drugs moderately prolong it, class Ib drugs slightly shorten it, and class Ic drugs have no effect, but widen the QRS complex.

Class Ia agents

- Disopyramide (Rhythmodan) decreases the firing rate of ectopic pacemakers and lengthens the effective refractory period in atrial and ventricular muscle. It thus has both ventricular and supraventricular activity.
- Quinidine (Kinidin) has been used in the prevention of ventricular tachycardia and fibrillation, but is not commonly used now because it is unpleasant to take (nausea and vomiting) and can cause severe side effects, such as ventricular fibrillation and heart block. An estimated 2–8% of patients develop marked QT prolongation that may precipitate torsades-de-pointes.
- Procainamide (Pronestyl) is derived from the local anaesthetic procaine and is occasionally used in the treatment of ventricular ectopics, ventricular tachycardia and paroxysmal atrial tachycardia. Gastrointestinal side effects are common, and lupus syndrome (SLE) has been described with long-term usage.

Class Ib agents

- Lidocaine (lignocaine) has been used for many years for the control of ventricular dysrhythmias complicating acute myocardial infarction, although amiodarone is now preferred. Lidocaine by infusion may be of value following ventricular fibrillation arrest to prevent recurrence, although the trend these days is to give smaller doses for shorter periods (up to 12 hours) than in the past. The incidence of side effects is then very much reduced, without an apparent increase in further episodes of ventricular fibrillation.
- Mexiletine (Mexitil) is very similar in action to lidocaine, but can also be given orally. It is used in the treatment of ventricular dysrhythmias.
- Phenytoin (Epanutin) is of particular value in ventricular dysrhythmias, especially those that are digitalis induced. This is because it shortens prolonged QT intervals, increases AV nodal conduction and suppresses ventricular ectopic activity. An intravenous dose of 250 mg produces an effect in 5–20 minutes.

Class Ic agents

- Flecainide (Tambocor) is effective in a wide range of chronic dysrhythmias, including atrial fibrillation and re-entry tachycardias. Because it slows conduction through the His–Purkinje system and prevents retrograde conduction through accessory pathways, it is especially valuable in the Wolff–Parkinson–White syndrome.
- Propafenone (Arhythmol) is an oral agent used in the treatment and prophylaxis of supraventricular and ventricular dysrhythmias. It must be given three times daily, which makes it inconvenient. It has a beta-blocker-like action and should be used with care in asthma.

Class II: Beta-blockers (examples: propranolol, bisoprolol, atenolol)

These drugs block catecholamine stimulation of the myocardial cells which might induce cardiac dysrhythmias. There is relatively little effect on heart rate and contractility at rest, but they slow the heart and decrease contractility when the sympathetic nervous system is activated, for example during exertion or stress. Beta-blockers also produce direct membrane-stabilising effects, similar to those of class I drugs. The refractory period in the AV node is increased, and the discharge rate of ectopic pacemakers is slowed.

Class III: Drugs prolonging repolarisation (examples: amiodarone, sotalol)

The major action of these drugs is to prolong the duration of the action potential, with consequent lengthening of the effective refractory period. The membrane responsiveness, conduction velocity and rate of rise of the action potential in phase 0 are not affected. They suppress ventricular ectopic activity, ventricular tachycardia and ventricular fibrillation.

Class IV: Calcium channel blockade of the SA and AV nodes (examples: verapamil, diltiazem)

These agents inhibit the slow inward calcium current and depress phases 2 and 3 (plateau phase) of the action potential. These actions are of particular importance in the upper part of the AV node and will block circus movements during re-entry tachycardias.

Adverse effects are common in all antidysrhthmic drugs, including proarrhythmia, brady-dysrhythmias and negative inotropic effects.

Proarrhythmic activity may vary from increasing ectopic beats to causing life-threatening dysrhythmias. Most antidysrhythmic drugs may potentially cause abnormalities of cardiac rhythm, even when the underlying rhythm disturbance is benign. The CAST Investigators (1989) showed that post-infarction patients were more likely to die if treated with certain antidysrhythmic agents than with placebo, an effect attributed to the pro-arrhythmic effect of the agents used.

Brady-dysrhythmias often occur because of effects on the AV and sino-atrial (SA) nodes, and are more common where there is underlying disease of the conducting tissue.

Negative inotropic effects occur by various mechanisms and are most marked in patients with known left ventricular dysfunction.

ASPIRIN

Aspirin irreversibly blocks the enzyme *cyclo-oxygenase*, and reduces the synthesis of various prostanoids, including *thromboxane A_2*, a potent vasoconstrictor and platelet aggregant. The beneficial dose is in the range of 75–300 mg daily. This effectively inhibits the ability of the blood platelets to synthesise thromboxane A_2 during their lifespan in the circulation of 7–10 days, and is responsible for their antithrombotic effect.

Aspirin is a safe and worthwhile intervention in the primary prevention of cardiovascular disease at a 10-year event risk of 15%, but is unhelpful and/or unsafe at a lesser risk (Sanmuganathan et al, 2001). Aspirin is recommended in all people with established atherosclerotic disease, and produces significant reduction in all-cause mortality, vascular mortality, non-fatal reinfarction of the myocardium and non-fatal stroke in people with unstable angina, acute myocardial infarction, stroke, transient ischaemic attacks (TIAs) or other clinical evidence of vascular disease (Anti-thrombotic Trialists' Collaboration, 2002). Following acute myocardial infarction, aspirin reduces the risk of subsequent

non-fatal myocardial infarction, reinfarction, stroke and cardiovascular death by up to 25%. In patients with unstable angina, it reduces the risk of myocardial infarction by at least 50%, and may also be used to reduce the risk of graft occlusion in those who have undergone coronary artery bypass grafting.

'Disprin CV' is aspirin specifically designed for cardiovascular disease. This formulation is micro-encapsulated for sustained release, and does not cause as much gastrointestinal upset, reducing blood loss by half in comparison with standard aspirin. It is, of course, more expensive and no more effective. The 100-mg formulation is recommended for prevention for coronary graft occlusion, while the 300-mg size is used for the other cardiovascular indications (TIA, post-myocardial infarction, unstable angina, etc.).

Dose

The dose is 75–325 mg/day for acute myocardial infarction; an initial loading dose of at least 150 mg should be chewed rather than swallowed whole to ensure rapid absorption. This is particularly important prior to thrombolysis. Doses of under 150 mg associate with fewer gastrointestinal side effects.

Side effects

True aspirin allergy is rare, but hypersensitivity may cause bronchospasm. The risk of a major gastrointestinal bleed is increased by about 1 in 250 patient–years even with low-dose or modified release aspirin. The beneficial antithrombotic effects of aspirin generally outweigh the adverse effects, and use in at-risk patients is strongly advised (JBS-2, 2005).

ATROPINE

Atropine is an acetylcholine antagonist that gives rise to parasympathetic blockade. It thus reverses effects on heart rate, systemic vascular resistance and blood pressure mediated by parasympathetic (vagal) activity. Atropine may be useful for treating symptomatic sinus bradycardia and heart block, which often occurs within 6 hours of acute myocardial infarction related to ischaemia or reperfusion (Bezold–Jarish reflex). High or repetitive doses of atropine should be avoided following acute myocardial infarction, because increased parasympathetic tone protects against ventricular fibrillation. Small doses should be used to achieve minimally effective heart rate, to a maximum dose of 3.0 mg. Doses of less than 0.5 mg occasionally elicit a paradoxical slowing of heart rate (Dauchot & Gravenstein, 1971).

Atropine blocks the effect of the vagus nerve on both the SA node and the AV node, increasing sinus automaticity and facilitating AV node conduction. Because cardiac arrest caused by asystole is a condition that could be exacerbated or precipitated by excessive vagal tone, atropine is given at a dose that will provide maximum vagal blockade (3 mg). It is also recommended if there is pulseless electrical activity (PEA) with a ventricular rate of less than 60 beats/minute.

Dose

A dose of 0.5 mg is given intravenously for bradycardia with symptoms (doses under 0.5 mg may worsen the bradycardia). A single dose of 3 mg is for cardiac arrest (asystole or PEA).

Side effects

Dry mouth, confusion, tachycardia and urinary retention.

BETA-ADRENERGIC BLOCKING AGENTS

Beta-blockers antagonise the effects of catecholamines by competitively occupying both alpha- and beta-adrenergic receptors.

- *Alpha-receptors* are associated with most of the usual adrenergic excitatory functions, such as vasoconstriction and dilatation of the pupils. Stimulation is excitatory in the heart, causing positive inotropic and chronotropic effects.
- *Beta-receptors* are usually inhibitory, resulting in vasodilatation (inhibition of vasoconstriction) and bronchodilatation (inhibition of bronchial constriction).

The heart and the bronchi have only beta-receptors (beta-1 receptors are cardiac, and beta-2 receptors are bronchial), and blockade of the cardiac sites reduces heart rate (particularly exercise-related tachycardia), myocardial contractility and systemic blood pressure.

The various mechanisms of action on the cardiovascular system are not fully understood, and probably vary within the group. Important effects of beta-blockers include:

- Antihypertensive action associated with a decrease in cardiac output and blockade of alpha-adrenoreceptors, producing peripheral vasodilatation. In addition, release of renin, angiotensin-II and aldosterone is reduced by blockade of beta$_1$-adrenoceptors on renal juxtaglomerular cells.
- Anti-ischaemic actions produced by reducing the heart rate, cardiac contractility, systolic blood pressure, leading to reducing oxygen consumption. In addition, by lowering the heart rate, the time for coronary flow is increased by prolongation of diastole, improving myocardial perfusion.
- Antidysrhythmic effect produced by slowing the heart rate, decreasing spontaneous firing of ectopic pacemakers, slowing conduction and increasing the refractory period of the AV node.
- Beta-blockers may also reduce the likelihood of an acute coronary syndrome by an antiplatelet effect, inhibition of vascular smooth muscle cell proliferation and reduction in the mechanical stress imposed on vulnerable plaques, preventing rupture.

The different beta-blockers have differing pharmacological properties (Table 17.1) that may affect choice.

Half-life

Unlike the plasma half-life, the pharmacological half-life depends on the dose. Most beta-blockers can be prescribed twice daily, providing a big enough dose is given. Hydrophilic agents have longer plasma half-lives, and may usually be taken once daily. Esmolol hydrochloride is a cardiospecific beta-blocker with a very short duration of action, which may be used in the treatment

Table 17.1 Properties of beta–adrenoceptor blocking drugs.

Generic name	Cardioselectivity	Intrinsic sympathomimetic activity	Membrane-stabilising activity	Potency (propranolol = 1)	Eliminating half-life (h)	Predominant route of elimination	Lipophilicity
Acebutolol	+	+	+	0.3	3–4	Renal	Low
Atenolol	+	0	0	1.0	6–9	Renal	Low
Labetalol	0	0	0	0.3	3–4	Hepatic	Low
Metoprolol	+	0	0	1.0	3–4	Hepatic	Moderate
Nadolol	0	0	0	1.0	14–24	Renal	Low
Oxprenolol	0	++	+	0.5–1.0	2–3	Hepatic	Moderate
Pindolol	0	+++	+	6.0	3–4	Renal (40%)	Moderate
						Hepatic	
Propranolol	0	0	++	1.0	3–4	Hepatic	High
Sotalol	0	0	0	0.3	8–10	Renal	Low
Timolol	0	0	0	6.0–8.0	4–5	Renal (20%)	Low
						Hepatic	

0, no effect; +, small effect; ++, moderate effect; +++, strong effect.

of supraventricular tachycardias, sinus tachycardia and hypertension, especially postoperatively.

Cardioselectivity

Beta-blockers differ in their relative affinity for beta-1 or beta-2 sites. Timolol, propranolol and sotalol act on both sites and are termed 'non-specific'. However, atenolol, bisoprolol, metoprolol and nebivolol act predominantly on the beta-1 cardiac sites, and are therefore termed 'cardioselective'. Cardioselectivity is relative and is lost at high doses. No beta-blocker is completely safe in patients with asthma (Salpeter et al, 2003).

Intrinsic sympathomimetic activity

Intrinsic sympathomimetic activity (ISA) implies that the drug partially stimulates the beta-sites, and thus reduces the degree of cardiodepression. Oxprenolol, acebutolol and celiprolol all have ISA, but it is doubtful whether this confers any advantages.

Lipid solubility

The pharmacokinetics of beta-blockers depends in part upon whether they are soluble in fat (lipophilic) or water (hydrophilic).

Lipophilic agents (e.g. propranolol, metoprolol, timolol) are well absorbed orally and have a short half-life. Variation in oral bioavailability is largely influenced by 'first-pass' metabolism of lipid-soluble compounds by the liver and gut wall, so oral bioavailability of lipophilic agents is low. In addition, lipophilic beta-blockers may accumulate in patients with reduced hepatic blood flow (e.g. elderly, chronic heart failure, cirrhosis) and cause toxicity. Lipophilic beta-blockers can cross the blood–brain barrier and may be responsible for central nervous system side effects (e.g. nightmares). Alcohol, phenytoin, rifampicin and smoking induce hepatic enzymes and decrease the plasma concentrations and elimination half-lives of lipophilic beta-blockers.

Hydrophilic beta-blockers such as atenolol, celiprolol, esmolol and sotalol are not so well absorbed orally, and most are excreted unchanged by the kidneys, so care is required in patients with renal impairment. They have a long plasma half-life,

do not easily cross the blood–brain barrier and are thus less likely to associate with sleep disturbance and nightmares.

Balanced clearance drugs are excreted by both the liver and the kidneys (e.g. bisoprolol, carvedilol). Esmolol is an ultrashort-acting intravenous drug that is rapidly hydrolysed by red cell esterases (half-life 9 min).

Vasodilating beta–blockers

Several beta-blockers have peripheral vasodilator activity mediated via a1-adrenoceptor blockade (carvedilol, labetalol), beta 2-adrenergic receptor agonism (celiprolol) or via mechanisms independent of the adrenoreceptor blockade (nebivolol).

Side effects

Common side effects include bradycardia, heart failure, bronchospasm, nightmares, insomnia, depression and peripheral coldness. Cold extremities are caused by unopposed alpha-adrenergic action and partly as a result of a fall in cardiac output. Central nervous system side effects are common with beta-blockers that cross the blood–brain barrier (lipid-soluble agents), especially propranolol. These may produce sedation, depression and nightmares. Beta-blockers adversely affect serum lipid profiles, although this may not be so marked in agents with ISA (Jowett & Galton, 1987). Chronic obstructive pulmonary disease and peripheral vascular disease are not absolute contraindications to beta-blocker therapy, and high-risk cardiac patients may derive greater benefits from beta-blockade even if they suffer from these co-morbidities (Heintzen & Strauer, 1994; Andrus et al, 2004).

Sudden withdrawal of beta–blockade

Following sudden withdrawal of beta-blockade, there may be an increase in both the number and the availability of beta-receptor sites (upregulation). Increased sensitivity to catecholamines causes an increase in myocardial work, heart rate and oxygen consumption. Angina, hypertension or even myocardial infarction may result. Patients should be warned of the dangers of suddenly stopping medication, because of this rebound effect. Beta-blockade should always be reduced slowly.

Therapeutic uses

Apart from treatment of hypertension, the major role of beta-blockers is in the treatment of stable angina, where 90% of patients will have improved exercise tolerance and reduced chest pain. Beta-blockers also have class II antidysrhythmic activity, and are recommended for the treatment of supraventricular tachycardias and in atrial fibrillation to control heart rate, to revert atrial fibrillation to sinus rhythm and to maintain sinus rhythm. Beta-blockers are effective in the control of ventricular dysrhythmias related to sympathetic activation, including stress-induced dysrhythmias (including ectopic beats), acute coronary syndromes, heart failure and for the prevention of sudden cardiac death. Sotalol has additional class III antidysrhythmic activity at high doses (> 160 mg/day).

Beta-blockers are contraindicated in dysrhythmias associated with Wolff–Parkinson–White syndrome, as they have no effect on the accessory pathway and may encourage rapid ventricular rates. They are also contraindicated in patients with the bradycardia/tachycardia syndrome, as sinus arrest with syncope may occur.

Beta-blockers reduce catecholamine concentrations in ischaemic myocardium, decrease platelet stickiness and have been shown to modify type A behaviour.

Beta–blockers and acute myocardial infarction

Beta-blockers should be given to all patients during the acute phase of an acute coronary syndrome, unless there are definite contraindications.

Intravenous administration should be considered in patients with ischaemic pain resistant to opiates, recurrent ischaemia and for the control of hypertension, tachycardia and dysrhythmias. They will limit infarct size, reduce life-threatening arrhythmias, relieve pain and reduce mortality including sudden cardiac death. Acute administration of beta-blockers should not be used if there is hypotension or heart failure.

Oral beta-blockers are recommended for indefinite long-term use in all patients who recover from an acute coronary syndrome to reduce morbidity and mortality (Freemantle et al, 1999). Patients at highest risk of further cardiac events are often denied beta-blocker therapy, but benefit most. This group includes those with large and anterior infarcts, those with heart failure, the elderly and those with diabetes. It is not known whether all beta-blockers are valuable for cardioprotection. Reduction in heart rate seems to be important, which is possibly why using beta-blockers with intrinsic sympathomimetic activity (e.g. pindolol and oxprenolol) does not confer benefit. Oral treatment with agents licensed for prophylaxis should be started when the patient is haemodynamically stable, and continued for at least 2–3 years if tolerated. The evidence for continuation of beta-blockers beyond 2–3 years after myocardial infarction is not clear, but most physicians would continue the drug indefinitely.

Patients with chronic, stable angina also benefit from therapy with beta-blockers. Apart from symptom relief, they also prevent infarction and improve survival.

Beta–blockers and cardiac failure

There is substantial evidence for the beneficial role of beta-blockers in heart failure. Metoprolol, bisoprolol and carvedilol all reduce mortality and morbidity in patients with stable New York Heart Association (NYHA) class II and class III systolic heart failure (McMurray, 1999). Nebivolol is a long-acting, cardioselective beta-blocker that is an effective and well-tolerated treatment for heart failure in the elderly (Flather et al, 2005). Metoprolol is not licensed for heart failure in the UK.

All patients with stable chronic heart failure from ischaemic or non-ischaemic cardiomyopathies in NYHA classes II–IV should be treated with beta-blockers, unless there is a contraindication. In addition, in patients with left ventricular systolic dysfunction, with or without symptomatic heart failure following acute myocardial infarction, long-term treatment is recommended in addition to ACE inhibition to reduce mortality. The beta-blockers should be started at very low doses and titrated up every 2–4 weeks to target doses, providing the heart failure remains stable (Table 17.2).

Table 17.2 Doses of beta-blockers used in heart failure.

Drug	Starting dose	Target dose
Bisoprolol	1.25 mg od	10 mg od
Carvedilol	3.125 mg bd	25 mg bd[a]
Nebivolol	1.25 mg od	10 mg od

a For patients weighing over 85 kg, without severe heart failure, the dose may be titrated up to 50 mg bd.

The response to beta-blockade is often biphasic, with improvement often preceded by an initial worsening of symptoms. Uptitration should be adapted to the patient's individual response.

BIVALIRUDIN (ANGIOX)

Bivalirudin is a direct, specific and reversible inhibitor of thrombin, used as an anticoagulant in patients undergoing percutaneous coronary intervention (PCI). It may be used instead of heparin and glycoprotein IIb/IIIa receptor inhibitors to decrease the risk of acute ischaemic complications during PCI, and associates with less bleeding.

Dose

Initially *by intravenous injection*, 750 μg/kg, then *by intravenous infusion* of 1.75 mg/kg/h, for up to 4 hours after PCI.

Side effects

Bleeding, nausea, vomiting, tachycardia, bradycardia, hypotension, angina, dyspnoea, headache.

CALCIUM CHLORIDE

Calcium ions can cause the asystolic heart to beat, as well as strengthening contractility. They may also counteract the effect of hyperkalaemia. However, routine administration of calcium salts during cardiopulmonary resuscitation is no longer recommended, as calcium may cause coronary and cerebral vasospasm, as well as increasing ventricular irritability in patients taking digoxin.

Small doses may be useful for cardiac arrest complicated by hypocalcaemia or hyperkalaemia, or for patients on high doses of calcium channel-blocking agents (e.g. nifedipine, verapamil or nicardipine). Calcium may be of value in the treatment of PEA, especially if the QRS complex is widened.

Dose

The dose is 10 mL of 10% calcium chloride solution by slow intravenous injection. Calcium can slow the heart rate and precipitate rhythm disturbances. In cardiac arrest, calcium may be given by rapid intravenous injection.

Side effects

Sudden death may occur if the patient is taking digoxin. Intramuscular or subcutaneous administration can cause tissue necrosis.

CALCIUM CHANNEL-BLOCKING AGENTS

Calcium channel-blocking agents interfere with the inward displacement of calcium ions through the slow channels of active cell membranes. They act on myocardial cells, the cells within the specialised conducting system of the heart, and the cells of vascular smooth muscle. This results in reduced myocardial contractility, inhibition of conduction and vasodilatation.

There are three main groups of calcium channel-blocking agents:

- dihydropyridines (e.g. nifedipine, amlodipine, nicardipine);
- phenylalkylamines (e.g. verapamil);
- benzthiazepines (e.g. diltiazem).

Calcium channel-blockers differ in their predilection for the various possible sites of action and, therefore, have differing therapeutic effects (Table 17.3). Different agents are therefore used in the treatment of hypertension, angina and supraventricular dysrhythmias.

Dihydropyridines

Nifedipine reduces peripheral and coronary vascular resistance. It has a mild negative inotropic effect,

Table 17.3 Cardiovascular effects of the calcium channel blockers.

	Verapamil	Diltiazem	Amlodipine
Heart rate	Reduced	Reduced	No effect
AV node conduction	Reduced	Reduced	No effect
Myocardial contractility	Marked reduction	Reduced	No effect
Peripheral vasodilatation	Increased	Increased	Marked increase

which is usually offset by increasing sympathetic activity secondary to its vasodilator effect. Amlodipine, nicardipine and isradipine are similar, although cardiodepression is not so marked.

Phenylalkylamines

The most striking effect of verapamil is on AV nodal conduction, making it very useful for the treatment of supraventricular tachycardias. Following an intravenous injection (5–10 mg), AV conduction is quickly reduced, and re-entry tachycardias at the AV node are terminated. Orally, it is not so effective, because much is metabolised by the liver.

If given to a patient taking beta-blockers, verapamil may cause profound hypotension, bradycardia or asystole. Verapamil is useful for controlling the ventricular rate in atrial fibrillation and atrial flutter, with or without digoxin. It is contraindicated in atrial fibrillation complicating the Wolff–Parkinson–White syndrome, as it gives rise to preferentially accessory conduction, which may result in ventricular fibrillation.

Dose

The recommended dose is 5–10 mg intravenously over 2–3 minutes, which may be repeated after 30 minutes. Asystole may result if the patient is taking beta-blockers. Oral therapy is 40–120 mg three times a day. Higher doses are required for the treatment of angina (40–120 mg three times daily) and hypertension (120–240 mg twice daily).

Benzthiazepines

Diltiazem inhibits transmission in cardiac conducting tissue and gives rise to a mild resting bradycardia. It vasodilates coronary arteries and peripheral arteries. While it is used predominantly in the treatment of angina, it may also be used in higher doses for hypertension. In patients without cardiac failure, once-daily long-acting diltiazem can be used following acute myocardial infarction where beta-blockers are contraindicated. It may then reduce recurrent ischaemia and the need for coronary revascularisation (Purcell & Fox, 2001). Diltiazem is useful in the prophylaxis of recurrent supraventricular tachycardia, and is useful in controlling the ventricular rate in patients with atrial fibrillation, with or without digoxin.

Side effects of calcium channel blockers

Vasodilator effects (flushing, headache and dizziness) sometimes occur at the start of therapy, and these are most pronounced with nifedipine. Fluid retention is common, often resulting in ankle oedema. Verapamil can produce constipation and also reduces digoxin excretion. If these two drugs are given together, the dose of digoxin should be halved. Diltiazem appears to produce fewer side effects than the other calcium blockers, as it has less effect on the heart than verapamil and less effect on the peripheral vessels than nifedipine.

CLOPIDOGREL (PLAVIX)

Clopidogrel is an antiplatelet agent used as an alternative to aspirin to prevent thromboembolic events (CAPRIE Steering Committee, 1996). Clopidogrel is a potent and irreversible adenosine diphosphate (ADP) receptor antagonist that inhibits ADP-induced platelet aggregation. For patients presenting to hospital with an acute coronary syndrome, clopidogrel (300 mg bolus followed by 75 mg daily) should be given in addition to aspirin (Walsh et al, 2005). Combination treatment should be continued for 12 months. Benefits occur as early as 2 hours following an oral loading dose of 300 mg, and thus aspirin 300 mg plus clopidogrel 300 mg should be given immediately to all patients with chest pain suspected of being of cardiac origin. The drugs may be discontinued if the diagnosis was subsequently not cardiac.

After percutaneous coronary intervention (PCI) with bare metal stent implantation, clopidogrel is given with aspirin for 4 weeks. Because drug-eluting stents delay endothelialisation of the struts, aspirin and clopidogrel should be continued for at least 12 months. If bypass surgery is planned, clopidogrel should be discontinued at least 5 days before surgery.

There is no value in adding clopidogrel to aspirin in patients with either clinically evident cardiovascular disease or multiple risk factors unless there has been an acute coronary event (Bhatt et al, 2006).

Dose

The dose is 75 mg daily.

Side effects

Similar to aspirin. Clopidogrel monotherapy has a superior gastrointestinal safety profile to aspirin monotherapy.

COLCHICINE

Colchicine is used to terminate an attack of acute gout. While very effective, gastrointestinal symptoms, including nausea, vomiting and especially diarrhoea, are very common. However, because gout usually complicates the treatment of heart failure, non-steroidal drugs cannot be given, and colchicine is a very good drug for terminating the attack. Colchicine is also of value in recurrent pericarditis.

Dose

The dose is 1 mg orally, and then 0.5 mg every 2–3 hours until the pain subsides (or vomiting and diarrhoea occur). The dose should be reduced in renal failure.

Side effects

Gastrointestinal and, rarely, bone marrow suppression.

DIGOXIN (LANOXIN)

Digoxin increases the force of myocardial contraction and exerts a slowing of conduction at the sinus and AV nodes. Therapeutic doses cause shortening of the QT interval, and flattening (or inversion) of the T waves with ST segment sag. False-positive ST changes may develop during exercise stress testing.

The principal use of digoxin is for controlling the ventricular rate in atrial fibrillation, especially when it occurs with heart failure. Digoxin has an acute positive inotropic effect, although whether this is maintained chronically is debatable. It is of little value in cases of high-output failure, cor pulmonale and restrictive cardiomyopathy. Long-term use in congestive heart failure without rhythm disturbance is controversial, and many patients in sinus rhythm remain well after therapy with digoxin is discontinued. In patients with thyrotoxicosis, very large doses, often supplemented with propranolol, may be required to slow the ventricular rate.

Digoxin following myocardial infarction

The role of digoxin in acute myocardial infarction is controversial. In patients with left ventricular failure following acute myocardial infarction, digoxin is effective, but concern surrounds the increased myocardial work caused by the positive inotropic effect of the drug, which may extend the area of myocardial necrosis. Beneficial haemodynamic effects are greatest in patients with moderate left ventricular failure, and the risk of extending myocardial damage is probably least in these patients. Post-infarction survival in patients with congestive heart failure and with multifocal ventricular ectopics may be improved by withholding or discontinuing digoxin.

Doses

Digoxin is very irritant to the tissues and should only be given orally or intravenously. Oral digoxin is rapidly and almost entirely absorbed. A loading dose is required at approximately 15 µg/kg in divided doses, with a maintenance dose of about 5 µg/kg in those with normal renal function. Digitalisation will take about 1 week if no loading dose is given. Effects are not directly correlated with blood levels of the drug because of variable protein binding, penetration and uptake by the myocardium and other factors. It is primarily metabolised by the kidneys within 2–3 days, but may accumulate in renal impairment. In some patients, digoxin is inactivated by gut flora, necessitating large oral doses to achieve satisfactory blood levels. If these patients are given broad-spectrum antibiotics that affect the gut flora, digoxin toxicity may be precipitated.

Where there is uncertainty, assessment of blood levels is helpful, although levels should not be measured within 6 hours of the last oral dose.

Digoxin toxicity

A major drawback to treatment with digoxin is the narrow margin between therapeutic doses and toxicity. Hence, adverse drug actions are very common, and many patients show toxicity at some time. Therapeutic levels are quoted as 0.5–2.5 ng/mL, but the diagnosis of digoxin toxicity is clinical, and too much reliance should not be placed on laboratory results. For example, digoxin toxicity can occur within the therapeutic range if there is concomitant electrolyte upsets, thyroid disease, renal impairment or hypoxia. Patients with blood levels >2.5 ng/mL may display no signs of toxicity.

The early symptoms of overdose are nausea, vomiting and diarrhoea. Headache and confusion, often with visual disturbances, are more serious. Classically, *xanthopsia* (yellow vision) is reported, but flickering dots, haloes and scotomata are more frequent visual symptoms. Digoxin toxicity can produce any rhythm disturbance, including ventricular fibrillation. More often, there are ventricular ectopics (especially ventricular bigeminy), sinus bradycardia, heart block and paroxysmal atrial tachycardia with block. The ECG usually shows other signs of toxicity such as ST/T wave changes or increased PR interval.

Treatment of toxicity

If stopping digoxin is inadequate, potassium supplementation is very effective, even in the absence of hypokalaemia. Propranolol (2 mg intravenously) is especially useful for supraventricular dysrhythmias, and phenytoin, amiodarone and lidocaine are effective in digitalis-induced ventricular dysrhythmias. Digibind (antidigoxin antibody fragments) can be used in serious cases (Jowett, 2002).

In the case of digoxin-related brady-dysrhythmias, potassium supplements should be stopped, because they potentiate heart block. Symptomatic bradycardias may require intravenous atropine, isoprenaline or even temporary cardiac pacing.

DIPYRIDAMOLE (PERSANTIN)

Dipyridamole inhibits ADP-induced platelet aggregation. It is often used as an adjunct to aspirin, and to oral anticoagulation in patients with prosthetic heart valves to prevent emboli. Dipyridamole is sometimes used to increase coronary perfusion during nuclear scanning, where it diverts blood away from areas of poor perfusion (dipyridamole–sestamibi stress test).

The combination of dipyridamole and aspirin is recommended for secondary prevention following ischaemic stroke or a TIA for a period of 2 years (NICE, 2005).

Dose

The dose is 300–600 mg/day in three or four divided doses. A modified release (MR) preparation is available.

Side effects

Dipyridamole may worsen coronary ischaemia, and interacts with adenosine to produce an enhanced effect.

DIURETICS

Loop diuretics (furosemide, bumetanide, torasemide)

Loop diuretics inhibit reabsorption from the ascending limb of the loop of Henlé in the renal tubule and are powerful diuretics. When given intravenously for left ventricular failure, symptom relief is almost immediate and occurs before a diuresis has taken place. This suggests that the primary value in acute heart failure is due to a vascular effect causing increased venous capacitance, and that the diuretic effect is secondary. The diuresis starts within a few minutes of intravenous administration, reaching a maximum within 15–30 minutes, and the effect is proportional to the dose. Orally, loop diuretics act within 1 hour, and the diuresis is complete within 6 hours. Bumetanide has a shorter diuresis that continues for about 3–4 hours. One milligram of bumetanide is about equivalent to 40–60 mg of furosemide but, at high doses, direct comparison of doses is not possible. In patients with impaired renal function, very large doses may occasionally be needed.

Side effects

Transient or permanent deafness may result if furosemide is injected too rapidly, particularly in those with renal impairment. Large doses must be diluted, and intravenous infusion is then a preferable method of administration. Potassium depletion, myalgia and cramps, and skin rashes are commoner side effects.

Thiazides

Thiazides inhibit sodium reabsorption at the beginning of the distal convoluted tubule. They have a slower onset (1–2 hours) and a more prolonged action (12–24 hours).

Bendroflumethiazide (bendrofluazide) is probably the most widely used drug, usually prescribed for hypertension. A dose of 2.5 mg daily produces a maximal or near-maximal blood pressure-lowering effect at 24 hours, with very little biochemical disturbance. Higher doses cause more marked changes in plasma potassium, sodium, uric acid, glucose and lipids, with little advantage in blood pressure control. *Indapamide* is said to lower blood pressure with less metabolic disturbance. *Chlortalidone* (chlorthalidone) has a longer duration of action than the thiazides and may be given on alternate days to control oedema.

Other thiazide diuretics (e.g. *cyclopenthiazide*, *hydrochlorothiazide* and *hydroflumethiazide*) do not offer any significant advantage over bendroflumethiazide and chlortalidone.

Metolazone is particularly effective when combined with a loop diuretic (even in renal failure), and may be used in resistant heart failure. A profound diuresis may result, and patients should be monitored carefully, usually on an inpatient basis.

Side effects

Hypokalaemia may occur with both thiazide and loop diuretics, but is more frequent with thiazides. Hypokalaemia should be avoided in patients with coronary artery disease, particularly in those taking digoxin. Many patients will be taking ACE inhibitors, which will conserve potassium, but others may need potassium-sparing diuretics or potassium supplements.

Potassium–sparing diuretics

Amiloride and *triamterene* are weak diuretics that act directly on the distal renal tubules. Diuresis occurs over 24 hours, but full activity may be delayed for 2–3 days. These drugs are seldom prescribed alone, and are usually co-prescribed with loop diuretics to prevent hypokalaemia. They should be used with great care in renal failure or when used with potassium supplements. Serum potassium must be closely monitored.

Aldosterone antagonists

Spironolactone (Aldactone) is an aldosterone antagonist and potassium-sparing diuretic. It also reduces cardiac fibrosis in both acute and chronic heart failure, and improves left ventricular function (Pitt et al, 1999). Spironolactone 25 mg should be added to standard therapy with a diuretic, ACE inhibitor and beta-blocker in patients with NYHA class III or IV heart failure with severe left ventricular systolic dysfunction (ejection fraction of no more than 35%).

Eplerinone (Inspra) is an aldosterone blocker but, unlike spironolactone, it selectively blocks the mineralocorticoid receptor, but not the glucocorticoid, androgen and progesterone receptors, thus reducing side effects, particularly gynaecomastia.

Aldosterone blockade helps to prevent ventricular remodelling following acute myocardial infarction (Struthers, 2005), and reduces cardiovascular morbidity and mortality in post-infarct patients with diabetes, overt heart failure or an ejection fraction under 40% (Pitt et al, 2003).

Because eplerinone is co-administered with an ACE inhibitor or ARB, there is a major risk of significant hyperkalaemia, particularly in those with impaired renal function, such as those aged 65 years or older. Close monitoring of serum potassium and renal function is needed.

More than half of the deaths avoided with eplerinone treatment in the EPHESUS trial were in the first 30 days, but benefits do continue in the longer term (Pitt et al, 2005). Patients should be reassessed after no longer than 12 months, with a view to either discontinuation or a switch to spironolactone, which is much cheaper.

Doses

Initiate at 25 mg once daily and, if the serum potassium concentration is below 5.0 mmol/L, titrate to the recommended target dose of 50 mg once daily within 4 weeks provided the serum potassium concentration remains below 5.5 mmol/L.

FISH OIL SUPPLEMENTS (MAXEPA, OMACOR)

Eating oily fish reduces mortality due to coronary heart disease, and several trials have shown a benefit of fish and fish oil supplements on coronary heart disease, particularly after myocardial infarction (Din et al, 2004). EPA (eicosapentaenoic acid) and DHA (docosahexaenoic acid) are essential polyunsaturated fatty acids that are part of the omega-3 family necessary for prostaglandin synthesis, and oily fish is the best source. Patients should consume about 1 g/day of EPA and DHA, by increasing their intake of oily fish to at least two servings per week, but fish oil supplements may be considered for those unable to tolerate fish or change their diet effectively.

Omacor capsules contain purified omega-3-acid esters with 46% EPA and 38% DHA, and are licensed for the treatment of hypertriglyceridaemia and secondary prevention after myocardial infarction. Omega-3 fatty acids have several potentially cardioprotective effects, although the relative contribution of each of these is not fully understood. Possible mechanisms include effects on the atherosclerotic process (anti-inflammatory, antithrombosis or improved endothelial function), effects on blood pressure and triglyceride levels or perhaps an antidysrhythmic effect.

Maxepa capsules are natural triglyceride marine concentrates containing 1 g of concentrated fish oils (18% EPA and 12% DHA), and are used for the treatment of hypertriglyceridaemia.

It should be noted that 'fish oil capsules' in health shops are not made of free-living fish, but mainly of farmed fish. Food for farmed fish contains grains and other starchy foods, and these fish oil capsules deliver large amounts of n-6 fatty acids. Omega-3 fats provide little, if any, benefit if there are excessive dietary omega-6 fats. Chronic excessive ingestion of omega-6 EFAs associates with heart attacks, thrombotic stroke, dysrhythmias and cancer. Furthermore, coronary heart disease mortality has been demonstrated to be proportional to plasma levels of omega-6 fatty acids (Lands, 2005).

Dose

Omacor capsules: 1–2/day; Maxepa capsules: 5 twice daily.

Side effects

These are mostly gastrointestinal.

GLYCOPROTEIN (GP) IIB/IIIA RECEPTOR ANTAGONISTS

These agents block the fibrinogen receptor on the surface of activated platelets, inhibiting platelet aggregation and reducing the risk of arterial thrombosis. They are more potent than other currently available antiplatelet drugs (e.g. aspirin), with an almost immediate onset of action when given intravenously.

Abciximab (ReoPro) is a monoclonal antibody that binds irreversibly to the GP IIb/IIIa receptor, prolonging platelet aggregation. It is not receptor specific and may affect other vascular receptors. It is indicated as an adjunct to aspirin and heparin for the prevention of ischaemic complications in patients during PCI, especially following an acute coronary syndrome. It is expensive, with the cost per course ranging from £840 to £1120, depending on the duration of treatment.

Eptifibatide (Integrilin) and *tirofiban (Aggrastat)* are synthetic 'small-molecule' GP IIb/IIIa inhibitors that reversibly inhibit binding to the GP IIb/IIIa receptor. They are not so expensive at around £500 per treatment.

The GP IIb/IIIa inhibitors are generally well tolerated, although bleeding is a major complication, usually at the puncture site. They are administered by initial bolus, followed by infusion over 12–96 hours because of their short half-lives. Abciximab acts for much longer, and thus only needs a 12-hours infusion. They are given in combination with aspirin and heparin.

The glycoprotein inhibitors are of benefit in high-risk acute coronary syndromes in the prevention of death and myocardial infarction at 30 days, but are of greatest benefit in those undergoing PCI. NICE (2002) guidance currently advises intravenous glycoprotein inhibitors with heparin and aspirin in high-risk acute coronary syndromes, as well as during emergency or elective PCI. Diabetic patients derive particular benefit from glycoprotein inhibitors.

Doses

- *Abciximab.* An initial intravenous bolus dose of 250 µg/kg body weight started within an hour of PCI followed by a maintenance dose of 0.125 µg/kg/minutes (maximum 10 µg/minutes) over 12 hours. In unstable angina, therapy may start up to 12 hours before PCI and continue for 36 hours after PCI.
- *Eptifibate.* Initially 180 µg/kg by slow intravenous injection, then by infusion 2 µg/kg/minute for up to 72 hours, or 96 hours with PCI.
- *Tirofiban.* Initially 0.4 µg/kg/minutes intravenously for 30 minutes, followed by a maintenance dose of 0.1 µg/kg/minutes for at least 48 hours to a maximum of 108 hours.

HEPARIN

Heparin is a naturally occurring, high-molecular-weight mucopolysaccharide with marked anticoagulation properties when given subcutaneously or intravenously. Intramuscular injection may produce large haematomas. Heparin is used to prevent thromboembolism and in the treatment of deep vein thrombosis and pulmonary emboli.

Heparin works by combining with antithrombin III in the coagulation cascade, preventing the formation of factor Xa. It also reduces platelet adhesion. Unlike warfarin, it does not block prothrombin formation in the liver.

The activated partial thromboplastin time (APTT) is used as an index of efficacy and should be maintained at about twice normal. Thrombocytopenia often complicates therapy, and platelet counts should be checked on alternate days.

Overdose, producing prolonged coagulation times, should be corrected by reducing the dose or stopping the drug altogether (the half-life is only 1.5 hours). More urgent cases can be treated with protamine sulphate (1 mg neutralises 100 U of heparin within 5 minutes). However, as protamine is a weak anticoagulant itself, doses exceeding 50 mg should not be given.

Heparin regimens (unfractionated heparin)

- *Low dose* (prophylaxis): 5000 units twice daily, subcutaneously. APTTs are not required.
- *Medium dose* (treatment of deep vein thrombosis or disseminated intravascular coagulation): 30 000–45 000 units daily by infusion or 4-hourly by intravenous injection. After 48 hours, the dose is reduced by about 50% and adjusted according to APTTs. Warfarin is usually started at the same time.
- *High dose* (pulmonary embolism, systemic embolisation): a bolus loading dose of 5000–10 000 units should be given, followed by intravenous infusion, but there should be no reduction in dose at 48 hours as above. Warfarin is usually not started acutely.

Low-molecular-weight heparins (LMWH) are obtained by modifying unfractionated heparin (UFH), reducing the molecular weight by about two-thirds. They are weaker inhibitors of thrombin (factor IIa), and essentially work by inhibiting enzyme Xa. The potency of the different LMWHs is expressed in international units (IU) for anti-Xa activity. After subcutaneous injection, they are better absorbed than UFH, and regular monitoring of anticoagulation is not required. Enoxaparin is used extensively in the treatment of acute coronary syndromes and as an adjunct to thrombolysis.

Fondaparinux is a synthetic factor Xa inhibitor that prevents thrombin generation and clotting. Fondaparinux is as good as, or better than, LMWH for the prophylaxis of postoperative deep venous thrombosis, treatment of deep vein thrombosis and pulmonary embolism (Turpie, 2005). Results from the OASIS-5 trial suggest that fondaparinux is as effective as enoxaparin in reducing cardiovascular events in the short term in acute coronary syndromes, while causing half the amount of bleeding, thus reducing mortality (Yusuf et al, 2006).

HORMONE REPLACEMENT THERAPY

Estrogen replacement is associated with a 35–50% lower risk of cardiovascular disease, but this does not seem to be the case when co-prescribed with progestogens, as is usual in hormone replacement therapy (HRT). The Heart and Estrogen/progestin Replacement Study (HERS) showed no benefit of hormone replacement in post-menopausal women with coronary disease. In fact, there was a slight increase in cardiac events in the first year of therapy (perhaps due to an immediate prothrombotic effect), but a subsequent decreased risk. Combined HRT is not currently recommended for cardioprotection, but decisions regarding HRT must be individualised, depending on the competing risks of coronary heart disease, osteoporosis, menopausal symptoms and endometrial and breast cancer. Following acute myocardial infarction, HRT may be continued without any apparent adverse effect (Grodstein et al, 2001).

HYDRALAZINE (APRESOLINE)

Hydralazine is an arteriolar vasodilator used in the treatment of hypertension. It increases heart rate and cardiac output by reducing afterload, and also increases renal and cerebral perfusion. However, myocardial work and oxygen consumption are also increased, and angina may be precipitated unless it is co-prescribed with a beta- blocker or diltiazem.

Dose

The oral dose is 25–75 mg three or four times daily.

Side effects

Side effects result from vasodilatation and include postural hypotension, headache and flushing. Long-term therapy may cause a lupus syndrome.

INOTROPIC SYMPATHOMIMETIC AGENTS

Depending on haemodynamic status, cardiac output may be improved by the use of sympathomimetic inotropes, but use should be confined to high-dependency units, with invasive haemodynamic monitoring (Jowett, 1997). In cardiogenic shock, peripheral resistance is frequently high, and these agents usually raise it further, worsening myocardial performance and exacerbating tissue ischaemia. Volume replacement is essential before these agents are used.

Dopamine (Intropin) is the natural precursor of noradrenaline and has similar alpha- and beta-stimulatory actions, particularly at beta-1 sites. Stroke volume is increased, with little effect on heart rate. It causes peripheral vasoconstriction, which raises blood pressure but, unlike other sympathetic agents, it produces selective renal and cerebral arterial vasodilatation, depending on dose (Table 17.4). At low doses, the renal effects

Table 17.4 Effects of dopamine at different doses.

Dose (µg/kg/min)	Effect
1–5	Dilates renal and mesenteric arterioles to produce increased renal blood flow and glomerular filtration rate and urine output
6–20	Direct inotropic effect on the heart, with dose-related increase in cardiac output and heart rate
> 20	Direct alpha-action leads to peripheral vasoconstriction, which raises blood pressure. There are further inotropic and chronotropic effects on the heart

are most marked but, as the dose increases, vasoconstriction and positive inotropic and chronotropic effects are more marked. Dopamine is of major value in cardiogenic and other types of shock, and prolonged low-dose infusion is useful in heart failure.

Dopamine is given by continuous intravenous infusion, preferably by a central line, because profound localised tissue ischaemia may result with extravasation. Should signs of tissue necrosis develop, the area should be infiltrated with phentolamine (10 mg in 10 mL of saline).

Dobutamine (Dobutrex) is a synthetic adrenergic agent, modified from isoprenaline. It stimulates beta-adrenergic cardiac receptors and thereby directly increases the force of myocardial contraction, with only small increases in heart rates. Unlike dopamine, there is little systemic vasoconstriction, because dopamine acts indirectly (by causing noradrenaline release), whereas dobutamine acts directly. Infusion rates are usually in the range 2.5–20.0 μg/kg/minutes. At doses of over 20 μg/kg/minutes, increases in heart rate may induce or exacerbate myocardial ischaemia, although some patients may need up to 40 μg/kg/minutes. Dobutamine is often given in combination with low-dose dopamine, which is used to promote renal perfusion.

Dopexamine (Dopacard) is similar to dopamine with positive inotropic effects, and also peripheral dopamine receptor stimulation to increase renal perfusion. It may not induce vasoconstriction.

Isoprenaline has often been used to stabilise patients with profound bradycardia, heart block and hypotension, while awaiting pacemaker insertion. It is currently only available on special order, and adrenaline infusions or transcutaneous pacing are more usual if atropine is ineffective.

Noradrenaline (norepinephrine) stimulates cardiac beta-1 receptors to produce a positive inotropic effect, and alpha-adrenergic vasoconstriction takes place in vascular beds, except in the cerebral and coronary vessels, which dilate. Cardiac output may increase or decrease, depending on vascular resistance and the functional state of the left ventricle.

While useful in septic shock, noradrenaline is not helpful for cardiogenic shock, because peripheral vasoconstriction increases myocardial work without increasing cardiac output. It may also constrict renal capillary beds, leading to renal hypoperfusion.

IVABRADINE (PROCORALAN)

Ivabradine is the first selective sinus node inhibitor. Blockade of the I_f ('funny') channels reduces heart rate with no effect on cardiac contractility or atrio-ventricular conduction. It is used for symptomatic treatment of stable angina in patients with normal sinus rhythm who have contraindications to or are intolerant of beta-blockers and/or diltiazem.

Dose

Initially 5 mg bd increasing to 7.5 mg bd after 1 month if required.

Side effects

Bradycardia, first-degree heart block and visual disturbances.

LEVOSIMENDAN

Levosimendan is one of a new class of drugs known as calcium sensitisers. The drug enhances cardiac contractility and produces vasodilatation ('inodilator' actions). In addition, the drug has the potential to reverse contractile dysfunction caused by acidosis or myocardial stunning. Levosimendan works by increasing the sensitivity of the cardiac myofilaments to calcium, rather than increasing intracellular concentrations of free calcium as other inotropic agents do (Table 17.5), an undesirable effect because it causes a marked increase in myocardial energy consumption and encourages disturbances in cardiac rhythm.

Levosimendan has been used as an injectable preparation for acute heart failure, but oral preparation has not yet been examined in clinical trials. In patients with decompensated CHF, levosimendan significantly reduced the incidence of worsening CHF or death, and improved cardiac indices.

Table 17.5 Features of different inotropic agents.

Drug	Dobutamine	Milrinone	Levosimendan
Class	Catecholamine	Phosphodiesterase inhibitor	Calcium sensitiser
Vasodilator action	Mild peripheral	Peripheral	Coronary and peripheral
Cardiac contractility	Increased	Increased	Increased
Myocardial oxygen demand	Increased	No	No
Dysrhythmias	Ventricular (5%)	Supraventricular (4%) Ventricular (12%)	None
Route	Intravenous	Intravenous/oral	Intravenous

Dose

The usual dosage is 6–12 μg/kg as a loading dose over 10 minutes followed by 0.05–0.2 μg/kg/minute as a continuous infusion. Haemodynamic responses are generally observed within 5 minutes of commencement of infusion of the loading dose. Peak effects are observed within 10–30 minutes of infusion; the duration of action of levosimendan is about 1–2 hours.

Side effects

Headache and hypotension are dose related and arise from vasodilatory action.

LIPID–REGULATING AGENTS

There are seven groups of drugs that may be used.

1 *HMGCoA inhibitors* (e.g. pravastatin, simvastatin). The hydroxy-methylglutaryl coenzyme A reductase inhibitors ('statins') competitively inhibit the rate-limiting enzyme in cholesterol synthesis. As endogenous synthesis of cholesterol is prevented, circulating cholesterol is taken up by the low-density lipoprotein (LDL) receptor on the surface of cells, and circulating LDL cholesterol concentrations fall. The statins are very potent, with reductions in total serum cholesterol of 40% sometimes being achieved. Side effects are myositis and hepatic dysfunction.

2 *Anion exchange (bile sequestrant) resins* (e.g. cholestyramine, colestipol). These bind bile acids, preventing reabsorption. Cholesterol is diverted into making more bile acids, so is progressively excreted. While LDL cholesterol concentrations are reduced, triglyceride levels may increase. Absorption of drugs, particularly digoxin and diuretics, is sometimes impaired. They should be taken 1 hours before or 4–6 hours after the resins. Anticoagulant action may be enhanced or depressed. Fat-soluble vitamins may need supplementation (A, D, E and K).

3 *Fibrates* (e.g. bezafibrate, ciprofibrate, gemfibrozil, fenofibrate). These are isobutyric derivatives that inhibit cholesterol synthesis in the liver and increase very-low-density lipoprotein (VLDL) removal from the blood. They predominantly reduce triglycerides, but also reduce LDL cholesterol and increase high-density lipoprotein (HDL) cholesterol. They also have the side effect of myositis, and should be used with caution in those with renal impairment and also those taking statins. Fibrates potentiate the actions of warfarin.

4 *Nicotinic acid group* (e.g. nicotinic acid, acipimox). Nicotinic acid (niacin) is a member of the B group of vitamins normally eaten in the diet. Large doses of nicotinic acid produce effects unrelated to its role as a vitamin that can be used to inhibit the breakdown of apolipoprotein A-1, the major protein component of HDL. Lipolysis is inhibited in adipose tissue, and predominantly reduces VLDL and thus triglyceride synthesis. There are decreases in LDL cholesterol, triglycerides and lipoprotein Lp(a), with an increase in HDL cholesterol. Nicotinic acid causes vasodilatation, and associates with flushing or pruritis. Angina may be worsened. An extended release form of nicotinic acid (Niaspan) has been marketed in the UK, which seems to reduce these side effects. *Acipimox* has

fewer side effects than nicotinic acid, but is less effective.

5 *Fish oils*. Omega-3 fatty acids are essential fatty acids that cannot be manufactured by the body and must be obtained from food. Regular consumption of fish and other marine foods is recommended to provide over 200 mg of these essential fatty acids daily (WHO, 2002). Concentrated omega-3 marine triglycerides in Maxepa capsules can reduce severely elevated triglyceride levels by inhibiting VLDL synthesis in the liver. Omocor capsules have higher concentrations of omega-3 esters, and can also be used in hypertriglyceridaemia, but have also been shown to reduce major cardiac events following myocardial infarction (Marchioli et al, 2005).

6 *Cholesteryl ester transfer protein (CTEP) inhibitors.* CETP is a plasma glycoprotein that is secreted from the liver and circulates in plasma, bound mainly to HDL. It promotes the redistribution of cholesteryl esters and triglycerides between plasma lipoproteins. By inhibiting transfer of cholesteryl esters from HDL_2 cholesterol to the ApoB lipoproteins, HDL cholesterol concentrations rise and LDL levels fall, an effect that is enhanced by co-prescription of a statin (Brousseau et al, 2004). The first drug in this group, torcetrapib, was withdrawn by Pfizer in December 2006 because of an increased risk of death.

7 *Ezetimibe* (ezetrol). Ezetimibe selectively inhibits transport of cholesterol across the wall of the small intestine, thereby reducing the delivery of cholesterol to the liver. It is used to treat primary hypercholesterolaemia either alone or, more commonly, co-prescribed with statins. There are no outcome data on cardiovascular morbidity and mortality. It is a reasonable option in the treatment of homozygous familial hypercholesterolaemia or familial sitosterolaemia.

Statins are the first choice in hypercholesterolaemia, with the addition of ezetimibe or bile acid sequestrant resins in refractory cases. On average, the statins will reduce LDL cholesterol by 20–60%, while increasing the HDL cholesterol by 5%. The degree of cholesterol lowering is greater in those with high initial concentrations, although reduction to target levels will be more difficult. Fibrates are usually the first choice in hypertriglyceridaemia, with the addition of nicotinic acid derivatives or Omacor if necessary.

Those with mixed hyperlipidaemia are usually responsive to statin therapy, with the addition of fibrates if the triglyceride levels remain elevated.

MAGNESIUM

Hypomagnesaemia is common, and has been reported in 7–11% of hospitalised patients and in over one-third of patients with CHF who use diuretics (Connolly & Worthley, 1999). Legumes and whole grains are excellent sources of magnesium, as are green vegetables, nuts, shellfish and dried fruit, and should be recommended in CHF patients.

ECG changes associated with hypomagnesaemia include prolongation of the QT interval, appearance of U waves and dysrhythmias. Magnesium should be considered for patients with symptomatic or life-threatening dysrhythmias even when serum magnesium levels are normal, and are the treatment of choice in digoxin-induced tachy-dysrhythmias and torsades-de-pointes. When used to supplement other standard rate-reducing therapies for rapid atrial fibrillation, magnesium sulphate enhances rate control and conversion to sinus rhythm (Davey & Teubner, 2005).

Dose

The dose is 2 g of magnesium sulphate (8 mmol) in 100 mL of 5% dextrose over 10–20 minutes, repeated once if required.

Side effects

Intravenous magnesium sulphate may cause unpleasant flushing, nausea and vomiting, particularly if it is administered too rapidly.

METOCLOPRAMIDE (MAXOLON)

Metoclopramide is a centrally acting anti-emetic agent, which also promotes gastric emptying. Oesophageal reflux is reduced, and small bowel transit time is increased.

Dose

The dose is 10 mg orally or intravenously.

Side effects

Drowsiness, dizziness and dystonic movements of the head and neck.

MINOXIDIL (LONITEN)

Minoxidil is a direct action arterial vasodilator that is useful in resistant hypertension. It causes fluid retention, and should be co-prescribed with diuretics (often high-dose loop diuretics). It may cause T wave changes on the ECG and, rarely, a pericardial effusion.

Dose

Initially 5 mg od orally, increasing to a maximum of 50 mg.

Side effects

Apart from fluid retention, increased hair growth is the commonest side effect.

NALOXONE (NARCAN)

Naloxone is a specific opiate antidote and is indicated if there is coma or respiratory failure following administration of diamorphine or morphine. It has a short intravenous half-life and needs repeated doses, depending upon the respiratory pattern.

Dose

The dose is 0.8–2.0 mg, repeated every 2–3 minutes intravenously or by infusion.

Side effects

Dysrhythmias.

NICORANDIL (IKOREL)

Nicorandil is a potassium channel-opening drug used in the treatment of angina. It increases membrane conductance to potassium ions, which hyperpolarises vascular smooth muscle to produce vasodilatation. It also has some nitrate-like properties. It thus reduces both cardiac pre-load and afterload, while dilating both the epicardial vessels and smaller resistance vessels.

Dose

The dose is 10–30 mg twice daily.

Side effects

Headaches, flushing, hypotension and tachycardia.

NITRATES

Organic nitrates have been the mainstay in the treatment of angina pectoris for over 100 years. The benefits arise from the combination of coronary and non-coronary actions, and different forms of coronary heart disease may respond differently. Nitrates relax vascular smooth muscle, mainly in the venous system, to increase capacitance and thus reduce pre-load to the heart. Arteriolar relaxation also occurs, with a fall in peripheral resistance (afterload). Although not a main action, coronary dilatation probably occurs, which may improve regional myocardial blood flow. These effects are most marked when the coronary arterial stenosis is due to spasm rather than a fixed lesion, but they are less effective than calcium antagonists. Sublingual glyceryl trinitrate (GTN) is accepted as the standard treatment for acute episodes of angina, and the longer acting variants are used as prophylaxis against attacks. Tolerance may develop rapidly after the initiation of therapy, but disappears quickly after discontinuing the drug, and appears to be a function of constant plasma levels of nitrates. Reduction of blood nitrate concentrations to low levels for 4–8 hours each day usually maintains effectiveness, so the second of the twice-daily doses should be taken at 8 hours rather than after 12 hours. Modified release formulations of isosorbide mononitrate do not produce tolerance if used once daily.

Uses

Apart from the treatment of angina, bolus therapy is of major value in the emergency treatment of left ventricular failure.

Choice

The haemodynamic effects of GTN are short lasting, and many different preparations have therefore been developed to prolong their effect and make them useful as prophylactic agents.

Sublingual GTN (0.3-, 0.5- or 0.6-mg tablets or spray)

These should be used as early as possible after the onset of angina or, prophylactically, before physical activity. If the pain persists, the dose may be repeated at 5-minute intervals until relief is obtained. It must always be explained that the drug is neither addictive nor to be reserved only for emergencies. Headache and hypotension are common and may be avoided if the pill is swallowed or spat out as soon as relief is obtained. The tablets are deactivated by heat and light and must, therefore, be kept cool and in a dark bottle. The activity of the drug after opening lasts only 8 weeks, and old tablets should be discarded. Tablets are also deactivated if cotton wool is placed in the bottle.

Oral nitrates

Because of hepatic inactivation, there is an extensive 'first-pass' effect on nitrates when taken orally, and as little as 10% of the drug may reach the circulation. Prolonged action can be achieved by using higher or more frequent doses. Isosorbide dinitrate (Isordil, Sorbitrate, Cedocard) is swallowed whole in doses of 10–60 mg at 4- to 6-hour intervals. The onset of action is after about 30 minutes, but sooner if the tablet is chewed. Isosorbide mononitrate (ISMO, Elantan) is thought not to be so extensively removed on first pass, which allows smaller doses to be given (20–40 mg twice daily).

Buccal nitrates

Sublingual GTN, Sorbichew and Nitrolingual sprays are rapidly acting oral preparations that are absorbed in the mouth, and bypass the liver, leading to improved efficacy. Suscard buccal is a form of nitrate that has been impregnated into an inert polymer matrix, allowing slow diffusion of the drug across the buccal mucosa. The pill is tucked under the top lip without chewing, and a gel-like coating forms around the drug, allowing it to adhere to the buccal mucosa. Slow absorption can then take place as long as the pill remains intact (usually 3–5 hours).

Transdermal nitrates

Slow-release skin preparations that hold a reservoir of GTN circumvent the first-pass metabolism of swallowed nitrates, and therapeutic blood levels are achieved within 1 hour, but may last for up to 24 hours if the patch is not removed. Tolerance will then develop.

The patches are applied to any clean, dry, non-hairy part of the skin. Absorption depends upon site and blood flow, and large amounts are sometimes required to produce therapeutic blood levels. The extremities should be avoided. Skin irritation and variable absorption limit their use, but there is a high placebo effect, especially if patches are applied over the heart.

Intravenous nitrates

Intravenous GTN (Tridil) and isosorbide dinitrate (Isoket) are useful in the management of unstable angina, prolonged infarction pain and left ventricular failure. The dose required for pain relief varies widely, and the infusion rate (1–10 mg/hour) must be titrated against pain and blood pressure.

Side effects

The major side effects of nitrates are due to vasodilatation, which may give rise to hypotension, tachycardia and headache. Alcohol will potentiate the effects. Side effects will not be as prominent with continued use, if the patient can be persuaded to persevere. Beta-blockers given at the same time may help to slow the heart and relieve the headache.

OPIATE ANALGESICS

Narcotic analgesics (opiates) are used to relieve moderate to severe pain. Drugs in the group all have similar effects and side effects, but differ in their duration of action. Although opiates are primarily analgesics, they also have sedative effects at high doses, particularly when used in combination with other centrally acting drugs (e.g. tranquillisers). Opiates stimulate the vomiting centres in the brain, so must be given with an anti-emetic drug.

Narcotic analgesics are usually given by slow intravenous injection or infusion following acute myocardial infarction, as intramuscular absorption is unpredictable and usually contraindicated. *Diamorphine* is the analgesic of choice as it produces vasodilatation, thus reducing myocardial work and oxygen consumption. It is also much more soluble and allows the injection of smaller volumes of fluid.

Dose

- Diamorphine: 2.5–10.0 mg intravenously, repeated as required.
- Morphine and cyclomorphine: 5–10 mg intravenously, repeated as required.
- Papaveretum (Omnopon) is a mixture of the alkaloids of opium (20 mg is roughly equivalent to 12.5 mg of morphine).

Side effects

Nausea, vomiting, constipation, urinary retention, bradycardia and respiratory depression.

PHOSPHODIESTERASE INHIBITORS

Phosphodiesterase inhibitors block one or more of the five subtypes of the enzyme phosphodiesterase (PDE), preventing the inactivation of the intracellular cyclic adenosine monophosphate (AMP) and cyclic guanosine monophosphate (GMP). The cardiovascular effects increase cardiac output and reduce systemic vascular resistance.

Non-selective phosphodiesterase inhibitors (e.g. caffeine and theophylline) cause adrenaline release from the adrenal glands. Theophylline is usually given as *aminophylline*, a mixture of theophylline with ethylenediamine, and is 20 times more soluble than theophylline alone. Beta-2 stimulation relieves bronchospasm, and beta-1 effects increase the heart rate and the force of myocardial contraction. More often used in the treatment of asthma, it has been used for heart failure to augment cardiac output but, as it may produce serious ventricular dysrhythmias, it is best avoided.

Endogenous adenosine is thought to cause or perpetuate profound bradycardias and asystole. Aminophylline antagonises adenosine antagonists, and has been suggested in the treatment of asystolic cardiac arrest or atropine-resistant AV nodal block complicating inferior myocardial infarction, although evidence is lacking (Abu-Laban et al, 2006).

Selective PDE-5 inhibitors such as sildenafil (Viagra), tadalafil (Cialis) and vardenafil (Levitra) are the mainstay of drug treatment for erectile dysfunction. Because of embarrassment, their use may not be volunteered. However, this group of drugs may be contraindicated in patients taking nitrates and nicorandil, as they can produce unpredictable and severe vasodilatation, leading to profound hypotension. The drugs may also interact with non-selective alpha-blockers, such as doxazosin, leading to postural hypotension.

Selective PDE-3 inhibitors (milrinone, enoximone) exert their major effect on the myocardium. They slow the breakdown of myocardial cyclic AMP, which results in an increased rate and force of myocardial contraction. Cyclic AMP also relaxes vascular smooth muscle to effect vasodilatation. As a consequence, phosphodiesterase inhibitors will improve cardiac output, and there is usually no change in blood pressure, heart rate or oxygen consumption. There is no evidence that these drugs improve survival, but they may be used for the short-term treatment of severe heart failure refractory to conventional treatment, providing the patient is monitored invasively.

RIMONABANT (ACOMPLIA)

Rimonabant is a selective cannabinoid-1 receptor (CB1) antagonist used as an adjunct to diet and exercise for the treatment of overweight and obese patients with associated risk factors, such as type 2 diabetes or dyslipidaemia. The endocannabinoid system is a physiological system present in brain and peripheral tissues (including adipocytes) that affects energy balance, glucose and lipid metabolism and body weight. It is also operative in neurons of the mesolimbic system that control the intake of highly palatable, sweet or fatty foods (Carai et al, 2005). Treatment with rimonabant associates with significant reductions in waist circumference, so it tends to antagonise features of the metabolic syndrome.

Dose

The dose is 20 mg taken in the morning before breakfast.

Side effects

Depression with disturbance in attention, gastrointestinal disorders (stomach discomfort, dry mouth). Infections may be more common.

SODIUM BICARBONATE

Intravenous sodium bicarbonate has been widely used in the past for correcting the metabolic acidosis that follows cardiac arrest. However, there is little evidence that this therapy improves outcome, and its use is no longer recommended because of the frequent occurrence of deleterious side effects, including increasing carbon dioxide levels, hyponatraemia, inactivation of concurrently administered catecholamines and tissue necrosis if accidentally given extravascularly. Sodium bicarbonate 50 mmol (50 mL of an 8.4% solution) may be helpful if cardiac arrest is associated with hyperkalaemia or tricyclic antidepressant overdose, with repeat of the dose according to the clinical condition and the result of repeated blood gas analysis.

Critically ill patients in hospital may warrant early therapy with sodium bicarbonate if there is developing hyperkalaemia or acidosis (pH < 7.1) that might precede a cardiac arrest, but these occasions are now the exception rather than the rule.

SODIUM NITROPRUSSIDE (NIPRIDE)

Sodium nitroprusside is a potent parenteral vasodilator, which may be employed in hypertensive emergencies and severe left ventricular failure. It relaxes both arteriolar and venous smooth muscle. It acts rapidly (within 2 minutes) and is given by controlled intravenous infusion. The drug is light-sensitive. Solutions are normally red/brown in colour, and deterioration is marked by a colour change to blue.

Dose

The drug should be freshly prepared (in 5% dextrose) and used within 4 hours. The normal adult dose for heart failure is 10–15 μg/minute, adjusted as required. Doses should normally not exceed 400 μg/minute. The maximal dose is 700–800 mg in 24 hours, and the drug is best not given for periods exceeding 72 hours because of the build up of plasma cyanide metabolites. If therapy is needed for more than 3 days, blood thiocyanate levels should be assayed.

Side effects

Nausea, sweating, dizziness and twitching denote toxicity. Sodium thiosulphate is an antidote if signs persist. Unexplained cyanosis may be due to the formation of methaemoglobinaemia. Large doses of hydroxocobalamin (vitamin B12, 1.5 mg/kg) may be used prophylactically to reduce plasma cyanide levels.

STATINS

Statins inhibit 3-hydroxy-3-methylglutaryl coenzyme A (HMGCoA) reductase, an enzyme involved in cholesterol synthesis. Inhibition of HMGCoA reductase lowers LDL cholesterol levels by slowing down the production of cholesterol in the liver and increasing the liver's ability to remove the LDL cholesterol already in the blood. The statins are very potent, with reductions in cholesterol of around 30–40% being achieved. In patients with raised triglycerides, statins reduce hepatic secretion of VLDL, and triglyceride levels fall by 20–40%. There may be minor increases in HDL cholesterol (5–10%).

There are currently five statins licensed in the UK (atorvastatin, fluvastatin, pravastatin, rosuvastatin and simvastatin). Cerivastatin (Lipobay) was withdrawn in 2001 because of 31 deaths associated with rhabdomyositis. Lovastatin is not available in the UK. The statins differ in their absorption, excretion, solubility and potency.

On average, a reduction of a third in the cholesterol concentration may be achieved by simvastatin 40 mg, pravastatin 40 mg, atorvastatin 10 mg, rosuvastatin 10 mg and fluvastatin 80 mg.

Who should be treated with statins?

Statins are safe and effective for a wide range of patients, and treatment should be considered for anyone with an increased risk of an occlusive vascular event (Cholesterol Treatment Trialists' Collaborators, 2005). A 1-mmol/L drop in serum concentration of LDL cholesterol reduces overall mortality by 12% over 5 years, the risk of coronary death or heart attack by 23%, need for coronary vascularisation by 24%, risk of stroke by 17% and risk of any major vascular event by 21%. Benefits start within the first year of treatment and increase with time. The absolute benefit relates mostly to the individual's absolute risk of such events as well as the size of reduction in LDL concentration, rather than the baseline values before treatment began. They are largely independent of the patient's age, sex or any pre-existing disease. Statins even reduce cardiovascular events in the elderly (over 75 years) and for people with LDL cholesterol concentrations under 2.6 mmol/L. The goal of treatment should therefore shift away from target concentrations of LDL cholesterol, and focus more on reducing the serum concentration by as much as possible (and keeping it down). All patients should receive advice on non-drug measures before committing them to lifelong drug therapy (Jowett & Galton, 1987).

Doses

In general, the LDL cholesterol is only reduced by an additional 7% for every doubling of the statin dose (Roberts, 1997) so, although the smallest dose of pravastatin and simvastatin is 10 mg, a starting dose of 40 mg is recommended. Because endogenous production of cholesterol takes place at night, short-acting statins such as simvastatin and pravastatin should be taken at bedtime. Atorvastatin and rosuvastatin are longer acting and more potent, and can be taken at any time of the day. The dose of atorvastatin is in the range 10–80 mg and 10–40 mg for rosuvastatin. Because the pharmacokinetics of rosuvastatin in Asian,

Japanese and Chinese patients differ, higher blood concentrations result, and the maximal dose should be 20 mg.

Zocor Heart-Pro (simvastatin 10 mg) is the first stain in the world to be sold across the counter without a prescription. It is indicated for primary prevention of coronary heart disease in those at 'moderate' risk, but there is no evidence that it is beneficial. Furthermore, because it is obtainable without prescription, there may be no assessment of other risk factors, risk/benefit analysis of the medication or monitoring for side effects or other drug interactions (see below). It cannot be recommended.

Side effects

Adverse events associated with all statins include headache, altered liver function tests, paraesthesia and gastrointestinal effects (including abdominal pain, flatulence, diarrhoea, nausea and vomiting). Rash and hypersensitivity reactions have been reported, but are rare. There is no evidence of a link between statins and cancer, even among older patients. Various muscle effects have been reported (see Box 17.1).

Overall, myopathy only affects 1–5% of patients, with fatal rhabdomyolysis occurring in one in a million patients. Muscle toxicity is relatively more common when fibrates are co-prescribed with statins (especially gemfibrozil).

Creatine phosphokinase (CK) concentrations should be checked prior to starting statin therapy, but do not need to be repeated unless there are symptoms. Statins should be discontinued if symptoms of myalgia are severe, the CK exceeds five times the upper limit of normal or transaminases (aspartate aminotransferase, alanine aminotransferase) persist at about three times the upper limit of normal.

Liver function tests should be carried out before and within 1–3 months of starting statin therapy, and then 6-monthly for 1 year unless signs or symptoms suggestive of hepatotoxicity indicate that they should be carried out sooner.

Interactions

A number of important drug interactions have been described that increase the risk of toxicity,

Box 17.1   Muscle effects of statins.

Myalgia (common)

Diffuse muscle ache (mostly proximal)
Creatine kinase (CK) levels normal or slightly
  elevated
Disappears on withdrawal of statin

Myositis

Muscle weakness
CK normal or elevated
Dose related

Myopathy

Muscle pain and necrosis
CK over 10 times the upper limit of normal
Dose related
Produces changes on an electromyogram (EMG)

Rhabdomyolysis (very rare)

Muscle destruction with pain and swelling
CK levels very high (and myoglobin)
May be fatal
Predisposing risk usually present (trauma, liver or
  renal failure, amiodarone or fibrate therapy,
  muscle enzyme defect)

Table 17.6   Summary of recommendations for
avoiding drug interactions with statins.

Interacting drug	Prescribing advice
Erythromycin Clarithromycin Azole antifungals	Avoid simvastatin, lovastatin and atorvastatin
Gemfibrozil	Do not exceed simvastatin 10 mg
Niacin Ciclosporin	Avoid atorvastatin and lovastatin
Verapamil Amiodarone	Do not exceed simvastatin 20 mg or atorvastatin 10 mg
Diltiazem	Do not exceed simvastatin 40 mg or atorvastatin 10 mg
Grapefruit juice	Avoid grapefruit juice

and muscle side effects in particular. The cytochrome P450 isoform CYP3A4 serves as the major pathway for metabolism of the statins, except for pravastatin and rosuvastatin. Inhibition of this pathway will increase statin concentrations, with the potential for toxicity. Drugs that may have an important clinical interaction include amiodarone, calcium channel blockers, some antibiotics, ciclosporin and itraconazole. Grapefruit juice can inhibit CYP3A4 for several hours, and is best avoided. A summary of recommendations is shown in Table 17.6.

Extensive evidence, excellent safety and high efficacy have resulted in an exponential rise in prescriptions for statins, now representing the largest drug cost to the NHS (£738 million in 2004). In May 2003, the UK simvastatin patent expired, and the cost has fallen substantially. If generic simvastatin were universally prescribed, statin costs would fall by £185 million a year (Moon & Bogle, 2006).

THROMBOLYTIC (FIBRINOLYTIC) AGENTS

Fibrinolytic drugs are used to break up thrombus within coronary arteries, and thus reduce mortality following myocardial infarction (Fibrinolytic Therapy Trialists' Collaborative Group, 1994). They work by activating plasminogen to form plasmin, which degrades fibrin and so breaks up thrombi ('thrombolytic'). There are currently four agents in common use [streptokinase, alteplase (tPA), reteplase and tenecteplase].

Streptokinase has to combine with plasminogen to form an activator complex, which acts on other circulating plasminogens to form plasmin, which acts directly on fibrin, breaking it down. Streptokinase is not thrombus specific, and conversion of plasminogen also takes place systemically, making haemorrhage more likely. *Alteplase, tenecteplase* and *reteplase* are genetically engineered versions of naturally occurring tissue plasminogen activator (tPA), and are much more clot specific. They bind preferentially to the fibrin within the clot and thus do not activate circulating plasminogen (i.e. they are plasminogen independent). This reduces the risk of systemic haemorrhage. Reteplase and tenecteplase are given by intravenous bolus, rather than infusion. Streptokinase should not be given to patients who have had the drug before and those presenting in under 6 hours, when other agents are more effective. The use of fibrinolytic agents in coronary thrombosis is discussed in detail in Chapter 7.

TRANEXAMIC ACID (CYKLOKAPRON)

Tranexamic acid inhibits plasminogen activation and fibrinolysis, and may be given in addition to fresh frozen plasma for severe haemorrhage complicating thrombolytic therapy.

Dose

The dose is 0.5–1.0 g by slow intravenous injection every 8 hours.

Side effects

Dizziness may follow rapid intravenous injection.

WARFARIN (MAREVAN)

Warfarin inhibits the action of vitamin K in the liver and so slows the synthesis of four plasma procoagulants (II, VII, IX and X). Its effect commences at about 12 hours and lasts for 2–5 days. The dose is titrated against the results of the prothrombin time. Because the prothrombin ratio of treated patients to control subjects varies from laboratory to laboratory, the World Health Organization system for international standardisation of prothrombin times has allowed comparison of anticoagulant control regimens, based upon common systems of reporting, termed international normalised ratios (INRs).

The decision to anticoagulate must take into account the benefits and potential hazards in each patient. The most worrying unwanted effect is bleeding, usually gastrointestinal, into the soft tissues or via the oropharynx. Intracranial haemorrhage is uncommon. Factors increasing the risk of bleeding include immobility, uncontrolled hypertension and serious co-morbidities. Overanticoagulation is treated by reducing the daily dose or stopping the drug altogether. If there is active bleeding, fresh frozen plasma may be given. Intravenous vitamin K_1 (phytomenadione) works more slowly (10 mg over 2–3 minutes).

Many factors affect the potency of warfarin:

- *increased potency*: heart failure, liver disease, fever, alcohol, aspirin, cimetidine, diuretics, antibiotics and oral hypoglycaemics;
- *decreased potency*: diabetes, hypothyroidism, hyperlipidaemia, sedatives, oral contraceptives, cholestyramine and antacids.

Anticoagulant therapy after acute myocardial infarction

Most trials on anticoagulation after myocardial infarction were undertaken when patients were treated by strict and prolonged bedrest, and deep vein thrombosis and pulmonary embolism were frequent complications. While the role of aspirin following acute myocardial infarction is clear, the use of anticoagulants as an alternative method of secondary prevention is still debated. Even the more recent trials were carried out before thrombolysis.

In contrast to aspirin, warfarin will interrupt the coagulation cascade and can prevent thromboembolic complications such as deep vein thrombosis, pulmonary embolism and systemic emboli originating from intracardiac thrombus associated with large anterior infarctions, atrial fibrillation or heart failure. Nearly three-quarters of symptomatic systemic emboli produce stroke, and cause significant mortality and morbidity. Most systemic embolisation occurs within 3 months, with the maximal risk being in the first 10 days. In the absence of prophylaxis, 2–6% of patients with anterior myocardial infarction suffer a stroke within 28 days. Patients with anterior Q wave infarction should be fully anticoagulated with warfarin for 3 months to prevent thromboembolism. Rates of thromboembolism in heart failure vary from 2.5% with mild heart failure to 20% per annum in those with dilated cardiomyopathy. There is no evidence to recommend routine anticoagulation in all patients with heart failure in sinus rhythm (Hardman & Cowie, 1999). Concomitant low-dose aspirin should be considered for high-risk patients, despite the inherent dangers of bleeding. Target INRs are shown in Table 17.7.

The oral direct thrombin inhibitor *ximelagatran* is the first new oral anticoagulant agent since warfarin was introduced more than 50 years ago.

Table 17.7 Targets for international normalised ratio (INR).

	Target	Range
1. Mechanical valves[a]		
a) *First generation* (e.g. Starr–Edwards, Björk–Shiley)	3.5	2.5–3.5
b) *Second generation* (e.g. St Jude Medical, Medtronic Hall)		
Mitral position	3.0	2.5–3.5
Aortic position	2.5	2.0–3.0
2. Bioprosthetic valves[b]	3.0	2.5–3.0
3. Valve repair	2.5	2.0–3.0
4. Atrial fibrillation		
a) In rheumatic heart disease	3.0	2.5–4.5
b) Non-valvular	2.5	2.0–3.0
5. Deep vein thrombosis/pulmonary embolism	2.5	2.0–3.0
6. Recurrent DVT/emboli despite good INR control[c]	3.5	3.0–4.5

a If the INR falls below 2.5 in patients with mechanical heart valves, there is a marked increase in the thromboembolic risk.
b As long as patients remain in sinus rhythm, anticoagulation is only used for 3 months, changing to low-dose aspirin.
c Plus aspirin 75 mg.

Unlike warfarin, ximelagatran exerts its anticoagulant effect almost immediately, has no known drug or food interactions and does not require frequent laboratory monitoring. Unfortunately, uncertainty about performance against warfarin, coupled with doubts regarding drug-related liver injury, has prevented licensing in the UK.

Outpatient anticoagulation

For patients who do not require immediate anticoagulation, a slow loading regimen is safe and may be carried out on an outpatient basis. This avoids over-anticoagulation and bleeding associated with more rapid loading. Patients may be started on 3 mg of warfarin daily for a week, and subsequent doses can be determined by weekly INR measurement (Janes et al, 2004). Therapeutic anticoagulation is achieved in the majority of patients within a month. If patients require a faster initiation of oral anticoagulation, regimens that start with 5-mg doses or a single 10-mg dose followed by 5-mg doses may be preferable to regimens that start with repeated 10-mg doses in certain patient groups, e.g. the elderly, those with liver disease or cardiac failure and those at high risk of bleeding (British Society of Haematology, 2005).

Near-patient testing

Near-patient testing with meters and testing strips has made self-monitoring of anticoagulation with warfarin feasible. The patients may both self-test and self-adjust treatment according to a predetermined dose schedule, or call a clinic to receive the appropriate dose adjustment. Self-monitoring and self-adjustment of oral anticoagulation with warfarin by patients is associated with improved outcomes of all-cause mortality, thromboembolic events and major haemorrhage (Heneghan et al, 2006). It is also more convenient for patients, and leads to better treatment compliance. However, self-monitoring is not feasible for all patients and requires the prior identification and education of suitable candidates.

References

Abu-Laban C, McIntyre J, Christenson C et al (2006) Aminophylline in brady-asystolic cardiac arrest: a randomised placebo-controlled trial. *Lancet* 367: 1577–1584.

ACE Inhibitor Myocardial Infarction Collaborative Group (1998) Indications for ACE inhibitors in the early treatment of acute myocardial infarction: systematic overview of individual data from 100,000 patients in randomized trials. *Circulation* 97: 2202–2212.

Al-Mallah MH, Tleyjeh IM, Abdel-Latif AA et al (2006) Angiotensin-converting enzyme inhibitors in coronary artery disease and preserved left ventricular systolic function: a systematic review and meta-analysis of randomized controlled trials. *Journal of the American College of Cardiology* 47: 1576–1583.

Andrus MR, Holloway KP, Clark DB (2004) Use of beta-blockers in patients with COPD. *Annals of Pharmacotherapy* 38: 142–145.

Anti-thrombotic Trialists' Collaboration (2002) Collaborative meta-analysis of randomised trials of anti-platelet therapy for prevention of death, myocardial infarction, and stroke in high risk patients. *British Medical Journal* 324: 71–86.

Bhatt DL, Fox KAA, Hacke W for the CHARISMA investigators (2006) Clopidogrel and aspirin versus aspirin alone for the prevention of atherosclerotic events. *New England Journal of Medicine* 354: 1706–1717.

British Society of Haematology (2005) British Committee for Standards in Haematology guidelines on oral anticoagulation (warfarin): third edition – 2005 update. *British Journal of Haematology* 132: 277–285.

Brousseau ME, Schaefer EJ, Wolfe ML et al (2004) Effects of an inhibitor of cholesteryl ester transfer protein on HDL cholesterol. *New England Journal of Medicine* 350: 1505–1515.

Brown B, Hall AS (2005) Renin–angiotensin system modulation: the weight of evidence. *American Journal of Hypertension* 18: 127S–133S.

CAPRIE Steering Committee (1996) A randomised blinded trial of clopidogrel versus aspirin in patients at risk of ischaemic events – CAPRIE. *Lancet* 348: 1329–1339.

Carai MA, Colombo G, Gessa GL (2005) Rimonabant: the first therapeutically relevant cannabinoid antagonist. *Life Sciences* 77: 2339–2350.

CAST Investigators (1989) Effect of encainide and flecainide on mortality in a randomised trial of arrhythmia suppression after myocardial infarction (the Cardiac Arrhythmia Suppression Trial). *New England Journal of Medicine*, 321: 406–412.

Cholesterol Treatment Trialists' (CTT) Collaborators (2005) Efficacy and safety of cholesterol-lowering treatment: prospective meta-analysis of data from 90,056 participants in 14 randomised trials of statins. *Lancet* 366: 1267–1278.

Connolly E, Worthley LIG (1999) Intravenous magnesium. *Critical Care and Resuscitation* 1: 162–172.

Dauchot P, Gravenstein JS (1971) Effects of atropine on the electrocardiogram in different age groups. *Clinical Pharmacology and Therapeutics* 12: 274–280.

Davey MJ, Teubner D (2005) A randomised controlled trial of magnesium sulfate, in addition to usual care, for rate control in atrial fibrillation. *Annals of Emergency Medicine* 45: 347–353.

De Smet PA (2002) Herbal remedies. *New England Journal of Medicine* 347: 2046–2056.

Din JN, Newby DE, Flapan AD (2004) Omega 3 fatty acids and cardiovascular disease – fishing for a natural treatment. *British Medical Journal* 328: 30–35.

Fibrinolytic Therapy Trialists' Collaborative Group (1994) Indications for fibrinolytic therapy in suspected acute myocardial infarction: collaborative overview of early and major mortality from all randomised trials of more than 1000 patients. *Lancet* 343: 311–322.

Flather MD, Shibata MC, Coats AJ et al (2005) Randomized trial to determine the effect of nebivolol on mortality and cardiovascular hospital admission in elderly patients with heart failure (SENIORS). *European Heart Journal* 26: 215–225.

Freemantle N, Cleland J, Young P et al (1999) Beta-blockade after myocardial infarction: systematic review and meta-regression analysis. *British Medical Journal* 318: 1730–1737.

Grodstein F, Manson JE, Stampfer MJ (2001) Postmenopausal hormone use and secondary prevention of coronary events in the nurses' health study: a prospective observational study. *Annals of Internal Medicine* 135: 1–8.

Hardman SMC, Cowie MR (1999) Anticoagulation in heart disease. *British Medical Journal* 318: 238–244.

Heintzen MP, Strauer BE (1994) Peripheral vascular effects of beta-blockers. *European Heart Journal* 15: 2–7.

Heneghan C, Alonso-Coello P, Garcia-Alamino J et al (2006) Self-monitoring of oral anticoagulation: a systematic review and meta-analysis. *Lancet* 367: 404–411.

Janes S, Challis R, Fisher F (2004) Safe introduction of warfarin for thrombotic prophylaxis in atrial fibrillation requiring only a weekly INR. *Clinical and Laboratory Haematology* 26: 43–47.

JBS-2 (2005) Joint British Societies' guidelines on prevention of cardiovascular disease in clinical practice. *Heart* 91: 1–52.

Jowett NI (1997) *Cardiovascular Monitoring*. London: Whurr.

Jowett NI (2002) Foxglove poisoning. *British Journal of Hospital Medicine* 63: 368–369.

Jowett NI, Galton DJ (1987) The management of the hyperlipidaemias. In: Hamer J (ed.) *Drugs for Heart Disease*, 2nd edn. London: Chapman and Hall.

Lands EM (2005) Dietary fat and health: the evidence and the politics of prevention. *Annals of the New York Academy of Sciences* 1055: 179–192.

McDowell SE, Coleman JC, Ferner RE (2006) Systematic review and meta-analysis of ethnic differences in risks of adverse reactions to drugs used in cardiovascular medicine. *British Medical Journal* 332: 1177–1181.

McMurray JJV (1999) Major beta-blocker mortality trials in chronic heart failure: a critical review. *Heart* 82(suppl IV): IV14–IV22.

Marchioli R, Levantesi G, Macchia A et al (2005) Antiarrhythmic mechanisms of n-3 PUFA and the results of the GISSI-Prevenzione trial. *Journal of Membrane Biology* 206: 117–128.

Moon JC, Bogle RG (2006) Switching statins. *British Medical Journal* 332: 1344–1345.

NICE (2002) *Guidance on the Use of Glycoprotein IIb/IIIa Inhibitors in the Treatment of Acute Coronary Syndromes.* Technology appraisal no. 47. London: NICE. www.nice.org.uk.

NICE (2005) *Clopidogrel and Modified Release Dipyridamole in the Prevention of Occlusive Vascular Events.* Technology appraisal no. 90. London: NICE. www.nice.org.uk.

Pitt B, Zannad F, Remme WJ et al for the Randomised Aldactone Evaluation Study Investigators (1999) The effects of spironolactone on morbidity and mortality in patients with severe heart failure. *New England Journal of Medicine* 341: 709–717.

Pitt B, Remme WJ, Zannad F for the Eplirinone Post-acute Myocardial Infarction Heart Failure Efficacy and Survival Study Investigators (2003) Eplerinone, a selective aldosterone blocker, in patients with left ventricular dysfunction after myocardial infarction. *New England Journal of Medicine* 348: 1309–1321.

Pitt B, White H, Nicolau J et al (2005) Eplerinone reduces mortality 30 days after randomization following acute myocardial infarction in patients with left ventricular systolic dysfunction and heart failure. *Journal of the American College of Cardiology* 46: 425–431.

Purcell H, Fox K (2001) Diltiazem comes in from the cold. *European Heart Journal* 22: 185–187.

Roberts WC (1997) The rule of 5 and the rule of 7 in lipid lowering by statin drugs. *American Journal of Cardiology* 80: 106–107.

Salpeter SR, Ormiston TM, Salpeter EE et al (2003) Cardio-selective beta-blockers for chronic obstructive pulmonary disease: a meta-analysis. *Respiratory Medicine* 97: 1094–1101.

Sanmuganathan PS, Ghahramani P, Jackson PR et al (2001) Aspirin for primary prevention of coronary heart disease: safety and absolute benefit related to coronary risk derived from meta-analysis of randomised trials. *Heart* 85: 265–271.

Shukla R, Jowett NI, Thompson DR et al (1994) Side effects with amiodarone therapy. *Postgraduate Medical Journal* 70: 492–498.

Struthers AD (2005) Aldosterone: an important mediator of cardiac modelling in heart failure. *British Journal of Cardiology* 12: 211–218.

Turpie AGG (2005) The safety of fondaparinux for the prevention and treatment of venous thromboembolism. *Expert Opinion on Drug Safety* 4: 707–721.

Vaughan Williams EM (1984) A classification of anti-arrhythmic actions reassessed after a decade of new drugs. *Journal of Clinical Pharmacology* 24: 129–147.

Walsh SJ, Spence MS, Crossman D et al (2005) Clopidogrel in non-ST segment elevation acute coronary syndromes: an overview of the submission by the British Cardiac Society and the Royal College Physicians of London to the National Institute for Clinical Excellence, and beyond. *Heart* 91: 1135–1140.

World Health Organization (2002) *Reducing Risks, Promoting Healthy Life.* Geneva: WHO.

Yusuf S, Mehta SR, Chrolavicus S for the OASIS 5 investigators (2006) Comparison of fondaparinux and enoxaparin in acute coronary syndromes. *New England Journal of Medicine* 354: 1464–1476.

Index

Note Page numbers in *italics* refer to figures, tables and boxes.